Health and Welfare
for Families
in the 21st Century

The Jones and Bartlett Series in Nursing

Health and Welfare for Families in the 21st Century

Senior Editor

HELEN M. WALLACE, MD, MPH

Editors

GORDON GREEN, MD, MPH
KENNETH J. JAROS, MSW, PhD
LISA L. PAINE, CNM, DrPH
MARY STORY, RD, PhD

JONES AND BARTLETT PUBLISHERS

Sudbury, Massachusetts

BOSTON   TORONTO   LONDON   SINGAPORE

World Headquarters
Jones and Bartlett Publishers
40 Tall Pine Drive
Sudbury, MA 01776
978-433-5000
info@jbpub.com
www.jbpub.com

Jones and Bartlett Publishers Canada
P.O. Box 19020
Toronto, ON M5S 1X1
CANADA

Jones and Bartlett Publishers International
Barb House, Barb Mews
London W6 7PA
UK

PRODUCTION CREDITS
ACQUISITIONS EDITOR Greg Vis
ASSOCIATE EDITOR Karen McClure
PRODUCTION EDITOR Lianne B. Ames
MANUFACTURING DIRECTOR Therese Bräuer
DESIGN UG Production Services
EDITORIAL PRODUCTION SERVICE UG Production Services
TYPESETTING UG
COVER DESIGN Dick Hannus
PRINTING AND BINDING Malloy Lithographing, Inc.
COVER PRINTING Malloy Lithographing, Inc.

Library of Congress Cataloging-in-Publication Data
Health and welfare for families in the 21st century / edited by Helen
  Wallace ... [et al.]
      p.   cm.
    Includes bibliographical references and index.
    ISBN 0-7637-0867-4
    1. Family—Health and hygiene   2. Family policy.   I. Wallace,
Helen M.
  RA418.5.F3H428 1998 *1999*

  362.1—dc21   98-8557
                                                                  CIP

The selection and dosage of drugs presented in this book are in accord with standards accepted at the time of publication. The authors and publishers have made every effort to provide accurate information. However, research, clinical practice, and government regulations often change the accepted standard in this field. Before administering any drug, the reader is advised to check the manufacturer's product information sheet for the most up-to-date recommendations on dosage, precautions, and contraindications. This is especially important in the case of drugs that are new or seldom used.
Printed in the United States of America

02 01 00 99   10 9 8 7 6 5 4 3 2

Contents

II Social Welfare, 113

IV Health Issues and Policy Implications, 345

List of Tables

List of Figures

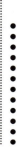

Preface

PHILIP R. LEE, MD

The restructuring in social welfare, medical care, and public health in the United States is producing dramatic changes in the health and welfare systems. These changes, which began in the 1980s, are now having major impacts, not only on institutions and organizations but also on families and children. The changes are affecting government agencies, as well as private and nonprofit organizations and institutions. The changes have been driven by a number of factors—rising costs; the growing role of the ideology in policy, particularly the role of the marketplace in medical care; the impact of technology, including information systems; the need to make these systems more responsive to consumers; and fiscal pressures, including the recent drive to balance the federal budget. These forces have affected particularly the government agencies and nonprofit agencies, with the result that downsizing, budget cuts, and privatization of many public health, social welfare, and medical care services have occurred, particularly affecting vulnerable populations.

Medicine, social welfare, and public health are at a critical crossroads as we enter the 21st century. It is not only the move from the industrial age to the information and knowledge age and the globalization of the economy that provide the broad context for these changes, but the more immediate consequences of the shift in values and the stress on market values that is affecting policies, programs, services, and people. Services that many of us have long viewed as public goods are not viewed as market goods.

Abraham Flexner's famous report, *Medical Education in the United States and Canada*, was published in 1910. In that report, Flexner described the sorry state of medical education in the United States and Canada. At the time, proprietary medical schools flourished and university-based medical education was rare. What made the commercial schools so despicable to Flexner was that they placed their owner's interests above those of the public. In his view, medical schools were public service corporations, not profit-making businesses. He felt that in medical education the interest of the public was paramount. It is important to consider the wealth of material presented in *Health and Welfare for Families in the 21st Century* from this public interest perspective.

This book provides professionals both practical and academic, and policymakers with a rich but practical framework for thinking about the needs of families and children, as well as a wide range of options. In clear, well-documented terms, *Health and Welfare for Families in the 21st Century* provides the essential information that is needed to make informed judgments about how best we can meet the needs of families and children in the 21st century. For me, one of the clearest themes to emerge is the need for collaboration both within sectors such as public health, but more importantly across the sectors of medicine, public health, and social welfare. This theme is also made very powerfully in the recent monograph by Dr. Roz Lasker, *Medicine and Public Health: The Power of Collaboration*.

I hope the book will be widely read and its ideas put to practical use. The issues and the action we take are vital to the health and well-being of the nation in the 21st century.

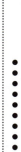

Preface

Audrey H. Nora, MD, MPH

As a nation, we demonstrate our commitment to the future through our efforts to ensure the health and well-being of our children, youth, and families. During this century, the rates of maternal and child death have fallen dramatically, yet new challenges such as substance abuse, HIV/AIDS, and increased violence have resulted in new morbidities.

As the 21st century begins, the major social, economic, and demographic changes of the last two decades will continue, including changes in family composition. Increasing numbers of children are living with a single parent, and more women are joining the work force, expanding the need for out-of-home child care and decreasing the amount of time families can spend together.

The number of children who have no health insurance has been increasing annually and is often associated with poverty. Among all children younger than 18 living in the United States in 1995, 66.1% were insured privately, 26.4% received their insurance through public assistance, and 13.8% were uninsured. Nearly 30% of uninsured children are eligible for Medicaid but are not enrolled in the program.

The good news is that Congress passed Title XXI as part of the Balanced Budget Act of 1997, which provides $24 billion in federal funds for the next 5 years for children's health insurance through state programs. This is the first major health program for children enacted in this century since Medicaid was passed in 1965 and is an exciting opportunity to craft state child and health insurance programs that are responsive to the changing health needs of children.

This book, *Health and Welfare for Families in the 21st Century*, is timely and comprehensive. The Bright Futures Children's Health Charter appears in the very beginning to restate the guiding principles, our vision for the 21st century of comprehensive health supervision of children and families. The chapters provide a logical organizational framework for outlining the complex, yet intertwining, issues involved in providing this kind of comprehensive care. The authors recognize the changing political environment relating to welfare and also address separate populations of children, including children with special health needs, homeless children, foster children, children with HIV, and adolescents.

Preventive care for children emerges as an important component of family needs. Injuries have become the leading cause of death for children aged 1 to 19 years. Adolescents have identified mental health services as their greatest need, yet accessible mental health services for children and adolescents are extremely sparse.

The diversity of our population creates the necessity for individualizing programs to meet the needs of communities and for multiple professions to work together in partnership to integrate services at the federal, state, and community levels.

Throughout this book, the authors focus on the rapid changes occurring in our health care system and the resultant need for all professionals dedicated to the improvement of the health of children, mothers, and families to be vigilant, flexible, and committed to keeping pace with these changes.

Foreword

Helen M. Wallace, MD, MPH, Gordon Green, MD, MPH,
Kenneth Jaros, MSW, PhD, Lisa L. Paine, CNM, DrPH,
Mary Story, RD, PhD

PRIOR TO 1900

Adoption of human legislation in the 1800s in the United States slowly followed that of England. It consisted of slow awakening of identification of the special conditions and needs of poor children, frequently orphaned in poor families, and the adoption of "poor laws" for poor children and poor families. Private charity played an important beginning role in providing some assistance for poor families, especially in New York City and other large cities. Milk stations were developed in New York City to prevent and control "summer diarrhea" and to promote the safe growth and development of children.

THE EARLY 1900S

During the period of the early 1900s, steps were slowly taken to recognize and pay special attention to the special needs of disadvantaged children and families. The first Bureau of Child Hygiene, with Dr. Josephine Baker as Director, was created in 1908 as the prelude to the Maternal and Child Health movement in the United States. The U.S.

Children's Bureau was set up in 1912. Child labor was recognized as a special hazard for children of poor families; federal legislation was enacted in 1919 to prevent and ameliorate it. Pioneers, predominantly women such as Lillian Wald, Jane Addams, and Florence Kelley, continued the tradition of special assistance to poor families through the establishment of Visiting Nurse Associations.

The federal Sheppard Towner Act in 1921 made it possible to provide prenatal care to poor pregnant women and child health supervision to children of poor families. The deaths of women during childbirth pointed out the need for special protection and care of women of childbearing age.

The Great Depression, beginning in 1929, created the circumstances of lack of jobs, clothing, food, and housing, as well as health care, with individuals selling apples on the streets of New York. All together, it made people realize that the United States was not able to care for its poor, disadvantaged people. Thus, the Social Security Act of 1935 was enacted.

SIXTY YEARS OF THE SOCIAL SECURITY ACT (1935–1995)

The 60-year period of the Social Security Act (1935–1995) and related legislation represents our country's efforts to identify some of the major social, health, education, nutritional, housing, and vocational needs of people in the United States—to prevent them and to rectify them. This can best be described as a period of identifying, testing, and trying out new measures of the federal, state, and local governments, and public and private sectors of our society, to create new methods to help people and families who need assistance. Specific measures were devised; some of the experimental efforts were shared around the country. Professional organizations had a role in attempting to set and raise standards, as did universities and training programs.

The era of the Social Security Act consisted of a series of steps to identify the human problems occurring for people and families who need help and how to help them. Some of these specifics include the following:

- The federal Emergency Maternity and Infant Care (EMIC) program, set up in 1943 to provide health care to pregnant wives and infants of men in the four lowest pay grades of the Armed Forces (the first national health care program in the United States)

- Maternity and Infant Care and Children and Youth legislation of the early 1960s, to assist vulnerable women, children, and families
- Medicaid and Medicare legislation of 1965, to assist the poor and the elderly with the costs of health care
- Augmentation of part of Title V of the Social Security Act for handicapped children and youth in the 1970s and continuing thereafter, through special legislation for handicapped children, and subsequent efforts to reach the younger handicapped through early intervention
- The Head Start Program, initiated in 1965 to provide a combination of health, education, and social services to 4-year-old-children of disadvantaged families, to give them a "head start" to get ready for school
- Special efforts to provide improved nutrition for pregnant women, infants, and young children through the Supplemental Food Program for Women, Infants, and Children (WIC) in 1974
- The 1970 family planning legislation to provide information and services to couples
- A myriad of Title IV-A and IV-E social legislation to assist with family support and child care needs of poor disadvantaged families, children, and women (part of this is the Aid to Families with Dependent Children [AFDC] Program)
- Expansion of the federal Medicaid program to include additional thousands of childbearing women and children in eligibility for Medicaid benefits in the early 1990s
- Expansion of the Social Security Income Program to include an additional thousands of handicapped children in eligibility for Supplemental Security Income (SSI) benefits, through the Zebley Court Decision in 1990

This 60-year period represents an enormous effort to make it possible for the United States to help people who need help, to help individuals to reach their maximum potential, and to help individuals to achieve a better life for themselves and others.

The 21st century represents a new beginning and opportunity to improve on these prior efforts.

It is evident that the 60 years of the Social Security Act, including Title V, produced an impressive list of accomplishments, especially for mothers, children, youth, and families. As some major unmet needs were identified, facts were collected about the extent of the individual problem, and plans were made to provide services and programs to eliminate the problem and to provide care for those mothers, children, youth, and families who were in need of help.

Thus, the changes in legislation that were introduced beginning in 1996 and 1997 in federal and state legislatures may represent new opportunities. We need to be innovative and creative about the needs for today and for the future. It is hoped that this new book will help.

Bright Futures Children's Health Charter

Throughout this century, principles developed by advocates for children have been the foundation for initiatives to improve children's lives. Bright Futures participants have adopted these principles in order to guide their work and meet the unique needs of children and families into the 21st century.

Every child deserves to be born well, to be physically fit, and to achieve self-responsibility for good health habits.

•

Every child and adolescent deserves ready access to coordinated and comprehensive preventive, health-promoting, therapeutic, and rehabilitative medical, mental health, and dental care. Such care is best provided through a continuing relationship with a primary health professional or team, and ready access to secondary and tertiary levels of care.

•

Every child and adolescent deserves a nurturing family and supportive relationships with other significant persons who provide security, positive role models, warmth, love, and unconditional acceptance. A child's health begins with the health of his parents.

•

Every child and adolescent deserves to grow and develop in a physically and psychologically safe home and school environment free of undue risk of injury, abuse, violence, or exposure to environmental toxins.

•

Every child and adolescent deserves satisfactory housing, good nutrition, a quality education, an adequate family income, a supportive social network, and access to community resources.

•

Every child deserves quality child care when her parents are working outside the home.

•

Every child and adolescent deserves the opportunity to develop ways to cope with stressful life experiences.

•

Every child and adolescent deserves the opportunity to be prepared for parenthood.

•

Every child and adolescent deserves the opportunity to develop positive values and become a responsible citizen in his community.

•

Every child and adolescent deserves to experience joy, have high self-esteem, have friends, acquire a sense of efficacy, and believe that she can succeed in life. She should help the next generation develop the motivation and habits necessary for similar achievement.

Source: Green M (ed.). *Bright Futures,* Arlington, VA: National Center for Education in Maternal and Child Health, Rockville, MD: Maternal and Child Health Bureau.

Contributors

GREG R. ALEXANDER, RS, MPH, ScD
Professor, Department of Maternal and Child Health
University of Alabama, School of Public Health
Birmingham, Alabama

JEAN L. ATHEY, PhD
Director, Emergency Medical Services and Children's Program
Maternal and Child Health Bureau
Rockville, Maryland

DONALD A. BARR, MD, PhD
Coordinator, Curriculum in Health Policy
Stanford University Program in Human Biology
Stanford, California

A. E. BENJAMIN, PhD
Professor
University of California, School of Public Policy and Social Research
Los Angeles, California

G. ALLEN BOLTON, MPH, MBA
Director
Greater Dallas Injury Prevention Center
Dallas, Texas

PAUL J. BOUMBULIAN, DPA, MPH
Senior Vice President, Strategic Planning & Population Medicine
Parkland Health and Hospital System
Dallas, Texas

BRADLEY R. BRADEN
Health Care Financing Administration
Office of the Actuary
Baltimore, Maryland

MARY CARRASCO, MD
Children's Hospital of Pittsburgh
Pittsburgh, Pennsylvania

PAUL S. CASAMASSIMO, DDS, MS
Professor and Chair, Pediatric Dentistry Section
Ohio State University College of Dentistry
Columbus, Ohio

MARY ELIZABETH COLLINS, PhD
Assistant Professor of Social Welfare Policy
Boston University School of Social Work
Boston, Massachusetts

VALIRE CARR COPELAND, PhD, MPH, MSW, BSW
Assistant Professor
University of Pittsburgh School of Social Work
Pittsburgh, Pennyslvania

CATHY A. COWAN
Health Care Financing Administration
Office of the Actuary
Baltimore, Maryland

EUGENE DECLERCQ, PhD
Associate Chair, Maternal and Child Health Department
Boston University School of Public Health
Boston, Massachusetts

DAVID S. DE LA CRUZ, PhD, MPH
Project Director, Health Start National Resource Center
National Center for Education in Maternal and Child Health
Arlington, Virginia

CAROLYN S. DONHAM
Health Care Financing Administration
Office of the Actuary
Baltimore, Maryland

ANNE COHN DONNELLY, DPH, MPH, MA
Community Service Fellow, Kellogg School of Management
Northwestern University
Evanston, Illinois

MARIANNE E. FELICE, MD
Professor of Pediatrics and Psychiatry
University of Maryland Division of Adolescent Medicine
Baltimore, Maryland

ROBERT C. FELLMETH, AB, JD
Price Professor of Public Interest Law
Director, Children's Advocacy Institute
San Diego, California

CLAUDE EARL FOX, MD, MPH
Health Resources and Service Administration
US Dept. of Health and Human Services
Rockville, Maryland

ROBERT E. FULLILOVE
Associate Dean of Minority Affairs
Columbia University School of Public Health
New York, New York

SHELLY GEHSHAN, MPP
Program Manager
National Conference of State Legislatures
Washington, District of Columbia

THURMA MCCANN GOLDMAN, MD
Department Health and Human Services
Maternal and Child Health Bureau
Rockville, Maryland

FREDERICK C. GREEN, MD, FAAP
Retired Emeritus Professor
George Washington University School of Medicine and Health Sciences
Washington, District of Columbia

GORDON GREEN, MD, MPH
Dean, The Southwestern Allied Health Sciences School
University of Texas Southwestern Medical Center
Dallas, Texas

LISA HARNACK, DrPH, RD
Assistant Professor
University of Minnesota Division of Epidemiology
Minneapolis, Minnesota

CATHERINE A. HESS, MSW
Executive Director
Association of Maternal and Child Health Programs
Washington, District of Columbia

MUNEHIRO HIRAYAMA, MD, PhD
Director and Professor Emeritus
University of Tokyo Japan Child and Family Research
Institute
Tokyo, Japan

SANDRA L. HOFFERTH, PhD
Senior Research Scientist
University of Michigan Institute for Social Research
Ann Arbor, Michigan

JULIE HUDMAN, MPP
Doctoral Candidate, Department of Health Policy and
Management
Johns Hopkins University School of Public Health
Baltimore, Maryland

DANA HUGHES, DrPH
Assistant Adjunct Professor
Department of Family and Community Medicine
Institute for Health Policy Studies
University of California
San Francisco, California

ELLEN HUTCHINS, ScD, MSW
Health Care Administrator
Maternal and Child Health Bureau
Rockville, Maryland

VINCE HUTCHINS, MD, MPH
Distinguished Research Professor in MCH Policy
National Center for Education in MCH
Georgetown University Public Policy Institute
Arlington, Virginia

KENNETH JAROS, MSW, PhD
Director, Public Health Social Work
Training Program in MCH
Assistant Professor, Graduate School of Public Health
University of Pittsburgh
Pittsburgh, Pennsylvania

WOODIE KESSEL, MD, MPH
Director
Maternal and Child Health Bureau
Division of Science, Education, and Analysis
Rockville, Maryland

JOHN L. KIELY, PhD
Chief, Infant and Child Health Studies Branch
National Center for Health Statistics
Hyattsville, Maryland

MICHELE KIELY, DrPH
Chief Epidemiologist, Division of Science, Education and Analysis
Maternal and Child Health Bureau
Rockville, Maryland

RICHARD D. KRUGMAN, MD
Professor and Dean of Pediatrics
University of Colorado School of Medicine
Denver, Colorado

JOEL KURITSKY, MD
Immunization Services Division
Centers for Disease Control and Prevention
Atlanta, Georgia

CHARLES D. LAVALLEE
Vice President and Executive Director
Western Pennsylvania Caring Foundation for Children
Pittsburgh, Pennsylvania

HELEN C. LAZENBY
Health Care Financing Administration
Office of the Actuary
Baltimore, Maryland

PHILIP R. LEE, MD
Professor Emeritus
Senior Advisor to the School of Medicine
University of California
San Francisco, California

KATHARINE R. LEVIT
Health Care Financing Administration
Office of the Actuary
Baltimore, Maryland

ANNA M. LONG
Health Care Financing Administration
Office of the Actuary
Baltimore, Maryland

LENA LUNDGREN-GRAVERAS, PhD
Assistant Professor of Social Welfare Policy
Boston University School of Social Work
Boston, Massachusetts

JENNIFER C. MAEHR, MD
Clinical Instructor
University of Maryland Division of Adolescent
Medicine
Baltimore, Maryland

JAMES S. MARKS, MD, MPH
Director
National Center for Chronic Disease Prevention &
Health Promotion
Centers for Disease Control
Atlanta, Georgia

RALPH MARTINI, MS
Director, Office of Operations and Management
Maternal and Child Health Bureau
Health Resources and Services Administration
Rockville, Maryland

LOIS MCCLOSKEY, DRPH
Assistant Professor, Department of Maternal and Child Health
Boston University School of Public Health
Boston, Massachusetts

PATRICIA A. MCDONNELL
Health Care Financing Administration
Office of the Actuary
Baltimore, Maryland

MERLE MCPHERSON, MD
Maternal and Child Health Bureau
Health Resources and Services Administration
Rockville, Maryland

YASUHIDE NAKAMURA, MD, PHD
Associate Professor Department of Community Health
School of International Medicine
University of Tokyo
Tokyo, Japan

AUDREY H. NORA, MD, MPH
Director, Maternal and Child Health Bureau
Health Resources and Services Administration
Department of the Health and Human Services
Rockville, Maryland

LISA L. PAINE, CNM, DRPH
Chair, Department of Maternal and Child Health
Boston University School of Public Health
Boston, Massachusetts

JOAN M. PATTERSON, PHD
Associate Professor and Chair, Maternal and Child Health
Program
University of Minnesota, School of Public Health
Minneapolis, Minnesota

MAGDA G. PECK, SCD
Associate Chairperson for Community Health
Chief, Section on Child Health Policy
University of Nebraska Medical Center Department of
Pediatrics
Omaha, Nebraska

DONNA J. PETERSEN, MHS, ScD
Associate Professor, Assistant Dean for Academic Affairs
University of Alabama School of Public Health
Birmingham, Alabama

IRWIN REDLENER, MD
Director, Community Pediatrics
Professor of Pediatrics
Albert Einstein College of Medicine
New York, New York

JOHN REISS, PhD
Director, Policy and Program Affairs
Institute for Child Health Policy
Gainesville, Florida

LANCE RODEWALD, MD
Associate Director, Science and Immunization Services Division
Centers for Disease Control and Prevention
Atlanta, Georgia

PATTI R. ROSQUIST, MD
Instructor of Pediatrics
University of Colorado Health Sciences Center
Denver, Colorado

DONALD SCHIFF, MD
Professor of Pediatrics
The Children's Hospital
Denver, Colorado

PETER SHERMAN, MD
Medical Director
New York Children's Health Project
New York, New York

LEKHA SIVARAJAN
Health Care Financing Administration
Office of the Actuary
Baltimore, Maryland

LYNN SQUIRE
Legislative Officer
Maternal and Child Health Bureau
Rockville, Maryland

BARBARA STARFIELD, MD, MPH
University Distinguished Professor
Johns Hopkins School of Hygiene and Public Health
Baltimore, Maryland

MADIE W. STEWART
Health Care Financing Administration
Office of the Actuary
Baltimore, Maryland

JEAN M. STILLER
Health Care Financing Administration
Office of the Actuary
Baltimore, Maryland

MARY STORY, RD, PhD
Associate Professor of Nutrition
Division of Epidemiology
University of Minnesota
Minneapolis, Minnesota

MARTHA STOWE, MSW, LMSW
Coalition Manager
Greater Dallas Injury Prevention Center
Dallas, Texas

KEVIN D. SUNDERMAN
Vice President and Executive Director
Western Pennsylvania Caring Foundation for Children
Pittsburgh, Pennsylvania

MARY LOU VALDEZ
International Health Officer for the Americas
Office of International and Refugee Health
US Department of Health and Human Services
Rockville, Maryland

KAREN VANLANDEGHEM, MPH
Assistant Executive Director Policy and Programs
Association of Maternal and Child Health
Washington, District of Columbia

HELEN M. WALLACE, MD, MPH
Professor, Maternal and Child Health
San Diego University, Graduate School of Public Health
San Diego, California

SANDRA WEXLER, PhD, ACSW
Assistant Professor
University of Pittsburgh School of Social Work
Pittsburgh, Pennsylvania

LYNN E. WILCOX, MD, MPH
Director, Division of Reproductive Health
National Center for Chronic Disease Prevention and Health Promotion
Centers for Disease Control
Atlanta, Georgia

PAUL H. WISE, MD, MPH
Department of Maternal and Child Health
Boston University School of Public Health
Boston, Massachusetts

DARLEEN K. WON
Health Care Financing Administration
Office of the Actuary
Baltimore, Maryland

I

Foundations

1

The American Family: Changes and Challenges for the 21st Century

SANDRA L. HOFFERTH

DEMOGRAPHIC CHANGES

During the last third of the 20th century, enormous demographic and economic changes occurred in American families. These include

1. Increased incidence of single-parent families
2. Increased maternal employment outside the home
3. Declining labor-market prospects for less-skilled, especially male, workers
4. Increased incidence of childhood poverty, both within their families and in their neighborhoods

Although the numbers have stabilized, today it is estimated that two thirds of first marriages will end in divorce, more than twice as many as two decades ago.[1] Currently, almost one quarter of white and more than two thirds of black children are born to unmarried mothers.[2] These two changes lead to a very high proportion of children (60% according to recent estimates) who are expected to spend at least part of their childhood with only one parent.[3] Although many divorced parents remarry, three in five children in such families spend more than 5 years with only one parent.[4] Parental divorce has been identified as a risk factor for school failure, school drop-out, and early parenthood, as well as for females becoming single head of household.[5-7] One explanation for this is insufficient economic and social support from absent fathers.[8-10] However, having a stepparent does not necessarily increase resources to children up to the level experienced with the natural parent. In fact, research suggests that parental remarriage may also have risks for children.[6] New research also suggests that many problems experienced by the children of divorce actually existed before the family breakup occurred. Divorce per se may not be the cause of children's problems, but merely a marker for them.[11,12]

A second change in American families has been a sharp increase in levels of maternal employment.[13] Women are much more likely to be working in the 1990s than in previous periods. In the United States, married mothers have traditionally been least likely to work. While 32% of married mothers with children under age 18 were in the work force in 1965, 70% were in the work force in 1994.[2] These numbers are among the highest in industrial nations today. Attempts to identify the consequences that loss of maternal time may have for children have shown few effects,[14] It may be that the extra income brought into the family offsets the loss of maternal time.[9,10] Research has begun to sort out the mechanisms, such as the quality of the home environment,[15] child care,[16] or characteristics of the job,[17] through which maternal employment affects individual children or subgroups of children.

A third important trend is the declining real earnings of less-skilled labor. The extent of inequality in the distribution of earned income since the 1970s has dramatically increased,[18,19] Workers with higher schooling levels and more experience have enjoyed increases in their inflation-adjusted earnings, while the real earnings of younger and less-educated workers have fallen sharply. The real earnings drops have been particularly great for less-skilled men. There is continuing debate over the underlying causes of these developments. Many analysts point to the changing nature of workplace technology, which has spurred demand for workers with more analytical skills and consequent flexibility. More certain are the adverse consequences of these developments for the economic and time resources available to children in young families.

However, the good news is that the earnings of females continued to rise through the late 1980s.[20] Women's increased participation in the work force[21] and the increased demand for managerial/professional and service occupations in which women are well-represented[22] have contributed to the modest increase in women's wages between 1980 and 1990.[20] Low unemployment (5.4% in 1996) and low inflation rates characterized the U.S. labor market in the late 1990s.[23]

A fourth trend, in part a consequence of the rise in the number of mother-only families and the declining earnings of less-skilled workers, is a much higher incidence of childhood poverty in the 1980s than in the 1970s.[24,25] In 1969 only about 14% of U.S. children lived in families with incomes below the official poverty line. Throughout the 1980s and 1990s the incidence of childhood poverty exceeded 20%, and for blacks, childhood poverty appeared to have become more persistent as well.[26] Poverty rates of single mother households exceeded 50% in 1994. The increased poverty was a reflection of the growing number of mother-only families, lower real wages of young adult workers, and falling real benefits in transfer programs such as Aid to Families with Dependent Children. Particularly worrisome is evidence of the increased geographic concentration of urban poverty.[27–29] Because of the lower resources of their families and communities, poor children are at risk for decrements in cognitive, physical, and emotional well-being.

While these trends may work toward the detriment of children, two others may work toward their advantage:

1. Higher schooling levels of parents
2. Smaller family size

About one fifth of mothers completed some college in the 1950s, compared with 40% in the 1980s. Less than 10% of black mothers and fathers completed some college in the 1950s. In the 1980s, the incidence had climbed to one of three black fathers and one of four black mothers.[3] These changes suggest that a larger proportion of children are better off today than several decades ago. Fewer than 8% of families whose head had at least some college education were poor in 1994. This trend may be offset by the large number of immigrant children entering U.S. schools. In contrast to those born in the United States, immigrants often have lower educational levels. They also bring diverse cultural habits and languages. Besides monetary advantages, education also affects the values, knowledge, experience, time allocation, and aspirations that parents bring to child-rearing. Consequently, parental educational attainments have consistently been found to be related to those of their children.

Finally, reduced fertility might influence children and families in a positive way. The number of children born to the average woman has declined substantially. Each woman born after 1945 is expected to bear about two children by the time she completes childbearing.[30] In contrast, the average woman born between 1930 and 1939 had about three children. Children in small families do consistently better academically than those in larger families, and it has been argued that this is due to the greater time and resources that can be devoted to these children.[31–33] Family size is not independent of the other demographic changes. One-parent and working-couple families tend to have fewer children than two-parent, one-earner families.

POLICY CHALLENGES

On August 22, 1996, the United States formalized what had been a major shift in U.S. policy toward low-income families during the early 1990s. In signing the Personal Responsibility and Work Opportunity Reconciliation Act of 1996 (PRWORA), President Clinton approved legislation that fundamentally altered the pact that the federal government had with its citizens to maintain a safety net for low-income families. First and foremost, the new law repealed the 60-year-old program of Aid to Families with Dependent Children (AFDC), the Job Opportunity and Basic Skills (JOBS) program instituted in 1988, and emergency assistance programs. In place of this assistance, as of July 1, 1997, each state must operate a program of assistance to needy families funded under the Temporary Assistance for Needy Families (TANF) Block Grant. The major difference between this new legislation and previous legislation is that individuals and families are no longer entitled to assistance under the federal statute. Instead, states will decide how their own programs are run. Furthermore, such assistance is temporary—for example, TANF funds cannot be used to assist families in which an adult has received assistance for 60 months. Recipients are required to work after 2 years of receiving assistance. Current immigrants are banned from receiving food stamps and, at state option, from funds provided through Medicaid, AFDC, Title XX Social Services Block Grant, and state-funded assistance until citizenship. Future immigrants are banned for at least 5 years from most federal programs. Refugees and those granted asylum in their first 5 years in the United States, veterans, and those with 40 quarters of work experience are exempt.

These changes were implemented based on the premise that the previous system had not reduced child poverty and nonmarital childbearing, but had merely resulted in increased dependence on public assistance.[34] Consequently, how the new welfare reform bill will affect the well-being of children and families is a question to be addressed over the coming years. There are two major legislative changes that were made: time limits and work requirements. Although a 5-year limit was imposed by the federal legislation, with work required after 2 years, states vary in their policies, with many requiring employment immediately and some limiting assistance to 2 years.

Time Limits

Time limits may affect families in several ways. By reducing their eligibility for income support and services, time limits may reduce family resources for day-to-day living. This may increase the risk of either having to move in with others or becoming homeless, reducing children's security and safety and increasing stress. Such dire predictions assume that families will not adjust in other ways.

Resources. Low-income families have access to three resource systems: the market, public support, and a social network, including most importantly the immediate family members, but also family members in other households, such as absent fathers. These three systems combine to define access to overall resources for consumption and other purposes, and there is potential to substitute across the systems. More pervasive public support in the form of welfare benefits, child care assistance, and Medicaid is seen as substituting for the market and social networks and social capital. In particular, a weakening of the labor market for less-skilled workers and a scaling back of public sector support may lead to a combination of the market and the family as income support and an insurance system.[35,36] The ability and willingness of families to assist needy members have not been tested on a large scale.

Living Arrangements. If parents are unable to obtain alternative resources, they may simply be unable to care for their children and may seek an alternative caregiver to care for the children either full-time or for part of the day, or they may seek to limit fertility. Time limits may increase the incentives for parents to place their children with relatives, since those relatives may be able to obtain money (TANF, foster care, or child care), whereas the biological mother may have exhausted her benefit eligibility. For example, in Maryland, a kinship caregiver may become a licensed foster parent and collect about $525 monthly for a child younger than 12. If she is not a licensed foster parent, she may still qualify for welfare benefits, which are only one third of the foster care subsidy. Finally, she may qualify to receive child care subsidies. This could conceivably lead to networks of mothers caring for one another's children. We expect that kin care will be the dominant form of alternative living arrangements.[37]

Conservatives argue that AFDC provided incentives for women to head their own families; they might predict increased marriage and residence with two parents as a result of PRWORA. Research has shown that levels of welfare payments affect living arrangements, including female-headed households, although the effects are not substantial.[38] Other factors, such as levels of wages and employment for men, are likely to be crucial to living arrangements.[39]

Liberals argue that the proportion of children living with neither parent will increase as low-income single mothers become ineligible for public assistance and find themselves unable to support their children. Using data from the Survey of Income and Program Participation, research[40] shows that less generous state welfare payments are associated with more children living apart from their mothers. We may see more teenage mothers living with their mothers, since the new legislation requires minor parents to live at home or in an adult-supervised setting and participate in education or training to receive assistance.

Stress. Not working and receiving TANF may also be stressful, especially if the parent knows that time on public assistance is limited. Anecdotal evidence from ethnographic work being conducted by Cherlin and colleagues in Massachusetts showed Boston TANF recipients to be very nervous and distressed about what would happen to them given the limited amount of time (24 months) that they were permitted to receive benefits.[41] Not working and not receiving TANF is likely to be the most stressful situation of all. Research found that the probability of divorce was elevated among families that experienced a major loss of income in a prior year.[42] Therefore, an elevated level of depression and lowered self-esteem and self-efficacy can be expected among recipients who live in states with the shortest time limits and who have not yet begun to work. These characteristics may be associated with poor parenting practices, such as abuse or neglect, and, in extreme cases, removal of the children from the home and placement in foster care.

Work Requirements

The second important aspect of the new policy is how soon recipients will be required to work after the effective date of the legislation or entry into the program. We know that many welfare mothers are and have been working and earning money.[43,44] However, they probably have not been reporting income, and the work may have been sporadic or illicit. Employment may increase the mother's earnings, but most of the jobs these women obtain pay the minimum wage and offer no benefits.

Among those who do work, starting regular employment and managing time, children's care arrangements, transportation, and the demands of a new job may be stressful for both parents and their children. Therefore, the work requirement may initially result in some negative consequences, such as increased depression and lowered self-efficacy. Some parents initially have low cognitive skills and poor social-emotional functioning that may prevent them from getting and keeping a job.

For those who become and stay employed, initial difficulties may be offset by higher self-esteem and self-efficacy.[17] Employment lends structure and consistency to family lives through scheduling of time around work, which is hypothesized to improve self-efficacy. After some months of employment, higher self-esteem, greater self-efficacy, and lower depression would be expected. Besides the length of time, effects may be determined by the type of work and work environment into which these women enter, including their autonomy and control over their work.[17]

Other Features of PRWORA

Several features of PRWORA may benefit families. For example, the legislation includes features designed to increase pressure on non-custodial parents to pay child support, which will increase resources for children and families. A second measure, the Individual Development Account, permits families to keep more of their earnings, which would encourage savings and provide more resources to families. A number of states intend to subsidize jobs through providing funds to employers who hire recipients. This should increase the supply of jobs and wages to recipients. Finally, several states plan to extend transitional benefits such as Medicaid and child care to recipients for up to 2 years after they stop receiving public assistance. This should raise their resources and increase the ability of recipients to get and keep a job.[45]

CONCLUSION

In the late 20th century, family changes resulted in a large proportion of female-headed families, declining wages for men, increased opportunities and labor force participation for women, and increased child poverty, as well as increased levels of education, reduced family size, and increased opportunities for those at the top of the income distribution. Until August 1996, AFDC, a social assistance program begun in 1935 for needy children without fathers, allowed low-income mothers to stay home and raise their children through a combination of cash and noncash subsidies.[46] The program trained some mothers and helped them find work, but the proportion who succeeded in working, leaving welfare, and staying off welfare was relatively small.[43,47] Even in cases of abuse and neglect, family reunification was the major objective. Now, with the entitlement ended, there is increased concern that many mothers will not be able to meet the eligibility criteria, that they will lose income and services, and that, as a result, they will be unable to care for their children.

A reduction in long-term assistance provided by the public sector has two implications. First, the extended family as a potential source of assistance becomes crucial. Many families that are well off have members who are in need of assistance, whether young or elderly. As a result, the impact may not be limited to those at the lower end, but could, in fact, be more far-reaching.[48] Second, since mothers will be employed, they will no longer be able to care for their children full-time. Instead, the government will pay other people to care for children. Parental concern over child care arrangements may affect their employment stability.[45,49] The shift in emphasis from maternal care to other care may affect children in ways that are still unknown, but that is likely to depend on the development of a high-quality system of care and education for the youngest members of society.

References

1. Martin, T.C., and Bumpass, L.L., Recent trends in marital disruption. *Demography.* 1989;26:37–51.
2. U.S. Bureau of the Census. *Statistical abstract of the United States 1996.* Washington, DC: U.S. Government Printing Office, 1996.

3. Hernandez, D.J. *America's children: Resources from family, government and the economy.* New York: Russell Sage Foundation, 1993.
4. Bumpass, L. Children and marital disruption: A replication and update. *Demography.* 1984;21:71–82.
5. McLanahan, S. The reproduction of poverty. *American Journal of Sociology.* 1985;90:873–901.
6. McLanahan, S. The two faces of divorce: Women's and children's interests. Paper presented at the American Sociological Association Annual Meeting. San Francisco, CA, August, 1989.
7. McLanahan, S., and Bumpass, L. Family structure and dependency: Early transitions to female household headship. *Demography.* 1988;25:1–16.
8. Weiss, Y., and Willis, R. Transfers among divorced couples: Evidence and interpretation. *Journal of Labor Economics.* October, 1993;629–679.
9. Garfinkel, I., and McLanahan, S. *Single mothers and their children: A new American dilemma.* Washington, DC: The Urban Institute, 1986.
10. Furstenberg, D., Nord, C., and Zill, N. The life course of children of divorce: Marital disruption and parental contact. *American Sociological Review.* 1983;48:656–668.
11. Cherlin, A., Furstenberg, Jr., F., et al. Longitudinal studies of the effects of divorce on children in Great Britain and the United States. *Science.* 1991;252:1386–1389.
12. NICHD. *Children of divorce.* Bethesda, MD: Center for Population Research, 1993.
13. Hofferth, S. and Phillips, D. Child care in the United States, 1970–1995. *Journal of Marriage and the Family.* 1987;49:559–571.
14. Hayes, C., Palmer, J., and Zaslow, M. *Who cares for America's children? Child care policy for the 1990s.* Washington, DC: National Academy Press, 1990.
15. Desai, S., Chase-Lansdale, P.L., and Michael, R.T. Mother or market? Effects of maternal employment on the intellectual ability of 4-year-old children. *Demography.* November, 1989;26:545–562.
16. NICHD Early Child Care Research Network. Mother-child interaction and cognitive outcomes associated with early child care. Symposium presented at Biennial Meeting of the Society for Research in Child Development. Washington, DC: April, 1997.
17. Parcel, T., and Menaghan, E. *Parents' jobs and children's lives.* New York: Aldine de Gruyter, 1994.
18. Levy, F., and Murnane, R. U.S. earnings levels and earnings inequality: A review of recent trends and proposed explanations. *Journal of Economic Literature.* 1992;30:1333–1381.
19. Danziger, S., and Gottschalk, P. *Uneven tides: Rising inequality in America.* New York: Russell Sage Foundation, 1993.
20. Spain, D., and Bianchi, S. *Balancing act: Motherhood, marriage, and employment among American women.* New York: Russell Sage Foundation, 1996.
21. Rones, P., Ilg, R., and Gardner, J. Trends in hours of work since the mid-1970s. *Monthly Labor Review.* April, 1997;120:3–14.
22. Wootton, B. Gender differences in occupational employment. *Monthly Labor Review.* April, 1997;120:15–24.
23. Goodman, W.C., and Ilg, R.E. Employment in 1996; Jobs up, unemployment down. *Monthly Labor Review.* February, 1997;120:3–15.
24. Smith, J. Children among the poor. *Demography.* 1989;26(2):235–248.
25. Smolensky, E., Danziger, S., and Gottschalk, P. The declining significance of age in the United States: Trends in the well-being of children and the elderly since 1939. In J. Palmer, T. Smeeding, and B. Torrey (eds). *The vulnerable.* Washington, DC: The Urban Institute, 1988, pp 29–54.
26. Duncan, G.J., and Rodgers, W.L. Longitudinal aspects of childhood poverty. *Journal of Marriage and the Family.* 1988;50:1007–1021.
27. Wilson, W.J. *The truly disadvantaged.* Chicago: University of Chicago, 1987.
28. Bane, M.J., and Jargowsky, P. Urban poverty and the underclass: Basic questions. Paper presented at the Annual Meeting of the Association for Public Policy and Management. Washington, DC, 1987.
29. Jargowsky, P. Ghetto poverty among Blacks in the 1980s. *Journal of Policy Analysis and Management.* 1994;13(2):288–310.

30. U.S. Bureau of the Census. Fertility of American women: June 1987. *Current Population Reports.* 1988;P-20:427.
31. Blake, J. *Family size and achievement.* Berkeley, CA: University of California Press, 1989.
32. Polit, D. *Effects of family size: A critical review of literature since 1973.* Washington, DC: American Institutes for Research, 1982.
33. Zajonc, R.B., and Markus, G.B. Birth order and intellectual development. *Psychological Review.* 1975;82:74–88.
34. Sawhill, I. Overview. In I. Sawhill (ed). *Welfare reform: An analysis of the issues.* Washington, DC: The Urban Institute, 1995, pp xi–xx.
35. Rosenzweig, M., and Wolpin, K. Intergenerational support and the life-cycle incomes of young men and their parents: Human capital investments, coresidence, and intergenerational financial transfers. *Journal of Labor Economics.* 1993;11(1, pt. 1):84–112.
36. Rosenzweig, M., and Wolpin, K. Parental and public transfers to young women and their children. *American Economic Review.* 1994;84(5):1195–1212.
37. Fields, J. Predicting child fosterage experience: Kin versus non-kin residence. Paper presented at Annual Meeting of the Population Association of America. Washington, DC, March 28–30, 1997.
38. Bane, M.J., and Ellwood, D. *Single mothers and their living arrangements.* Cambridge, MA: Harvard University, 1984.
39. Smock, P., and Manning, W. Cohabiting partners' economic circumstances and marriage. *Demography.* 1997;34.
40. Brandon, P.D. *Social policy and the redistribution of preschool-aged children.* Unpublished manuscript. Amherst, MA: University of Massachusetts, 1997.
41. Cherlin, A. *Personal communication.* Discussion of ethnographic findings from Boston, MA. Madison, WI, April, 1997.
42. Yeung, W.J., and Hofferth, S. *Family adaptations to economic loss.* Ann Arbor, MI: 1997.
43. Harris, K.M. Work and welfare among single mothers in poverty. *American Journal of Sociology.* 1993;99:317–352.
44. Edin, K., and Lein, L. work, welfare, and single mothers' economic survival strategies. *American Sociological Review.* 1997;61:253–266.
45. Hofferth, S., and Collins, N. Child care and employment turnover. Paper presented at the Biennial Meeting of the Society for Research in Child Development. Washington, DC, April, 1997.
46. Cauthen, N., and Amenta, E. The formative years of Aid to Dependent Children. *American Sociological Review.* 1996;61:427–448.
47. Harris, K.M. Life after welfare: Women, work, and repeat dependency. *American Sociological Review.* 1996;61:407–426.
48. Lampman, R., and Smeeding, T. Interfamily transfers as alternatives to government transfers to persons. *Review of Income and Wealth.* March, 1983;29:45–66.
49. Meyers, M. Child care in JOBS employment and training programs: What difference does quality make? *Journal of Marriage and the Family.* 1993;55:767–783.

2

Health Care and Health Care Policy in a Changing World

PHILIP R. LEE, A. E. BENJAMIN, AND DONALD A. BARR

The organization of medicine is not a thing apart which can be subjected to study in isolation. It is an aspect of culture, whose arrangements are inseparable from the general organization of society.[1]
　　Walter H. Hamilton

Understanding the structure of a health care system first requires understanding the society in which that system exists. The health care system that has evolved in the United States reflects not only the impact of science and technology but also the politics, cultural values, and priorities that have deep historical roots. In other texts, we have described five characteristics of American society and policy that have had powerful influences on the evolution of the health care system, including the American character (e.g., individualism) federalism, pluralism, and incrementalism.[2,3] We will briefly describe each of these and will then offer a historical perspective of how they have shaped health care policies over time and how each of them has contributed to the problems our health care system now faces.

The American Character

The concept of autonomy and the ethical principle of respect for autonomy has been one of the fundamental building blocks of public policy since the founding of the nation. The policies that established the nation were built on the strongly held view that the right of individuals to their own beliefs and values should be protected by government and protected from the government. To this day the principles of individual choice, confidentiality, and privacy are strongly held. In 1990, the Patient Self Determination Act (P.L. 101-508) translated the concept of autonomy into public health policy concerning the individual's right to make decisions with respect to his or her own medical care, to refuse treatment, and to prepare advanced directives regarding care.

Along with the concept of autonomy has been a deeply held distrust of government. Although the distrust of government waxes and wanes, it is ever present and is reflected in the limited role of government in dealing with such issues as the financing of health care. Distrust of government was one of the factors that resulted in the lack of action by the United States Congress on the health care reforms proposed by President Clinton in 1993. In 1993, the President raised the issue of health care reform to the top of the domestic policy agenda, but the United States Congress ended more than a year of deliberation without taking any action. In this case, it was in part the concentrated interests of those who opposed reform (insurance industry, small business) that tapped the broad distrust of government to sap public support and generate opposition to the proposed reforms. The creation of three branches of government by the founding fathers reflected in part the distrust of government and the need to create the necessary checks and balances to prevent the abuse of power by any branch of government or by the majority of the populace.

Throughout the history of the country there have been shifts toward a strong federal role, originally advocated by Alexander Hamilton, and away from such a role. During the 20th century, periods of public action (1900s, 1930s, and 1960s) were preceded and followed by periods of private action (1890s, 1920s, 1950s, and 1980s).

FEDERALISM AND THE ROLE OF GOVERNMENT IN HEALTH CARE

Government at all levels plays an important role in planning, financing, organization, and delivering health services in the United States. At the federal level, Medicare is the dominant program for financing health care for the elderly. The Departments of Veterans Affairs, Defense, and Health and Human Services all maintain large, complex health care delivery systems to meet the needs of veterans, the military and their dependents, and American Indians and Alaska Natives.

The federal government, particularly through the U.S. Public Health Service, funds a range of categorical public health and medical care programs, largely through grants in aid to states and local governments.

At the state level, Medicaid has become the largest medical care program, financed with federal, state, and, in some cases, local government matching funds. The states have historically had the major role in public health programs in the financing and provision of care for the chronically mentally ill and in substance abuse prevention and treatment.

Local governments, particularly in urban areas, have often been major providers of medical care for the indigent, largely through public hospitals and clinics.

Much of the modern infrastructure for health care has been funded or subsidized with public funds during the past 50 years, including the construction of public and most voluntary hospitals, the training of most of the health professions, and the bulk of basic biomedical research. Currently, approximately 40% of all health care expenditures are provided by the federal, state, and local governments.

Although government's role in financing health care is a major one, this role is not the result of a consistent or comprehensive plan for the organization of health care services, but an episodic response to market failures (e.g., Medicare). Over time, as the private sector has been unable or unwilling to meet the health care needs of specific segments of the population, government has stepped in to fill the gap. Initially, the needs were met largely by local government and voluntary efforts. Later, states stepped in to meet the needs of the mentally ill. The federal government played a limited role, except for specific beneficiary groups such as veterans and specific public health problems (e.g., venereal disease, tuberculosis), until the enactment of Medicare and Medicaid in 1965. The Balanced Budget Act of 1997 includes some of the most significant changes ever made in the Medicare and Medicaid programs, providing states with greater flexibility in the administration of Medicaid and individuals greater choice of competing plans in Medicare. The result of this piecemeal approach to the development of health policy has been a proliferation of federal categorical programs administered by moire than a dozen government departments and agencies (e.g., Department of Health and Human Services, Transportation, Agriculture, Energy, and the Environmental Protection Agency).

The role of government, particularly the federal government, has been at the heart of this debate about the future of health care in the United States since President Truman proposed a program of federally financed national health insurance in 1947.

This evolving role of government in the financing organization and delivery of health care reflects the role of federalism in the United States. The concept of federalism, and the concomitant role of the federal government in social policy, has evolved in the 200 years since the American Revolution and the drafting of the U.S. Constitution. After the failure of the Articles of Confederation, the drafters of the Constitution saw a need for a central government with clear but delineated authority in areas of common concern such as national defense and foreign policy. Functions such as education, police protection, and health care were left under state and local authority. The lines between federal and state authority were clearly drawn. It was not until after the Civil War, however, that state governments began to play a significant role in health care and public health policy.

This arrangement worked well so long as two conditions were met:

1. There was consistency between the levels of administrative authority and financial accountability.
2. The various levels of government involved had the appropriate resources and other capacities to carry out their responsibilities.

In health care, it is clear that these conditions have not been consistently maintained. The result often has been an increase in federal responsibility for health care, particularly in the financing of care. In some areas, such as Medicare, the shift to federal responsibility has included both administrative authority and financial accountability. In others, such as Medicaid and family planning, the disjunction between authority (i.e., federal) and accountability (i.e., states) has led to dysfunctional outcomes, including funding cutbacks, eligibility restrictions, low levels of payment to providers of care, and programmatic restrictions. The success of the federalist system depends on maintaining this balance between administrative authority and financial responsibility and between federal, state, and local responsibility.

There have been a number of reasons why state and local governments were not able to maintain their historical authority over social policy, not the least of which has been the lack of political will to extend government authority into new or controversial areas (e.g., civil rights). In parallel with the variation among states in the political will to assume responsibility for social needs have been variations in the ability of states to generate sufficient revenue through taxation and in the capacity to plan and administer complex programs. An important pattern has emerged as to how states respond to health programs that are initiated by the federal government for vulnerable populations but left to states to establish local eligibility and funding criteria: states will vary widely around a median level of benefits. Any federal attempt to guarantee a basic level of benefits using this decentralized approach will succeed for only a certain segment of the intended population.

One final consequence of the approach to health policy that decentralizes responsibility over health care programs has been the vulnerability of local governments and agencies to state funding cutbacks. These local entities are important providers of many health services, particularly hospital, outpatient, and emergency services for the poor; mental health and substance abuse services; and a variety of public health services. When local governments are mandated to provide these services (either by regulation or court order) but are not provided the supplemental resources to do so, both the quality of the local programs and the fiscal health of the local agency can be compromised. Although this does not usually occur during periods of sustained economic growth and low unemployment, quality of programs can vary strikingly from one community to another during economic downturns.

PLURALISM AND THE ROLE OF SPECIAL INTERESTS

In addition to establishing a central government with delineated authority, the founders of this country established a legislative and regulatory system based on pluralism in order to protect the individual from the power of government. Decision-making power in a pluralistic society is spread among many groups so that no one group gains excessive power. Over time, pluralism has become not only a mechanism for making decisions but also an ideology that shapes our perceptions of the proper role of government. In order for their voices to be heard, individuals have increasingly organized into groups with interests as broad as the political parties and as narrow as single issues (e.g., abortion). These groups not only are allowed to influence the legislation process, they are encouraged to do so. During the first half of this century, the groups that dominated the health policy process were characterized as an iron triangle, including legislative committees, executive branch agencies, and private interest groups (e.g., the American Medical Association [AMA]). More recently, the process has become more complex and the iron triangles replaced by policy networks. Peterson has observed that the health policy community today "is heterogeneous and loosely structured, creating a network whose broad boundaries are defined by shared attentiveness of participants to the same issues in the policy domain."[4]

The influence of special interests as a manifestation of our pluralistic system is clearly seen throughout the health policy process. In this century, the American Medical Association has exerted a powerful influence on health policy, although its influence has diminished significantly since the enactment of Medicare. Other influential interests have been the hospitals, the insurance industry, and the pharmaceutical companies. Although groups representing patients (e.g., American Association of Retired Persons, organized labor) have exerted influence over specific programs, it has been these four general groups that have tended to shape health policy in the period after World War II. More recently, business interest groups (e.g., Business Group on Health) have begun to be more influential.

Since the late 1960s, as the cost of health care has become a predominant issue, power over health policy has shifted from the providers to the purchasers (e.g., large employers). Regardless of this realignment of power among interest groups, the power of special interests over the process of establishing and implementing health policy has remained intact. The effectiveness of many of these interest groups (e.g. small businesses, insurance) was very evident in President Clinton's ill-fated attempt at health care reform. It is extremely difficult to achieve broad consensus or to implement broad health policy—or even to convince Congress to make minor changes in policy—in the face of the power of special interests. This inhibition inherent in the pluralistic system in the United States has shaped and continues to shape the health policy process.

INCREMENTALISM AS THE PRINCIPAL MEANS OF HEALTH POLICY REFORM

Kingdon[5] and more recently Longest[6] have provided a model for understanding how policy decisions are made. In Longest's model, the process includes policy formulation and policy implementation phases, with both influenced by a policy modification phase. It is very clear that although President Clinton played the key role in placing national health insurance on the policy agenda in 1993, he did not control the process after that. When a policy issue rises to the top of the agenda, two other factors must then be present for successful reform to take place: a policy solution that is broadly seen as successfully addressing the issue, and political circumstances that allow for reform to take place. When all three (agenda, solution, political circumstances) are present simultaneously, a "window of opportunity" exists for significant policy reform. If any one of the three is absent, the potential for significant reform is diminished substantially. A number of analysts have suggested that just such a window for major health care reform existed in the early Clinton years, but his policy solution proved unacceptable to a majority in Congress and later the success of the "Republican Revolution" in 1994 fundamentally altered the political circumstances, thus removing one of the factors and dooming any efforts at major health care reform.

Once a policy has been enacted, a second process of implementation takes place, usually involving the executive branch agency responsible for establishing the necessary guidelines and regulations. In the case of Medicare, this is the Health Care Financing Administration (HCFA), Department of Health and Human Services (HHS). The HCFA also has a major role in approving state Medicaid regulations. For many categorical public health programs, although the authority is ultimately vested in the Secretary of HHS, the implementation is provided by the agencies (e.g., National Institutes of Health, Food and Drug Administration, Centers for Disease Control and Prevention). In addition to having the potential to influence all phases of the policy formulating phase, special interest groups can also play an important role in guiding policy implementation. Through ongoing relationships with the implementing agencies, they are able to influence the rules by which policy programs will operate. The AMA, for example, works closely with HCFA to influence Medicare regulations.

A third phase of the policy process as it affects health care—policy modification—has also been described by Longest.[6] Part of the responsibility of the legislative process is in oversight of the implementation of programs in achieving their intended goals. Oversight will become increasingly important in the future in view of the strict limits set on discretionary spending and in Medicare and Medicaid spending during the next five years. Although oversight has always been important in ensuring implementation, it is now being pursued vigorously because the Congress is in Republican hands and the Executive branch is controlled by the Democrats.

When policies either do not have clear goals by which to measure them or have not been successful in attaining their stated goals, they often enter back into the legislative process for further modification. From this perspective, the policy process becomes cyclical: policy formation leads to implementation, which leads to modification, which feeds back into the formation phase. In fact, many key health policies have been modifications to previously existing policies. For example, Medicare and Medicaid were amendments to the Social Security Act and were actually extensions of earlier programs (the Old Age, Survivors' and Disability Insurance program and the Kerr-Mills program to provide medical care for the elderly poor). Medicare, in turn, was shaped by major amendments affecting hospital payments (1983) and physician payments (1989), largely because of the rising costs of health care. The Balanced Budget Act of 1997 represented yet another major shift in Medicare policy, following years of oversight hearings.

The complexity of the policy-setting process, the susceptibility of policy implementation to outside influence, and the cyclical nature of policy modification all have led to a phenomenon that is characteristic of the United States government: the incremental approach to decision-making. Whether for health care or any other social issue, policy is usually made in this country in small steps (increments). An exception was welfare reform, which did call for sweeping changes. One of the reasons for the failure of Clinton's health care reform plan was that it did not propose an incremental approach to change.

Incrementalism has come to be understood by most of the players as the way things are to be done. There is a general hesitance to take anything but a small bite out of a major policy issue, both because of a general comfort with the status quo and because of the risk of unforeseen and unintended consequences of major policy modifications. It appears that only at times of crisis, when there is broad consensus that the need for major action overshadows the risk of unintended outcomes, is our governmental system able to adopt major policy reform. (It should be pointed out that the failed Clinton health care reforms were followed by incremental health insurance reform in the Kennedy-Kassebaum bill and the incremental expansion of health insurance coverage to a portion of uninsured children.)

HISTORICAL DEVELOPMENT OF AMERICAN HEALTH POLICY

Throughout most of the nation's history, the federal government played a minor role in health policy; most of the policy interventions in public health were at the state and local levels, and most of medical care was left to the private sector. At times of crisis, such as the Civil War, the Great Depression, or, more recently, the Civil Rights Movement, quantum shifts in authority from the state level to the federal level or from the private sector to the public sector take place.

In a series of earlier books,[1,2,7] we have reviewed the historical development of health policy in the United States. Others, including Rosemary Stevens[8,9] and Paul Starr,[10] have dealt with the sweeping changes in Medicare and Medical care, and Mullen[11] has provided a history of the U.S. Public Health Service.

We have described four distinct periods in the evolution of health policy:

1. A limited role for the federal government (1798–1862)
2. The emergence of a larger federal role (1862–1932)
3. The expansion of the federal role (1935–1969)
4. New federalism (1969–present)

In the early years of the republic, the Elizabethan poor laws of England were the foundation of most policies for the poor, the aged, and the infirm. In 1798, Congress passed the Act for the Relief of Sick and Disabled Seamen, imposing a twenty cent per month tax on seamen's wages to pay for their medical care. This legislation represented the first step in establishing the U.S. Public Health Service.11

After the Civil War, the development of the germ theory of disease by Pasteur was the most powerful force affecting both public health and medical care. In public health, progress was more rapid than in medical care, with policies related to environmental sanitation, clean water, the pasteurization of milk, and expanded programs of quarantine grounded largely in the police power of state and local governments. The first federal law directly related to public health broadly was the Biologies Control Act of 1902 (P.L. 57-244), followed by the Pure Food and Drug Act (P.L. 59-384) in 1906.

In addition to the gradual increase in federal authority during this period, significant shifts were taking place in the private sector's role in health care.

During the latter half of the 19th century, there was a rapid growth in the number and in the role of hospitals. During this period, there was also the establishment of proprietary medical schools (replacing apprenticeship training) and the development of state and local public health agencies. The fragmentation of the hospitals' governance and management began with the growing number of voluntary, nonprofit, often religious hospitals in addition to local public hospitals and the proliferation of proprietary hospitals, usually owned by physicians. As medicine began to be rooted in science, and physicians gained more respect, physicians began to replace the hospital trustees in determining who was and who was not admitted to the hospital.

Late in the 19th century and early in the 20th century, hospitals gradually shifted from places for the poor to come to die to centers of medical, but particularly surgical, care for the general public. Two general types of hospitals emerged: public hospitals financed largely at the local level, and private, community-based, nonprofit hospitals, many of them operated by religious institutions. Both the proprietary, hospital-based medical schools and physician-owned proprietary hospitals gradually disappeared in the early decades of the 20th century, largely due to the efforts of the American Medical Association, stimulated by the Flexner Report in 1910.[12]

It was also during this time that state governments, at the urging of state medical societies, became involved in licensing practitioners and supporting medical education. Thus, while government was becoming increasingly involved in guiding health policy during this period, most of this activity was at the state and local rather than the federal level, and the public role in health policy was still quite limited compared with that of the private sector.

Substitution of Public Services and Financing for Private Efforts (1935–1969)

The crisis presented by the Great Depression brought action by the federal government in areas that previously had been left to state and local control. From banking regulation to support for small businesses, from public employment to old age security, there was a broadly held perception that the federal government should do what state governments had been unable or unwilling to do to respond to the crisis. Over the span of a few years, the role of the federal government vis-à-vis the states changed fundamentally. American federalism evolved from a pattern of limited federal responsibility for domestic policy to a cooperative relationship between federal and state governments with a strong, often leading role for the federal government.

This new relationship is seen nowhere more clearly than in the Social Security Act. Included within the Act was the new principle of federal aid to the states for public health and welfare assistance, including grants for maternal and child health and crippled children's services (Title V) and for general public health programs (Title VI). The Old Age, Survivors' and Disability Insurance (OASDI) program included in the original Act provided the philosophical and fiscal basis for the Medicare program enacted 30 years later.

During this period of transformation, the National Cancer Institute was established (1938); the authority of the Food and Drug Administration (FDA) was greatly strengthened, requiring approval of drugs for safety before marketing (1938); and the Nurse Training Act was passed (1941), providing schools of nursing with direct federal aid to permit them to increase their enrollments and improve their physical facilities.

After World War II, there was a growing federal role in the support of medical research, mental health research and treatment programs, and the construction of community hospitals (Hill-Burnham Act of 1946). The establishment of the Department of Health, Education, and Welfare in 1953 (now the Department of Health and Human Services), including the U.S. Public Health Service, the then separate FDA, and the Social Security Administration, firmly established the federal government's role in the nation's health care system. This new role was not, however, the result of any comprehensive or coordinated plan to develop a national health care policy. Rather, it was the amalgamation of a variety of incremental steps taken for a variety of reasons at a variety of times.

In the 1960s, there was further expansion of this new federal role in health policy. Through the "creative federalism" followed by the Kennedy and Johnson Administrations, the federal government became increasingly involved in a number of areas, including environmental health (e.g., air pollution control), community mental health centers, neighborhood health centers, health professions training, family planning, and other efforts to improve health care delivery to underserved communities. Many of these programs were financed through direct federal support for local governments and local nonprofit agencies. One of the most important laws enacted in the 1960s was the Civil Rights Act of 1964, later used as the means to desegregate the hospitals in the south. A further extension of the federal government's direct regulatory authority came with the 1962 amendments to the Food, Drug, and Cosmetics Act, which specified that manufacturers must demonstrate that a drug is both safe and effective before marketing it. Congress, between 1965 and 1967, enacted more new health legislation than all the previous congresses in the nation's 175 years.

The most dramatic expansion of federal authority in health policy was through the Social Security Amendments of 1965, establishing the Medicare and Medicaid programs to finance health care for all people older than 65 and all people receiving cash welfare assistance. These policies marked one of the first times that major health care programs were enacted over the objection of the American Medical Association, fundamentally altering the power relationship between physicians and the federal government. Never again was the medical profession able to exercise veto authority over federal health policy.

These programs of the Kennedy and Johnson years had a profound effect on intergovernmental relationships and on federal expenditures for domestic social programs. The combination of direct federal payments for Medicare and Medicaid and federal grants-in-aid helped lead to a ballooning of the federal budget, which, in the face of the strain on the domestic economy caused by the Vietnam War, created a new crisis and a dramatic shift in the role of the federal government.

The trend away from community involvement in health care was temporarily reversed with an effort in the Great Society era to base health care for vulnerable, underserved populations in community-controlled programs (e.g., neighborhood health centers, community mental health centers). Other efforts to strengthen the communities' role in the 1970s include health planning and the beginning of the "health cities" movement. Market forces, which began to play an increasingly important role in health care in the 1970s and 1980s, can have either a positive or negative impact on the role of the community, but their initial impact has been to shift control away from communities.

Entering the Era of Limited Resources: The "New Federalism" (1969–1997)

First coined by President Nixon, the term *New Federalism* described a movement to reverse the swing of government power to the federal government, transferring authority over policy and program to the states. The Nixon and Ford administrations favored block grants to the states for the support of local policy initiatives, with relatively little federal oversight. Congress resisted this move, favoring instead the continued use of categorical grants requiring detailed provisions regulating the type and level of services to be provided.

While Congress and the President argued over the issue of block versus categorical grants in the 1970s, the federal government confronted the problem of skyrocketing health care costs, largely a result of the Medicare and Medicaid programs. Federal and state governments had become third parties that underwrote the costs of a fee-for-service-based health care system that included few if any mechanisms to constrain costs. Coupled with a growing physician work force and increasing specialization, the explosion of new technology catalyzed by the enactment of the Medicare and Medicaid systems and the rapid expansion of biomedical research funded by the National Institutes of Health helped lead to a rapid upward spiral in health care costs and thus in federal expenditures.

The federal response to rapidly rising health care expenditures assumed a variety of forms, ranging from the elimination of federal subsidies for hospital construction and health professions education to price controls for a limited period and more permanent limits on hospital and physician payments by Medicare.

Additionally, in a step that was to have profound effects on the direction later market-based reforms would take, the federal government stimulated the development and expansion of health maintenance organizations (HMOs) through the Health Maintenance Organization Act of 1972. Historically an anathema to most physicians and especially to the American Medical Association, HMOs had grown very slowly.

The movement away from federal responsibility for domestic social policy accelerated when Ronald Reagan was elected President in 1980. The most prominent changes enacted by the Reagan administration that directly affected health care included (1) a sharp reduction in federal expenditures for social programs, including elimination of the revenue-sharing program initiated by President Nixon; (2) decentralization of regulatory and programmatic authority to the states, particularly through the use or block grants that came with few strings attached; (3) an increasing reliance on market forces and private institutions to stimulate needed reforms and control rising costs; and (4) through across-the-board federal tax reductions, a substantial decline in the ability of the federal government to fund new health programs. Contrary to the "deregulatory" philosophy of the administration, it established the means to regulate hospital costs, using prospective payment through the diagnosis-related group (DRG) system as an alternative to Medicare's cost-based reimbursement for hospital costs.

No longer was the federal government to be the unquestioning payer for health services. No longer did the federal government have the capacity, even if the political will were present, to fund new health care programs. The rising budget deficit, not health care, became foremost on the national agenda. The Bush Administration followed in 1989 with its support for a congressionally initiated Medicare fee schedule, to be set by the government, to control Medicare payments to physicians specified in the Omnibus Budget Reconciliation Act of 1989 (P.L. 101-239).

At the state level, increasing policy authority brought with it increasing financial burdens. As states became more responsible for establishing and implementing their own programs, they also became increasingly responsible for the costs of those programs. In the area of health care, the spiral of rising costs of Medicaid continued largely unabated, leading to increasing strain on state budgets. Once again a situation was created in which there was a mismatch between authority over a policy program and the capacity to finance that program.

A number of states turned to the private market and to market-based competition as a means of holding down costs, both the costs of publicly financed programs and the costs of health care overall. An initial change that was to have profound effects on our system of health care was an increasing reliance on for-profit corporations to operate within the health care system. Traditionally functioning as nonprofit, community-based institutions, many hospitals were taken over by for-profit chains financed through the sale of stock. A number of organizations involved in the direct provision of care, such as home health agencies and kidney dialysis centers, shifted from community control or nonprofit status to a for-profit basis. The requirement that HMOs operate on a nonprofit basis, included in the original HMO Act, was removed, opening the market to for-profit companies to become directly involved in the financing and provision of care. A number of states chose to rely on private HMOs to provide care to Medicaid beneficiaries, leaving it to the HMO to determine what constitutes "medically necessary" care.

The continued increase in health care costs seen in the late 1980s coupled with the growing role of private markets in providing access to health care services led to a new awareness of what is really an old problem: the rising number of uninsured individuals and families. Currently as many as 44 million Americans have no insurance to pay for needed health care. The number of uninsured is increasing about 1 million per year despite the growing economy with its low levels of unemployment.

The dilemma that confronted the Clinton Administration when it took office in 1992 was that Americans want to have their health care cake and eat it too. They want health care made more available to the uninsured, and they want the cost of health care to come under control, but only if these actions don't diminish the ability of the average American to get whatever treatment he or she perceives to be necessary or appropriate in a timely manner. This perhaps is the fundamental American health policy dilemma. President and the Congress in 1993 faced conflicting needs and expectations with neither a mechanism to establish a broad-based consensus on how to reconcile them nor a mechanism to enact that consensus if it was achieved. President Clinton had campaigned on the need for the federal government to reassert itself in the area of health policy. With the broad goals of expanding coverage to the uninsured while simultaneously controlling health care costs, the Clinton health reform plan would have given broad new authority to the federal government to regulate the market for health insurance, while maintaining a reliance on market-based competition. It sought a new balance between the market-based delivery of care and a broad umbrella of federal oversight. The idea was an attempt to redefine the role of federalism in health policy, but it was seriously out of synch with the continued movement in the evolution of federal authority. As pointed out by Theda Skocpol,[13] the ebbing tide of federal authority over social policy had not yet run its course. With an irony that has not yet been fully appreciated, the country was ready for one part of the Clinton proposal but not the other. Although Congress rejected an increased role for the federal government in regulating the market for health insurance, the deliberations surrounding the Clinton proposal nevertheless opened the door even more widely for market-based competition among health plans to become the principal paradigm for American health care at the end of the 20th century. Although it is happening in some areas of the country more rapidly than others, there has been a clear shift to the evolving concept of managed care for the financing, provision, and oversight of health care to most Americans. The shift comes, however, without any organized system of oversight or regulation and with an increasing role for for-profit companies. As a reaction, many states are now proposing a variety of "consumer protective" laws (more than 400 bills introduced in state legislatures in 1997) to begin to place some limits on private sector managed care plans, and the President has proposed a "Consumer Bill of Rights." At the same time, states are increasingly mandating the enrollment of Medicaid beneficiaries (e.g., mothers and children) in managed care plans, and Medicare is poised to significantly expand the role of managed care plans.

Reductions in care, financial incentives that pit physicians' needs against those of patients, and a disavowal of responsibility for caring for the uninsured all are characteristics of this new American system of health care. In the words of one of the more vigorous advocates of for-profit health care plans,

Investor-owned health plans are a driving force behind this transformation [of the health care delivery system in America], and nonprofit health plans, in my view, are a byproduct of the past . . . There is an appropriate role for nonprofit plans, but it is not in the operation of competitive health plans.[14]

Was this the health care system that the American public intended to have? Did the United States get here as a result of a well-thought-out policy deliberation? As with much of the history of American health policy, the answer to both questions is "no." Once again the separation of the authority over health policy and the financial responsibility for it has led to an outcome that was unintended and, as many believe, is not in the best interest of the American people.

While the private sector was moving rapidly, without adequate federal or state ground rules to "level the playing field," there was paralysis of health policy making at the federal level after the failure of President Clinton's health care reform proposals in 1993–1994. The situation only grew worse after the Republicans captured both the Senate and the House of Representatives in 1994. What followed was 2 years of ideological debate with a standoff between the President and the Congress. After President Clinton's reelection in 1996 and the continued control of Congress by the Republicans, the Congress and the Clinton Administration began to work together to produce potentially constructive changes in the Medicare program. The result was the Balanced Budget Act of 1997, signed by President Clinton in August 1997.

The basic Medicare provisions, including a 5-year spending reduction of $115 billion below Congressional Budget Office (CBO) projections based on existing policies, were

- Coordinated care plans, including HMOs, preferred provider organizations (PPOs), plans offered by provider sponsored organizations (PSOs), and point-of-service plans (POSs)
- Private fee-for-service
- On a demonstration basis, high deductible plans with medical savings account

The balanced Budget Act of 1997 reflected a political consensus that had arisen from the ashes of the rancorous stalemate of 1995–1996 that followed the Republican capture of the Congress. The Medicare reform process reversed almost every aspect of the failed partisan debates of the previous 2 years. The Medicare reform process in 1997 was similar to the successful Medicare hospital and physician payment reform of 1983 and 1989 and the expansion of Medicaid eligibility for children in poverty in the early 1990s.

The direction for health care in the 21st century, at least in its early years, may well have been set by the Balanced Budget Act of 1997, just as it was set in the past 30 years by the Social Security Amendment of 1965, which established Medicare and Medicaid as public programs that bought into and reinforced the then dominant fee-for-service system. Times have changed and health care will change as well.

References

1. Hamilton, W.H. *Medical care for the American people: The final report of the Committee on the Cost of Medical Care.* Adopted October 31, 1932. Chicago: University of Chicago Press, 1932.
2. Lee, P.R., and Benjamin, A.E. Health policy and the politics of health care. In S.J. Williams and P.R. Torrens (eds). *Introduction to health services.* 4th ed. Albany: Delmar Publishers, 1993.
3. Lee, P.R., Benjamin, A.E., and Weber, M.A. Policies and strategies for health care in the United States. In *Oxford Textbook of Public Health.* 3rd ed. Oxford: Oxford University Press, 1996.
4. Peterson, M.A. Political influence in the 1990s: From iron triangle to policy network. *Journal of Health Politics, Policy and Law.* Summer, 1993;18:395–438.
5. Kingdon, J.W. *Agendas, alternatives, and public policies.* Boston: Little, Brown, 1993.
6. Longest, B. *Health policymaking in the United States.* Ann Arbor, MI: Health Administration Press, 1994.
7. Lee, P.R., and Silver, G.A. Health planning—A view from the top with specific reference to the U.S.A. In J. Fry and W.A.J. Farndale (eds). *International medical care.* Oxford: MTP Medical and Technical Publishing, 1972.
8. Stevens, R. *American medicine and the public interest.* New York: Basic Books, 1971.
9. Stevens, R. *In sickness and in wealth: American hospitals in the twentieth century.* New York: Basic Books, 1989.
10. Starr, P. *Social transformation of American medicine: The rise of the sovereign profession and the making of a vast industry.* New York: Basic Books, 1982.
11. Mullen, F. *Plague and politics.* New York: Basic Books, 1989.
12. Flexner, A. *Medical education in the United States and Canada.* New York: Carnegie Foundation for the Advancement of Teaching, 1910.
13. Skocpol, T. *Boomerang: Clinton's health security effort and the turn against government in U.S. politics.* New York: W.W. Norton, 1996.
14. Hassan, M. Let's end the nonprofit charade. *New England Journal of Medicine.* 1996;334:1055–1057.

3

Healthy American Families in a Postmodern Society: An Ecological Perspective

JOAN M. PATTERSON

Preparation of this chapter was supported by the Maternal and Child Health Bureau
Grant #MCJ000111.

The family is the primary social context affecting the health and well-being of children, adolescents, and adults. While there has long been implicit recognition of the centrality of the family in the lives of children, it is only since the 1980s that phrases such as "family-centered care" have been used to emphasize a recommended style of professional practice.[1] Professionals are expected to work collaboratively with families in meeting the needs of children, while paying attention to families' knowledge, expertise, values, beliefs, and preferences. Despite this avowed paradigm for practice, knowledge about family systems and the skills needed to work effectively with them are often assumed. Many maternal and child health (MCH) professionals are unaware of the expanding body of theoretical and empirical knowledge in the family field that can be applied to their work with children and families. The goal of this chapter is to present a perspective on understanding the family system that can be applied in professional practice environments, by policymakers, and in research studies.

CHILDREN AND FAMILIES ARE PART OF AN ECOSYSTEM

Traditionally, MCH has focused on meeting the health needs of children. The family, especially the mother, was seen as either supporting or undermining child outcomes. The effects were viewed primarily as occurring in one direction—from parent to child. It is important to recognize, however, that dyadic interaction does not occur in isolation, but rather in a social context that shapes its direction and quality. Social contexts present opportunities and risks for the development and well-being of those within them. While the family is the most proximate social context for children (and most adults), and thus has a powerful influence on behavior and health, there are other social contexts that also influence individuals and families: schools, workplaces, neighborhoods, peer groups, and churches, for example. Furthermore, these social systems are inextricably interconnected, and they mutually influence each other. For example, a job requiring an adult to travel extensively or work long hours can affect the pattern and quality of that person's relationships with children or with a partner. Conversely, parental worry about the adequacy of child care can affect work productivity. No matter which system one chooses to study, intervene with, or make policy about (e.g., child, parent, family, neighborhood, school, workplace, community), consideration must be given to its interconnections with other contexts to enhance effectiveness. In essence, this is the ecological perspective.[2,3]

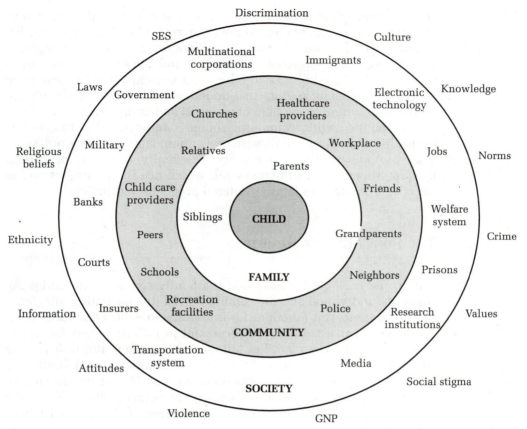

FIGURE 3.1

....

The ecosystem of the child and the family.

A schematic of the ecosystem of a child is presented in Figure 3.1. The child is viewed within the context of the family, which resides within a community context. Within each of these systems, there are subsystems, which have definable boundaries. A system's boundary sets it apart from its context and is important for maintaining the identity and integrity of the system. Without a boundary, a system merges into its surroundings and ceases to be a separate system.

The systems in which family members interact with others directly are called *microsystems* and are embedded in a larger ideological context, called the *macrosystem*. Components of the macrosystem are generally more abstract and include such things as values, norms, social policies, cultural patterns, institutional patterns, and social conditions. Most importantly, neither microsystems nor the macrosystem are static, but rather are dynamic and evolving as a result of the continuous reciprocal influences of these systems on each other. The way in which a family, a child, a community, or a school functions and the degree to which it can be considered "healthy," is influenced by the macrosystem as well as the linkages to other microsystems. It is this emergent property of dynamic systems that underlies the notion of development, which is so central to the field of maternal and child health.

In public health, community often is emphasized as the context for health promotion and disease prevention; family is more or less assumed to be part of the community. The family, however, has certain unique properties as a microsystem, which need to be understood to effectively implement family-centered programs and policies.

THE FUNCTIONS OF FAMILIES

Within the ecological framework, the family serves as the bridge between the individual and the community. In this mediating role, families fulfill important functions for individual members and for society. To the extent that families are successful in fulfilling these functions, society benefits; when families falter or are unable to fulfill them, it is costly to society. Four central functions of families are (1) family formation and membership, (2) economic support, (3) nurturance and socialization, and (4) protection of vulnerable members. In Table 3.1, the ways in which these functions serve the needs of individual family members and of society are presented.

The ability of families to successfully fulfill these functions depends to a great extent on the risks or opportunities in other social systems in the community and in the macrosystem. Public programs and policies, societal norms and values, and other community institutions all shape the style and degree of fulfillment of these functions. When schools do not educate young people and prepare them for jobs and careers, or when institutional policies limit employment opportunities for certain cultural, gender, or ethnic groups, many families are challenged in meeting their economic function. When pregnancies are unplanned or unwanted, the motivation to form and maintain a family is threatened. Furthermore, when this membership function is undermined, the economic, nurturant, and protective functions of the family may subsequently be challenged as well. The cumulative costs of a family's inability to fulfill these functions are significant.

In addition to external challenges, special needs of individuals within the family can challenge successful fulfillment of family functions. For example, a child with special health needs often requires

TABLE 3.1

Primary Functions of the Family for Individual Members and for Society

	What the Function Does For	
Family Function	*Individual Family Members*	*Society*
Membership and Family Formation	Provides a sense of belonging Provides personal and social identity Provides meaning and direction for life	Controls reproductive function Ensures continuation of the species
Economic	Provides for basic needs of food, shelter, and clothing and other resources to enhance human development	Contributes to healthy development of members who are/become contributing members of society (and who need fewer public resources)
Nurturance, Education, and Socialization	Provides for the physical, psychological, social, and spiritual development of children and adults Instills social values and norms	Prepares and socializes children for productive adult roles Supports adults in being productive members of society Controls antisocial behavior and protects society from harm
Protection of Vulnerable Members	Provides protective car and support for young, ill, disabled, or otherwise vulnerable members	Minimizes public responsibility for care of vulnerable, dependent individuals

greater levels of protection and specialized care over an extended period of the family's life cycle. The child with special needs may challenge the economic resources of the family or may need special education and different parental nurturance requiring specialized training. In these instances, public support and programs are needed to bolster the family's ability to successfully fulfill their functions. Such support can make a difference in outcomes, not only for the child with special needs, but for other family members and for maintenance of a healthy family unit. Healthy families contribute to society and reduce the likelihood of needing more costly services later.

The example of a child with special health needs can be used to further illustrate the dynamic interrelationships of other systems in the ecosystem. Within the past century, there has been an increase in the number of families caring for vulnerable family members because of (1) advances in biomedical knowledge and technology (linked to macrolevel social policies supporting scientific research) that sustain fragile lives at birth, in old age, and following major injuries and illnesses; and (2) social policies and norms (macro-level change resulting from research findings) favoring deinstitutionalization of those with disabilities and mainstreaming them into normative community and family contexts. This caregiving burden for families has been further exacerbated by the current national emphasis on controlling spiraling health care costs (macro-level beliefs, attitudes, and values influencing community-level health care payers and providers) by changing the way health care services are organized, paid for, and delivered. Thus, within the community context, health care services are increasingly being delivered by managed care organizations that often control costs by restricting and/or denying access to some services. Families are expected to pick up the pieces and directly provide more services or pay for services their vulnerable members need to survive and have a decent quality of life. Not all families have been able to absorb these added demands and simultaneously fulfill their other functions. Extensive caregiving may, for example, challenge fulfillment of their economic function or compromise their ability to nurture each other, or even undermine membership if the child must be placed in foster care or if the parents divorce.

This example draws attention to the need to understand why similar circumstances can lead to such different outcomes for families and why some families are able to fulfill their functions, even under extreme circumstances, while other families are not.

What Is a Family?

A family system is a group of individuals (two or more) and the pattern of relationships between them. Contained within this definition are two critical aspects of a family: family structure and family functioning. *Family structure* is defined as who is in the system. An invisible boundary marks who is in (and who is out) and sets the family apart from its social context. Family structure allows for the family within to create its own identity and sense of itself so that it can effectively carry out the functions already described. One of the important tasks of a family is to define and maintain this boundary—to be clear about who is part of its family unit.

In postmodern* America, there is considerable variability about who is considered "family." The U.S. Census Bureau definition of fam-

Postmodern refers to the contemporary era characterized by a multiplicity of structural forms and styles of interacting within social institutions (including the family), which continue to change more rapidly given the exponential increase in new knowledge that can be quickly and widely disseminated using electronic technology.

ily as two or more persons living together who are related by blood, marriage, or adoption does not allow for this variability. A postmodern definition of family might be "the nexus of two or more people, living in close contact, who care for one another, and provide guidance for their dependent members."[4] This definition validates diverse family forms, such as heterosexual and homosexual married, remarried, or co-habiting couples, with or without children; or separated, divorced, and always single adults with children. The definition also incorporates cultural and ethnic variability. For example, among African Americans, friends and neighbors who function as family members in providing support but who do not live in the household are called "fictive kin" and often are considered to be part of the family.[5]

Family functioning refers to the ongoing patterns of relationship connecting members of a family system to each other.[6] Functioning patterns are not the same as family functions; rather, functioning is a process variable and describes the way in which families fulfill their functions. There are, for example, family patterns for showing affection (hugs, kisses, smiles, verbal compliments), for showing anger and conflict (yelling, ignoring, pouting, banging things, denial), for accomplishing daily routines (preparing meals, shopping, assigning tasks), for disciplining children (stern language, withholding privileges, logical consequences), for celebrating holidays and birthdays (type of food served, who is invited, where celebration occurs), and so forth. It is important to note that family functioning refers to a property of the whole unit, not just a property of one or two members. Furthermore, family functioning is not unitary, even though it is often referred to this way. Rather, it is multidimensional; many different aspects of functioning can be considered, such as cohesion, flexibility, communication, and behavioral control. Deciding which dimensions of family functioning to pay attention to depends on the application (e.g., marital enrichment program, parent education, providing services to a child with special health needs). When family assessment or functioning is limited to a single dimension or is equated with the dimensions of a known self-report family questionnaire, the rich scientific basis for understanding family process is lost and so, too, is our ability to understand the strengths and needs of families.

VARIATIONS IN FAMILY STRUCTURE AND FUNCTIONING

Today, families in the United States are characterized by extraordinary variation in both structure and functioning. It is this variability that has given rise to so much controversy and so many negative judgments about families. The family as a unitary form does not exist. Rather, there are multiple family forms experienced by different individuals within our society, as well as by any given individual over his or her life span. Among the many ways this variability in families can be examined are by socioeconomic status, culture and ethnicity, historical time, and changes over an individual's life cycle.

Socioeconomic Status

Family structure both influences socioeconnomic status (SES) and is influenced by it. A family structure that includes two working adults generally has a higher level of family income. A two-parent family is usually associated with higher social status. The dramatic increase in the number of single-parent households (see Chapter 1) is a major factor associated with the increase in poverty among children in the United States.[7] Conversely, SES can influence family structure. For example, immigrant families, who struggle to access economic resources and who have lower social status, are more likely to live in extended families as a way to provide economic and emotional support to each other and increase their chances for a higher quality of life. Another example of how SES can influence family structure is the dramatic increase in the divorce rate beginning in the mid-1960s.[8] In addition to changing societal norms making divorce more acceptable, it has been noted that the relative increase in average family income made it more possible for many middle-class couples to divorce and create two viable economic units.

In addition to family structure, SES influences and is influenced by family functioning patterns. Most notable is the way a family's economic status influences its ability to maintain its sense of control over life choices. Families with a higher income maintain more closed external boundaries as evidenced in their having more privacy and experiencing less control from outside agencies. In contrast, families with lower SES, who are more dependent on public programs for support, are more subject to intrusion from outside "helpers." When helping systems are judgmental, are overly directive, and insist on certain behavioral criteria, families have a harder time maintaining a sense of direction for their lives. Their external boundaries are weakened, which increases the risk for dissolution of the family. (Remember that a family that cannot maintain boundaries around itself ceases to be a separate system.) When providing assistance, it is important for helping professionals to recognize the importance of supporting a family in maintaining its own sense of who they are as a family, what they value about themselves, and what they want for their future.

The desire to increase or even maintain their SES has led to more families with two employed adults. Depending on the reasons for dual employment, it can be associated with quite different family functioning patterns. When both adults feel forced to work to support the family, there is more conflict and less cohesiveness in the family than in those families in which both adults work by choice as a way to enhance their personal growth.

Another way that SES affects family structure is with regard to the increased scarcity of blue-collar jobs for those with less education. Fathers who are unable to obtain work and provide support for their families are more likely to leave the family, resulting in a single-parent family structure. With advances in technology, more jobs require specialized education and training, which has increased unemployment among lower SES groups. Historically, inability to get a job also has been associated with discrimination and racism. This is only one of several ways that race, ethnicity, and culture affect family structure and functioning.

Ethnicity and Culture

Differences in family structure between and within ethnic groups reflect both historical and cultural preferences, as well as responses to policies and attitudes of the larger macro environment. For example, the family structure of African Americans is characterized by more single-female households, which are bolstered by extensive ties to female kin and fictive kin. This matriarchal structure is, in part, related to a history of employment discrimination against African American males, making it difficult for them to enact the provider role and thus contributing to disconnectedness from their families.[9] In contrast to these single-parent families, Hispanic families are more likely to have two parents, and they often have more children as well, which reflects religious beliefs discouraging divorce and encouraging childbearing (macro-level influence). Ties to extended families are also strong among Hispanics.[10]

In addition to structure, a family's functioning style very often incorporates ethnic, cultural, or religious beliefs and traditions. For example, the person in the family who has the most power and authority is often shaped by religious, cultural, or ethnic beliefs. It may be the husband/father, an elder, or the husband's mother. Communication patterns are another way families are influenced by their culture. The quiet stoicism of Americans from Northern Europe stands in contrast to the intense expressions of anger, love, and other emotions characteristic of other Americans. Many Native American tribes proscribe talking with certain family members and some proscribe eye contact when talking with someone of higher status. Some cultures prefer using food rather than language to communicate, whereas others expect insightful dialogue as a way to ascribe meaning to life experiences.[11]

The degree to which any given family maintains a distinct ethnic, cultural, or religious identity in their structure and functioning varies within these groups. When a group has experienced a history of discrimination and has learned to band together against the mainstream culture as a way to survive, there may be an implicit expectation of loyalty to these distinct patterns. Many times, there is tension and conflict within families when some members choose to adopt the values and lifestyle of the dominant homogeneous culture. The family's functioning patterns reveal this conflict, which can pervade the family and even extend to neighborhood and community groups. The familiar play and movie *West Side Story* depicts these kinds of tensions, which are all too real for many families in our large inner cities today. Intergenerational conflict frequently occurs among new immigrant families when children acquire the language and cultural preferences for the American lifestyle. It is important that these conflicts be viewed as reflecting pressure from outside the family and not simply be labeled as something dysfunctional within the family.

Historical Time

Many of the critics of family life in the United States today draw from a romanticized view of family life in the past, as exemplified in former television programs such as *Ozzie and Harriet*, *The Waltons*, or *Leave It to Beaver*. Two idealized models of family life that persist today are the intact extended family of the distant past and the modern nuclear family of the recent past.[12] In actuality, these family forms are myths since they never were dominant for most American people of any era.[13] Before the industrial revolution, death precluded large numbers of multigenerational, intact families; infant mortality was high, parental death was common, and the average life expectancy was in the mid-40s. Family units were organized primarily around the economic function, with mothers and children contributing labor. Mothers and fathers shared in the education and socialization of their children. Generally a more patriarchal, authoritarian family functioning style prevailed. In addition, many households included non-kin boarders (e.g., immigrants, orphans, frail adults), suggesting considerable diversity in family arrangements.

The "modern" family usually refers to the forms that emerged after the industrial revolution. In many families, men went to work in factories and earned most of the family income; education of children was taken over by the community; and women were expected to cultivate a nurturing home environment for children who were now viewed as vulnerable and in need of protection. Emphasis was placed on families' nurturance and socialization function. Segregated family roles led to women's and children's economic dependence on male breadwinners and diminished men's involvement with their families. While this family form was viewed as the ideal, in actuality, only middle-class fathers could successfully compete for the jobs that would support their families with one income. Immigrants and ethnic minority families still required two wage earners. It was during the prosperity of the 1950s following World War II that the idealized family form of a breadwinner father and a stay-at-home mother became dominant. During this time, when women did have to work to support the family, it was viewed as demeaning, and they achieved lower pay and lower status. Working mothers were viewed as harmful to their husbands' self-esteem and to their children's healthy development. This period was short-lived, however. The percentage of mothers working has steadily increased since the 1960s because of increased divorce and female-headed households, fewer children, more educated women, and dual parent employment to improve economic status.[7] However, the pervasiveness of this idealization of the 1950s family has continued, perhaps because so many baby boomers (now in leadership roles) actually experienced it and because growth of the media, particularly television, introduced so many Americans to this ideology.[14]

As we move into the 21st century, families most likely will continue to show even greater variability in their structure and functioning because of the impact of ecosystemic changes such as encouragement of cultural diversity, the growing gap between those who have wealth and the poor, the globalization of the economy and other social institutions, the exponential increase in new knowledge generation, and the pervasiveness of telecommunications for information dissemination.

Changes Over the Life Cycle

Family development theory can be used to understand variability in family structure and functioning at different stages of the family life cycle. Normative family structure changes occur with the addition (birth, adoption) and departure (young adults leave home, death) of members. Family functioning patterns change as children grow and develop and become more independent. With more than half of marriages ending in divorce and with many of these adults remarrying, these structural changes call for different functioning patterns as new, often more complex, roles are negotiated. Many stepfamilies experience difficulty clarifying their structure (e.g., children are unsure who is in the family and who is not), which, in turn, can lead to problems in family functioning patterns (such as who makes decisions and about which things, how to show affection and to whom, methods for disciplining children).

In other words, all individuals experience many different forms of family structure and functioning over their life spans as they grow and develop, create and end relationships, and experience health problems, disability, deaths, and loss. It is likely that this normative variability will continue to increase as life expectancy continues to expand. Program planners and policymakers are encouraged to take these sources of variability into account in their work to support families' efforts to satisfactorily fulfill their functions. This work with and on behalf of families is ultimately directed at improving the health and well-being of individual family members as well as the family system. Given the sources and extent of variability in postmodern families, we can now examine what constitutes a healthy family.

FAMILY SYSTEM HEALTH

Assessing the health of any system is complex. At the individual level, health has been defined as the absence of illness (a dichotomy), as varying along a continuum from good to poor, or even as a dynamic state, expressed as the process of living.[15] The World Health Organization[16] definition emphasizes the multidimensional nature of health: physical, psychological, social, and spiritual well-being.

At the family level, there are at least two different ways to conceptualize health: (1) as the sum of the individual health statuses of all family members or (2) as the health of the family unit as a whole, that is, the health of the family system's functioning patterns. The second method acknowledges that a system is more than the sum of its parts. It examines the quality of the ongoing interaction patterns linking individual family members with each other. The focus is on family process.

Similar to the challenge in deciding what constitutes individual well-being, this systemic definition of family health calls for a judgment about what constitutes "quality." How should this judgment be made and by whom? Froma Walsh has examined this issue in her discussion of "normal family processes."[12] She notes that there are at least four different ways to conceptualize family normality: asymptomatic functioning, average functioning, optimal functioning, and transactional processes.

Asymptomatic functioning requires that there are no symptoms of disorder in any family member. It parallels the dichotomy applied to healthy versus ill individuals. However, it would be a rare family that has no problems, and furthermore, a family problem should not be equated with family pathology. It would also be erroneous to assume that all individual symptoms are indicative of family pathology and, conversely, that all healthy individuals live in healthy families.

Average family functioning is based on social norms defining what is most common across all families. In this view, family functioning patterns are viewed along a continuum. Self-report measures of family functioning are based on this approach. Statistically, any functioning dimension has a normal distribution with a measure of central tendency (mean, mode, median). The amount of deviation from this central measure is used to determine the degree to which a family is average and healthy. Sometimes, cut-off scores (e.g., the mean, plus or minus 1 to 2 standard deviations) are used to determine whether a family is unhealthy (even though the positive end of the distribution would have to be considered "super" healthy). Many questionnaires have published "norms" providing a basis for comparing one family or a sample of families. However, the norming group does not always represent the whole population and may be biased in favor of one cultural or ethnic group (e.g., white middle-class families that often are easier to recruit to collect these data). In addition to objective tests, averages often are implied in subjective judgments about a given family. A family that has a different structure and style of functioning is all too often labeled "dysfunctional." However, deviation from the average does not necessarily imply pathology. Given the range of family cultural beliefs and behaviors, as well as the range of circumstances within a family's ecological context, statistically or subjectively determined deviant behavior may, in fact, be the most adaptive and healthy. This, or course, begs the question of who should decide what is healthy and under what circumstances. Most importantly, we should be cautious in making judgments about family functioning, especially for those with different cultural, religious, and ethnic backgrounds than our own, without fully understanding contextual factors.

Optimal family functioning is based on the ability of a family to successfully accomplish family tasks and promote the development and well-being of individual members. Or alternatively, it can be viewed as successfully accomplishing family functions to meet the needs of individual members and of society. As was noted earlier, *who* decides what is optimal and for whom is an important consideration in any application of this basis for assessing family health.

Transactional family processes provide a basis for conceptualizing family normality or health relative to a family's context. From this perspective, it is recognized that family processes change over time in response to changes within the family and that these processes vary relative to interactions with other systems in the family's ecological context. There is a natural propensity for a family to interact in a way that allows for a satisfactory "fit" between individual members and the family unit and between the family unit and systems outside its boundaries. Achieving a fit does not imply that families must do all the changing; rather, larger systems often need to change to accommodate varying family needs and preferences. Sometimes families are labeled dysfunctional when they encounter a rigid community system that forces all families to fit into its established patterns and expectations. Recall the earlier discussion about the intrusiveness of many helping systems in overly directing families (especially those with multiple problems) about how to behave and interact.

The perspective offered here is that determination of whether a family is functional or dysfunctional must be made relative to the family's circumstances—stage of the life cycle; family structure; its cultural, religious, ethnic beliefs, values, and preferences; the unique needs and demands emanating from within the family (e.g., a child with special health needs); its socioeconomic status; and other social demographic factors. A family should be encouraged to establish its own goals and patterns for accomplishing its functions, without invoking harm to individual members or to others in society. When a family struggles to accomplish these functions, it should not automatically be assumed that the family is dysfunctional. Many times families are blamed for society's problems or failures or for shifts in societal expectations that the family is unable to accommodate (e.g., providing home care for a vulnerable member). This pejorative labeling of families is often encouraged by our deficit-based helping institutions, in which malfunctioning is the basis for receiving services. Unfortunately, these negative attributions often exacerbate the family's problem and contribute to their inability to develop self-sufficiency.

Assessing the lack of fit between individual members and their family unit or between the family and its community context requires an understanding of the needs and resources in all these systems. Achieving a better fit between two systems often calls for accommodation within both systems by increasing the flow of resources into the burdened system and/or reducing demands and expectations on it.

Whose Health Matters Most?

Many would argue that the bottom line is really the health and well-being of individuals; the family is only a means to that end. However, from a systems perspective, it is an arbitrary punctuation in a circular sequence of effects to focus only on whether the family does or does not contribute to individual health. Individual health (or lack of it) affects the functioning patterns in a family. For example, following divorce, a single parent who is economically and psychologically distressed may interact with her child in a way that meets the parent's needs. These expectations from the child may subsequently interfere with the child's accomplishment of his or her developmental tasks, such as difficulty developing peer relationships or problems with academic achievement. These child problems could, in turn, intensify the parent's distress and exacerbate the problematic relationship between the parent and child, and so on, in a circular sequence of effects. Another example of these mutual effects can be seen when a child is diagnosed with a chronic illness. An aberration in a biological system of one individual can lead to alterations in his or her developmental course, which affects relationships in the family and establishes new patterns of family functioning, which have an effect on the child's development, and so on. In Figure 3.2, this circular pattern of effects between a child with chronic illness and the family is diagrammed.

We could extend these reciprocal interaction patterns between child and family outward to include community interactions. For example, social stigma could lead to isolation of the child, with parents trying to compensate for this pain or loss, which could further inten-

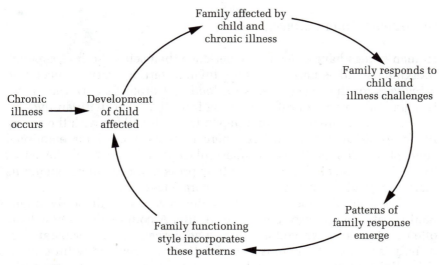

FIGURE 3.2

....

Circular sequence of effects between child with chronic illness and family functioning.

sify maladaptive patterns of family functioning. Or formal community systems of support and care (such as schools, health care providers, and insurers) may be inadequate to meet the child's needs, thereby adding to the burden of an already strained family system. From these examples, we can see how the health of individuals, families, and communities are inextricably intertwined. Rather than blaming or trying to "fix" families, programs and policies should be developed with these interconnections in mind.

PRIMARY SYSTEMIC ISSUES SHAPING FAMILY FUNCTIONING PATTERNS

Family scholars are frequently asked to describe the traits of healthy families. Given the previously described perspective on the wide variability in adaptive family structure and family functioning patterns, it is risky and perhaps a disservice to families to do this, because a list can easily become prescriptive or be used to make judgments. However, there are two processes in human development, which are enacted in a family context, that provide a window into a family's style of functioning. These processes involve achieving a balance (1) between separateness and connectedness and (2) between change and stability.[17]

Separateness and Connectedness

Human beings have a need to experience themselves both as separate individuals and as part of a group. Infants start out very connected to caregivers for their basic needs for food and protection. Development is a gradual process of differentiating from the other, with an increasing capacity to function as an independent being. Even with the capacity for physical independence, there remains a need for emotional connection. The family is a primary place this connection is enacted. Every family needs to find a way to express connectedness among its members, while allowing for some separateness too.

The desired amount of connectedness varies significantly among families at different ages and stages of life. A couple with a new baby often prefers to be very close; during adolescence, more separateness usually is preferred. There is also variation between and within different religious, cultural, and ethnic groups. The Amish, for example, emphasize strong connectedness to the family and community. In contrast, the dominant European American culture emphasizes individualism. Adolescents are encouraged to be independent from their parents. Many problematic behaviors observed in adolescents are manifestations of family conflict in renegotiating the balance between connectedness and separateness. Unfortunately, many professionals working with youth align with the adolescent against the parents. In so doing, a professional (whose contact with the youth is relatively brief) may inadvertently circumvent the resolution of this challenge between family members whose kinship connections extend over a lifetime.

While most families prefer neither extreme of disengagement or enmeshment,[19] even these extremes can be adaptive for a family if this is a shared functioning preference. It is disagreement about what is desired and expected of other members at different life cycle stages that can lead to problems in family functioning. The underlying tension in achieving a satisfactory balance between togetherness and apartness often underlies the symptoms in families seeking professional help for their problems.

Change and Stability

The second central process of family functioning is achieving a balance between change and stability in roles, rules, and patterns of interacting with each other. In contemporary America, there is a tendency to place a high value on the ability of individuals and families to change rapidly in response to changing circumstances. However, too much change can undermine the stability of most family systems. Families need to hold on to some core sense of place and identity and to have some continuity with their past and future if they are to maintain their integrity as a system. Family scholars point to daily routines and rituals as one important way in which families retain this sense of who they are.

Again, there is wide variability in how much any given family desires or needs to change. Traditional families are more likely to hold on to values and beliefs from their past; postmodern families, on the other hand, are more eager to create something new that integrates current circumstances. Both kinds of families can be healthy and adaptive. Professionals should be aware of these family differences whenever they are advocating for traditional behaviors or, conversely, encouraging families to change and adapt to new circumstances. Families in transition, such as immigrant families, new stepfamilies, and those suffering losses, moving up or down the SES ladder, or moving from one location to another, often struggle with how much and in what ways to change.

Communication skills, congruent with cultural expectations, are the facilitating dimension for expressing connectedness, for negotiating change, and for resolving conflicts about how much closeness or change is desired. Prevention programs designed for families, not just for individuals, that integrate an understanding of these two underlying processes and that teach culturally appropriate communication skills would be helpful to many families.

THE ROLE OF POLICYMAKERS AND PROFESSIONALS IN FACILITATING FAMILY HEALTH

Throughout this discussion, there have been several allusions to the role of professionals in helping or hindering families' pursuit of their own health. In advocating this position, it is important to emphasize its underlying assumption: families are capable of creating their own healthy systems. Many policymakers and professionals would disagree with this assertion because of the evidence they see of neglected, maltreated children and youth and the symptomatic behavior observed in the adults in their lives. Families often are blamed for causing social problems. From an ecosystems perspective, however, such behaviors are embedded in a larger social context in which transactions between systems have contributed to the development and/or maintenance of these maladaptive behaviors. Any lasting change in the structure and functioning of families will require multi-level, holistic thinking. A systems perspective also suggests the possibility that a relatively small change, leveraged at a critical entry point, can set in motion a ripple effect of changes across interconnected systems. Multi-level changes and leveraged changes should be considered at both the macro- and micro-levels.

Macrosystem Strategies

It is beyond the scope of this chapter to fully consider the many ways in which social policies have and could be used to strengthen the ability of families, especially those that are poor or otherwise marginalized from society's resources. Such policies are needed at federal, state, and local levels as well as in the private free enterprise sector. For example:

- Families' abilities to provide for the needs of their vulnerable members are profoundly influenced by legislation regulating public expenditures for health care, such as Medicaid, Supplemental Security Income (SSI), or the Children's Health Insurance Plan enacted in 1997.

- The stress on families caused by trying to balance work and family responsibilities could be helped by policies such as the Family and Medical Leave Act of 1993, which provided up to 12 weeks of unpaid leave (with job protection and medical benefits) for birth of a newborn, an adoption, or a family member's illness. However, more than half of all workers do not benefit because the law does not apply to employers with fewer than 50 employees nor to individuals employed at the same job for less than 12 consecutive months.

- Many employers have independently established family-supportive programs and policies, such as on-site child care, flextime, extended paid parental/family leave, good health care benefit packages, and work-at-home options. Generally, employers find that such programs increase worker satisfaction and productivity and hence are cost effective.

- Child care policies are needed to guarantee higher licensing standards, improved training for child care workers, and increased pay.

A fundamental issue that must be addressed at the macro-level is the growing gap between the rich and the poor in the United States, which significantly restricts the ability of families to provide for their members. The increasing number of children who live in poor families underlies much of the dysfunction observed in families today. Inability to provide economic support undermines family fulfillment of membership, nurturance, and protective functions as well. More equitable distribution of this country's wealth will require major changes in social policy. The policies of other developed countries are evidence that this is possible and suggest specific strategies for how this might be accomplished. (See Kamerman[19] for a discussion of some of these policies.)

Microsystem Strategies

There are numerous ways that the community systems in which family members interact directly can contribute to family health. Too many institutional settings are characterized by long-standing, dysfunctional patterns, which can undermine the health of those they attempt to serve. From an ecological and systemic perspective, this observation suggests an important strategy related to health promotion. It is critical that any individual or social system advocating and working for the health of others give equal attention to the health of their own system. This notion of congruence in practice and philosophy between multiple levels of systems is called *isomorphism*. Lizbeth Schorr[20] observed that human service agencies that were the most effective in serving children and families had developed organizational structures that respected and empowered the individuals who worked in them, thereby enabling them to be creative, effective, and competent in their work with others.

In addition to working in healthy organizations, many human service professionals could enhance their effectiveness with training in how to provide family-centered, culturally competent services. Skills such as de-centering, sharing power with others, observing and commenting on another's strengths, valuing and respecting differences, and facilitating natural network building can be developed. These process skills affect the quality of connections between systems. Professionals need to recognize that it is not only *what* information or skill they give or teach that matters, but also *how* it is given.

Family resource and support programs have been increasing as part of community building initiatives across the country. In the best circumstances, program needs and methods for delivering programs are identified by family members living in the community. Top-down resources should be increased so that these community-based, grassroots efforts can be expanded.

There are many programs being offered that educate family members to fulfill family functions, recognizing that not all adults have had the life experiences to prepare them for family roles and challenges. Programs such as couples communication, parenting (children of all ages), stress management, financial management, and the like are offered through many community education programs and increasingly by managed health care organizations through their community health outreach efforts.

For many families, education for family roles occurs informally among one's network of family and friends. However, other families may not be embedded in a natural network; they could benefit from professional support in establishing this kind of support. In all of these family education endeavors, it is critically important that cultural, ethnic, and religious variability be taken into account. Most importantly, a philosophy of adult education that empowers family members to discover their own strengths and capabilities has the potential for sustained effects.

CONCLUSION

While it may seem overwhelming and complex to think of human development and health promotion of children, youth, and families from this ecological perspective, our prior reductionist tendencies have often led to blame and despair. Particularly, this has been the case with regard to families. Rather than making negative judgments about the wide variety of family forms and functioning styles present in our society, this diversity can be seen as an advantage. Systems analysts have pointed out that complex systems that develop more requisite variety over time are ultimately more adaptive and capable of survival. They have a larger repertoire of possibilities for understanding and solving complex problems. As we approach the 21st century, the range of diversity among families in our society should be a source of hope and optimism for our future.

References

1. Hutchins, V. and McPherson, M. National agenda for children with special health needs. *American Psychologist.* February, 1991;141–143.
2. Bronfenbrenner, U. *The ecology of human development.* Cambridge, MA: Harvard University Press, 1979.
3. Garbarino, J. *Children and families in the social environment.* 2nd ed. New York: Aldine de Gruyter, 1992.
4. Wood, B. L. A developmental biopsychosocial approach to the treatment of chronic illness in children and adolescents. In R. Mikesell, D. Lusterman, and S. McDaniel (eds). *Integrating family therapy. Handbook of family psychology and systems theory.* Washington, DC: American Psychological Association, 1995.
5. Boyd-Franklin, N. *Black families in therapy: A multi-systems approach.* New York: Guildord Press, 1989.
6. Bateson, G. *Steps to an ecology of mind.* New York: Ballantine, 1972.
7. Hernandez, D. J. Children's changing access to resources: A historical perspective. *Social Policy Report.* 1994;8(1):1–23.
8. U.S. National Center for Health Statistics. *Advance report of final divorce statistics, 1988.* Vol. 39, No. 12, supplement 2. Washington, DC: Author, 1991.
9. McAdoo, J. L. The roles of African American fathers: An ecological perspective. *Families in Society: The Journal of Contemporary Human Services.* January, 1993;28–35.
10. Wilkinson, D. Family ethnicity in America. In H. McAdoo (ed). *Family ethnicity. Strength in diversity.* Newbury Park, CA: Sage, 1993, pp 15–59.
11. McGoldrick, M. Ethnicity, cultural diversity, and normality. In F. Walsh (ed), *Normal family processes.* New York: Guilford, 1993, pp 330–360.
12. Walsh, F. *Normal family processes.* New York: Guilford, 1993.
13. Hareven, T. American families in transition. Historical perspective onchange. In F. Walsh (ed). *Normal family processes.* New York: Guilford, 1982.
14. Stacey, J. *Brave new families: Stories of domestic upheaval in late twentieth century America.* New York: Basic Books, 1990.
15. Anderson, K., and Tomlinson, P. The family health system as an emerging paradigmatic view for nursing. *Image: Journal of Nursing Scholarship.* 1992;14(1):57–63.

16. World Health Organization. *Statistical indices of family health* (Rep. No. 589). Geneva, Switzerland: Author, 1996.
17. Olson, D., Sprenkle, D., and Russell, C. Circumplex model of marital and family systems I: Cohesion and adaptability dimensions, family types, and clinical applications. *Family Process.* 1979;18:3–28.
18. Olson, D. Circumplex model of marital and family systems: Assessing family functioning. In F. Walsh (ed). *Normal family processes.* New York: Guilford, 1993, pp 104–137.
19. Kamerman, S. Child and family policies: An international overview. In E. Zigler, S. Kagan, and N. Hall (eds). *Children, families and government. Preparing for the twenty-first century.* Cambridge: Cambridge University Press, 1996, pp 31–48.
20. Schorr, L. *Within our reach. Breaking the cycle of disadvantage.* New York: Doubleday, 1988

4

The Family and Health in the 21st Century

Claude Earl Fox

With an eye on the 21st century, the U.S. Public Health Service set out in 1979 to determine whether carefully defined health promotion and disease prevention objectives, purposefully pursued by health care providers and a nationwide consortium of community, federal, and state agencies, could effect measurable improvement in the health of the American population. First came a set of five national health targets, published in 1979 in *Healthy People: The Surgeon General's Report on Health Promotion and Disease Prevention*,[1] challenging the nation to reduce mortality among four different age groups and to increase independence among older adults within 10 years. Through prevention interventions and strategies that unified the nation's public health activities, three mortality targets—those for infants, children, and adults—were achieved.

Invigorated by this success, the Public Health Service launched a second, bolder prevention agenda: *Healthy People 2000*.[2] Healthy People 2000 and its midcourse review and revisions[3,4] generated 319 objectives and 319 special population targets, all directed toward achieving three goals: increasing the span of healthy life, reducing health disparities, and ensuring access to preventive services.[5] The national objectives cluster in 22 priority areas under the overarching approaches of health promotion, health protection, and preventive services (Fig. 4.1).

Health promotion	Health protection	Preventive services
1. Physical activity and fitness 2. Nutrition 3. Tobacco 4. Substance abuse: alcohol and other drugs 5. Family planning 6. Mental health and mental disorders 7. Violent and abusive behavior 8. Educational and community based programs	9. Unintentional injuries 10. Occupational safety and health 11. Environmental health 12. Food and drug safety 13. Oral health	14. Maternal and infant health 15. Heart disease and stroke 16. Cancer 17. Diabetes and chronic disabling conditions 18. HIV infection 19. Sexually transmitted diseases 20. Immunization and infectious disease 21. Clinical preventive services
22. Surveillance and data systems		

Goals

- **Increase the span of healthy life for Americans.**
- **Reduce health disparities among Americans.**
- **Achieve access to preventive services for all Americans.**

FIGURE 4.1

Healthy People Year 2000 priority areas.

The health status of American families in the 21st century will, in large part, reflect our national resolve to achieve these Healthy People 2000 objectives. By 1997, there was progress toward the *Year 2000* targets in more than half the objectives, with 13% meeting or surpassing their targets.[6] This picture of progress is an occasion for celebration of the collective success that collaborative efforts have made in improving the health of all Americans.[7] But conditions worsened in 18% of the objectives, 2% showed no change, and there were insufficient data to assess the status of 14%—evidence that much remains to be accomplished.

HEALTH STATUS OF CHILDREN, YOUTH, AND FAMILIES

Healthy People 2000 upholds a public commitment to building healthy American families launched in 1935 with the signing of the nation's maternal and child health legislation, Title V of the Social Security Act. More than 60 years later, we continue to see dramatic improvements in the health indicators of the country's children, youth, and families.[8] During the 1990s, the nation's infant mortality rate continued a slow but steady decline, even in communities with some of the highest infant mortality rates.[9] The proportion of women receiving prenatal care in the first trimester of pregnancy has increased, as have the numbers of women breast feeding their infants and the numbers of children receiving immunizations by the age of 3.

Yet progress toward the Year 2000 goals remains uneven and substantial health risks will continue to plague children and families into the next century. In its infant mortality rate, the United States ranks no better than 23rd among developed nations. Persistent problems include a mortality rate for black infants more than twice the rate for white infants. Children born into poor families have an infant mortality rate more than 50% higher than children in homes above the poverty line, according to the Annie E. Casey Foundation.[10] Mortality rates are also higher for children born to parents with low educational attainment or children in communities riddled with social problems.

To ensure successful birth outcomes and a healthy first year of life for their infants, women should begin prenatal care in their first trimester of pregnancy and avoid smoking, taking drugs, and drinking alcohol while pregnant. Yet nearly one of every five pregnant women receives no first-trimester care. An expectant mother with no prenatal care is three times as likely to have a low-birthweight baby, and these too-small babies are 5 to 10 times more likely than normal-weight babies to die within their first year. Although reducing the number of low-birthweight babies born each year is among the most important Year 2000 goals, there has been virtually no change in the low-birthweight rate since the early 1980s.

Approximately one in five women report use of alcohol during pregnancy, 22,000 of them at levels found to result in growth and neurodevelopmental defects in the offspring. There has been a rise in the number of babies born with fetal alcohol syndrome, the most severe of the adverse effects of prenatal alcohol exposure. Smoking is reported by approximately one in every five pregnant women. Illicit drug use occurs in 1 in 20 pregnant women, and use of psychotherapeutic drugs in about one in eight. Further reductions in infant mortality and morbidity in the 21st century will require a focus on strategies to modify these and other behaviors and lifestyles that affect birth outcomes.

An encouraging study from the National Center for Health Statistics[11] shows that the percentage of teens who have had sexual intercourse has begun to drop after increasing steadily for more than two decades. But teenage birth rates are rising, and the proportion of births to teenage unmarried females is substantially higher than in the mid-1970s. There is some evidence that the likelihood of unintended pregnancy may be reduced by educating teens about the long-term economic and social costs associated with teenage childbearing. Data from the School Health Policies and Programs Study[11] show that 80% of junior and senior high schools now have required classes that include discussion of human sexuality. Nearly 49% of the states require human sexuality to be taught in at least one grade.

PROGRESS THROUGH PUBLIC HEALTH INTERVENTIONS

In 1997, the Healthy People 2000 Review[6] reported an increase in years of healthy life for the total population, marking a halt in the steady decline of this key indicator of health status. For blacks, this was the first such increase since tracking began in 1990. Both measures, however, are still below their baselines and far from their Year 2000 targets.

A 1997 report from the National Center for Health Statistics,[12] examining the relationship between health status and family characteristics, found that such family traits as education, income, marital status, and family size have an important impact on the health of family members. In general, the report found that married men and women living with a spouse, families with higher education and income, and children in two-parent households were the healthiest. Yet, an estimated 43% of marriages still end in divorce, and the number of families with children headed by a single parent has risen steadily over the past few decades, a growing point of concern among policymakers and the public.

Children and adults alike show the impact of income; those living in the poorest families report a higher level of poor health and hospitalization. The long-term trend in the United States has been toward increasing income inequality, with increasing shares of household income received by already high-income households and declining shares by households where incomes are lowest.

Familial poverty seeds future morbidities—poor health, lowered school performance, delinquency—and deprives family members of access to services conducive to good health. Census data showing that median household income increased in the United States between 1994 and 1995 for the first time in 6 years and that the number of Americans living below the poverty level dropped for the second straight year present heartening news. But the nation's poor still numbered 36.4 million people, 40% of them children. The poverty rate for children is higher than for any other age group in the United States, and remains one of the highest in the developed world.

Other trends are more auspicious. The life expectancy rate, only 47.3 years at the turn of the century, had risen to 75.8 years by 1995. One study suggests that only 5 of those added years of life can be attributed to the work of the medical care system;[13] the greater portion of this improvement derives from public health interventions: cleaner water, less environmental pollution, decreases in cigarette smoking, control of infectious disease, and wider use of prenatal care. Demographers at the University of Pennsylvania have projected that half the population alive in 2000 will owe their existence to simple changes in hygiene and public health in the 20th century, without which their parents, grandparents, or earlier ancestors would have died before giving birth to succeeding generations.

Progress has been reported for more than 75% of objectives involving the nation's preeminent cripplers and killers—mortality rates for heart disease, cancer, stroke, accidents, and HIV/AIDS have slowed beyond all expectation, while potent three-drug cocktails, earlier detection, and refinements in symptomatic treatment extend survival and engender glimmers of optimism in a once bleak landscape.

Heart disease still kills nearly as many Americans as all other diseases combined. But since the late 1970s, the death rate for cardiovascular disease has declined significantly: 46% for all cardiovascular disease, 51% for coronary heart disease, and 60% for stroke. Some Year 2000 objectives addressing the major modifiable risk factors for cardiovascular disease are showing progress: Average blood pressure levels have dropped, as has the prevalence of high blood pressure and high blood cholesterol among adults.

The second leading cause of death in the United States is cancer, accounting for nearly one of every four deaths. There is evidence that the prospects for preventing and surviving cancer continue to improve. The age-adjusted rate of lung cancer mortality has dropped for the first time in at least 50 years, and the declining age-adjusted death rate for colorectal cancer has surpassed the Year 2000 target. Age-adjusted breast cancer rates declined to 21 per 100,000 women by 1995, and more women are receiving mammograms and Pap tests. Americans could prevent perhaps as much as 50% or more of cancer incidence through smoking cessation and prudent dietary changes, such as consumption of less fat and more fruits and vegetables.

Tobacco use is responsible for approximately one of every five deaths and is the single most important preventable cause of death and disease in our society. About one half of all regular smokers will eventually die as a result of this addictive behavior. Recent data show some progress toward achieving the Year 2000 objectives in the tobacco priority area. Cigarette smoking prevalence has declined somewhat since the 1987 baseline. An estimated 61 million Americans were current smokers in 1995, among them 4.5 million adolescents, but the average age of first use for cigarettes has increased. More schools are offering anti-tobacco education, and all 50 states and the District of Columbia have enacted laws prohibiting the sale and distribution of tobacco products to youth under 18 years.

Unintentional injuries are the fifth leading cause of death in the United States and a major cause of disabilities and hospitalization. Motor vehicle accidents remain the most costly unintentional injuries, but simple preventive measures have proven effective in reducing the toll of death and injury. Laws requiring use of safety belts and child safety seats save thousands of lives each year, and motorcycle and bicycle helmet use is associated with less severe injuries and lower health care costs.

Fires account for about 5% of all unintentional injury deaths. More than one quarter of these deaths are attributable to arson or children playing with fire. Seventy-five percent of fires started by children involved children aged 5 or younger playing with matches or lighters, and nearly half the arsons are traced to youth aged 18 and under. These data strongly emphasize the need to target fire prevention efforts at youth as a step toward reducing fire-related injuries in the 21st century.

Approximately 11% of preventable deaths are related to alcohol and illicit drug use. The 1995 National Household Survey on Drug Abuse (NHSDA)[14] reported that 12.8 million Americans—or 6.1% of the American population aged 12 years and older—were current users of illicit drugs, approximately the same level as has been reported annually since 1992. Survey data clearly showed a continuing increase in illicit drug use prevalence among youth, with increased use of marijuana reported in 1994 and continuing into 1995. Increases in hallucinogen and cocaine use among youth were consistent with findings of the Monitoring the Future Study, which showed statistically significant increases in drug use among 8th, 10th, and 12th graders from 1992 to 1995. Both studies showed that drugs are easily accessible to young people, while at the same time the perceived risk of harm in using drugs has decreased.

The NHSDA warns that the recent upturn in illicit drug use among youth has important implications for substance abuse prevention and treatment efforts, both now and in the 21st century.[14] In terms of prevention, there is an obvious need to focus immediate attention on children and adolescents. The increasing proportion of young people using illicit drugs will probably result in continuing pressure on the substance abuse treatment system in future years, as many new drug users progress to addiction and require intervention.

More than 2 million Americans become victims of violence each year. Although the homicide rate appears back on track toward the Year 2000 goal, with decreases reported for 1994 and 1995, the assault rate has increased 30% since 1986. Rapes and attempted rapes have more than doubled over that same period. Firearms play a major role in violence, especially among younger victims, with handguns used in 78% of all firearm crimes. A combined effort by law enforcement and public health services will be necessary to effectively address the problem of violence in the next century.

As the population in the United States grows older, problems posed by chronic and disabling conditions increasingly demand the nation's attention. Already nearly 40 million Americans have functional limitations that interfere with their daily activities. It is encouraging, then, that several measures of chronic disability have declined in recent years. These include people whose activity is limited because of chronic conditions or asthma and people with significant hearing or visual impairment.

A growing proportion of U.S. children, adolescents, and adults are overweight. The third National Health and Nutrition Examination Survey, conducted by the National Center for Health Statistics in 1988–1997,[15] showed substantial increases in obesity in all age groups; approximately 14% of children, 24% of adolescents, and 35% of adults are overweight. Although diet and physical activity are the two primary behavioral factors believed to be associated with overweight, caloric intake has increased and recreational activity is limited for many Americans.

In July 1996, the U.S. Department of Health and Human Services issued the first Surgeon General's Report on Physical Activity and

Health,[16] recommending 30 minutes of moderate physical activity each day. The report found that regular moderate physical activity can substantially reduce the risk of heart disease, diabetes, colon cancer, and high blood pressure. On average, physically active people outlive those who are inactive. Regular physical activity can also help maintain the functional independence of older adults and enhance the quality of life for people of all ages.

HEALTH GOALS FOR THE YEAR 2010

The foundation is now being laid for the third generation of Healthy People objectives: Healthy People 2010. To ensure broad-based support for the objectives, 200 members of the Healthy People 2000 Consortium from the private, voluntary, and business sectors met with federal and state representatives in November 1996 to review lessons learned from the 1990 and 2000 objectives and to build the prevention agenda for the first decade of the next millennium.

A supportive social environment may be one of the key factors in successfully changing behaviors that contribute to many of today's leading health threats. Consequently, leadership, collaboration, and initiatives at the community level are fundamental to progress. Community-based programs are increasingly recognizing the importance of addressing the social and physical environments in which behaviors occur and are reinforced. Educational and community-based interventions are designed to reach groups of people outside traditional health care settings through programs targeted for people who come together in various settings, such as students within a school, employees at a work site, or members of civic or religious groups that meet regularly. Other programs are best planned as community-wide health promotion initiatives to reach large numbers of people with highly visible and more easily implemented interventions.

Outcomes must have a sufficient scientific base. We need better data collection and improved analytical capability. We need to fully document the nation's unmet health needs, related both to health status indicators and to the capability of our health service delivery system. We need more attention to the body of knowledge on intervention, and continued research to understand the specific contributions of prevention strategies in achieving target outcomes.

We need to enlist private partners in our cause to make sure health promotion and disease prevention messages are heard—for instance, pediatricians talking in their community about bicycle safety; or nurses on the ward talking with patients about breast examination. With proper tools and information, an array of private partners could be marshaled to carry health promotion messages into the community, especially to hard-to-reach and high-risk adolescents. For that we need a diverse, community-based health work force, trained in the community, accessible to the community, and able to recognize and respond to the community's unmet needs.

Finally, as a nation, we must remain vigilant to emerging health problems—a lesson driven home in this century by the onslaught of HIV/AIDS.

Those of us who work in public health know there will always be more need than resources. Healthy People 2000 and its Year 2010 successor point our collective energies toward results of greatest consequence. Our national commitment to achieving the Healthy People objectives will prove a powerful force for ensuring healthy families in the 21st century.

References

1. U.S. Department of Health and Human Services. *Healthy people: The Surgeon General's report on health promotion and disease prevention.* Washington, DC: Public Health Service, 1979.
2. U.S. Department of Health and Human Services. *Healthy people 2000: National health promotion and disease prevention objectives.* Washington, DC: Public Health Service, 1991.
3. U.S. Department of Health and Human Services. *Healthy people 2000 midcourse review and 1995 revisions.* Washington, DC: Public Health Service, 1995.
4. U.S. Department of Health and Human Services. *Healthy people 2000 review: 1995–96.* Washington, DC: Public Health Service, 1996.
5. U.S. Department of Health and Human Services. *Health U.S. prevention profile.* Washington, DC: Public Health Service, 1992.
6. U.S. Department of Health and Human Services. *Healthy people 2000 review, 1997.* Washington, DC: Public Health Service, 1997.
7. U.S. Department of Health and Human Services. *For a healthy nation: Returns on investment in public health.* Washington, DC: Public Health Service, 1997.
8. U.S. Department of Health and Human Services. *Child health USA '95.* Washington, DC: Public Health Service, Health Resources and Services Administration, Maternal and Child Health Bureau, September, 1996.
9. White, K.M., and Preston, S.H. How many Americans are alive because of twentieth-century improvements in mortality? *Population and Development Review.* September, 1996;22(3):415–429.
10. Annie F. Casey Foundation. 1997 Kids Count summary and findings. Online. Available URL: http://www.accf.org/kc1997/summary.htm.
11. National Center for Health Statistics. Teen sex down, new study shows. Released May 1, 1997. Online. Available URL: http://www.cdc.gov/nchswww/releases/97news/97news/nsfgteen.htm.
12. National Center for Health Statistics. Family environment affects health of family members. Released January, 1997. Online. Available URL: http://www.cdc.gov/nchswww/releases/97facts/97sheets/famhealt.htm.
13. Bunker, J.P., Frazier, H.S., and Mosteller, F. Improving health: Measuring effects of medical care. *Milbank Quarterly.* 1994;72(2):225–258.
14. Substance Abuse and Mental Health Administration. Highlights of 1995 National Household Survey on Drug Abuse: Trends in initiation of drug abuse. Released 1996. Online. Available URL: http://www.samhsa.gov/oas/nhsda/ar18txt.htm//A1.

15. Update: Prevention of overweight among children, adolescents, and adults—United States 1988–1994. *MMWR*. March 7, 1997;46(9):199–202.

16. U.S. Department of Health and Human Services. *Physical activity and health: A report of the Surgeon General*. Washington, DC: Center for Disease Control and Prevention; National Center for Chronic Disease Prevention and Health Promotion; President's Council on Physical Fitness and Sports, July, 1996. Online. Available URL: http://www.cdc.gov/nccdphp/sgr/sgr.htm.

5

The Health and Welfare Policy Process: The Case of the 1996 Welfare Reforms

Eugene Declercq

This legislation is the best hope we have today to provide some real hope for a future for those families and children in our society who, in many instances, are totally without hope.[1]

    Senate Budget Committee Chairman Pete Domenici

The bill that President Clinton signed is not welfare reform. It does not promote work effectively, and it will hurt millions of poor children by the time it is fully implemented.[2]

    Former Department of Health and Human Services Assistant Secretary Peter Edelman, describing the reasons for his resignation

On August 22, 1996, President Clinton signed legislation (P.L. 104-193) that brought to an end a 6-decade guarantee by the national government to provide support to any low-income mothers and children who met eligibility requirements. The above quotes suggest the gulf that separated supporters and opponents of this legislation, and the debate surrounding the passage was intense, with the President promising to "fix" the legislation on reelection. The provisions of the new law are described elsewhere in this volume (see Chapters 8 and 10) and are not repeated here. Rather, this chapter uses the process by which welfare reform became law to examine the health and welfare policy process in general.

THE POLICY PROCESS IN THE UNITED STATES

The Context of Policymaking

Contemporary health and welfare policymaking in the United States occurs in a constitutional, historical, political, and social context that shapes the parameters within which individual policy decisions are made. This chapter examines how two constitutional and historical contexts (federalism and separation of powers) and three contemporary political implications of that context (the role of constituencies, compromise, and incrementalism) particularly shape health and welfare policymaking. There are many more elements to the policy process, and interested readers should consult the sizable literature on the topic,[3] but this chapter addresses those five factors of particular importance to health and welfare policy. The nature of a policy will be the result of the blending of these contextual factors with contemporary political considerations and the individual needs of the decision makers. For example, although those of us on the outside might consider a policy such as the 1996 welfare reform as a discrete decision, for those who must make policy decisions, each choice:

- Sets a precedent for later decisions (e.g., should other national programs be turned over to the states?)
- Is related to a history of the given policy (e.g., how has welfare policy evolved over the years?)
- Influences their personal future in general (e.g., how will voters react?) and within the institution (e.g., what will my colleagues think?)
- Affects real people (e.g., how does this influence those receiving welfare?)

The process that results from mixing these personal considerations with societal need all within a constitutional framework is seldom predictable and very frustrating to observe for those passionate about a policy. However, examination of this process will provide readers with some tools by which they may better understand the health and welfare policymaking process, not only in the case of the 1996 welfare reform, but for future policies as well.

Historical and Constitutional Context
Federalism and Separation of Powers

In establishing the structure of the new government, the Founding Fathers faced a series of decisions concerning how close the government would be to "the people." Should they establish a government that was more responsive to the will of the people or one that was more distant, but likely more stable? In virtually every instance, they chose stability over responsiveness. They accomplished this largely by dividing power between the national and state governments in a federal system, and within the national government power was further subdivided among the executive, legislative, and judicial branches. These decisions, more than two centuries old, created a system that still strongly favors the status quo and makes it very hard for new policies to be enacted. We'll look first at federalism.

A federal system has been described as ". . . the mode of political organization that unites smaller political units in a manner designed to protect the existence and authority of both national and subnational systems enabling all to share in the overall system's decision making and executing processes."[4] The extraordinary division of political power in the United States is exemplified by the existence of more than 85,000 governmental units in the United States,[5] with most having some role in health and welfare policy. A long-term trend toward greater centralization of governmental powers has been challenged of late with ideological conservatives seeking to return more power to the states and localities through a process termed *devolution.*[6] Marquis and Long aptly summarize the arguments for increasing state responsibilities:

The heterogeneity of the population, values and institutions among the states, such that state government can be more responsive to the needs of the people; that the states can serve as laboratories for developing and testing new ideas and programs; and that placing responsibility for the costs of the program closer to the beneficiaries promotes better decision making.[7]

Advocates for a stronger national role typically emphasize the need for equity in the protection of rights and delivery of services across different governmental levels.

For purposes of analysis of health and welfare policy, one can see debates over federalism as involving elements of both policy choice and symbolism. From a policy perspective, the current welfare reforms shift the balance of responsibility back to the states after more than 6 decades as a national entitlement, and the result may be wide interstate variations. Opponents see this as leading to inequity, whereas reform advocates applaud the chance to test alternative models of service delivery. The degree to which the reforms also cap the national government's fiscal responsibilities for the program obviously attracted the support of national policymakers as well. Advocacy for a stronger state role has also historically been used by elected officials to avoid direct opposition to a popular program. Given the symbolic importance of women and children, those advocating program cuts for them may well be inclined to invoke a federalism argument against "centralized control," rather than directly attack welfare programs.

Separation of powers within the national and state levels of government has also enhanced stability and slowed policy change. The need to gain agreement across executive, legislative, and judicial branches has required advocates for change to form coalitions and engage in compromise to build a sufficient consensus around their initiatives. A system in which power is divided across levels (federalism) and then divided again among institutions at each level (separation of powers) and then further divided within institutions (e.g., committees with overlapping jurisdictions within each house of Congress) provides a substantial advantage to advocates with the resources and commitment to engage in the policy process over the long term. Not surprisingly, large institutional interests, such as business and trade organizations, can fare quite well in this system, whereas groups advocating for consumers, particularly those with little political power, struggle.

The Role of Constituencies, Compromise, and Incrementalism

Policymakers will invoke the need to serve their constituents as a justification for a controversial vote. Who are these constituents? Although we typically think of constituents as the people in a legislative district, constituencies build up around programs as well, and these often play the critical role in the policy process. What often emerges in health and welfare policy is the development of a "provider constituency" of service providers whose advocacy involves both commitment to actual program consumers (e.g., children with special health care needs) and the furtherance of their own agendas (e.g., more funding for rehabilitation centers). Actual program constituents, such as low-income mothers or children in need, have neither the financial resources nor the time to follow the workings of such a complex process. Their fate is therefore largely left to the good will of policymakers (there is such a thing), the efforts of those that provide services to them, and a handful of consumer advocacy groups. It is not surprising, therefore, that policies that should help groups at risk often appear to serve other agendas.

The principle of majority rule typically necessitates coalition building to achieve sufficient support for passage. The formation of a coalition, however, requires that the parties to the coalition compromise on points of disagreement in order to achieve some consensus. The likelihood for compromise is also enhanced by the understanding by the participants that they may need each other's support again in the future. The final result of this apparently glacial pace of policymaking is that major policy changes are typically incremental, making marginal changes on past practices. Even when there is a major change, as in the case of welfare reform (or in the 1960s civil rights policy), it is preceded by years of smaller changes that set the stage for a more fundamental reform. The failure of the Clinton health reform package was in part because it represented too much change for the policy process to address, and subsequent national reforms (e.g., targeted extensions of health insurance coverage) are examples of a more incremental approach.

Where are "the people" in this process? Mostly on the outside, more concerned with matters they perceive as closer to their lives. It is, therefore, to the advantage of those on the inside of the system to maintain the complexity of the process to discourage too much direct citizen input. Theoretically, the will of the people is manifested through political parties and interest groups. In theory, parties can build coalitions among the disparate interests in the society, and organized groups can provide ongoing representation to policymakers of the concerns of their members. However, interest group resources are concentrated in major groups representing labor, business, and trade associations, not the public at large. Political action committees (PACs) representing these three sources gave more than $186 million to candidates in the 1996 elections, representing 85.5% of all PAC money donated.[8] Parties in turn have become increasingly beholden to big money interests while serving as a conduit for "soft money" (contributions that avoid the limits established by the Federal Election Commission) funneled to candidates. In the 1996 election cycle, both Republicans (more than $69 million) and Democrats (almost $28 million) set records for party income.[9] Despite rhetoric to the contrary, the degree to which either the parties or interest groups can be seen as representing the average person, let alone the interests of the poor, is doubtful. Party differences can also contribute to stalemate, and in a situation of government divided by party, as we have faced in 24 of the 30 years from 1969 to 1998, the potential for compromise and incremental change, as well as inaction, increases.

How can the context for health and welfare policymaking be summarized? For those for whom the political structure has granted past privileges, the preservation of those privileges (that is, maintenance of the status quo) is their paramount goal. The fragmentation of the U.S. political system across (federalism) and within (separation of powers) levels of government abets their efforts. Policy change requires overcoming not only the active opposition of those who benefit from current policy but the tremendous inertia inherent in such a system. Ironically, it was just such inertia that helped preserve a welfare system so long out of favor with large portions of the public.

The constituents (consumers) of health and welfare policy have limited resources to engage in the policy process, and so their "position" is often represented by an activist constituency of service providers. The needs of service providers and consumers obviously do not always coincide, but a policymaker may well see the opinions of those activist constituents as not just their own position but that of the constituency as a whole. As described later in the case of welfare reform, opinions of "the people" often form only the broadest boundaries within which the policy process takes place.

MAKING HEALTH AND WELFARE POLICY IN THE UNITED STATES: THE POLICY CYCLE

The policy process in the United States involves several stages. The exact delineation of the stages is a matter of debate among policy analysts, but most of these models involve some form of the following stages: an initial state defined by the analyst, followed by agenda placement, policy adoption and formulation, implementation, and evaluation. Each is briefly described here, followed by an application of the model to welfare reform legislation.

Initial State

This stage simply reflects the current status of outcomes, policies, and opinions at the time one chooses to begin the analysis. In the case of welfare reform legislation, the initial state could be determined by using early 1996 as an arbitrary starting point and describing, as later, the status of welfare policy at that point, combined with relevant trend data and public attitudes toward the issue. See the related chapters in this volume for a more complete description of the state of welfare policy prior to the most recent successful movement for reform.

Agenda Placement

Agenda placement is the process by which issues draw the attention of the media and public at large and, more importantly, those who make policy. In his influential analysis, John Kingdon argues that items reach the agenda of policymakers as a result of the confluence of three process "streams": (1) problem recognition, (2) the formation and refining of policy proposals, often by "policy entrepreneurs," and (3) the political mood of the times.[10] The initial definition of a problem being "recognized" is less a fixed reality than a dynamic social construct created by those advancing or opposing an issue[11] with the goal of setting the parameters for a possible solution. For example, was welfare reform about "getting people back to work," "returning power to the states," "cutting the size of government," or "punishing the poor?" Problems may get recognized as meriting governmental attention through the publication of a regularly measured indicator (e.g., monthly or annual reports on the size of the welfare caseload), the occurrence of a "focusing event" usually drawing widespread attention to an existing problem (e.g., the prosecution of a case of welfare fraud), or the generation of routine feedback (systematic and anecdotal) that highlights an implementation problem with an existing policy. Central to agenda building are "policy entrepreneurs" who advance problem definitions and solutions that serve their organization's interests.[9] In health and welfare policy, the "provider constituency" described earlier often serves as policy entrepreneurs, seeking to define problems in a fashion that suggests their own remedy (e.g., educational, training, or health care programs) as its solution.

Policy Adoption and Formulation

Policy formulation is described in *The Future of Public Health* as "the process by which society makes decisions about problems, chooses goals and the proper means to reach them."[12] Once an issue has reached the agenda of policymakers, the policy adoption and formulation stages determine what form the issue will take and which institutions—legislative, bureaucratic/regulatory, or judicial—will shape the policy. The particular decision-making mechanism of the branch that has direct responsibility for the issue becomes paramount in this stage, be it a court hearing, a regulatory review panel, or most commonly, a legislative committee.

Legislative committees, although initially established to provide legislative bodies with a reasonable means by which to divide the workload, have added many other roles (including quietly keeping items off the policy agenda) in their evolution over the past two centuries.[13] In addition to the advantages of specialization inherent in a committee structure, the smaller size of committees facilitates negotiations and compromise on proposed language for the legislation. Once a bill has secured committee support, it proceeds to a floor vote, which will determine its fate. For many bills, particularly those seen as technical and narrow, the floor vote is simply a ratification of committee action, as legislators defer to the specialized knowledge of committee members.[14] However, in health and welfare legislation, the nature of the issues more clearly symbolizes members' own ideological positions, their own constituents are more likely to have expressed their opinion on the issue, and floor debate and voting become less tied to committee action. In floor voting, legislators are likely to be focused less on reaching an ideal long-term solution than simply finding a more immediately satisfactory one, an incentive for them to seek only incremental change.

The chief executive's role in policy adoption and formulation is usually limited, but in this final stage, the option of vetoing legislation (with a typically two-thirds majority necessary for override) gives them the opportunity to bargain for changes in legislation. Actual vetoes are comparatively rare, but that is in part because legislatures often compromise with the executive on final language. What are the consequences of a policy process in which every step apparently involves compromise? The reliance on compromise means support coalitions for policies can usually be built only for small incremental changes that often lack clear language in the legislation, which causes confusion when the next stage, implementation, occurs.

Policy Implementation

After the legislative, judicial, and/or executive branches have established a policy, it is still left up to those in the field to administer it. The law, judicial opinion, or regulatory ruling must be interpreted by those bureaucrats who actually provide the services described in the policy. It is those charged with implementation who clients actually deal with on a regular basis, and given the repeated compromises often involved in policymaking, these bureaucrats may have considerable discretion in deciding which clients will receive particular benefits. In health and welfare policy, the fragmented and heavily institutionalized nature of past programs, with national funding and guidelines but implementation responsibility at the state and local levels has placed a premium on understanding the myriad rules and regulations that guide the system.

Policy Evaluation

The implementation of a policy does not guarantee it will have the expected (or any) effect on the targeted population. The analysis of policy impact is the subject of the applied field research termed *policy evaluation*, and its work can greatly enhance the policy process. The results of such evaluations are considered with other evidence (letters to policymakers, public opinion polls, anecdotes) in establishing the climate for an initial state. In health and welfare policy, because evaluations typically focus on complex human behaviors, conclusions linking specific policy initiatives (e.g., a decrease in welfare benefits) to individual behaviors (e.g., reduced unmarried childbearing) often reflect ideology more than research.

WELFARE REFORM AND THE POLICY CYCLE

Initial State

The initial state for welfare policy prior to the 1996 reforms has been described in more detail in other chapters in this volume (see Chapters 8 and 10). Nationally, Aid to Families with Dependent Children (AFDC), the main target of reform efforts, totaled more than 5 million families and 11.8 million recipients in 1994, almost two-thirds of whom (62%) were younger than 18 or older than 65 and 78% of whom lived below the poverty level.[5] Expenditures and caseloads for AFDC had been rising dramatically for more than two decades, with a 24%

growth in caseload between 1990 and 1994 and a corresponding 22% rise in expenditures to $25.9 billion. Interestingly, in the same period, Medicaid, with more than double the caseload in 1990 (25.3 million), nonetheless grew at a much faster rate, with a 34.8% caseload increase and a virtual doubling (98.1%) in expenditures to $143.6 billion in 1994.[5] However, in many states, caseloads had been leveling off or decreasing in recent years (e.g., Massachusetts' caseload went down every month for 4 years). These overall figures also mask enormous interstate differences, which in 1995 resulted in an average benefit in New York almost six times higher than that in Mississippi.[15]

Agenda Placement

After years of complaints about welfare, what brought it to the policy agenda in 1996? In one sense it had been there for years, with annual debates over financing, regulations, and relationships with states. As in many federal programs, the national government's response came after most states had already enacted reforms, in this case with the support of the national government. There had also been significant national reforms, most notably the Family Support Act in 1988.[2] This law may be seen as an important incremental step toward the 1996 reforms because Democrats (including then Governor Clinton) agreed to the principle of work requirements. However, 1996 agenda placement was primarily dictated by three factors: (1) President Clinton's 1992 campaign pledge to "end welfare as we know it," (2) the failure of the Clinton health plan in 1994, and (3) the subsequent election of a Republican Congress and their "Contract with America." This third factor was the most important, because Republicans consciously attempted with the "Contract" to set the policy agenda for the 104th Congress, and item 3 of the contract was welfare reform. Their insistence on placing welfare reform on the agenda and moving responsibility for it to the states, combined with the President's generalized support for change, created a confluence of Kingdon's problem and policy streams. What was needed to place the item on the policy agenda, applying Kingdon's model, was the right political environment. In this case, that meant public support.

Was the public anxious to have welfare reform on the political agenda? The best way to characterize public opinion on the issue might be "angry but disinterested." The disinterest is seen in polls in which the public is asked, in an open-ended question, to identify the most important problems facing the United States. As the country approached the debate over welfare reform in the Spring of 1996, a national *LA Times* poll found only 10% of the public thinking it should be the country's highest priority, ranking it fourth overall.[16] The same question in earlier years shows a slow growth in concern for the issue (2% in 1993; 4% in 1994) but hardly raging concern.[17] A similar finding is seen in responses to national surveys reported by *Times Mirror* in five surveys in 1993 and 1994, in which welfare reform consistently ranked fourth or fifth as a national concern. The anger is shown in response to specific questions that ask about welfare and those who receive it. Much of the following discussion draws on Weaver and coworkers' analysis of public opinion polls on welfare, in which they note, "One of the most stable elements of American public opinion is the unpopularity of welfare."[18] As far back as 1976, a majority (52%) of respondents to national surveys felt that most people who receive money from welfare could get along without it, a figure that has declined somewhat, but in 1994 was still at 46%. By 1995, the proportion of the public that felt our system of public assistance was not working had risen to 72%. Including the term *welfare* in a question appeared to cause a more negative response than simply asking about the "poor" or "people in need," as the public attitudes toward government assistance became more negative.[18]

With regard to welfare reform itself, the public had more faith in Republicans than President Clinton to reform the system, providing more impetus for their leadership on this issue. The public favored work programs, training programs, fixed time periods, and a cap on payments for welfare mothers who have additional children. In 1996, by more than a 4-to-1 margin, the public favored providing child care so women can work rather than have the mother stay home with her children.[19] Perhaps the strongest example of public anger was seen in the response by the 78% of the public who favored limits on welfare. One third of these respondents indicated that they favored the limits even if it meant that many children would be living in households with no income at all.[19]

As with many issues that reach the political agenda, the public generally supported the welfare reform initiative, but they were not the driving force that placed the item on the agenda. The public, rather than driving the policy process, establish the parameters within which policy initiatives can develop. This result is important when we discuss policy adoption and formulation, because the public's generalized support, combined with inattention, provides policymakers with considerable discretion in creating specific policy initiatives.

Policy Adoption and Formulation

As noted in the earlier description of policy adoption and formulation, this stage is generally dominated by politics and process, and the case of the welfare reform bill was no exception. Passage of a major piece of controversial legislation relatively late in a presidential election year is extremely difficult. Partisan lines are drawn more sharply as each legislative vote is seen as a potential campaign issue for an adversary, and neither party wants to give its opponents the credit for passing a major bill. Although there was general public support for welfare reform, the specific items sought by voters (e.g., child care, training programs) would undercut a secondary (perhaps primary for some) goal of cutting costs. Therefore, supporters of proposed reforms needed symbolic cover to overcome concerns about harming children. Devolution, giving states much more responsibility for welfare programs, provided an ideological justification that fit the public's general distrust of government. As a fiscal issue, the restructuring of the funding as a block grant limited federal responsibility and made future national expenditures more predictable.

A key element in this process was the support of state governors (many of whom came to office in the 1994 "Republican Revolution") for having the primary responsibility for welfare.[1] A February 6, 1996, proposal by the National Governors' Association called for even more state control of both welfare and Medicaid than an earlier Republican proposal that had been one of two Republican bills vetoed by President Clinton (the first on December 6, 1995 and the second on January 9, 1996).[20] The President condemned the first House version of welfare reform, calling it, "weak on work and tough on children";[21] however, he did have kind words for a Senate version of reform and that became part of the basis for later revisions. A major issue is the joining of welfare reform with Medicaid cuts, a linkage President Clinton referred to as a "poison pill" that would prevent him from signing any reform legislation. Although Medicaid represented a far greater financial commitment by the national and state governments, it retained higher levels of public support, perhaps in part because of its role in financing long-term care for the middle-class elderly. By spring of 1996, support for bipartisan legislation was building as Democrats wanted to pass something that at least let them symbolically say they voted for welfare reform, whereas Republicans continued to press for an ending of the entitlement to support. Congressional Democrats were also fearful that the President, himself up for reelection and not wanting to provide Senator Dole with a campaign issue, might end up supporting a Republican version of the bill[20] and leave them having voted against reform. The legislation had been designated as a deficit-reducing budget reconciliation bill, which prevented a Senate filibuster against it.[21]

Each House passed new versions in the summer, and a conference committee met in late July to work out the now relatively minor differences in language. Two key amendments, both protecting Medicaid coverage for the poor, added during the Senate floor debate, made the bill more palatable to Democrats and moderate Republicans. Most members of the conference committee, dominated by Republicans, sought a version that would be acceptable to the President so they could run for reelection based on a successful welfare reform bill.[21] A study was released by the Urban Institute and used the same assumptions as earlier Department of Health and Human Services studies that had been cited in justifying the President's two previous vetoes of Republican bills. It predicted the new law would move 1.1 million children into poverty.[2] Nonetheless, the conference committee's version passed both Houses with ease and in a press conference on July 31st, the President indicated he would sign it, saying "even though the bill has serious flaws that are unrelated to welfare reform, I believe we have a duty to seize the opportunity it gives us to end welfare as we know it."[22] He signed it into law on August 22, 1996, 10 weeks before his resounding reelection.

Policy Implementation and Evaluation

It is premature to assess the implementation process and evaluate the overall impact of the new law. The Census Bureau announced in April 1997 that it was beginning a 10-year project to study the impact of the welfare reform legislation.[23] President Clinton did work with Congress to change some provisions of the bill and blocked several Republicans proposals. These changes reduced some of the negative impact of the bill on legal immigrants and provided more funding for job placement for long-time welfare recipients but did not alter the fundamental nature of the 1996 law.[24] A strong economy has helped buffer some of the immediate effects of the law, including providing more opportunities for former welfare recipients seeking jobs, but successful job placement is not inexpensive or easy to implement and often involves substantial training, a state responsibility under the new law.[25]

IMPLICATIONS FOR THE FUTURE

Several themes emerge when examining the health and welfare policy process.

   1. The Problem with Constituencies. The nature of health and welfare policies is that they largely deal with politically vulnerable populations. The most notable exception, Medicare, is also the most generously funded program. Welfare policies in particular serve a constituency that is not now, nor likely to be, politically active or in command of important political resources. Therefore, the fate of these policies will be subject to larger political forces that shape the general policy process such as generalized movements to the right or left. These forces influence the entire policy process, but in other areas activists protect the status quo through their understanding and constant involvement with the political process. The major activists on behalf of health and welfare policy are those who provide associated services (e.g., training programs), whose interests might not always intersect with those of the disenfranchised. There are also the smaller number of individuals and groups that seek to protect the vulnerable (e.g., Children's Defense Fund). These groups are often politically savvy but simply do not have the resources necessary to significantly and consistently influence the policy process. The other group that may advocate in the future for the vulnerable may be state leaders, not out of a newly discovered concern for the poor, but to protect their own interests as the full impact of the welfare block grant system causes local pressure to improve support.

2. Limited National Role. For the foreseeable future, the role of the national government in welfare policy is likely to be limited. The major benefit to the national government of the welfare reforms is that, by shifting to a block grant approach, they have made their fiscal planning more predictable. Costs at the national level are not now directly linked to the caseload of recipients entitled to support and will not automatically rise in a bad economy. The result may be harsh on the poor and place new burdens on the states, but there is no incentive for the federal government to go back to its previous role. If the system of relatively fixed block grants is seen as working by the national government, with limited opposition from the vulnerable (see #1), there will be a great temptation to extend this approach to other areas where there is a weak constituency to oppose it.

3. Incremental Changes Based on Compromise. Major policy changes come about rarely and usually only after a series of smaller steps. There had been considerable public dissatisfaction with the welfare system dating back to the 1970s, but major change did not occur until 1996. It is not likely that there will be a major shift back. It is more probable that small changes will be enacted, with additional federal funding for specific targeted initiatives (e.g., state innovations in training). The advantage of these largely symbolic approaches is that they allow elected leaders to claim credit for policy initiatives without having to make tough choices about resource allocation.

4. A Lack of Concern with Implementation and Evaluation. It is not clear what will happen if the welfare reforms do not work. Perhaps more importantly, assessment of the results of welfare reform will not be simple. There will be evaluations and studies of the implementation, but such studies are very complex and seldom have clear-cut findings. Therefore, both proponents and opponents of reform will likely find elements that support their view. The interpretation of the impact of reform will also depend on which of the multiple goals of the reform one chooses to address. If it was to help individuals move from a life of dependency to independence, how easily can that be systematically measured, and if it fails in this regard, who will complain? If it was to cap the national government's expenditures for welfare, how can it fail? If it was to reduce a problem (e.g., out of wedlock birth) that systematic studies showed it was not related to in the first place, how will we know what made a difference? In an area like health and welfare policy, in which assessment of process and outcome is so strongly linked to one's ideological predisposition, we cannot expect clear assessment of policy impact.

5. Recommendations. What's the appropriate action for an advocate? There is no quick answer in a system that favors those with time, persistence, and resources. The key point to keep in mind is that policymakers tend to project the communications they have with "activist constituents" to the population as a whole. How do you become an activist constituent? By regularly contacting those in positions to influence the policy of choice and speaking with an understanding of the process, thus avoiding being marginalized. It will also help to support those already involved in the fray at the national and state levels. It is now possible to keep reasonably informed about policy at any of the stages described earlier through websites or newsletters. The latter are helpful but often quite expensive and aimed at insiders. Regularly consulting the websites that deal with health and welfare issues can keep one abreast of important actions. Simply enter "welfare policy" into a web search engine and begin finding the sites most appropriate for you. Keep in mind that if the goal is to influence policy, the commitment must be long term and sensitive to the norms of the often frustrating process this chapter has described.

References

1. Katz, J.L. Voter call for revamped welfare poses problem for Democrats. *CQ Weekly Report.* April 20, 1996;1027–1029.
2. Edelman, P. The worst thing Bill Clinton has done. *The Atlantic Monthly.* 1997;279: 43–58.

3. Dye, Thomas. *Understanding Public Policy.* 9th ed. Upper Saddle River, NJ: Prentice Hall, 1998.

4. Elazar, D.J. *American federalism: A view from the states.* New York: Thomas Y. Cromwell, 1966.

5. U.S. Bureau of the Census. *Statistical abstract of the United States 1997: The national data book.* Washington, DC: U.S. Government Printing Office, 1997.

6. Staeheli, L.A., Kodras, J.E., and Flint, C. *State devolution in America.* London: Sage Publications, 1997.

7. Marquis, M.S., and Long, S.H. Federalism and health system reform: Prospects for state action. *JAMA.* 1997;278(6):514–517.

8. Federal Election Commission. Press Release, August 22, 1997.

9. Federal Election Commission. Press Release, September 22, 1997.

10. Kingdon, J. *Agendas, alternatives and public policies.* 2nd ed. New York: HarperCollins, 1995.

11. Rochefort, D.A., and Cobb, R.W. (eds). *The politics of problem definition: Shaping the policy agenda.* Lawrence, KS: University of Kansas Press, 1994.

12. Institute of Medicine. *The Future of Public Health.* Washington: National Academy Press, 1989.

13. Smith, S., and Deering, C. *Committees in Congress.* 2nd ed. Washington, DC: CQ Press, 1990.

14. Kingdon, J. *Congressmen's voting decisions.* 3rd ed. Ann Arbor, MI: University of Michigan Press, 1989.

15. Tanner, M., Moore, S., Hartman, David. *The work versus welfare trade-off: an analysis of the total level of welfare benefits by state.* Cato Policy Analysis No. 240 (September 19,1995) Washington, DC: Cato Institute.

16. LA Times Poll. April, 1996.

17. LA Times Poll. October, 1994.

18. Weaver, R.K., Shapiro, R.Y., and Jacobs, L.R. The polls—trends: Welfare. *Public Opinion Quarterly* 1995;59:606–627.

19. Bowman, K. (ed). Opinion pulse: Welfare reform update. *The American Enterprise.* March/April, 1997;8:91.

20. Katz, J.L. Welfare showdown looms as GOP readies plan. *CQ Weekly Report.* July 27, 1996;2115–2119.

21. Katz, J.L. After 60 years, most control is passing to states. *CQ Weekly Report.* August 3, 1996;2190–2196.

22. Congressional Quarterly. *For the record: Presidential news conference.* August 3, 1996;2216–2218.

23. U.S. Department of Commerce. 1997. Census Bureau launches 10-year study to follow effects of welfare reform legislation (press release). April 29, 1997.

24. Congressional Quarterly. Issue: Welfare. *CQ Weekly Report.* December 6, 1997;3013.

25. Grunwald, M. How she got a job. *The American Prospect.* 1997;33:25–29.

6

The Childrens' Health Care Safety Net: A Changing Environment

LYNN SQUIRE AND RALPH MARTINI

The United States has had a long-standing commitment to maintenance of a health care safety net for persons who are uninsured, difficult to serve, discriminated against, or who cannot get care elsewhere. Although any provider can participate, local health departments that contain maternal and child health clinics, community health centers, urban public hospitals, and some inner-city teaching hospitals are generally considered to be the core safety net institutions.

The populations served by safety net providers range from the uninsured and Medicaid populations to a broader array of the vulnerable. Children, including those with disabilities, and pregnant women were the earliest groups protected by the safety net. They have been joined more recently by persons with acquired immunodeficiency syndrome (AIDS), the frail elderly, the homeless, the mentally ill, and substance abusers.

In the absence of universal health insurance, concern has grown that the rise to preeminence of a competitive, market-driven health care market may destroy the viability of the safety net. This concern was heightened in 1996 by rollbacks in Medicaid for immigrants and for children receiving Supplemental Security Income (SSI) that were passed by Congress in the Personal Responsibility and Work Opportunity Act of 1996 (P.L. 104-193),[1] which threatened to put greater pressure on safety net resources.

Offsetting some of this pressure was the enactment of the Health Insurance Portability and Accountability Act of 1996 (P.L. 104-191),[2] which is expected to improve continuity of coverage for special needs populations in the individual and group insurance markets when it goes into effect in 1998. With this legislation in place, attention refocused in 1997 on options to further reduce the number of uninsured. After the rejection in 1994 of global approaches to covering the uninsured, interest in incremental approaches, especially health insurance for children, increased. By the summer of 1997, this interest culminated in the largest expansion of child health coverage in recent history.

On August 5, 1997, the Balanced Budget Act of 1997 (P.L. 105-33)[3] became law. Title XXI—was added to the Social Security Act, establishing a State Children's Health Insurance Program (SCHIP). This capped entitlement program will phase in almost $48 billion to the states by formula over the next 10 years and is expected to sharply decrease the number of children without health insurance. Each state will have considerable discretion to determine how to spend its allotted funds, choosing from such options as expanding its current Medicaid coverage, enrolling children in certain "benchmark" private group health and managed care plans, or developing new plans that meet certain criteria. The law precludes denial of benefits based on a pre-existing medical condition. In addition, Medicaid benefits were restored for disabled children who will lose their SSI eligibility as a result of P.L. 104-193. State Child Health Plans are subject to approval by the Secretary of Health and Human Services. Implementation of SCHIP began on October 1, 1997.

With major changes expected to continue unabated in the financing and delivery of health care services, federal and state governments will be compelled to reassess the role of public sector safety net providers, organizations, and financial sources of support. In this environment, there have as yet been few signals as to what direction public sector provided care for pregnant women or children may take.

Currently, federal and state governments, particularly through Medicaid, play a crucial role in financing the safety net for children and families. Medicaid[4] serves as the nation's leading health insurer for low-income women and children; in 1995 it covered nearly 18 million children and 8 million women of childbearing age. As a result of program expansions, children and pregnant women account for the greatest growth in the number of Medicaid beneficiaries since 1988. By 1994, Medicaid paid for health care services for more than one third of all children under age five.

The bulk of the service needs of women and children is for preventive and primary care and other acute care services. Pregnant women primarily need prenatal and obstetric care. Relatively healthy women need preventive and primary care services such as annual gynecological exams, family planning services, and care for minor illness or injury. Medical screenings for children also are a well-established and recommended practice in this country. Medicaid's Early and Periodic Screening, Diagnosis and Treatment (EPSDT) program, established as a mandatory service under Medicaid in 1967, remains the nation's primary source of well-child care for low-income youth. Medicaid EPSDT services are a particularly vital funding source for children with special health care needs. Also, since 1988, the Medicare Catastrophic Coverage Act of 1988 (P.L. 100-360),[5] has allowed the use of Medicaid funding, at state option, for the cost of "related services" in a school-age child's individualized educational plan (IEP) or an infant's or toddler's individualized family service plan (IFSP). As a result, early intervention programs and school districts in 35 states have been designated as Medicaid providers and receive reimbursement for a variety of health education and rehabilitative services or therapies.

Although women and children in the Medicaid program tend to require fewer services than other recipients who need more expensive care, many recipients have socioeconomic problems or behaviors that affect their health status and access to adequate medical care, including prenatal care. Certain program elements most often made available through safety net programs—such as outreach, education, and non-medical support services—are critical to producing real improvements in prenatal care usage and birth outcomes.

As the most frequent strategy used by states to control Medicaid costs, managed care has the potential to improve access to health care for maternal and child health (MCH) populations. If these programs are planned and implemented with careful attention to detail, a number of benefits can be realized, including coordination of medical services by a single provider, reduced reliance on emergency rooms for non-emergency care, fewer hospitalizations, and predictable (and reduced) costs through capitation. On the other hand, capitation can provide an incentive to underserve clients. Thus, the expansion of managed care to Medicaid populations can threaten the survival of traditional safety net providers by squeezing them out of existing systems of public medical assistance.

Medicaid's movement toward managed care seems certain to undermine even its indirect support role in the operation of the safety net for children. Supplemental payments to traditional providers are generally not a Medicaid plan responsibility. The contracts vest extraordinary discretion in managed care organizations (MCOs) to select and pay their network providers and allocate patients among them. To the extent that Medicaid support has been tied to patient care, this funding may disappear under managed care, leaving safety net providers to look elsewhere for operating funds.

Further, many federal and state policymakers are just beginning to consider the broader issues that flow from the relationship between MCOs and the larger health care system within which they function. For example, states have only recently begun to explore relationships between MCOs and public health agencies in the areas of coverage, service provision, and data collection.

Advocates for primarily adult oriented public hospitals and health clinics have long sought to highlight the changing environment for public sector safety net providers.[6] This chapter looks at the impact of this changing environment on public MCH safety net providers in particular. It presents an overview of publicly supported maternal and child health service programs and briefly describes three possible scenarios—the *fully vested public sector*, the *residual public sector*, and the *divested public sector*—as possible future roles for maternal and child health providers in a changing health care environment. It raises some questions for communities and governments to weigh as they determine the future role of these providers.

SAFETY NET PROGRAMS

At present, federal and state government roles in the delivery of safety net health services to children, including children with special health care needs, may take the form of providing, funding, organizing, promoting, or coordinating services. Some of the major federal and federal-state programs are described here.

Maternal and Child Health Services Block Grant

Charged with primary responsibility for promoting and improving the health of the nation's mothers and children, the Maternal and Child Health Bureau (MCHB) draws on nearly a century of commitment and experience. Early efforts are rooted in MCHB's predecessor, the Children's Bureau, which was established in 1912. In 1935, Congress enacted Title V of the Social Security Act, which authorized the Maternal and Child Health Program and the Crippled Children's Program (referred to since 1986 as Children with Special Health Care Needs), providing a foundation and structure for ensuring MCH efforts for more than 60 years.

When the Title V program was converted to a block grant in 1981, seven categorical programs were consolidated. States were given considerable discretion to determine how to use federal funds to implement the legislation. Amendments enacted as part of the Omnibus Budget Reconciliation Act of 1989 (P.L. 101-239)[8] introduced strict requirements for the use of funds and for state planning and reporting. States exercise authority in priority setting, allocating funds, and delivering services to fit state and local needs and characteristics. They are required, however, to use at least 30% of Title V funds on preventive and primary care services for children and at least 30% on services for children with special health care needs (CSHCN). They may spend no more than 10% of Title V funds on administrative costs and must maintain the state contribution to at least the fiscal year (FY) 1989 funding level.

Today, Title V is administered by the MCHB, Health Resources and Services Administration (HRSA), and the U.S. Department of Health and Human Services (HHS). The program has three components: formula block grants to 59 states and territories, grants for special projects of regional and national significance (SPRANS), and community integrated service systems (CISS) grants.

The annual Title V appropriation is allocated in the following manner: Of the amount appropriated annually up to $600 million, 85% is for allotment to the states and 15% is for the SPRANS federal set-aside program. Of the amount appropriated over $600 million, 12.75% is for the CISS federal set-aside program, and the remaining amount is distributed 85% to the states and 15% for SPRANS.

Funds are allotted to states using a percentage method based on (1) FY 1981 funding levels for MCH-related programs that were combined into the block grant when it was initiated and (2) the number of low-income children in the state. States must match three dollars for every four federal dollars they receive. This results in more than $1 billion available annually for MCH programs at the state and local levels. Historically, many states have "overmatched," i.e., provided funding significantly in excess of the required match. Tables 6.1 through 6.3 set forth

TABLE 6.1

Federal Funding* for Selected Federal and Federal-State Programs Serving Women or Children, 1984, 1990, and 1993–1997 (in millions)

Program	Federal Fiscal Year						
	1984	1990	1993	1994	1995	1996	1997
Medical Assistance (Medicaid) Program[†]	$20,061	$41,103	$75,774	$82,034	$89,070	$91,990	$98,503 (Est.)
Maternal Child Health Services Block Grant	399	554	665	687	684	678	681
Healthy Start	—	—	79	98	104	93	96
Supplemental Security Income (SSI) Program[†]	8,498	12,568	22,642	26,281	26,488	26,674	28,696 (Est.)
WIC	1,360	2,126	2,860	3,210	3,470	3,730	3,730
Emergency Medical Services for Children	—	4	5	8	10	11	12
Pediatric AIDS	—	15	21	22	26	29	36
Health Centers	373	457	616	663	757[‡]	758[‡]	802[‡]
Family Planning (Title X)	140	139	173	181	193	193	198
Head Start	996	1,448	2,779	3,326	3,534	3,569	3,981
Early Intervention	—	80	213	253	316	316	315
Vaccines for Children	—	—	—	81	420	204	523 (Est.)

*The figures for the Medicaid and SSI programs, which are entitlement programs, represent annual outlays of federal funds. The figures for other programs represent annual appropriations of federal funds.
[†]The figures for the Medicaid and SSI Programs represent total expenditures for beneficiaries, including but not limited to children.
[‡]Consolidated Health Center Program: includes CHC/MHC, Health Care for the Homeless, Health Care for Residents in Public Housing.
From Office of Management and Budget. *Budget of the United States Government, appendix, for fiscal years 1986, 1992, and 1995–1998.* Washington, DC: U.S. Government Printing Office.

TABLE 6.2

Maternal and Child Health Appropriation Levels by Type of Grant, 1982–1997 (in millions)

Federal Fiscal Year	Total	Block Grants to States	Children with Special Health Care Needs Allocation//	Discretionary Grants
1982	$373.8	$316.2		$57.6
1983	478.0	422.1*		55.9
1984	399.0	339.2		59.8
1985	478.0	406.3		71.7
1986	457.4†	388.8		68.6
1987	496.8‡	421.1		75.7
1988	526.6§	444.3		82.3
1989	554.3§	465.3		89.0
1990	553.6	470.6	$141.2	83.0
1991	587.3	499.2	149.8	88.1
1992	649.7	547.1	164.1	102.6¶
1993	664.4	557.9	167.4	106.7¶
1994	687.0	574.5	172.4	112.5¶
1995	684.0	572.2	171.7	111.8¶
1996	678.2	568.0	170.4	110.2¶
1997	681.0	568.0	170.4	130.0¶**

*Includes $105 million designated funds from the Jobs Bill Urgent Supplement Legislation (P.L. 98-8).
†Reflects a $20.6 million reduction stemming from the Gramm-Rudman Act (P.L. 97-216).
‡Includes a supplemental appropriation for $18.8 million.
§Includes funds for projects to screen for sickle cell anemia and other hemoglobinopathies as well as new child health demonstration projects for primary care services and community network and case management services for children with special health care needs.
//Minimum 30% of allocation for children with special health care needs.
¶Includes $6.4 million for the first year, $8.2 million for the second year, $11.1 million for the third year, $10.7 million for the fourth year, and $10.0 in fifth and sixth year of Community Integrated Service System (CISS) Projects.
**Includes $2.857 for the Traumatic Brain Injury Program (P.L. 104-208).
From Maternal and Child Health Bureau, HRSA, PHS, U.S. Department of Health and Human Services. *Summary of federal appropriation for MCH Bureau Program.*

TABLE 6.3

SPRANS *Grant Funding Levels by Category of* SPRANS *Grant,*
1982–1997 *(in millions)*

Year	Total	Research	Training	Genetics	Hemophilia*	TBI	Other
1982	$57.55	$2.35	$27.92	$7.25	$2.60	—	$17.43
1983	55.95	3.70	26.66	7.33	2.60	—	15.66
1984	59.85	4.70	27.50	7.40	3.03	—	17.22
1985	71.70	6.00	29.50	8.00	3.60	—	24.60
1986	68.62	5.35	28.28	7.50	3.45	—	24.04
1987	75.62	6.20	28.40	8.81[†]	3.69	—	30.97
1988	82.28	7.20	29.43	10.89[†]	3.69	—	30.97
1989	88.98	7.20	30.33	13.87[†]	4.70	—	32.88
1990	83.04	7.60	30.86	7.00	4.70	—	32.88
1991	88.10	7.60	32.87	7.50	4.70	—	35.43
1992	96.19	7.75	33.67	9.10	5.20	—	40.47
1993	98.37	7.00	35.19	9.29	5.36	—	41.53
1994	101.39	6.72	37.09	9.29	5.30	—	42.99
1995	101.00	8.10	35.10	9.00	5.30	—	43.50
1996	100.20	7.10	41.00	9.20	5.30	—	37.60
1997	103.10	7.10	40.50	9.30	5.30	2.86	38.10

*Does not include transfer of funds from CDC for AIDS service programming in hemophilia, 1986–1995 ($2.5, $3.5, $6.3, $7.2, $7.5, $8.5, $7.6, $7.6, $7.6, and $6.0 million in successive years).
†Includes funds for projects to screen for sickle cell anemia and other hemoglobinopathies as well as new child health demonstration projects for primary care services and community network and case management services for children with special health care needs.
From Maternal and Child Health Bureau, HRSA, PHS, U.S. Department of Health and Human Services. *Summary of federal appropriations for MCH Bureau Programs.*

the MCH Block Grant appropriations for selected years and the allocation of these appropriations among different components of the Block Grant.

The Title V program provides flexible funding to States to plan and implement programs to improve the health status of all mothers and children consistent with national health objectives. The services must be provided free of charge to people with incomes below federal poverty guidelines. States often use their block grant funds to strengthen the safety net:

supplementing other services, filling in identified gaps, and providing population-based prevention services. Title V is required by federal law to coordinate with other related federal programs (including Medicaid) to enhance program effectiveness and plays a key partnership role in developing services for pregnant women on Medicaid. A number of state initiatives to improve access to prenatal care and improve the health of newborns are administered jointly by Medicaid and the Title V programs.

Over the years, state CSHCN programs have extended their coverage beyond their original focus on orthopedic problems to children with a variety of other physical disabilities, impairments, and chronic illnesses. Because Title V does not define the term *children with special health care needs*, state CSHCN agencies are free to determine their own eligibility requirements and to design and implement their programs to meet these children's specific needs. There is, thus, wide variation among state CSHCN programs in the services funded and provided as well as other program functions and activities. All state CSHCN programs are required, however, "to provide and promote family-centered, community-based, coordinated care (including care coordination services as defined in the legislation) for children with special health care needs and to facilitate the development of community-based systems of services for such children and their families."

At the state level, MCH programs are usually administered by the state health agency, although a few state CSHCN programs are administered by other state entities. State MCH programs play a key partnership role in developing services for pregnant women on Medicaid. A survey of state programs indicates that states use their Title V funds in the following ways: (1) about 35% pays for "enabling services," such as outreach, transportation, referral to other existing services, home visiting, translation services, and nutrition counseling; (2) about 30% funds infrastructure and capacity building, such as operating programs and clinics, funding local health care providers, and supporting school health services and education programs; (3) about 25% is spent on direct services, such as providing prenatal care, immunizations, and preventive and primary care for children; and (4) about 10% is used for population-based services such as conducting community needs assessments, developing standards and monitoring compliance with them, and providing technical assistance to providers and programs.

Title V's two federal project grant programs enhance the program's capacity to assist state and local governments in providing a safety net for poor mothers and children. Activities supported by SPRANS include MCH research, training, genetic services and newborn screening, hemophilia diagnostic and treatment centers, and maternal and child health improvement projects (MCHIPs) that support a broad range of innovative demonstration strategies. In FY 1997, the Bureau funded 500 SPRANS grants at a total of $103 million.

The CISS program, funded since 1992, seeks to reduce infant mortality and build infrastructure to improve the health of mothers and children by funding projects for the development and expansion of integrated services at the community level. In FY 1997, 112 CISS grants were awarded, totaling $10 million.

Healthy Start

The Healthy Start Initiative,[9] authorized under section 301 of the Public Health Service Act, funds the development of programs and strategies to reduce infant mortality in targeted high-risk communities and the replication of program successes across the nation. Healthy Start was initiated in 1991 as a demonstration program. It is administered by HRSA's MCH Bureau.

Healthy Start grants offer a vital lifeline to the youngest, smallest, most vulnerable Americans before and after their births. They stress innovation, personal responsibility, community commitment, increased access to services, and service integration to decrease infant mortality and low birthweight. Twenty-two communities with infant mortality rates 1.5 to 2.5 times higher than the national average have participated in the 5-year Phase I program. Projects have developed community consortia, conducted needs assessment, and formulated comprehensive action plans to implement health care and social support services intended to reduce infant mortality by 50% in their respective communities in 5 years. Services to children, women of childbearing age, and their families have also broadened the knowledge base of successful strategies for reducing infant mortality. The Healthy Start program has an aggressive public information and education component to raise awareness in local communities concerning the problem of infant mortality, promote healthy behaviors, and motivate mothers to enter prenatal care early.

For FY 1997, the Healthy Start program was funded at $96 million. Phase II of the Healthy Start Initiative will replicate the best models from the demonstration phase in an additional 40 communities with unacceptably high rates of infant mortality. For the future, intensive coordination between Healthy Start and welfare-to-work initiatives stemming from 1996's welfare reform legislation is planned. Table 6.1 displays Healthy Start's funding history. The lessons learned from Healthy Start are intended to be shared extensively with the wider MCH community. An extensive outcomes and process-oriented national evaluation, to be completed in mid-1998, is being conducted in the original Healthy Start communities. Each grantee is also conducting evaluations of some of its unique interventions.

Supplemental Security Income

Title XVI of the Social Security Act, enacted in 1972, created the Supplemental Security Income (SSI) Program for the Aged, Blind, and Disabled.[10] SSI provides cash benefits to low-income blind and disabled children and adults who meet the Act's definition of disability and income eligibility requirements.

SSI is administered by the Social Security Administration (SSA) and, like Medicaid, is an entitlement program. Table 6.1 summarizes federal SSI funding for selected years. A close relationship between the SSI program and the state CSHCN programs has existed since 1976, when the SSI/Disabled Children's Program was established through amendment of the SSI legislation. This amendment required SSI recipients under age 16 to be referred to the state Crippled Children's Services programs for counseling, establishment of individual service plans and referrals for needed services, and monitoring of compliance with individual service plans. In addition, the state programs were directed to provide medical, social, developmental, and rehabilitative services for children under age 17 and for children age 7 and over who had never attended school. The SSI/Disabled Children's Program was consolidated into the MCH Block Grant in 1981.

There is also a strong link between SSI program eligibility and Medicaid eligibility. In most states, children determined to be eligible for SSI benefits are eligible for Medicaid. Thus, the SSI program is of significance especially to children with special health care needs not only because it can provide needed financial assistance but also because it may enable them to obtain needed health services.

Determining whether a child is disabled for purposes of SSI eligibility has been a continuing and controversial problem. In a 1990 decision, Sullivan v. Zebley,[11] the United States Supreme Court ruled that the process used by SSA for determining disability of children violated the Social Security Act because children were subject to a more restrictive standard than adults and did not receive the same kind of individual assessment that adults received. In response to Zebley, SSA issued regulations under which children applying for SSI were to receive individual functional assessments of how their claimed impairment limits their ability to act and behave in an age-appropriate manner.

In the wake of expanded SSI eligibility and outreach efforts by SSA, the population of children receiving benefits under the SSI program grew rapidly. From 1989 to 1994 the number of SSI child recipients increased from 300,000 to 900,000, and the proportion of children making up the SSI recipient pool increased from 6.5% to 14.2%. In 1996, the increase in child SSI recipients and the corresponding increase in the cost of the program, together with widely publicized claims that fraud had added children on the SSI rolls, led to sweeping changes in SSI law as part of welfare reform. Public Law 104-193 required SSA to issue new regulations that eliminated eligibility based on individualized functional assessment and "maladaptive behavior."[12]

In 1997, families of more than 260,000 children receiving SSI benefits were notified by SSA that their eligibility would be reviewed. About 50,000 of these children were considered likely to lose their Medicaid coverage along with their SSI eligibility. Responding to alarmed advocates for disabled children, the President, in his Budget Message for FY 1998, proposed to restore Medicaid coverage for those disabled children whose SSI benefits would be terminated because of the SSI program changes. This proposal was adopted as part of P.L. 105-33.[13]

Special Supplemental Nutrition Program for Women, Infants and Children (WIC)

The WIC program,[14] authorized under the Child Nutrition Act of 1966, as amended, and administered by the U.S. Department of Agriculture, provides no-cost, supplemental nutritious foods, nutrition education, and referrals to health care to low-income pregnant, breastfeeding, and postpartum women; infants; and children to age 5 determined to be at nutritional risk and financially in need. Individuals are certified as meeting an income standard or as participating in certain other means-tested federal programs. Certification regarding nutritional need for supplemental foods is determined by local level professionals.

Grants are made by statutory and regulatory formulas to state health departments, comparable agencies, or Indian tribal organizations. These agencies distribute funds to participating local public or nonprofit private health or welfare agencies. Funds pay for supplemental foods, nutrition education, and health care referrals for participants, as well as specified administrative costs, including certification services. Only local agencies qualifying under state agency applications may operate WIC programs. Most state WIC programs are administered by the Title V director in the state health agency. Federal WIC appropriations do not require a state match, but some states contribute non-federal funds to augment the program.

Table 6.1 presents the funding history for the WIC program for selected years. In FY 1997, funding for WIC was about $3.9 billion. The program operated in 88 state agencies, including 50 states, 33 Indian agencies, Puerto Rico, the Virgin Islands, Guam, American Samoa, and the District of Columbia. In FY 1996, an average of 7.2 million women, infants, and children received WIC benefits every month, at an average food package cost of $31.17 per person.

Emergency Medical Services for Children

The Emergency Medical Services for Children (EMSC) program[15], established in 1984 under section 1910 of the Public Health Service Act, funds grants to the states to develop or enhance emergency medical services (EMS) programs for children with critical illnesses and life-threatening injuries. The purpose of the EMSC program is to reduce morbidity and mortality among children by expanding and improving emergency transportation and medical services. The creation of this program was a response to the fact that EMS systems around the country had largely ignored the special needs of children in emergency treatment for trauma or acute illnesses. Not all emergency medical personnel had adequate training necessary to care for children, and the necessary special pediatric equipment was not widely available.

The EMSC program is jointly administered by the MCHB and the National Highway Traffic Safety Administration. Table 6.1 displays the history of federal appropriations for this program. Since the late 1980s, the EMSC program has assisted nearly all states, the District of Columbia, and Puerto Rico in incorporating pediatric components into their emergency medical systems. During this period, the program has also furnished support to two resource centers for information dissemination and technical assistance and consultation activities.

Ryan White Title IV Pediatric AIDS Program

In 1987 Congress appropriated funds for the MCHB to develop the Pediatric AIDS Health Care Demonstration Program, later expanded to the Pediatric/Family HIV Health Care Demonstration Program. This program was subsequently incorporated into the Ryan White CARE Act as Title IV,[16] authorized under Title XXVI of the Public Health Service Act. This program was directed toward a relatively new population of children with special health care needs—children infected with human immunodeficiency virus (HIV) that produces acquired immunodeficiency syndrome (AIDS). Today, the Ryan White Title IV Program combines the goals of pediatric AIDS research with family-centered health and support services to meet the unique needs of adolescents, children, and their mothers for HIV care.

In the 1990s, HIV infection has become a leading cause of morbidity and mortality among children. The vast majority, nearly 90%, of reported pediatric AIDS cases are attributable to perinatal transmission of the virus from an infected woman to her fetus or newborn. It is estimated that between the years 1988 and 1992 there were 1,000 to

2,000 HIV-infected infants born annually, and by 1995 there were more than 5,500 reported AIDS cases of children under age 13.

The Ryan White Title IV Program is administered by HRSA. Table 6.1 lists the federal appropriations for this program. The program represents the federal government's principal effort to respond to the challenge posed by pediatric AIDS. The projects funded under the program have demonstrated effective ways to prevent HIV infection among children and to deliver family-centered, community-based, co-ordinated care for infants, children, adolescents, and their families affected by HIV/AIDS.

These projects provide comprehensive health services to children infected with HIV, have successfully integrated research findings into their actual clinical care, and provide social support for affected families. They stress the identification of HIV-positive pregnant women through outreach, counseling, and testing, which in turn enables better follow-up care. Title IV grantees have supported provision of AZT to mothers and infants during pregnancy, delivery, and post partum to reduce perinatal transmission of HIV. The projects also stress the link of families whose members have HIV infection or are at risk of HIV infection with other sources of prevention, health, and social support services.

Consolidated Health Centers

Consolidated Health Centers[17]—centers for community health, migrant health, health care for the homeless, and health services for residents of public housing—provide comprehensive primary medical care services with a culturally sensitive, family-oriented focus. These services include preventive health and dental services, acute and chronic care services, and appropriate hospitalization and specialty referrals.

Targeted to medically underserved, low-income, and disadvantaged populations, health centers serve large numbers of minority populations, women of childbearing age, infants, people with HIV infection, substance abusers, and homeless individuals and their families. Anyone may receive services, and charges are assessed on a sliding scale based on ability to pay. In FY 1995, health centers served more than eight million people. Of this total, approximately 3.5 million, or 44% were infants, children and youth under age 19. The history of Federal funding for health centers for selected years is displayed in Table 6.1.

Health center services are prevention-oriented and include such children's services as immunizations, well-baby care, and developmental screenings. Health centers also provide ancillary services such as laboratory tests, x-rays, environmental health services, and pharmacy services. In addition, many centers provide enabling health and community services, such as transportation, health education, nutrition, counseling, and translation services. The National Health Service Corps provides a significant proportion of the total number of providers employed by health centers.

Health centers emphasize case management, i.e., the coordination of the center's services with community social and economic services appropriate to the needs of the patient. Health centers also link with services provided by other safety net providers, such as WIC, Title V, and substance abuse and other health and social service programs, which may be located on-site to provide "one-stop shopping."

Health centers are supported through a variety of sources, including federal health center grants, Medicaid, Medicare, third-party insurance, patient fees, and state and local contributions. Most states also use Title V funds to support their health centers. Around the country, health centers are actively exploring opportunities to network with other public and/or private providers in order to participate in local provider arrangements increasingly dominated by Medicaid managed care.

Family Planning

Medicaid funds about half of all publicly funded family planning services[18] for low-income women and adolescents; however, many low-income women and sexually active teenagers do not qualify for Medicaid. The other major source of family planning funds is Title X of the Public Health Service Act, the only Federal program devoted solely to family planning services. Within HHS, the Title X program is administered by the Office of Population Affairs/Office of Public Health and Science. The program provides grants to public and private, nonprofit agencies to provide voluntary family planning services. In FY 1996, more than 4 million clients, primarily women, received family planning services at over 4,000 clinics funded in part by Title X. Title X is the only federal program focused solely on family planning, decreasing unintended pregnancy, and decreasing adolescent pregnancy. While other programs, such as Medicaid, provide funding for family planning, Title X serves as a safety net for populations largely unserved by Medicaid, including teens, nulliparous women, and the working poor. Programs must give priority to clients who are members of low-income families. Title X clinics provide free care to members of low-income families and charge fees on a sliding scale to those with higher incomes.

For many clients, the family planning clinic has been the primary, or sole, point of contact with the health care system, providing basic gynecologic care, contraception, diagnosis and treatment for sexually transmitted diseases, breast and cervical cancer screening, and education and referral information. Title X also supports training and research that focus on improving family planning service delivery.

In FY 1996, there were 83 family planning grantees, of which 33 were state or territorial health departments. In an additional 11 states, the state health department was one of two or more grantees receiving funds. Table 6.1 details the history of funding for this program.

Title V and the Social Services Block Grant also help fund some state and local family planning services. In addition, state and local governments contribute funds to public family planning services.

Other Programs

A host of categorical federal and federal-state health programs serve pregnant women and/or children, including those with special health care needs. Many of these programs focus on preventive and primary care for low-income individuals, medically underserved individuals, or both. In addition, there are programs that target various categories of disadvantaged children and include a health component along with other types of service components. Examples include the following.

Head Start. Head Start[19] is a national program that provides comprehensive developmental services for low-income, preschool children ages 3 to 5 and social services for their families. Specific services for children focus on education, socio-emotional development, physical and mental health, and nutrition. Head Start began in 1965 in the Office of Economic Opportunity as an innovative way in which to serve children of low-income families and is now administered by the Administration for Children and Families, HHS. The cornerstone of the program is parent and community involvement, making it one of the most successful preschool programs in the country. Approximately 1,400 community-based nonprofit organizations and school systems develop unique and innovative programs to meet specific needs.

Head Start's health component emphasizes the importance of the early identification of health problems. Every child is involved in a comprehensive health program, which includes immunizations, medical, dental, and mental health, and nutritional services. The majority of Head Start children are eligible for Medicaid, and coordination between the programs helps reduce duplication and identify children for such needed services as immunizations, well-child screenings, and referral for follow-up services.

Grants for Head State programs are awarded to local public or private nonprofit agencies. Twenty percent of the total cost of a Head

Start program must be contributed by the community. Head Start programs operate in all 50 states, the District of Columbia, Puerto Rico, and the U.S. territories. In FY 1997, almost $4 billion was available for enrolled children in more than 37,000 Head Start classrooms. About 13% of the enrollees were children with disabilities. Recent funding for Head Start is displayed in Table 6.1.

Early Intervention. Special Education Grants for Infants and Toddlers with Disabilities,[20] originally authorized in 1987 under Part H of the Individuals with Disabilities Education Act (IDEA), assist each state in developing a statewide, comprehensive, coordinated, multidisciplinary, interagency system to provide early intervention services for infants and toddlers with disabilities and their families. The program was revised most recently in 1997 under P.L. 105-17, which reauthorized it under a new Part C of IDEA.

At the federal level, Part C funds are administered by the Department of Education. In many states, Part C funds are administered by state Title V agencies that also administer programs for children with special health care needs.

Funds are awarded by formula to help states, territories, and tribal governments in planning, developing, and implementing statewide systems of early intervention services. Funding may also be used to provide direct services for infants and toddlers with disabilities and their families that are not otherwise provided by other public or private sources, to expand and improve on services for infants and toddlers with disabilities that are otherwise available, and to provide a free appropriate public education to children with disabilities. The funding history for the Early Intervention Program is displayed in Table 6.1.

Vaccines for Children Program. The federal Vaccines for Children (VFC) program[21] was created under the Omnibus Budget Reconciliation Act of 1993 (P.L. 103-66) to improve childhood immunization rates. As an entitlement program, it covers children under 18 who are Medicaid-eligible, uninsured, or Native American. It also provides free vaccines to children whose insurance plans do not pay for immunizations, if those children obtain them in federally qualified health centers or rural health centers. The federal government purchases vaccine from manufacturers at discounted prices for distribution to states. States have the option to purchase additional vaccine at the lower federal contract prices.

The VFC program is administered by Health Care Financing Administration. The Advisory Committee on Immunization Practices of the Centers for Disease Control and Prevention (CDC) is responsible for recommending what vaccines to include in the Childhood Immunization Schedule. The CDC is also responsible for determining which vaccines are provided through the VFC program. This joint responsibility streamlines implementation of immunization recommendations and inclusion of appropriate vaccines.

States must establish a distribution network, which includes both public clinics and private physicians who choose to participate. Involving private pediatricians in the VFC program is intended to increase the number of children who receive adequate immunizations and foster continuity of care. As of December 1996, 10,377 public provider sites and 31,468 private provider sites were enrolled in the VFC program, for a total of 41,845 sites.

Table 6.1 presents the funding history for the VFC program. The program became operational in all 50 states in 1996. By September 1996, only Indiana and New Jersey were not receiving vaccine delivery to enrolled public and private providers. Vaccines purchased under CDC contracts are substantially lower in price than those that are privately purchased at retail cost. State Medicaid programs have realized substantial savings from the VFC program. For example, California is reinvesting savings of about $20 million a year to improve childhood immunization rates. Prior to VFC, Medicaid providers in most states purchased vaccine at commercial prices and waited for reimbursement from Medicaid.

EMERGING SAFETY NET PROVIDER SCENARIOS

The sharp changes in the health care environment leave many state and local governments questioning whether, how, and in what way the public sector safety net providers should be involved in health care.

The three scenarios suggested by Andrulis for defining the public sector's role in health care appear to be evolving for MCH safety net providers. The distinguishing feature of the *fully vested public sector* is the full engagement of the public sector in the marketplace. Under this scenario, the public sector would gain sufficient financial and governmental support to compete with private sector managed care entities. The primary characteristic of the *residual public sector* is a reorientation to promote and depend on significantly greater private sector involvement in carrying out many traditional public sector responsibilities. Under this scenario, public health would play primarily a charity role in patient care and an oversight role in community health. The primary attribute of the *divested public sector* is the virtual takeover by the private sector of traditional public sector responsibilities, such as running public hospitals and absorbing community health centers, with public health agencies retaining population-based roles of monitoring and surveillance.

Safety net provider status remains fluid in many communities. Thus, these scenarios represent more of an evolution than an existing end point. All safety net providers, however, are struggling with the potential or real impact of managed care. The struggle varies depending on the stage of managed care development and penetration in their state and community, the type of organization and the services it provides, and the capability of its leadership and management. But all safety net providers, regardless of type, are faced with responding to this major upheaval in the health care system and the change in traditional ways of serving their populations. Some are still at the strategic planning point and others are well into implementation as they work to make often massive changes in their infrastructure and operations.

Federal, state, and local government agencies are playing critical roles throughout this transition of the public sector provider community. For example, state MCH and CSHCN programs have approached managed care in a variety of ways that reflect their broad mandate and the evolutionary nature of their role in the changing health care environment. A review of the role of state Title V programs in managed care, covering the activities of nearly 30 states, illustrates the breadth of these roles and partnerships.[22] Among them are providing outreach, enrollment, and education; ensuring quality services through contracting; ensuring appropriate provider networks and settings; planning services and care coordination; developing standards and guidelines; linking resources; monitoring and evaluation; providing training and technical assistance; and collecting and reporting data.

The sheer range of current roles being undertaken by Title V agencies in managed care goes far to address questions about whether traditional children's safety net programs still have a role to play in the managed care environment. Clearly, Title V is pursuing a number of critical and innovative functions regarding managed care. While in some states, such as Rhode Island and Arkansas, the Title V program is divesting its direct service delivery role to focus more on other core public health functions, in other states, such as Louisiana, Title V programs continue to be fully vested in providing direct services both within and outside of managed care settings.

Many state Title V programs are now functioning as part of the residual public sector, reflecting the wholesale reorientation of the existing health care system. The range of roles that state Title V programs are playing is a demonstration of the program's flexibility and evolving role in managed care. However, the continued effectiveness of the efforts of state Title V programs depends on partnerships with Medicaid agencies, employers, local health departments, managed care organizations, families, and others. The nature and needs of these partnerships as well as state politics, resources, and existing systems will affect how managed care is approached by each state.

BEYOND MANAGED CARE

None of the scenarios described in this chapter represents a "best case." In communities in which the private sector has a historical commitment to caring for the poor, a potentially effective relationship may very well include a streamlined public sector and a broader recognition of obligation among MCOs and other providers. In other circumstances, integration of the public and private sectors may achieve the most beneficial outcome. What seems clear, however, is that failure to assess the impact of public sector shifts or reductions could have serious adverse effects on vulnerable populations and essential community services. Even as alliances between such public health agencies as Title V and managed care plans occur, market forces unleashed by the managed care revolution could very well lead to fewer public resources being available for remaining uninsured MCH populations. This could leave such populations further alienated from the mainstream service system, with serious implications across a community.

Particularly now, as they move to implement the newly enacted SCHIP program, states must weigh the efficacy of the various public-private sector scenarios to meet their child health objectives. State and local governments should carefully determine the course they want their safety net providers to take in this era of instability and uncertainty. While this process is occurring, communities will benefit from information on emerging models and designs for assessing the most beneficial approach for their circumstances and other experiences. Charting the best course will require more than resources and regulatory oversight. Rather, it calls for a vision—one that reaches beyond managed care—to apply both public and private resources for defining, achieving, and sustaining community health in the broadest sense.

CONCLUSION

For more than half a century, federal and federal-state health programs have been at the forefront of the improvement and expansion of health services for mothers and children. These programs have become an integral part of the health care infrastructure, and they fund and provide many of the health services poor women and children receive.

The health care system is currently in flux, with both public and private health care sectors being fundamentally restructured. Within this context, Title V agencies across the country are already evolving and forming partnerships that are addressing managed care in a variety of innovative ways.

As a consequence of passage of SCHIP in 1997, state and local governments are being called on to make critical decisions that could affect allocation of resources considered vital to the health of mothers and children for years to come. Implementing vastly broadened children's coverage and ensuring children appropriate access to care will require unprecedented efforts on the part of providers and public-private sector community partnerships to ensure that the changes now taking place in federal and federal-state health programs continue to promote high quality. In the current environment, the federal leadership role for maternal and child health remains of critical importance.

References

1. 110 STAT.2105.
2. 110 STAT.1936.
3. 111 STAT.251.
4. Catalog of Federal Domestic Assistance (CFDA) 93.778 (Medicaid; Title XIX): 42 U.S.C. 1396 et. seq., as amended. Washington, DC: U.S. Government Printing Office, 1997.
5. 102 STAT.683.
6. Andrulis, D.P. The public sector in health care: evolution or dissolution? *Health Affairs.* July–August, 1997;131–139.
7. CFDA 93.994; 93.110 (Maternal and Child Health Block Grant; MCH Consolidated Federal Programs): 42 U.S.C. 701, et. scq., as amended.
8. 103 STAT.2470.
9. CFDA 93.926 (Healthy Start Initiative): 42 U.S.C. 241.
10. CFDA 96.006 (Supplemental Security Income): 42 U.S.C. 1381–1383d.
11. Sullivan v. Zebley, 493 US 521, 1991.
12. 62 FR 28 (February 11, 1997), 6407–6432.
13. P.L. 105-33, Section 4913.
14. CFDA 10.557 (WIC): 42 U.S.C. 1786.
15. CFDA 193.127 (EMSC): 42 U.S.C. 2426.
16. CFDA 93.153 (Ryan White CARE Act Title IV): 42 U.S.C. 300ff-71.
17. CFDA 93.224 (Primary Health Centers): 42 U.S.C. 254b; 254c.
18. CFDA 93.217 (Family Planning): 42 U.S.C. 300.
19. CFDA 93.600 (Head Start): 42 U.S.C. 980I et. seq.
20. CFDA 84.181 (Special Education for Disabled Infants and Families): 20 U.S.C. 1471–1488.
21. CFDA [n/a] (VFC): 42 U.S.C. 256c.
22. Association of Maternal and Child Health Programs. *Partnerships for healthier families: Roles for state Title V programs in assuring quality services for women, infants, children and youth in managed care.* Washington, DC: 1997.

7

Evaluation, Performance Monitoring, and Health Status Surveillance

Donna J. Petersen and Greg R. Alexander

This work was supported in part by DHHS, HRSA, MCHB grant MCJ-9040.

The ongoing emphasis on welfare, health care, and public health reform provides a crucial and timely opportunity to strengthen public health's capacity to monitor and evaluate the effects of various system-level reforms and initiatives on populations, families, and in particular children, including children with special health care needs. Although evaluation has long been seen as a critical element to program development and management, state maternal and child health programs are hindered by the lack of a framework for identifying and using data to assess the effects of their own efforts, much less those of greater system change occurring around them. It is essential that maternal and child health professionals enhance their understanding of evaluation principles and their application to program performance assessment and system-level monitoring if they are to continue to pursue success in ensuring the health of the nation's children and families.

EVALUATION

Evaluation is indispensable to the accomplishment of the core assessment and assurance functions of public health. Evaluation is a logical and important component of any type of public health activity, serving as the objective assessment of whether or not a particular service, intervention, program, or system succeeded in achieving its intent. Evaluation facilitates an understanding of whether a mission was achieved by comparing actual accomplishments of an intervention or program to the original expectations or a targeted desired state; evaluation also provides feedback for continuously improving operations and performance.[1]

The basic steps in evaluation are inextricably linked to program planning and include (1) articulating measurable objectives, (2) planning and implementing specific activities to achieve those objectives, and (3) collecting information to determine whether the planned activities were carried out and whether the pre-selected objectives were reached.[1] In public health, needs assessment is typically the initial step in establishing objectives and is a fundamental part of evaluation, taking the form of a comparison of current health status and health care utilization indicators against stated objectives or goals. The national Year 2000 health objectives provide for such comparisons and allow public health programs to assess discrepancies between current levels of health status and stated national goals and to plan activities to reduce discrepancies.[2]

Evaluations can be relatively simple or can involve sophisticated and complex designs. The issues involved in the design and conduct of evaluation research have been elegantly described in several outstanding texts and will not be addressed here.[1,3-5] However, it is important to note that in addition to clearly stated and measurable objectives, any good evaluation design also considers both the nature and scope of activities conducted as part of the intervention or program (i.e., process evaluation) and the results of those activities (i.e., outcome evaluation).[1] A good design will also assess the accuracy of the implementation of the program plan (i.e., implementation evaluation: did we do what we said we were going to do?). Finally, evaluation should be viewed as an ongoing process that provides feedback on the headway made toward attaining our long-term program objectives and goals (i.e., progress evaluation: are we on course and do we need midcourse corrections?).

PERFORMANCE MONITORING

The importance of evaluating specific interventions has been well understood in public health and other related fields. The recognition that evaluation at the level of broad-based programs is also important has been manifest most recently by the federal inclusion of required performance measures to improve accountability across states for their use of federal grant funds. Performance monitoring is rooted in the basic concepts of evaluation—assessing progress against stated objectives. Indeed, growing interest on the part of Congress in understanding the results of their legislative and allocation decisions resulted in the passage of the Government Performance and Reporting Act of 1995, which requires each federal agency to establish performance measures that can be reported as part of the budgetary process, thus linking funding decisions with performance. In response to this movement, several federal agencies have created Performance Partnership grants, blocking several categorical programs in exchange for states' agreeing to meet performance goals. In the latest revision of guidance material for state Maternal and Child Health (MCH) Block Grant applications, states are directed to list program priorities derived from required needs assessments and to describe their planned efforts to address their identified needs.[6] These plans must specify capacity, process, risk factor, and outcome indicators. States are further required both to develop a set of negotiated performance measures specific to their needs, data capacity, and priorities and to report on a set of outcome measures reflecting overall MCH goals.[7] Finally, states must report annual budgets according to expenditures by specific categories of activity. Together, reporting progress toward performance measures, reporting budgets according to service categories, and monitoring progress toward national health goals create three levels of accountability for state MCH programs. A 1997 report by The Institute of Medicine reinforces the importance of community performance monitoring in overall efforts to improve community health. This report further notes that "... although many performance monitoring activities are focused on specific health care organizations, only at the population level is it possible to examine the effectiveness of health promotion and disease prevention activities and to determine whether the needs of all segments of the community are being addressed."[8]

As in any evaluation effort, the selection of measurable objectives and the indicators of whether or not they have been achieved is a critical exercise that is further dependent on the availability of relevant and accurate data. This is also true for performance monitoring. Although specific criteria for selection of public health–related performance indicators have yet to be specified, some basic tenets can be proposed for selecting health status indicators as performance measures. Such measures should reflect health conditions for which (1) the etiology of the disease is fairly well understood; (2) there is a well-established prevention or intervention approach that is cost-effective, affordable and socially acceptable; and (3) improvement in the indicator can be reasonably anticipated within 3 to 5 years. Health status indicators that do not meet these basic criteria may still be important items for ongoing monitoring and surveillance efforts.

EVALUATION OF SYSTEMS

Although much attention has been placed on service, intervention, and program evaluation and performance monitoring, the evaluation of entire systems of care is an important and emerging area for public health in general and MCH in particular. There are limited examples of attempts to evaluate the impact of systems. Assessment of regional systems of perinatal care and their impact on birthweight-specific neonatal mortality rates is the most evident example of systems evaluation in the MCH area.[9] From community-based coalitions that use outreach and education to promote optimal use of health care services; to the health professionals that utilize the skills of collaboration, quality assurance, and professional education to continuously improve the level of health care; to reforms of publicly funded health care coverage enrolling clients into managed care arrangements that seek to promote greater access and quality at reduced costs, each of these system-level initiatives contributes to the infrastructure that supports population-based improvements in health outcome indicators. Documenting the elements of these system components that facilitate successful interventions and articulating the interrelationships among the component parts that support achievement of targeted outcome objectives are essential to systems evaluation. Not unexpectedly, the availability of timely, high-quality data is also critical for the success of system-level evaluation. A strong monitoring system not only helps assess the level to which desired outcomes were achieved and sustained, it also provides a systems-based data system, providing information on emerging needs, trends, declining needs, and targeted evaluations of specific interventions.

A major barrier to the evaluation of systems is the establishment of the characterization and measurement of the purpose, attributes, structure, provision, and interactions of the system. In addition to descriptives of the personnel, facilities, and range and availability of services, the following dimensions have been proposed as attributes of primary care systems for children: continuous, coordinated, comprehensive, community-oriented, family-centered, accessible, culturally competent, developmentally appropriate, and accountable.[10-13] As primary care systems for children exist within a larger system of health care that in turn operates within the public health system, attributes of the overall system, the level of development, the interrelationships, and the level of coordinated functioning are important added characteristics. Hence, systems evaluation also entails the development of a taxonomy for the characterization of the functioning of the entire health system and the other social systems that exist within a community and state. Platt has proposed the following dimensions for use as a framework for analyzing the functioning of systems: communication, decision-making, boundary-setting, conflict resolution, mutual support, resource distribution, and external relations.[14]

In all, the evaluation of the emergence, reformulation, and impact of systems represents a complex undertaking. Notwithstanding the inherent difficulties in systems evaluation, increasing efforts in this area are needed to help guide policy during this period of health care and welfare reform. The evaluation of the impact of a system can take the form of comparison against stated target objectives, a historical comparison of outputs of a system at two points in time, or comparison of the outputs of two different systems. Given that it is the overall system that is being assessed along various dimensions, it is important to determine whether or not the system collectively and its component parts individually are to be judged against the stated goals, against past performance, or against another system or system components. Several possibilities exist for designing a system evaluation.

Historical comparisons of health status and health care utilization indicators depend on the availability and quality of trend data. Pre–post contrasts require knowledge of the factors that may have led to changes in the selected process and outcome measurements, independent of changes in the particular system or system components under study. Because historical comparison studies are among the weakest evaluation designs and are subject to numerous biases that threaten the validity of results,[1] they may be among the least attractive approaches for evaluating systems.

Contemporary comparisons between operating systems represent another possible approach for systems evaluation, although this design may be difficult because of the growing statewide and multi-state operations of many health care organizations. Given that large and integrated systems will possess singularly unique characteristics, the opportunities to compare systems with similar characteristics and service populations may be increasingly limited. A design that monitors progress toward stated goals and objectives may be the most fruitful starting place for system evaluation. As such, *system monitoring* is best undertaken prospectively, given the weaknesses of historical designs.

Rossi and Freeman define monitoring as "a set of quality assurance activities directed at maximizing a program's conformity with its design."[3] Unlike program evaluation, which seeks to determine whether or not a particular intervention in fact achieved its intended goals, monitoring is broader and complements and supports program implementation. The function of monitoring is also entirely consistent with public health responsibilities, as it provides the means to continually assess needs and changes in those needs, the availability and accessibility of resources, the short- and long-term products of those resources, and the effects, positive or negative, on health outcomes of interest.

Monitoring is a data-driven effort, dependent on the timely availability of high-quality data that directly relate to and reflect the original hypotheses that led to system-level or programmatic interventions. Rossi and Freeman also note that ". . . a few items of data gathered consistently and reliably are generally much better for monitoring purposes than a more comprehensive set of information of doubtful reliability and inconsistent collection."[3]

As in any evaluation, monitoring requires the development of clearly articulated objectives, reasonable data collection strategies, and consistent and accurate data reporting. Monitoring within a systems context encompasses the basic notion of a system: a set of component parts that regularly communicate and interrelate toward a common purpose or shared goal. Articulating these goals and the objectives that flow from them; identifying and defining the component parts, explicating the communication pathways among the parts, and placing the overall system in its appropriate context all are necessary to ensure successful and useful monitoring.

As illustrated in the model described by Donabedian, the overall system, and to some degree each of the entities within it, consists of components that can be categorized into four domains: inputs, processes, outputs, and outcomes.[15] For purposes of developing and establishing a method for monitoring the system, the elements of each of these domains must be clearly explicated so that indicators and data measurement strategies can be devised for each activity. The general model has been described as follows.

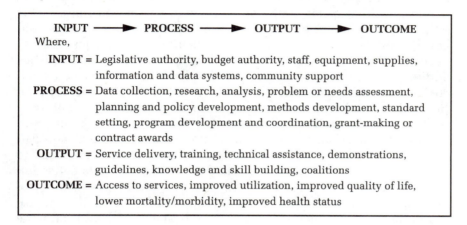

INPUT ──▶ PROCESS ──▶ OUTPUT ──▶ OUTCOME

Where,

INPUT = Legislative authority, budget authority, staff, equipment, supplies, information and data systems, community support

PROCESS = Data collection, research, analysis, problem or needs assessment, planning and policy development, methods development, standard setting, program development and coordination, grant-making or contract awards

OUTPUT = Service delivery, training, technical assistance, demonstrations, guidelines, knowledge and skill building, coalitions

OUTCOME = Access to services, improved utilization, improved quality of life, lower mortality/morbidity, improved health status

HEALTH STATUS SURVEILLANCE

Monitoring and surveillance are fundamental functions of public health and have become well-established tools to support health promotion, disease prevention, and epidemiologic research efforts, in addition to being important to program planning, implementation, evaluation, and advocacy. These activities provide the means to ensure that health status is maintained or improved within populations and communities; that emerging health problems are identified early; that necessary health and related services are available, accessible, and of high quality; and that expenditures are justified by documented results in the form of process, output, and outcome objectives achieved.[16] The basic elements of monitoring and surveillance include the *ongoing* and *systematic:* (1) collection of data; (2) evaluation, consolidation, analysis, and interpretation of data; and (3) prompt dissemination of the synthesized results to the public, relevant stakeholders, and decision/policymakers.[16,17]

It has been pointed out that the critical element to surveillance is the establishment of an ongoing effort with established data systems and data analysis and dissemination procedures. These elements and the emphasis on timely and regular data dissemination distinguish this monitoring activity from one-time epidemiologic surveys and other sporadic research studies that may be more directed at hypothesis testing or the detailed investigation of disease etiology.

Although public health surveillance has traditionally been used in efforts to control infectious disease, there has been growing appreciation of its use for the broad domains of public health: describing and measuring shifts in population demographic structures and dynamics, health systems, and a broad array of health outcomes.[17] This larger view of public health surveillance encompasses an expanded conceptualization of public health as extending beyond just disease occurrence and risk exposure to include population characteristics and the "services, resources and policies that constitute the organized social response to health conditions."[17] A broad-based model for public health monitoring and surveillance should describe not only health status and individual and family predictors of health outcomes but also characteristics of the health system, broadly defined, and patterns of health care utilization. In some instances, databases exist to provide insights into these areas; in others, traditional data collection methods are needed (e.g., surveys); while in still others, qualitative and empirical methods should also be explored for their utility in providing critical information on the overall status of health and the health system.

Ironically, public health has an immensely rich supply of vital record and other population-based data on births, deaths, immunizations, newborn screening, and communicable diseases, amidst a persistent dearth of information on many other important aspects of family life and child development. Despite decades of efforts to develop stronger, more comprehensive data systems, we continue to mainly rely on existing databases, patching together weak assemblages of program management data created for the administration of public health service programs. Obviously, the time and expense involved in developing and implementing reliable and valid survey instruments are the limiting factors for states embarking on systematic and ongoing surveillance efforts. Few, if any, states are fortunate in having available population-wide surveillance systems that provide the breadth of data needed to fully assess health status within the state. This continues in spite of numerous efforts to focus attention on this blind spot in our nation's focus on health. In regard to child health surveillance, Dr. Mary Grace Kovar made the following, still relevant, observation in the mid-1980s: "A great deal of data has been gathered, but there has not been a research plan or a coordinated plan to direct what was being collected and why. As a result, there are gaps and missing pieces; data have not been tabulated to investigate a set of hypotheses; information is not presented in a unified body of knowledge so that the public, the legislature, and the administrative bodies can use it."[18]

CASE EXAMPLES

In Arizona and Minnesota, efforts are under way to develop state-wide surveillance systems to monitor the health status of children. In 1995, the Arizona MCH agency assembled a group of leaders, experts, and stakeholders in an effort to identify a set of measurable indicators of child health. A model of child health surveillance was developed (Fig. 7.1) that articulated four domains: child health status, health care uti-

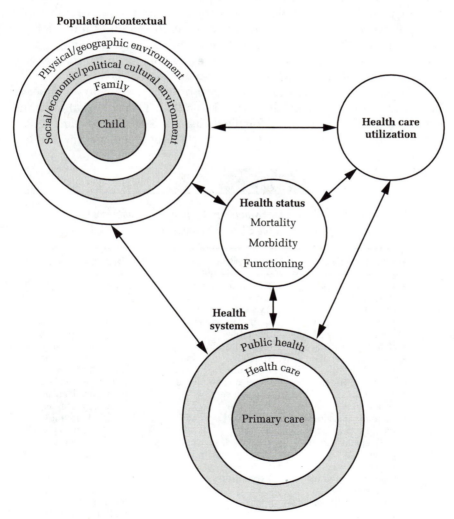

FIGURE 7.1

Child health surveillance system model.

lization, the health care system, and population/contextual factors.[19] Using this model, they considered a variety of potential indicators that could be drawn from available databases.

In 1996, following several years of state- and market-driven health care reforms and facing welfare reform, the Minnesota Department of Health embarked on a process to strengthen its capacity in the surveillance and monitoring of the health of children. The envisioned monitoring system was intended to be dynamic and modified over time as population characteristics, system elements, and priorities change. State health leaders recognized that a real-time monitoring system would be essential to the success of efforts to provide input into policy decisions potentially affecting children and their families. Given the varying levels of timeliness and quality within the data available, this problem was not easily resolvable, but it is one that will remain a top priority in the years to come.

Using the Arizona model, a group of experts developed a set of indicators within the four domains (Table 7.1). The potential uses and interpretations of these data for needs assessment and systems development include, but are not limited to, (1) documenting various fac-

---

TABLE 7.1

Proposed Child Health Indicators for Evaluation, Performance Monitoring, and Surveillance in the State of Minnesota

Health Status	Health Utilization	Health Systems	Population/Contextual
• Mortality rates • Incidence of communicable diseases • Mental health • Youth risk behavior • Adolescent pregnancy • Low birthweight • Confirmed cases of child abuse and neglect • Incidence of injuries • Nutritional deficiency	• Immunizations • Barriers to utilization • Emergency room visits • School screening • Well-child visits • EPSDT • School clinic use • Mental health service use • Specialty services used by children with special health care needs • Community resources used by children with special health care needs	• Health insurance coverage • Type and number of pediatric providers available • Type and number of specialty providers available • Type and number of support services available • Perceived availability of care • Denials of service • Uncompensated care • Out-of-pocket expenditures	• Children in poverty • Children in special education • School drop-out rate • Adolescent arrest rate • Community violence • Pre-1970 housing units • Housing costs as percentage of income • Urgent care facilities • Public libraries, books • Law enforcement level • Adult continuing education programs • Youth vocational education • Open/green spaces • Bike and walking paths • Voting in elections • Alcohol outlets • Food shelf use

EPSDT, early periodic screening, diagnosis, and treatment.

tors related to the child, the family, the community, and the environment that individually or collectively impact health status, regardless of health care utilization or system factors; (2) documenting various health care system factors that affect utilization; (3) documenting various utilization measures that affect health status and that also have an impact on the health system itself; (4) monitoring trends in indicators of interest over time and across geographic areas; (5) providing preliminary evidence regarding the potential impact of various program interventions operating currently or in the future; (6) advocating for needed policy initiatives as indicated and supported by these data; (7) advocating for program initiatives across various sectors, both public and private; and (8) supporting the public health role in fostering accountability across the health system for health outcomes and health service availability and quality.

CONCLUSION

Given the growing emphasis on needs assessment and health status monitoring as essential components of public health practice and on performance measurement as a way to ensure system- and unit-level accountability, it is critical that public health professionals become well-versed in the design and implementation of health status and performance monitoring and surveillance systems. While evaluation has long been considered an essential component of good program planning and should be built into any program development and implementation effort, the profuse systemic changes currently occurring in welfare, public health, and health care systems suggest an equally critical need for broad-based performance and health status monitoring and surveillance strategies. These efforts are needed to support the continuation within the evolving larger U.S. health system of a population-based health approach and to enhance the ability of public health programs to be accountable for their overall performance. Indeed, a strengthened capacity in the area of public health performance and health status monitoring and surveillance, as well as further emphasis on program and system evaluation, is fundamental to ensure the vitality of the health care system and the optimal health status of populations.

References

1. Isaac, S., and Michael, W.B. *Handbook in research and evaluation.* San Diego, CA: EdITS, 1990.
2. Public Health Service. *Healthy people 2000: National health promotion and disease prevention objectives.* DHHS Publication No. (PHS) 91-50212. Washington, DC: U.S. Government Printing Office, 1991.

3. Rossi, P.H., and Freeman, H.E. *Evaluation: A systematic approach.* Newbury Park, Sage Publications, 1993.

4. Shadish, W.R., Cook, T.D., and Leviton, L.C. *Foundations of program evaluation.* Newbury Park, Sage Publications, 1991.

5. Weiss, C.H. Evaluation research. Englewood Cliffs, NJ: Prentice Hall, 1972.

6. *Maternal and Child Health Services Block Grant application guidance.* Rockville, MD: Maternal and Child Health Bureau, Health Resources and Services Administration, US DHHS, August, 1997.

7. *Systems indicators: Development of definitions and state performance measures* [draft]. Rockville, MD: Maternal and Child Health Bureau, HRSA, US PHS, DHHS, 1995.

8. Institute of Medicine. *Improving health in the community: A role for performance monitoring.* Washington, DC: National Academy Press, 1997.

9. Hulsey, T.C., Heins, H.C., Marshall, T.A., Martin, M.L., McGee, T.W., et al. Regionalized perinatal care in South Carolina. *Journal of the South Carolina Medical Association.* 1989;85(8):357–384.

10. Grason, H., Wigton, A. *Review of the literature and measurement strategies related to key principles in the development of systems of care for children and youth.* Baltimore, MD: Child and Adolescent Health Policy Center, The Johns Hopkins University, 1995.

11. *Primary health care for children and adolescents: Definitions and attributes.* Rockville, MD: Maternal and Child Health Bureau, HRSA, US PHS, DHHS, 1994.

12. Starfield, B. *Primary care: Concept, evaluation and policy.* New York, Oxford University Press, 1992.

13. Johansen, A.S., Starfield, B., and Harlow, J. *Analysis of the concept of primary care for children and adolescents: A policy research brief.* Baltimore, MD: Child and Adolescent Health Policy Center, The Johns Hopkins University, 1994.

14. Platt, L.J., and Hill, I. *Measuring systems development in Wyoming: Instruments to assess communities' progress.* Washington, DC: Health Systems Research, June, 1995.

15. Donabedian, A. Explorations in quality assessment and monitoring. In *The definition of quality and approaches to its assessment,* Vol. 1. Ann Arbor, MI: Health Administration Press, 1980.

16. Thacker, S.B., and Berkelman, R.L. Public health surveillance in the United States. *Epidemiologic Reviews* 1988;10:164–190.

17. Sepúlveda, J., López-Cervantes, M., Frenk, J., de León, J.G., Lezana-Fernández, M.A., and Santo-Burgoa, C. Keynote address: Key issues in public health surveillance for the 1990s. Proceedings of the 1992 Symposium on Public Health Surveillance. *MMWR* 1992;41(Suppl):61–76.

18. Walker, D.K., and Richmond, J.B. (eds). *Monitoring child health in the United States: Selected issues and policies.* Cambridge, MA: Harvard University Press, 1984.

19. Alexander, G.R. *A population-based maternal and child health status surveillance system for the State of Arizona.* Technical report prepared for Health Systems Research, Inc. and the Community and Family Health Section of the Arizona Department of Health Services, January, 1996. (Available on HRS WWW site.)

II

Social Welfare

8

Children and Welfare Reform: What Are the Effects of this Landmark Policy Change?

Julie Hudman and Barbara Starfield

The Personal Responsibility and Work Opportunity Reconciliation Act of 1996 is a compre-
hensive bipartisan welfare reform plan that will dramatically change the nation's welfare sys-
tem into one that requires work in exchange for time-limited assistance. The law contains
strong work requirements, a performance bonus to reward states for moving welfare recipients
into jobs, state maintenance of effort requirements, comprehensive child support enforcement,
and supports for families moving from welfare to work—including funding for child care and
guaranteed medical coverage. President Clinton (Press Release, August 22, 1996)

On August 22, 1996, President Clinton signed into law a welfare
reform bill that he claimed would provide support and guarantee medical coverage for families moving from welfare to work. Closer analysis
of this landmark legislation suggests an alternative outcome, as well as
concern regarding the well-being of children. The Personal Responsibility and Work Opportunity Reconciliation Act of 1996 (P.L. 104-193)
eliminated the Aid to Families with Dependent Children program
(AFDC),* a cash entitlement to individuals with open-ended funding
provided by states with matching funds from the federal government.[1]
In its place, the Act created the Temporary Assistance to Needy Families (TANF), a block grant program that provides a capped amount of
funding to each state, regardless of increases in unemployment or
number of applications for welfare.

Although Medicaid, the joint federal-state medical assistance
program, was left as an entitlement to those individuals categorically
eligible by virtue of their low-income, Congress and the President enacted changes to the health care safety net in the context of welfare reform. The most direct effect of the Act on children's health care is
through changes in eligibility for these safety net programs. For example, the law alters how eligibility is determined for Supplemental Security Income (SSI)† for both children and immigrants and significantly cuts funding for food stamps and other nutrition programs
serving children and their families.

Other less known provisions of the welfare law that are discussed
in this chapter may also have significant effects on access to Medicaid
services. Perhaps the most important of these changes is the delinking
of welfare and Medicaid. Although the link was previously weakened
in the 1980s with the expansions of Medicaid-eligible groups, welfare

---

*Aid to Families with Dependent Children (AFDC) was established by the original So-
cial Security Act in 1935 as a cash grant program to enable states to aid needy children
without fathers. States define the need by setting their benefit levels, establishing
(within federal guidelines) income and resource limits, and administering the program.
†Supplemental Security Income (SSI), authorized by Title XVI to the Social Security
Act, is a means-tested, federally administered income assistance program. The program,
established in 1972, provides monthly cash payments to the needy aged, blind and disabled populations using uniform nationwide eligibility standards.[1]

reform fully severed the two programs. This change may remove the "welfare stigma" from Medicaid, but it also could have a significant negative impact on access to Medicaid for vulnerable children and families. Other indirect effects include positive or negative health outcomes that may result from the repeal of this federal entitlement of cash benefits for 5 million very poor families, which include 9.8 million children.[2] Research indicates strong correlations between poverty and poor health outcomes for children.[3-6]; withdrawal of cash benefits is likely to increase poverty. Other research indicates that maternal employment can have a positive effect on children's health in situations where mothers previously on welfare moved to employment, but only if they earn at least $5.00 an hour.[7]* It is not at all clear that employment obtained will guarantee this income.

This chapter first discusses why children are a vulnerable population and how various government programs, such as welfare and Medicaid, are important to children's health. This is followed by a discussion of the new welfare reform law, how it affects Medicaid, and the direct and indirect effects of the law on children's access to health programs. Finally, future concerns and current research projects regarding welfare reform's effects on children are described.

WHY BE CONCERNED WITH CHILDREN'S HEALTH?

Concerns about the health effects of welfare reform on children stem primarily from three associations: (1) the link between children and poverty, (2) the link between poverty and poor health outcomes, and (3) the uncoupling of welfare and eligibility for Medicaid. Poor mothers and infants are often identified as a "vulnerable population,"[8] probably because, of all age cohorts, children younger than the age of 6 and their families are at the greatest risk of being poor. In 1994, 20.2% of all children were living in poverty.[9] The strongest predictor of poverty is the breakup of families or single women having children; other contributing factors include inadequate child support, low or non-existent welfare payments, and low earnings of single mothers.[10]

There are several reasons why poor families are at a greater risk of poor health outcomes relative to other families. They use less or lower quality services critical to personal development and well-being, such as food, shelter, medical care, and education, usually be-

---

*One caveat of this research is that these mothers voluntarily moved from welfare to work. Results from this research might not apply to mothers involuntarily working and also might be confounded by the job skills or family situations of women who voluntarily left the welfare rolls.

cause they have less money to invest in them.[11] Poor children are specifically at risk of poor health outcomes because they live with parents who are under relatively high levels of stress and depression, which can lead to fewer emotional resources available to nurture their children.[11] Furthermore, poor families tend to live in neighborhoods with relatively less social capital with fewer resources, jobs, and connections to mainstream economic activity. Regardless of the cause, the research is clear that poverty is related to poor health outcomes.[10,12–14]

One of the most established connections of negative health outcomes and poverty status is low birthweight.* In the United States, poor women have been shown to be at a higher risk of preterm delivery and low-birthweight infants even when controlling for other risk factors such as substance abuse and source of prenatal care.[11,15] Children born at a low weight and living in high-risk environments are at an increased risk for poor health outcomes compared with normal birthweight children in similar environments. These effects are long lasting and can be measured by excessive bed days, restricted-activity days, and school-loss days; school failure; low school ranking; behavior problems; and maternal perception of child health status as fair or poor.[16]

Researchers agree that class or poverty-related differences in health outcomes exist, but controversy remains regarding the mechanisms of these effects.[10,13] The child's social environment is strongly related with health status throughout the early years of life.[17] Children in poverty are at a higher risk for poor health outcomes than other populations living in poverty, and various government programs are intended to alleviate some of the problems associated with this adversity.[3,18]

For all of the reasons noted, welfare reform is likely to directly and indirectly influence children's health. To date, only a few studies have analyzed the specific impacts on children's health resulting from public policy changes in health services,[19] and specific state welfare reform efforts have not yet been properly studied.[20†] To the extent that welfare reform increases poverty among children with or without re-

---

*Other negative health outcomes associated with persons of lower socioeconomic status are higher rates of mortality, cardiovascular diseases, infant and maternal mortality, unintended injury, homicide, and suicide and prevalence of other diseases such as arthritis, heart disease, ulcers, diabetes, hypertension, and chronic bronchitis.[11]

†However, since the enactment of the Personal Responsibility and Work Opportunity Reconciliation Act of 1996, there has been significant interest in the area of welfare reform's effects on children. Projects such as the Urban Institute's New Federalism Study and the U.S. Department of Health and Human Services' Project on State-Level Child Outcomes are just two of the many research studies under way to monitor the effects of welfare policy changes on children's well-being.

ducing access to medical assistance, we can expect the effects to be disproportionately negative.

PROGRAMS IMPORTANT TO CHILDREN'S HEALTH

Recognizing the vulnerable position of children, the federal government has developed several programs to reduce the economic burden of poverty and to supplement services available to families in poverty. For example, the Aid to Families with Dependent Children (AFDC) and Supplemental Security Income (SSI) programs were intended to alleviate financial stressors associated with poverty and disability. Established by the Social Security Act in 1935, AFDC was a means-tested (based on need) cash grant program that enabled states to aid needy children. As a means-tested program, SSI provided monthly cash payments to the needy aged, blind, and disabled. Other programs, such as the Food Stamp program, directly improve the nutritional status of children and families. Programs such as Medicaid and the Supplemental Food Program for Women, Infants and Children (WIC) aim to improve health outcomes. These programs or portions of them also facilitate receipt of prenatal care services, which have been shown to improve birth outcomes.[21]

Each of these programs, along with others, are critical to providing children a healthy start on life and protection from some of the negative health outcomes associated with poverty. Although each of these programs is vital, the discussion here focuses on the main program that affords children access to health care—Medicaid. Health insurance coverage alone, including Medicaid, does not reduce socioeconomic differences in health;[22] however, researchers have shown that public and private insurance does affect one's ability to access health care services, including preventive services.[23,24] The U.S. General Accounting Office[25] conducted a literature review and found that children's access to, and use of, health care was greatly increased by the presence of health insurance. Reported access to care and lack of barriers to care have been shown to decrease the likelihood of preventable hospitalizations.[26]

Medicaid

Created through an amendment to the Social Security Act (Title XIX), Medicaid is a health program for categorically eligible groups and is rooted in the welfare system.[27] Before welfare reform, participants in federal cash assistance programs such as AFDC or SSI were almost always automatically eligible for Medicaid.* For example, when a family applied for welfare and other cash assistance, it was automatically considered also for Medicaid, and if enrolled, received health benefits.

Because welfare-eligible families rarely have health insurance, Medicaid is an important facilitator of receipt of health services for children. The net result of Medicaid expansions significantly expanded the proportion of children with health insurance beyond those eligible for welfare. Prior to 1984, Medicaid coverage for the most part was tied to receipt of cash assistance—either through AFDC or SSI.[29] Between 1984 and 1990, several major legislative changes were made to Medicaid to "delink" the AFDC program, with the intent of expanding eligibility for Medicaid through the budget reconciliation process. These changes included provisions that required states to provide Medicaid to pregnant women and children up to age 6 whose family income was below 133% of the poverty level, permitted states to extend coverage to pregnant women and infants with income to 185% of the poverty level, and phased in coverage for children in families with income under 100% of the poverty level. In addition, eligibility for mothers was expanded to 60 days post partum to permit women to obtain family planning services as well as other services following delivery.[21] Other changes affecting pregnant women included allowing a more liberal eligibility standard by permitting states to disregard some of the recipient's income and assets; allowing states and providers to assume eligibility (presumptive eligibility) immediately for pregnant women; and adding reimbursable services such as health education and case management to the Medicaid benefit package.[21] The aim of these policy changes has been to loosen the link between welfare receipt and Medicaid eligibility so that women and children's access to health care services could be expanded.[30] Previously, states wanting to increase eligibility limits for Medicaid had to similarly increase their eligibility for AFDC, thus making the Medicaid expansion nearly impossible politically.

Nearly one quarter of all children younger than age 18 (17.1 million) had Medicaid coverage in 1995, although only about 52% were on welfare. Approximately two thirds of all children whose family income was below the poverty level were covered by Medicaid in 1995.[31] Changes in the federal law providing continued annual phase-in of Medicaid coverage by age will bring Medicaid eligibility to all children (to age 19) in poverty born after September 1983. By 1995, Medicaid was the health insurance source for 27% of children with family incomes between 100% and 199% of the poverty level.[31] (The

---

*Certain states (called 209b states) do not base Medicaid on SSI eligibility, but instead use a more restrictive eligibility criteria. The current 209b states are Connecticut, Hawaii, Illinois, Indiana, Minnesota, Missouri, New Hampshire, North Dakota, Ohio, Oklahoma, and Virginia.[28]

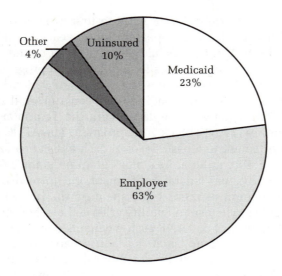

FIGURE 8.1

Health insurance coverage of children, by source of coverage, 1995.

1997 poverty guidelines of the U.S. Department of Health and Human Services [HHS] for a family of three at poverty is $13,330.)

Despite the increase in Medicaid coverage over time, the total share of children with health insurance coverage has stayed relatively constant over the past several years owing primarily to a decline in employer-provided health insurance (Fig. 8.1). As of 1997, 10 million children lacked any health care coverage.[32] In addition, individuals eligible for programs do not always enroll and, thus, do not have access to health care services to which they are otherwise entitled. The Urban Institute estimated that 2 million uninsured children were eligible for Medicaid coverage in 1994.[33] The new State Children's Health Insurance Program (CHIP), enacted as part of the Balanced Budget Act of 1997, targets this group of uninsured children. The Congressional Budget Office (CBO) estimates that CHIP will cover 2.8 million previously uninsured children, and another 660,000 children eligible for Medicaid will be enrolled in that program because of outreach and screening efforts associated with CHIP.[34]

The Personal Responsibility And Work Opportunity Reconciliation Act of 1996

The Personal Responsibility and Work Opportunity Reconciliation Act was signed into law by President Clinton on August 22, 1996, following nearly 4 years of debate after Clinton first promised to "end welfare as we know it." The Act repealed the 61-year-old AFDC program created by Title IV-A of the Social Security Act. It contains broad provisions and changes to numerous federal laws and programs. The CBO estimated that the Act would generate savings of $2.9 billion in fiscal year 1997 and $54.2 billion in savings between 1997 and 2002.

The AFDC program was replaced with the Temporary Assistance for Needy Families (TANF) block grant program. The AFDC program had created an entitlement to a basic level of cash assistance for any family meeting the eligibility criteria. As a block grant program, TANF does not operate as an individual federal entitlement, but instead provides each state with the amount of funds to be spent on the poor. Under TANF, states can establish whatever eligibility criteria they choose; for instance, a state can make receipt of TANF cash payments contingent on the nonreceipt of other forms of aid, such as Medicaid and child support.[35] Recipients may not receive benefits for more than a total of 5 years and must go to work after 2 years on assistance, with few exceptions.[36] Because cash assistance is no longer an entitlement, states are not required to provide cash assistance coverage for all categorically eligible individuals. Each state may determine its own eligibility criteria and cap the number of recipients. Furthermore, the state may choose to use the block grant funds in other ways, such as expanded child care or job training.[36]

IMPACT OF WELFARE REFORM ON ELIGIBILITY FOR CHILDREN'S HEALTH PROGRAMS

Although welfare reform appears at first to make relatively few changes that could directly have an impact on children's access to health programs, the implementation of the law is likely to do so. Changes to the AFDC and SSI programs and their relationship to Medicaid will significantly affect access to health care services for children. Furthermore, changes in benefits for immigrant and nutrition programs may have a negative impact on children. Other changes to programs, such as child support, may counterbalance some of these negative effects, but the extent to which this is the case is unclear.

Welfare Reform and Medicaid Coverage

The Act attempts to maintain the health care safety net for low-income children and their families by maintaining Medicaid. States are still required to provide Medicaid coverage for 1 year for families that become ineligible for cash welfare assistance as a result of increased employment-related earnings.[36]* The Act also requires that families be provided Medicaid coverage for 4 months if they become ineligible because of increased earnings from child support. However, families that leave welfare because of sanctions for non-compliance are not eligible for transitional Medicaid. The Act explicitly states that "families that would have been eligible for AFDC because of their low-income as of July 16, 1996 must be provided Medicaid" as long as their income remains at this low level. However, the law allows states to lower this "frozen" income standard as part of welfare reform to the state's previous income standards on May 1, 1988.[36] Although the Act should not alter the Medicaid eligibility standards for most pregnant women and children, 1.3 million children aged 13 and older and more than 4 million parents currently receiving Medicaid because of categorical eligibility could be at risk for losing their coverage by not abiding by new welfare work or administrative requirements.[37] Other persons at risk of losing benefits include both unmarried minors who live outside an adult-supervised home and individuals† who fail to stay in school or do not attend other equivalent training programs.[35] Furthermore, families that leave welfare for work are likely to be in low-income jobs that provide an income above Medicaid eligibility levels yet do not offer health insurance. One study found that 17% of children are uninsured 1 year after their family left welfare; this amount rose to 27% uninsured after 2 years and then dropped to 12% after 3 years.[38] The same study found that Medicaid covered 59% of the children in the first year after welfare, then dropped to 38% in the second year and covered about 33% of children 3 years after leaving welfare.[38] Welfare reform, with the stigma and political rhetoric surrounding the issue, might have the effect of deterring potential eligible families from accessing other safety net programs, including Medicaid.

The Act will affect many different populations; Table 8.1 summarizes the Medicaid qualifications for women and children before welfare reform and how these have changed after welfare reform.

Supplemental Security Income (SSI)

The Act also reduces SSI assistance to disabled children through more stringent eligibility standards. The Act replaces the Individualized Functional Assessment (IFA) test for determining disability

---

*The Act stipulates that states must provide 6 months full Medicaid benefits and 6 months subsidized Medicaid benefits for families that leave welfare for work.
†Once the adolescent either graduates from school or refuses to attend school or equivalent training, he or she is subject to the state's work requirements and time limits to continue to receive TANF cash grants.

TABLE 8.1

Women and Children's Medicaid Eligibility Before and After Welfare Reform

Persons at Risk for Loss of Cash Assistance (AFDC/TANF or SSI)	Medicaid Eligibility Criteria Before Welfare Reform	Estimated Number that May Lose Coverage	New Medicaid Eligibility Criteria After Welfare Reform
Women	*Mandatory* for cash recipients (AFDC/SSI) *Mandatory* for pregnant women with family income to 133% of poverty level *Optional* eligibility for pregnant women with family income to 185% of poverty (34 states) *Optional* medically needy* eligibility (34 states)	4.5 million	*Mandatory* eligibility under 7-16-96 AFDC eligibility criteria or SSI recipients *Mandatory* eligibility for pregnant women with family income to 133% of poverty level *Optional* eligibility for pregnant women with family income to 185% of poverty level (34 states) *Optional* medically needy eligibility (34 states) *Optional* medically needy coverage for women who are qualified aliens *Mandatory restriction* of benefits for 5 years to any immigrants entering the country after 7-16-96
Children	*Mandatory* eligibility to age 6 with family income to 133% of poverty level *Mandatory* eligibility from age 6 to 13 with family income below 100% of poverty level *Mandatory* eligibility for age 14 to 19 if eligible for AFDC (state income levels average 41% of poverty level) *Mandatory* eligibility for children with family income under 100% of poverty level is being phased in annually. By 2002, all poor children younger than 19 years will be eligible for Medicaid. *Mandatory* eligibility for children who receive SSI *Optional* medically needy eligibility (34 states)	1.3 million	*Mandatory* eligibility under 7-16-96 AFDC eligibility criteria *Mandatory* eligibility from age 6 to 13 with family income below 100% of poverty level *Mandatory* eligibility for age 14 to 19 if eligible for AFDC (state income levels average 41% of poverty level) *Mandatory* eligibility for children with family income under 100% of poverty level is being phased in annually. By 2002, all poor children younger than 19 years will be eligible for Medicaid. *Mandatory* eligibility under SSI using new disability test *Optional* medically needy eligibility (34 states)

*This group is eligible for Medicaid coverage at a state option, targeted at individuals who incur high medical bills, yet have too high an income for cash assistance programs. Certain groups are automatically medically needy groups if the state exercises this optional program, such as pregnant women and children who would have been eligible except for excess income or resources.[35]

Data from references 29, 35, and 37.

Thomas Rock of Alabama, Teddy Stone of Vermont, and Judy Hall of Connecticut are all 15 years old. They all apply for SSI benefits after welfare reform with the new, stricter standards. Alhough they all would have received SSI, and thus Medicaid, under the old Individualized Functional Assessment method, none is determined eligible for SSI after welfare reform. But are they still eligible for Medicaid? It depends on the state.

- Thomas Rock does not qualify for Medicaid benefits because he was born before 1983 and the family income is above the Alabama 1996 AFDC level, although below the poverty line.

- Teddy Stone does qualify for Medicaid benefits even though his family income is above the Vermont 1996 AFDC level. Vermont has elected to cover all children younger than 18 to 225% of the poverty level using the methodology allowed under Section 1902 (r)(2) of Title XIX.

- Judy Hall's family income (for Judy, her mom and her sister) is approximately 50% of the poverty level. Connecticut chose to "freeze" its AFDC income level at 54% of the poverty level; therefore, Judy will qualify for Medicaid under the state's 1996 AFDC standards.

Adapted from the National Governors' Association: *Welfare reform joint briefing.* 1997.

FIGURE 8.2

Case Example: Impact of New SSI Eligibility on Medicaid Coverage for Children in Different States.

among children with a test that requires children to meet certain specified impairments in order to qualify for aid.[35] An estimated 135,000 children would have lost SSI benefits and automatic Medicaid eligibility by the year 2002 because of these changes in determining disability.[39] The Balanced Budget Act of 1997 (BBA) reinstated Medicaid eligibility, but not SSI eligibility, for children who were receiving SSI at the time of welfare reform's enactment as long as these children continued to meet previous disability and financial criteria. However, the BBA does not protect future children that would have received SSI under the old eligibility determination. According to the CBO, some children who do not qualify for SSI under the stricter eligibility standards will probably continue to qualify for Medicaid as poverty-level children because of their families' low income or their high medical bills (Fig. 8.2).

Nutrition Programs For Children

Welfare reform significantly cut the Food Stamp program. Through various program reductions, the Act reduced Food Stamp program outlays by $23.1 billion between 1997 and 2002.[35] Food stamp benefits are projected to drop 20% by the year 2002, with average benefits falling from about 80 cents to 66 cents per person per meal.[40] Families with children will absorb close to two thirds of the food stamp cuts, with families below half of the poverty line ($6,250 for a family of three in 1996) absorbing half of the cuts. The welfare reform law also reduced federal funding for school breakfast and lunch programs, as well as making significant reductions in funding for child and adult care food programs, including aggregate limits on the number of meals that can be reimbursed in a given day in child care centers. Start-up funding for school breakfast and summer food service programs has been eliminated.[35] Willis and associates[41] argue that welfare reform could create a higher demand for various food programs. Currently, there are more eligible individuals for these programs than can be served at present-level funding without this added pressure from the newly eligible population.

Child Support and Child Care

Several new provisions of the Act may benefit children and low-income families, such as new child support laws and child care funds. State child support enforcement systems have been expanded,[36] and the law also increased for 1 year the level of federal financial contributions to the cost of administering state child welfare programs. The Act created a new child care block grant, replacing the entitlement to AFDC Work-Related Child Care, Transitional Child Care, and At-Risk Child Care. Total funding is nearly 50% greater than under the combined programs without the reforms.[36] In general, assistance to foster care children was not changed.

Immigrants

The Act made significant cuts in benefits to both legal and illegal immigrants that could have effects on children's health. Benefit restrictions for immigrants reach beyond what is traditionally thought of as welfare programs, and affect access to health care, housing, and nutritional assistance. Although immigrants use benefits at a rate comparable to most U.S. citizens (about 5%), cuts to immigrants account for 44% of the projected savings in the new welfare law.[42] Some analysts predict that children will be harmed more by the immigrant-related cuts from the welfare reform law than by any other provision of the law.[42] Other effects include a possible trend of immigrants not applying for any government benefits, even if their children are legal citizens, because they fear this would jeopardize their own immigration status.

The Act retained existing rules regarding Medicaid treatment of undocumented persons and non-legal immigrants. They remain ineligible for most forms of means-tested public assistance but are still entitled by law to coverage for emergency care paid for by Medicaid.[33] Prior to the passage of welfare reform, most persons who were legal immigrants and all permanent U.S. residents were entitled to full Medicaid coverage if they were categorically eligible by receiving benefits from SSI or AFDC. The welfare reform law terminated SSI for legal residents, which also terminated their Medicaid coverage. The BBA restored SSI and Medicaid benefits to all elderly and disabled (including children) qualified aliens who received SSI and Medicaid as of August 22, 1996. Furthermore, the BBA permits legal residents in the United States as of August 22, 1996, to receive SSI, and thus Medicaid, if they subsequently become disabled and qualify for coverage under the new definition of disability.

For the purposes of determining the rights of legal residents, the Act identifies a new category, *qualified aliens*, which includes persons lawfully admitted for permanent residence, persons granted asylum, deportees, refugees, persons paroled into the United States for at least 1 year, persons whose deportation has been withheld, and persons granted conditional entry.[35] Qualified aliens in the United States before August 22, 1996, are eligible for Medicaid coverage at state option. As of Spring of 1997, seven states had not extended Medicaid coverage to the legal residents who lost coverage because of welfare reform.[43] The exceptions to this provision include legal immigrants who are working more than 40 quarters, veterans, refugees, and others who were granted conditional entry into the United States and persons for whom deportation has been delayed. These legal immigrants are still entitled to full Medicaid benefits.[43]

After August 22, 1996, except for emergency care services, no federal funds classified as federal means-tested public benefits may be used to serve future legal entrants (including qualified aliens) into the United States for a period of 5 years beginning on their date of entry. Even for those who qualify, states must consider the income and resources of sponsors in determining qualified aliens' eligibility for benefits after the 5-year ban and must obtain affidavits of support from the sponsors.[35]

IMPACT OF WELFARE REFORM ON ENROLLMENT IN AND USE OF CHILDREN'S HEALTH PROGRAMS

The direct effects (such as eligibility changes and program reductions) of welfare reform on children's health are apparent and numerous;

however, the effects on participation in health programs are harder to assess and may have a more far-reaching impact on the entire socially deprived population. The concern for children's health relates to the link between welfare and Medicaid. With the implementation of welfare reform, Medicaid administration and enrollment procedures will go through major changes that require monitoring.

The welfare reform law stipulates that the actual receipt of benefits under Title IV-A (welfare) no longer results in automatic Medicaid coverage, because, for the purposes of Medicaid coverage, Title IV-A effectively has been repealed.[36] The new law continues to provide Medicaid coverage to poor families if they meet the state's previous AFDC income standard as of July 16, 1996 (or a state may choose to lower the standard to the May 1988 level), regardless of whether they qualify for TANF. States can determine eligibility for Medicaid either through the TANF application process or through a separate mechanism.[36] Because AFDC recipients have previously automatically qualified for Medicaid without a separate application, a state that separates the two applications may have significant loss of Medicaid coverage among former AFDC recipients, including non-pregnant women and older children, with no alternative mechanism to become eligible for Medicaid.[35] However, early reports from some states indicate that they are using one application form (a cash assistance form), and if someone is eligible for cash assistance, then they are eligible for Medicaid.[29]

Although the states (at this time) are using one application and maintaining Medicaid for most of the current eligible populations, the separation of Medicaid eligibility from receipt of welfare, as well as the increase in families leaving welfare, could prove a barrier to families' access to primary care services, especially when and where the recipient accesses the health system. Families with Medicaid coverage use health care services at rates comparable to privately insured populations.[44] However, the new law may cause a drop in families with Medicaid because they are not eligible or they are unaware that they remain eligible. Early reports from states' welfare reform programs found a decrease in Medicaid receipt among families leaving welfare—from 84% to 100% coverage with welfare benefits to 26% to 61% coverage after leaving welfare.[45] To receive Medicaid benefits, an individual first must be eligible, then must enroll in the program, and finally must use the benefits. Although the welfare law does not necessarily change the eligibility levels for Medicaid, it does change the nature of the enrollment process and how people find out they are eligible for various social programs. For example, the rate at which eligible individuals enroll in the Medicaid program (referred to as the take-up rate) is significantly higher for persons who automatically qualify because of cash assistance receipt (AFDC or SSI).* Individuals categorically eligible for Medicaid owing to AFDC receipt, must then still separately enroll in the Medicaid program to receive benefits. Although not all AFDC recipients immediately enroll in the Medicaid program, the take-up rate for this group significantly exceeds the rate for persons eligible for Medicaid based on other eligibility criteria (such as their low income, pregnancy status, or high medical bills). In the case of persons who are only eligible for Medicaid but not cash assistance, the take-up rate is much lower. One study found that pregnant women applying for cash assistance benefits had an 81% take-up rate for Medicaid in their first trimester as opposed to 51% to 61% of the pregnant women who were eligible only for Medicaid benefits.[46] Furthermore, enrollment for individuals not automatically eligible for Medicaid tends to occur when medical care is already needed, so that opportunities for prevention and early detection are missed.

As states move to manage care for their Medicaid populations, this delinking of welfare and Medicaid could have a tremendous impact on continuity of care and enrollment into managed care plans. Currently, welfare caseloads for cash assistance have been dropping rapidly, with few new cases opening. Although many of these families might still be eligible for Medicaid, they may not be signing up for Medicaid benefits because of a lack of knowledge that they are still eligible for the program or because of the stigma created by welfare reform. If Medicaid enrollment drops among the "healthy" patients who were previously receiving AFDC, and patients enroll in Medicaid only when they are sick, managed care organizations will be receiving a sicker, more expensive population. How will the plans react to Medicaid recipients who do not seek access to the health care system until they most need it? This question will need to be addressed by each state when implementing welfare reform.

Medicaid administrative issues will help determine the scope of Medicaid coverage for poor families, composed typically of women and children. States must decide whether or not to continue to use a single application for TANF and Medicaid eligibility. Some researchers view the delinking of Medicaid and welfare as positive because it will remove the "welfare stigma" from Medicaid and confirm its status as a health insurance program for low-income and working people.[33] In addition, states must decide how aggressively to conduct outreach to identify people, especially children, who are eligible for Medicaid but

---

*In addition, recent analysis by the General Accounting Office found that approximately 3 million children who were currently eligible for Medicaid had not enrolled. Various reasons include lack of awareness and enrollment barriers such as requalifying every 6 months or in-person interviews (33 states).[29]

not TANF. Because eligibility criteria for TANF may change with the provision of time limits and work requirements, it is likely that more poor families will be eligible for Medicaid but not TANF. In the past, these families were identified by the welfare office; the Medicaid agency now will be responsible for outreach to this population.

As families move off welfare to low-paying jobs, many children will qualify for Medicaid on the basis on family income rather than as TANF recipients. However, many families may become "working poor" families that make too much money to qualify for social program benefits, such as Medicaid, but too little to afford certain necessities. Additionally, Heymann and Earle[47] found that one in three working poor families needed at least 2 weeks time off in a year to care for their sick children, and one in four working poor families needed 3 weeks off. However, 28% of mothers in these families did not have sick leave, and the 1993 Family and Medical Leave Act does not alleviate this situation in many instances. Thus, even when families do succeed in being enrolled in Medicaid, their working circumstances may prevent them from seeking needed care for their children. The new State Children's Health Insurance Program (CHIP) targets the children of these families. CHIP will provide more than $20.3 billion dollars in new federal funds to families below 200% of the poverty level.[34] However, other issues that could have a major impact on children's health in working poor families or in families that leave welfare but are not working are not currently being addressed.

THE FUTURE FOR CHILDREN'S HEALTH

The effects of welfare reform on children's health are unknown; descriptive, analytical, and evaluative research is needed to determine these effects. When studying vulnerable populations such as women and children, evaluators should address topics such as public policies, health needs, resources, access to care, type and adequacy of care received, and its cost.[8,20] Many organizations, including the Department of Health and Human Services, are monitoring the effects on children. One such evaluation is the Urban Institute's New Federalism project (privately funded at $25 million), which is monitoring the impact on children and families for many social programs in four areas: health care, income and employment, social services, and well-being of children and their families. More indirect or subtle differences such as welfare reform's effects on health outcomes for children will require more resources and time in order to fully determine. Surveys will also be needed to examine the specific effects on enrollment in and use of health services (including high-quality primary care) and their impact on health. Even though the results from various research projects will not be known for some time, adverse effects for children might be more immediate. The Child Health and Illness Profile is one instrument that could be used to measure such effects. It was developed to assess health in surveys, to determine the existence of systematic differences in health of socioeconomically disadvantaged subpopulations, and to provide a basis for assessing the impact of changes in health services or health policies.[48]

Passage of the Personal Responsibility and Work Opportunity Reconciliation Act of 1996 reversed more than 50 years of efforts to provide a core safety net for families at high social risk. The negative effects from possible increases in poverty in families will be debated and researched for years to come, as will the positive effects associated with leaving welfare for work. Welfare reform's effects on children will be both immediate, as in the case of loss of cash assistance and other benefits, and subtle and not evident for some time, as in the case of enrollment in and use of Medicaid. Only time and evaluation will tell the story of welfare reform's impact on children's health.

References

1. *Green Book: Overview of entitlement programs*, United States House of Representatives, Committee on Ways and Means, 1996.
2. Mannix, M., Freedman, H., Cohan, M., and Lamb, C. Implementation of the Temporary Assistance for Needy Families Block Grant: An overview. *Clearinghouse Review: Journal of Poverty Law.* 1997;30(9–10):868–902.
3. Brooks-Gunn, J., and Duncan, G. The effects of poverty on children. *The Future of Children.* 1997;7(2):55–71.
4. Corcoran, M., and Chaudry, A. The dynamics of childhood poverty. *The Future of Children.* 1997;7(2):40–54.
5. Sherman, A. *Poverty matters: The cost of childhood poverty in America.* Washington, DC: Children's Defense Fund, 1997.
6. Montgomery, L., Kiely, J., and Pappas, G. The effects of poverty, race and family structure on U.S. children's health: Data from NHIS 1978 through 1980 and 1984 through 1991. *American Journal of Public Health.* 1996;86(10):1401–1405.
7. Moore, K., and Driscoll, A. Low-wage maternal employment and outcomes for children: A study. *The Future of Children.* 1997;7(1):122–127.
8. Aday, L.A., *At risk in America: The health and health care needs of vulnerable populations in the United States.* San Francisco: Jossey-Bass, 1993.
9. Annie E. Casey Foundation. *Kids Count data book: State profiles of child well-being.* Baltimore: Annie E. Casey Foundation, 1997.
10. Haan, M.N., Kaplan, G., Syme, S., and O'Neil, A. Recent publications on socioeconomic status and health. In Bunker, et al (eds). *Pathways to health: The role of social factors.* Menlo Park, CA: Kaiser Family Foundation, 1989.
11. Hughes, D., and Simpson, L. The role of social change in preventing low birth weight. *The Future of Children.* 1995;5(1):87–102.
12. Feinstein, J., The relationship between socioeconomic status and health: A review of the literature. *The Milbank Quarterly.* 1993;1(2):279–322.

13. Krieger, N., Rowley, D., Herman, A., Avery, B., and Phillips, M. Racism, sexism, and social class: Implications for studies of health, disease and well-being. *American Journal of Preventive Medicine.* 1993;9:82–122.

14. Marmot, M., Bobak, M., and Smith, G. Explanations for social inequalities in health. In Amick, et al (eds). *Society and Health.* New York: Oxford University Press, 1995, pp 172–210.

15. Starfield, B., Shapiro, S., Weiss, J., Liang, K.Y., Ra, K., Paige, D., and Wang, X.B. Race, family income and low birth weight. *American Journal of Epidemiology.* 1991;134(10):1167–1174.

16. McGauhey, P.J., Starfield, B., Alexander, C., and Ensminger, M. Social environment and vulnerability of low birth weight children: A social-epidemiological perspective. *Pediatrics.* 1991;88(5):943–953.

17. McGauhey, P.J., and Starfield, B. Child health and social environment of white and black children. *Social Science Medicine.* 1993;36(7):867–874.

18. Devaney, B., Ellwood, M., and Love, J. Programs that mitigate the effects of poverty on children. *The Future of Children.* 1997;7(2):88–112.

19. Starfield, B., Motherhood and apple pie: The effectiveness of medical care for children. *Milbank Memorial Fund Quarterly.* 1985;63(3):523–546.

20. Willis, E., and Kliegman, R. Wisconsin's welfare reform and its potential effects on the health of children. *Journal of Health Care for the Poor and Underserved.* 1997;8(1):25–35.

21. Hughes, D., and Runyan, S. Prenatal care and public policy: Lessons for promoting women's health. *Journal of the American Medical Women's Association.* 1995;50(5):156–159.

22. Adler, N., Boyce, T., Chesney, M., Folkman, S., and Syme, S.L. Socioeconomic inequalities in health: No easy solution. *JAMA.* 1993;269:3140–3145.

23. Schoen, C., Lyons, B., Rowland, D., Davis, K., and Puleo, E. Insurance matters for low-income adults: Results from the Kaiser/Commonwealth Five State Low-Income Survey. *Health Affairs.* 1998;16(5):163–171.

24. Cunningham, P., and Hahn, B. The changing American family: Implications for children's health insurance coverage and the use of ambulatory care services. *The Future of Children.* 1994;4(3):24–42.

25. U.S. General Accounting Office. *Health insurance: Coverage leads to increased health care access for children.* GAO/HEHS-98-14. Washington, DC: GAO, November, 1997.

26. Bindman, A., Grumbach, K., Osmond, D., Komaromy, M., Vranizan, K., Lurie, N., Billings, J., and Stewart, A. Preventable hospitalizations and access to health care. *JAMA.* 1995;274(4):305–311.

27. Starr, P. *The social transformation of American medicine.* Basic Books, 1982.

28. Yates, T., Changes in children's Supplemental Security Income disability program may spell loss of benefits for tens of thousands of children. *Clearinghouse Review: Journal of Poverty Law.* 1997;30(9–10):1026–1043.

29. Kaiser Commission on the Future of Medicaid. *Medicaid facts: Medicaid's role for children.* Washington, DC, May 1997.

30. Weissert, C., and Weissert, W. *Governing health: The politics of health policy.* Baltimore, MD: Johns Hopkins University Press, 1996.

31. Liska, D., Bruen, B., Salganicoff, A., Long, P., and Kessler, B. *Medicaid expenditures and beneficiaries: National and state profiles and trends, 1990–1995.* 3rd ed., Washington, DC: The Kaiser Commission on the Future of Medicaid, November, 1997.

32. U.S. General Accounting Office. *Health insurance for children: Declines in employment-based coverage leave millions uninsured; State and private programs offer new approaches.* GAO/T-HEHS-97-105. Washington, DC: GAO, 1997.

33. Koppleman, J. *Impact of the new welfare law on Medicaid.* Issue Brief: No. 697. Washington, DC: National Health Policy Forum, February, 1997.

34. Rosenbaum, S., Johnson, K., Sonosky, C., Markus, A., and DeGraw, C. The children's hour: The State Children's Health Insurance Program. *Health Affairs.* 1998;17(1):75–89.

35. Rosenbaum, S., and Darnell, J. *An analysis of the Medicaid and health-related provisions of the Personal Responsibility and Work Opportunity Reconciliation Act of 1996.* Washington, DC: Center for Health Policy Research, February, 1997.

36. Committee on Ways and Means. *Committee report of the summary of the welfare reforms made by Public Law 104-193.* U.S. Congress, Washington, DC. 1996.

37. Center for Budget and Policy Priorities. *An analysis of the AFDC-related Medicaid provisions in the new welfare law.* Washington, DC: Center for Budget and Policy Priorities, September, 1996.

38. Moffitt, R., and Slade, E. Health care coverage for children who are on and off welfare. *The Future of Children.* 1997;7(1):87–98.

39. Daniels, S. Statement of Associate Commissioner for Disability. Baltimore, MD: Social Security Administration, February 6, 1997.

40. Lewis, C. The impact of the Personal Responsibility and Work Opportunity Reconciliation Act of 1996 on food and nutrition programs. *Clearinghouse Review: Journal of Poverty Law.* 1997;30(9–10):950–963.

41. Willis, E., Kliegman, R., Meurer, J., and Perry, J. Welfare reform and food insecurity: Influence on children. *Archives of Pediatric and Adolescent Medicine.* 1997;151:871–875.

42. National Immigration Law Center. Preserving services for immigrants: State and local implementation of the new welfare and immigration laws. *Clearinghouse Review: Journal of Poverty Law.* 1997;30(9–10):964–987.

43. Rosenbaum, S., and Darnell, J. *A Comparison of Medicaid provision in the Balanced Budget Act of 1997 (P.L. 105-33) with prior law.* Washington, DC: The Henry J. Kaiser Family Foundation, October, 1997.

44. Marquis, M.S., and Long, S.H. Reconsidering the effect of Medicaid on health care services use. *Health Services Research.* 1996;30(6):791–808.

45. U.S. General Accounting Office. *Welfare reform: States early experiences with benefit termination.* GAO/HEHS-97-74. Washington, DC: GAO, May, 1997.

46. Ellwood, M. and Kenny, G. Medicaid and pregnant women: Who is being enrolled and when. *Health Care Financing Review.* 1995;17(2):7–28.

47. Heymann, S.J., and Earle, A. Working conditions faced by poor families and the care of children. *Focus.* 1997;19(1):56–58.

48. Starfield, B., Bergner, M., Ensminger, M., Riley, A., Ryan, S., Green, B., McGauhey, P., Skinner, A., and Kim, S. Adolescent health status measurement: Development of the child health and illness profile. *Pediatrics.* 1993;91(2):430–435.

9

Combating Family Poverty: A Review of the American Welfare System

SANDRA WEXLER AND VALIRE CARR COPELAND

The authors thank Donald Brieland and Kenneth Jaros for their helpful comments on this manuscript.

For much of this century, public health and social work practitioners have been major players in efforts to combat poverty and its effects on mothers and children. Research demonstrates a strong, consistent relationship between poverty and negative maternal and child health outcomes.[1-5] Discussion of this complex relationship requires an understanding of the fundamental link between health and welfare at both macro- and micro-levels. A review of the development of the American welfare state provides insight into how our country has moved from a priority of relieving poverty to one of eliminating dependency.

The history of American efforts to alleviate poverty is one of shifting attitudes, beliefs, interventions, and loci of responsibility. The programs and policies formulated, both now and in the past, have reflected explicit or implicit theories of causation and have incorporated answers to such questions as: Who are the poor?; Why are they poor?; and What type of assistance is needed?[6] Responses also have both mirrored and influenced societal views of gender, race, and social class.[7,8] Central to any discussion of poverty and public policy is the issue of whether assistance is an act of charity or an entitlement of citizenship.

This chapter examines American policy responses to poor mothers and their children. It begins with a brief historical review of the forms of aid available before 1935. The chapter then describes the Social Security Act of 1935 that created the modern American welfare state. Next, it traces the debates about and the modifications in the income maintenance system through the mid-1990s. Finally, it offers some thoughts about public health and social practice in the new, "post-welfare" context.

ASSISTANCE FOR POOR FAMILIES BEFORE 1935

American responses to poverty are rooted historically in the Elizabethan Poor Law of 1601, from which the distinction between worthy and unworthy poor derives.[9-12] From the colonial period through the end of the 1700s, "outdoor" relief—that is, assistance provided in the home—was the common way of assisting worthy, poor families.[13] Although other methods (i.e., poorhouses, auction, contract) also were used,[14] outdoor relief was especially favored in the United States.[7] Outdoor relief, administered locally by an appointed overseer of the poor and funded through local taxes, included the provision of clothing, food, coal, other supplies, and sometimes an allowance.[11,13]

Poor families were much like their neighbors, sharing common heritage, religion, and hardships. "Distinctions between the family and the community were often vague; in many ways, the home and the community were one."[15] Being poor, in itself, was not a cause for shame; rather, neediness was seen as beyond the control of the individual, as a result of unavoidable circumstances—unfavorable weather, death of the provider, old age, or injury—and as an inevitable feature of society.[13]

Not all needy residents, however, were deemed worthy of aid. Drunkards, loafers, and "sturdy beggars"[13] were defined as unworthy and were thought to deserve their fate. "Strangers" (i.e., non-residents), Native Americans, and African Americans were denied relief, too.[10,12] And whereas widows merited assistance, unmarried mothers were viewed as unfit and unworthy. Children were placed with local families—boarded out if they were younger than age 6 and indentured or apprenticed if they were older.[7]

The 19th century was a time of ideological and political debate, rapid population growth, and geographic expansion.[16] The Civil War revealed deep national divisions and produced massive social dislocation. Urbanization and industrialization were transforming American society. Ideas about how to provide assistance also began to change, paralleling and reflecting these other societal changes.[13]

Outdoor relief was criticized for fostering laziness, for contributing to immorality, and for increasing public costs.[14] "Social provision," it was argued, "would validate debased manhood by servicing it."[17] Outdoor relief as a public function was said to create dependency; aid by private charities was thought to avert this problem.[18]

"Indoor" relief—almshouses, poorhouses, workhouses, and orphanages—became the preferred response. Institutions were proposed as a less costly alternative, providing care more cheaply and making assistance less attractive to those who might apply.[14] The number of institutions rose sharply in the pre–Civil War years,[13] with some designated for specific racial, ethnic, and religious groups. A variety of specialized institutions, such as reformatories, homes for unwed mothers, orphanages, schools for the disabled, and asylums for the mentally ill were created as well.[19]

The poor of the 1800s no longer necessarily shared the characteristics of their better-off neighbors. The 6 million European immigrants who arrived between 1800 and 1860 and congregated in the growing northern industrial cities[13] differed from the majority in their religion, customs, and language. Institutions, it was believed, could reform their immoderate ways and instill in them the virtues of work;[14] as well as impose a degree of social control[20] on these potentially "dangerous classes."[21]

Whereas being poor had been thought to be a matter of God's will, it was now considered to be evidence of deficits in one's character and family-of-origin.[18] Reformers attempted to distinguish poverty from pauperism: those in poverty—widows, the orphaned, the aged, and the incapacitated—suffered from misfortune and were worthy of aid, whereas paupers were unworthy, having brought about their own downfall.[11,14] Relief efforts embraced the 1834 English Poor Law Reform concept of less eligibility: benefits should be less than that earned by the poorest laborer.[12,22] Thus, even the worthy poor faced lives of enormous hardship and deprivation.

Criticisms of indoor relief mounted during the second half of the 19th century. Some "child-saving" activists challenged the use of large institutions, arguing that children's development required a family environment.[14,19] Women's associations pressed for social reforms and for legislation to protect mothers and children from the vagaries of the industrial system.[23]

Reform in the late 1800s involved two contrasting approaches: charity organization societies, whose friendly visitors adjudged the eligibility of the poor for aid and offered them moral guidance to change their ways; and settlement houses, which stressed direct involvement with communities as a way to improve individual situations and environmental conditions.[24] The emergent Progressive movement, which has been called a "uniquely American movement,"[12] set out a diverse reform agenda that influenced turn-of-the-century social and political thought.[10,20]

Further momentous changes were sweeping the country at the beginning of the 20th century. Industrial capitalism and large corporations dominated the economic landscape. Wealth and income became more concentrated, and labor unrest grew.[18] Rural to urban migration and the immigration of 22 million people between 1890 and 1920 dramatically changed America's cities.[10] Following the 1896 Supreme Court decision in Plessy v. Ferguson, which upheld the doctrine of "separate but equal,"[25] the segregation and repression of African Americans went unchecked.[16]

Progressive reformers promoted the idea that children should not be removed from their family because of poverty alone. To preserve families, the 1909 White House Conference on the Care of Dependent Children recommended providing financial assistance by means of mothers' pensions.[14,19,26] Recognizing the societal service performed by married women who remained at home to raise children,[13] mothers' pensions were designed to limit the intrusions on motherhood caused by employment and poverty.[17]

The appropriateness of mothers' pensions was vigorously debated, with proponents arguing for public sponsorship and opponents countering that assistance was better provided by private charities.[16] Public sponsorship ultimately prevailed, although private charities often delivered the programs locally. Illinois and Missouri passed the first mothers' pension laws in 1911, and enactment of such statutes spread rapidly among the states. By 1935, all but two states—South Carolina and Georgia—had authorized mothers' pensions.[13,14,23,26]

Each state's legislation set its own level of benefits and conditions for assistance.[26] Within the state, the decision to provide aid, along with administrative and financial responsibilities for the program, was vested in the counties.[13] Wide variation resulted, with some counties in a state providing financial assistance and some not. In fact, before the 1935 Social Security Act, less than half of the nation's counties provided mothers' pensions.[18]

Potential beneficiaries had to meet behavioral as well as economic criteria.[8,23,26] Applicants typically had to show proof of residency and citizenship. "Suitable home" provisions were common, and mothers had to demonstrate that they were "fit"—that they did not drink or smoke, kept a tidy home, went to church, did not have boarders, and maintained proper hygiene.[13] Charity workers exercised discretion in determining fitness and suitability, and many impoverished families were excluded on these grounds.

Mothers' pensions were principally intended for widows, who were regarded as the deserving poor.[7,26] Unmarried mothers, African Americans, and Mexican Americans often were excluded[17] or were granted lower amounts.[8] Although amendments broadened many of these statutes,[13] marital status remained a criterion in all but 10 states.[23] Yet despite their limitations, mothers' pension programs served to legitimate the government's role in providing financial assistance to poor families.[8]

THE 1935 SOCIAL SECURITY ACT—THE CREATION OF THE WELFARE SYSTEM

The Great Depression, which began in 1929, plunged the United States into social and economic crisis. Mothers' pension programs were never adequate to provide aid to all who could qualify or to allow those who received assistance to give up employment completely.[16,23] The Depression caused some of these programs to shrink significantly and led others to suspend the distribution of aid periodically.[8] Temporary financial support for these programs came in 1933 from the Federal Emergency Relief Act,[8] one of President Franklin D. Roosevelt's first New Deal enactments.[16]

Swept into the office by a landslide in 1932, President Roosevelt instituted a variety of emergency relief programs to help individuals and state governments, many of which were themselves almost bankrupt. While these emergency efforts helped relieve the immediate crisis, the Roosevelt administration moved to formulate more permanent measures. In June 1934, the President appointed a Committee on Economic Security to draft legislation.[20]

The result was the Social Security Act of 1935, characterized as "the Magna Carta of the American welfare state."[20] It included two major programmatic areas: social insurance (e.g., Old Age Insurance and Unemployment Compensation) and public assistance (e.g., Old Age Assistance, Aid to Dependent Children, and Aid to the Blind). The Act also contained provisions for maternal and child health, crippled children, and child welfare programs, and state and local public health services.[16]

The public assistance programs of the Social Security Act were state-administered and financed through a combination of federal and state funds. To be eligible for assistance, an individual had to belong to one of the defined categories and had to demonstrate need. In contrast, the two social insurance programs were federally administered and funded through a payroll tax to which both employers and employees contributed.[16] Farm laborers, domestic workers, government employees, however, were not covered by these social insurance programs, resulting in the exclusion of many women and persons of color.[18] Moreover, the distinctions drawn between the social insurance and public assistance programs in many ways reified the historical division of worthy and unworthy poor: social insurance program beneficiaries merited coverage by virtue of their work histories, whereas public assistance program recipients had not necessarily earned their benefits.[12]

Title IV of the Social Security Act created the Aid to Dependent Children (ADC) program, commonly termed "welfare." ADC replaced the state-sponsored, locally administered mothers' pensions with an expanded federal-state program.[8] To reduce the intra-state variability common to the mothers' pension programs, the ADC program had to be offered statewide.[18]

ADC grants were based on the number of children in a family, with federal funds matching up to a maximum of $18 for the first child and up to $12 for each additional child.[8,16] These allowances were based on the amounts given to families of servicemen who had lost their lives in the World War but did not include the additional $30 monthly stipend received by veterans' widows.[11]

ADC incorporated many of the elements and assumptions of the mothers' pension programs, including the belief that worthy mothers should be occupied fully raising their young children.[8,18] Many of its original architects viewed ADC as a short-term program that would become obsolete as families qualified for social insurance benefits.[6,9]

Starting in 1939, many widows and their children did leave ADC to become beneficiaries of Survivors' Insurance.[18]

Compared with the 50% share it paid under Old Age Assistance, the federal government originally contributed a third of the funding for ADC, with the states responsible for the rest.[20] In 1939, the federal contribution was raised to $1 for $1 of state money.[22] Each state had to designate a single agency to administer ADC and had to define a standard of need that reflected a subsistence budget.[8] Each state was also required to establish eligibility criteria and benefit levels within broad federal guidelines, although benefits did not have to be large enough to equal the state's standard of need. Not surprisingly, significant variation occurred among the states, and no state had payments high enough to lift a family out of poverty.[27]

By 1940, only a third of eligible children received ADC.[22] Public discourse in the 1940s focused on economic recovery, the situation in Europe, war production and World War II, and post-war prosperity, rather than on poverty.[12] Yet despite the more positive economic situation, low pay and joblessness among women, especially African American women, led them to ADC.[18]

The 1950s were characterized by economic growth, rising wages, and a pervasive sense of complacency; poverty was no longer a major problem in the new "classless" American society.[13,16] The Civil Rights movement was in its formative stages.[14] The 1950s were also an era of heightened social conservatism. The perceived threat of Communism was attacked domestically by the McCarthy hearings and internationally by increased military might. Over $40 billion a year (about 75% of the national budget) went to military spending.[20]

The number of ADC recipients rose steadily in the 1950s, increasing 13% during the decade. Program costs expanded more rapidly, exhibiting a 60% rise over the decade.[16] Moveover, the composition of ADC clientele began to change. By the mid-1950s, a program designed for white widows was serving increasing numbers of African American and unmarried mothers.[13,18]

The contradictions and tensions of the 1950s were reflected in the policies of the decade. In 1950, ADC was expanded to permit grants to the adult caretakers (most often the mothers of dependent children). That year, as well, Aid to the Permanently and Totally Disabled was created; in 1956, disability insurance was introduced. Social services were added to the ADC program in 1956, but funding was not appropriated.[13,18]

Parallel to these expansions, an attack on public welfare began to take shape.[16] Many states, particularly those in the South, implemented punitive administrative policies to reduce ADC rolls and to deter new applications. These policies commonly involved residency requirements, "suitable home" criteria, and "man-in-the-house" or "substitute father" rules (i.e., any man living in an ADC home was assumed to contribute financially to the family).[13,18]

THE WAR ON POVERTY AND THE BEGINNING OF THE WELFARE "PROBLEM"

"The relative quiet of the 1950s gave way to the quasi-revolutionary spirit of the 1960s."[10] Rural and urban poverty was rediscovered.[13] Various social movements demanded "rights" for African Americans, Mexican Americans, Native Americans, women, juveniles, and gays and lesbians.[16] Welfare recipients and their supporters formed the National Welfare Rights Organization in 1966 to advocate for the rights of welfare recipients.[22,28]

Two new explanations were offered for poverty. One argument, which drew on Oscar Lewis's anthropological work, cited a "culture of poverty," or a set of attitudes, beliefs, and behaviors among the poor themselves that distinguished them from mainstream society and that was transmitted intergenerationally. The other perspective, derived from Richard Cloward and Lloyd Ohlin's writings on juvenile delinquency, highlighted structural factors, particularly limitations to opportunities.[22]

President Kennedy's New Frontier and President Johnson's Great Society programs changed the social policy landscape dramatically. Major health, welfare, and economic development initiatives expanded the welfare state to an unprecedented degree. Legislation from this period include the Manpower Development and Training Act of 1962, the Community Mental Health Centers Act of 1963, the Civil Rights Acts of 1964 and 1965, the Food Stamp Act of 1964, and the 1965 Title XVIII (Medicare) and Title XIX (Medicaid) amendments.[13,29]

The ADC program was not immune from this groundswell of legislative activity. Significant changes were made by the Public Welfare Amendments of 1962, commonly referred to as the Social Service Amendments.[30] One thrust of the amendments was to respond to charges that the program contributed to family breakup by encouraging fathers to leave. States, therefore, were given the option of providing benefits to two-parent families in which the main earner was unemployed. Although no more than half the states at any given time offered AFDC-UP (UP standing for unemployed parent) benefits, those that did could require unemployed adult recipients (typically fathers) to "work off" their public assistance grant.[18] Moreover, ADC was renamed Aid to Families with Dependent Children (AFDC) to affirm the program's emphasis on the family unit.[9,31]

The second thrust of 1962 amendments, drawing on the culture of poverty thesis, expanded the scope and funding of social services to ameliorate the deficits of poor, multi-problem beneficiary families.[22,31] Smaller caseloads were recommended to complement this rehabilitative approach.[9] States could provide these social services not only to current AFDC recipients but also to former clients and to those deemed at-risk of becoming recipients. The federal share of funding was high—fully $3 for every $1 of state money—making provision of these services attractive to the states.[13,14,16] Demonstration funding also was provided to the Community Work and Training program to assist AFDC recipients in becoming self-supporting.[32]

The optimism of the early 1960s gave way to growing conflict and skepticism. Between 1965 and 1968, cities across the nation were shaken by riots.[33] Criticism of the Viet Nam War mounted, and thousands took to the streets in anti-war protests. Some liberal reformers argued that the war was being carried on at the expense of domestic anti-poverty programs.[20]

Meanwhile, the welfare rolls continued to rise, climbing from 3.5 million in 1961 to 5 million in 1967. Never-married mothers accounted for 40% of the increase. About half the recipients were members of racial or ethnic minorities. By 1967, AFDC costs had reached $2.2 billion.[18]

The 1967 Social Security Amendments marked yet another shift in societal attitudes about welfare.[34] The developers of ADC had recognized the societal function performed by mothers staying at home to raise their young children.[35] By the late 1960s, however, "as more mothers with infants entered the job market, the argument that welfare mothers should earn their living gained broad support."[27]

The 1967 amendments separated cash assistance from social services, which had been added only 5 years earlier. Welfare advocates applauded this change, reasoning that the separation would counter the pejorative assumption that all recipient families needed services.[9,36] "Soft" services, such as counseling, lost favor to "hard" services, such as day care or vocational rehabilitation, that could promote self-sufficiency. The amendments allowed the states to purchase services from nongovernmental sources.[13]

Two provisions of the 1967 amendments were designed to encourage employment. Prior to 1967, an adult recipient who obtained employment would have her or his grant reduced by a dollar for every dollar earned. To make work more attractive, the "30 plus one third" rule required states to exclude a portion of recipients' monthly income (i.e., the first $30 and a third of the remainder earned) and certain work-related expenses from the income/assets base used to compute the AFDC grant.[9,16,22,27]

Workfare, in contrast, required that employable adult recipients, except single parents with children younger than the age of 6 or those exempted for other reasons, engage in work or employment training.[16,29] The Work Incentive Program (WIN) was designed to assist recipients in learning job search skills, obtaining training, and gaining work experience.[27,32] Child care and other supportive services were to be made available to WIN participants.[30] Those who did not comply with WIN requirements could have their grants reduced or suspended for 3 months.[18]

A series of judicial rulings also significantly influenced AFDC policies and procedures. Between 1968 and 1970, the U.S. Supreme Court handed down three landmark decisions in AFDC-related cases.[37] Of greatest consequence was the opinion rendered in Goldberg v. Kelly (1970), in which the Court held that the Fourteenth Amendment's due process clause entitled AFDC recipients to an administrative hearing prior to being terminated from the program. Welfare, the Court wrote, "was a 'right' or ... a 'statutory entitlement' "; that is, welfare recipients "have a valid reason to expect that, if they meet certain requirements, they should get AFDC."[37]

By the close of the decade, public and political interest intensified to reform welfare, which was viewed as a failure and a mounting burden to taxpayers.[38,39] Critics charged that welfare discouraged work, fostered family dissolution, and encouraged childbearing outside of marriage, especially among teens.[9] Varying benefit levels allegedly contributed to migration from low- to high-benefit states.[40] Meanwhile, the welfare rolls continued to increase, spurred by liberalized eligibility requirements, more generous benefits, increased numbers of households headed by never-married and divorced mothers, and a new sense among the poor of their entitlement to benefits that was stimulated by the Welfare Rights Movement.

In 1969, the Nixon administration proposed the Family Assistance Plan (FAP) as a substitute for AFDC and AFDC-UP.[20] The FAP proposal guaranteed a minimum income to all poor American families with children.[29] It required participation in employment or job training by all able-bodied individuals whose children were older than the age of 3.[10,16] To encourage employment, families would have been allowed to keep the first $60 plus half of their monthly income without losing their governmental subsidy, until an income maximum (or breakeven point) was reached, when aid would end.[22]

The FAP proposal was controversial among liberals and conservatives alike. With little support in Congress, FAP was abandoned in 1972. However, a portion of President Nixon's general welfare reform plan was enacted that year: Old Age Assistance, Aid to the Blind, and Aid to the Permanently and Totally Disabled were combined into a new federally administered program, Supplemental Security Income.[9,20] Thus, of the Social Security Act's public assistance programs, only AFDC remained under state administrative control.

Legislative modifications to the WIN program in 1971 and 1975 heightened the emphasis on job placement over training and imposed additional penalties for nonparticipation.[30,32] Recognition of absent parents' financial obligations to their children led to the creation in 1974 of the Office of Child Support Enforcement, whose mission was to encourage states to pursue vigorously paternity establishment and child support collection.[9] That same year, the Earned Income Tax Credit was passed, representing the first use of the tax system as a vehicle for giving resources to the poor.[20]

President Carter, who took office in 1977, proposed to supplant the AFDC, SSI, and Food Stamp programs with the Better Jobs and Income Program. The proposal entailed a negative income tax and public jobs creation plan that applied to all poor individuals and families. Its controversial provisions and high annual costs—projected at $30.7 billion a year, or $2.8 billion above what was then spent[13]—contributed to its failure.[29,34,38]

THE REAGAN YEARS AND THE FAMILY SUPPORT ACT OF 1988

The economic growth of the 1950s and 1960s ended in the 1970s. Ronald Reagan's 1980 campaign themes of lower taxes, higher military spending, a balanced budget, and a return to "traditional" values struck a responsive chord among many voters.[20] Reagan's victory over Carter legitimated neoconservative politics and policies.

The Reagan administration profoundly transformed discourse on social policy issues.[41–43] The problem was no longer poverty, but dependency; the cause was neither structural features of the economic system nor characteristics of the poor, per se, but the very government programs that had been implemented to help the poor.[44] As President Reagan asserted: "In 1964, the famous War on Poverty was declared. . . . Poverty won the War. Poverty won, in part, because instead of helping the poor, government programs ruptured the bonds holding poor families together."[45]

Capitalizing on a growing popular disillusionment with the federal government's ability to resolve social problems,[16] President Reagan called for less "big government" in domestic matters. In the economic arena, this meant reduced federal regulation of business and decreased taxes, especially for the wealthy, supply-side prescriptions to stimulate economic growth.[20] In the social policy arena, the emphasis was on transferring social welfare authority to state and local governments and on reducing means-tested social programs.[43] The federal government's role in welfare-related matters was to be a "safety net," a last resort when charities, volunteerism, the private sector, and individual initiatives failed.[14]

President Reagan launched his effort to dismantle the liberal welfare state soon after assuming office.[22] The Omnibus Budget Reconciliation Act (OBRA) of 1981 eliminated some programs and replaced 57 other categorical programs with seven block grants, which were given reduced funding.[29] OBRA also restricted eligibility for food stamps.[20]

OBRA imposed stricter eligibility requirements for AFDC, broadened the definition of assets for eligibility and benefit-setting purposes, limited to 4 months the earned income disregard for employed recipients, capped child care and work-related deductions, added further work requirements, and reduced WIN training funds.[30,42,46] These changes reflected the Reagan administration's views of individual and public responsibility: "those who have children should support them" and "should be required to work,"[31] with government aid available only to the truly needy.[34]

"The impact of the 1981 amendments was immediate and dramatic. In the following year, during the worst recession since the Great Depression, the number of families receiving AFDC declined by 8%."[27] By 1983, OBRA had resulted in about $1.1 billion in federal and state savings and a 2% increase in poverty.[22] The percentage of families disqualified for AFDC benefits ranged from 8% to 60%, depending on the state, with an additional 8% to 48% having their benefits reduced.[46]

President Reagan, re-elected in 1984 by a decisive majority, continued to push for reductions in domestic spending, particularly in means-tested programs, as a way to alleviate the rising federal deficit.[20] Attacks on the AFDC system and its recipients were bolstered by "poverty-by-choice" theories, which posited that the poor choose values, attitudes, and behaviors that keep them impoverished.[41] Rhetoric focused on the question of "reciprocity"—what welfare recipients owed to society in return for public financial support.[42]

Welfare reform again became a political issue in 1987, and both the Senate and the House considered bills to restructure AFDC. The Family Support Act of 1988 was hailed as the most important revision in welfare policy since the Social Security Act.[47,48] The Family Support Act was favored by both liberals and conservatives, who, for different reasons, saw it as a way to resolve the welfare dilemma.[49,50]

The legislation changed AFDC from an income support to a mandatory work and training program,[48] emphasizing short-term cost savings over long-term human capital investment.[32] Its major thrusts were paternity establishment, child support collection, and mandatory work. These provisions reflected the Administration's arguments that the obligation to support children resides first with the parents[29,42] and that encouragement of economic self-sufficiency must replace dependency on public stipends.[50]

Mandatory work (i.e., workfare) provisions were the centerpiece of the legislation. WIN was replaced by the Job Opportunities and Basic Skills Training (JOBS) program, which states were to implement by October 1990.[49] JOBS required AFDC recipients whose children were at least 3 years of age (or, at the state's option, at least 1 year of age) to participate in a training or employment preparation program or to locate work.[18] The legislation identified three groups for special consideration: young parents (i.e., younger than age 24) who lacked a high school diploma and work experience, long-term recipients (i.e., with more than 3 years in any 5-year period), and those nearing the end of their eligibility based on the age of the youngest child.[51] States could exercise considerable latitude in the design of their JOBS programs.[29]

To encourage the transition from welfare to employment, the Family Support Act included provisions for supportive services for JOBS participants and for time-limited, post-AFDC child care services and Medicaid coverage.[51] The AFDC-UP program, which then existed in 27 states,[49] was made mandatory nationwide. Participation of one parent (or at the state's option, both) in workfare was required. Recipients who did not comply with JOBS program requirements would lose the parent's portion of the AFDC grant for a specified period, although aid to the children would continue.[51]

George Bush succeeded Ronald Reagan to the presidency in January 1989. President Bush called for a "kinder, gentler nation" and for volunteers to be "a thousand points of light" in eradicating domestic social problems. Like his predecessor, President Bush emphasized military spending, "no new taxes," and a transfer of responsibility for social programs to the states.[9,16,20] Bush also inherited "a staggering $2.6 trillion debt . . . a crisis in the scandal-ridden savings and loan industry . . . and an economy with various structural weaknesses that, by 1990, would lapse into an increasingly serious recession."[13]

President Bush did not initiate any major federal-level modifications to the AFDC program. He did, however, encourage state experimentation and characterized the states as "laboratories."[9] States, seeking to reduce their welfare expenditures, applied for and received waivers to institute policies and procedures that did not comply with the existing federal rules.[9] The "devolution revolution"[52] was set in motion, wherein ever greater authority for welfare programming shifted from the federal government to state and local governments.

THE 1990S AND THE END OF THE WELFARE ENTITLEMENT

The United States entered the final decade of this century facing a decline in economic productivity, continued unemployment and underemployment, and an increase in the concentration of income and wealth among the richest 5%.[16] The number of Americans living in poverty in 1992 was the highest it had been since 1962.[22] Members of racial and ethnic minorities, children, and single-parent, mother-headed families were especially vulnerable to impoverishment.[16]

Although the JOBS program was in the early stages of implementation and its impacts were far from certain, the dismantling of the welfare system became a prominent theme in the 1992 presidential campaign.[13] Bill Clinton, the Democratic challenger, promised to "scrap the current welfare system and make welfare a second chance, not a way of life."[22] Clinton's victory in the 1992 election placed a Democrat in the White House; the 1994 elections gave Republicans control of Congress, with many of those in the House claiming their victory as a mandate for the policies outlined in their Contract with America.[16]

Democrats and Republicans alike vilified AFDC and its beneficiaries.[53] Myths about welfare mothers became popular reality; scant attention was given to the realities of life on welfare or to the declining value of welfare grants.[16,44] Responsibility for everything from gang violence to drug addiction to teenage pregnancy to the changing composition of American families began to be attributed to the welfare system and to "dependent" welfare mothers.[54]

By the mid-1990s, welfare "reform" meant "reducing expenditures of public money, increasing labor-force participation of single parents (largely women), and changing the social and sexual behavior of women."[16] The Personal Responsibility Act, based on the Republican's Contract with America, was introduced in the House in 1995. After a year of political wrangling, a final welfare bill emerged that incorporated elements of the Personal Responsibility Act and suggestions made by the National Governors' Association.[16] President Clinton's promise to "end welfare as we know it" came to fruition on August 22, 1996 when he signed the Personal Responsibility and Work Opportunity Reconciliation Act.

The Act modified a number of long-standing U.S. social policies, as discussed in more detail in Chapter 10. It fundamentally changed the system of welfare that existed in America for 60 years, ending the entitlement status of public aid and imposing a 5-year lifetime limit on financial assistance. It replaced the AFDC and AFDC-UP programs with the Temporary Assistance for Needy Families (TANF) program.[55–57]

It is too early to tell how TANF will function in the various states. It is being implemented during a time of prosperity and low unemployment. Between March 1994 and October 1996, AFDC caseloads declined by at least 5% in every state but Hawaii.[58] This decrease has given states a short-term cushion of TANF funds (since the allocated amount is based on federal payments made during prior years in which there were higher welfare rolls) and has lowered the proportion of the states' caseload that has to be placed to meet the first federal work requirement.[57]

Predictions of immediate and dramatic increases in homelessness, food pantry usage, and immigration have not been realized. Yet, as Edin and Lein[59] have shown, low-wage, dead-end jobs that offer few, if any, benefits do little to promote the economic self-sufficiency of poor families. The survival of working-poor families, which is precarious at best, can easily be thrown into jeopardy without adequate, affordable, and stable child care and accessible and adequate medical care.

Two important tests of TANF are yet to come: What will happen when large numbers of recipient families reach the end of their 5 years' eligibility? and How will the TANF program and its beneficiaries fare when there is an economic downturn? Historical evidence suggests that states and localities may be ill-equipped to handle the needs of poor families without the infusion of federal dollars.

CONCLUSION

Much remains to be done as America prepares to enter the 21st century, and various suggestions for responding to post-TANF realities are beginning to appear in the literature.[35,52,60] Public health and social work students and professionals are uniquely qualified (1) to conduct research that gives voice to those most directly affected by the current changes and that provides policy-relevant evidence; (2) to document the effects of TANF on family well-being, including economic status, health status and health care utilization, and psychological and social functioning; (3) to conduct education in our communities that addresses the misconceptions about welfare and welfare recipients; and (4) to engage in local and state coalition-building and advocacy efforts. The expertise of social work and public health practitioners can contribute to future policy decisions and to the lives of those affected by them.

References

1. Copeland, V.C. Immunization among African American children: Implications for social work. *Health and Social Work.* 1996;21:105–114.
2. Kington, R.S., and Smith, J.P. Socioeconomic status and racial and ethnic differences in functional status associated with chronic diseases. *American Journal of Public Health.* 1997;87:805–810.
3. Montgomery, L.E., Kiely, J.L., and Pappas, G. The effects of poverty, race, and family structure on U.S. children's health: Data from NHIS, 1978 through 1980 and 1989–1991. *American Journal of Public Health.* 1996;86:1401–1405.
4. Sorlie, P.D., Backlund, E., and Keller, J.B. U.S. mortality by economic, demographic, and social characteristics: The national longitudinal mortality study. *American Journal of Public Health.* 1995;85:949–956.
5. *Maternal and Child Health Bureau.* Child Health USA '95 (DHHS Publication No. HRSA-M-DSEA-96–5). Washington, DC: U.S. Government Printing Office, 1996.
6. Plotnick, R.D. Income support for families with children. In P.J. Pecora, J.K. Whittaker, A.N. Maluccio with R.P. Barth, and R.D. Plotnick (eds). *The child welfare challenge: Policy, practice, and research.* New York: Aldine De Gruyter, 1992; pp 59–90.
7. Davidson, C.E. Dependent children and their families: A historical survey. In F.H. Jacobs, and M.W. Davies (eds). *More than kissing babies? Current child and family policy in the United States.* Westport, CT: Auburn House, 1994; pp 65–89.
8. Gordon, L. *Pitied by not entitled: Single mothers and the history of welfare.* New York: The Free Press, 1994.
9. DiNitto, D.M. *Social welfare: Politics and public policy.* 3rd ed. Englewood Cliffs, NJ: Prentice Hall, 1991.
10. Karger, H.J., and Stoesz, D. *American social welfare policy: A pluralist approach.* 3rd ed. New York: Longman, 1997.
11. Leiby, J. *A history of social welfare and social work in the United States.* New York: Columbia University Press, 1978.
12. Reid, P.N. Social welfare history. In *Encyclopedia of social work.* 19th ed., Vol. 3. Washington, DC: NASW Press, 1995, pp 2206–2225.
13. Trattner, W.I. *From poor law to welfare state: A history of social welfare in America.* 5th ed. New York: The Free Press, 1994.
14. Katz, M.B. *In the shadow of the poor house: A social history of welfare in America.* Rev. ed. New York: Basic Books, 1996.
15. Baker, P. The domestication of politics: Women and American political society, 1780–1920. In L. Gordon (ed). *Women, the state, and welfare.* Madison, WI: University of Wisconsin Press, 1990, pp 55–91.
16. Axinn, J., and Levin, H. *Social welfare: A history of the American response to need.* 4th ed. White Plains, NY: Longman, 1997.
17. Mink, G. The lady and the tramp: Gender, race, and the origins of the American welfare state. In L. Gordon (ed). *Women, the state, and welfare.* Madison, WI: University of Wisconsin Press, 1990, pp 92–122.
18. Abramovitz, M. *Regulating the lives of women: Social welfare policy from colonial times to the present.* Rev. ed. Boston: South End, 1996.
19. Liebmann, G.W. The AFDC conundrum: A new look at an old institution. *Social Work.* 1993;38:36–43.

20. Jansson, B.S. *The reluctant welfare state: A history of American social welfare policies.* 2nd ed. Pacific Grove, CA: Brooks/Cole, 1993.
21. Brace, C.L. *The dangerous classes of New York, and twenty years' work among them.* Washington, DC: National Association of Social Workers, 1872/1973.
22. Patterson, J.T. *America's struggle against poverty, 1900–1994.* Cambridge, MA: Harvard University Press, 1994.
23. Skocpol, T. *Protecting soldiers and mothers.* Cambridge, MA: The Belknap Press of Harvard University Press, 1992.
24. Brieland, D. Social work practice: History and evolution. In *Encyclopedia of social work.* 19th ed., Vol. 3. Washington, DC: NASW Press, 1995, pp 2247–2257.
25. Brieland, D., and Lemmon, J.A. *Social work and the law.* 2nd ed. St Paul, MN: West Publishing, 1985.
26. Nelson, B.J. The origins of the two-channel welfare state: Workmen's compensation and mothers' aid. In L. Gordon (ed). *Women, the state, and welfare.* Madison, WI: University of Wisconsin Press, 1990, pp 123–151.
27. Levitan, S.A. *Programs in aid of the poor.* 6th ed. Baltimore, MD: The Johns Hopkins Press, 1990.
28. Piven, F.F., and Cloward, R.A. *Poor people's movements: Why they succeed, how they fail.* New York: Vintage Books, 1977/1979.
29. Dickinson, N.S. Federal social legislation from 1961 to 1994. In *Encyclopedia of social work.* 19th ed., Vol. 2. Washington, DC: NASW Press, 1995, pp 1005–1013.
30. Abramovitz, M. Aid to families with dependent children. In *Encyclopedia of social work.* 19th ed., Vol. 1. Washington, DC: NASW Press, 1995, pp 183–194.
31. Mason, J., Wodarski, J.S., and Parham, T.M.J. Work and welfare: A reevaluation of AFDC. *Social Work.* 1985;30:197–203.
32. Goodwin, L. The work incentive years in current perspective: What have we learned? Where do we go from here? *Journal of Sociology and Social Welfare.* 1989;16(2):45–65.
33. Schram, S.F., and Turbett, J.P. The welfare explosion: Mass society versus social control. *Social Service Review.* 1983;57:614–625.
34. Gueron, J.M. Reforming welfare with work. *Public Welfare.* 1987;45(4):13–25.
35. Aaronson, S., and Hartmann, H. Reform, not rhetoric: A critique of welfare policy and charting new directions. *American Journal of Orthopsychiatry.* 1996; 64:583–598.
36. Miller, D.C. AFDC: Mapping a strategy for tomorrow. *Social Service Review.* 1983;57:599–613.
37. Levy, P.A. The durability of Supreme Court welfare reforms of the 1960s. *Social Service Review.* 1992;66:213–236.
38. Day, P.J. *A new history of social welfare.* Englewood Cliffs, NJ: Prentice Hall, 1989.
39. Karger, H.J., and Stoesz, D. Retreat and retrenchment: Progressives and the welfare state. *Social Work.* 1993;38:212–220.
40. Dear, R.D. What's right with welfare? The other face of AFDC. *Journal of Sociology and Social Welfare.* 1989;16(2):5–43.
41. Rose, N.E. The political economy of welfare. *Journal of Sociology and Social Welfare.* 1989;16(2):]87–108.
42. Stoesz, D., and Karger, H.J. Welfare reform: From illusion to reality. *Social Work.* 1990;35:141–147.
43. Stoesz, D., and Karger, H.J. Deconstructing welfare: The Reagan legacy and the welfare state. *Social Work.* 1993;38:619–628.
44. Funiciello, T., and Schram, S.F. Post-mortem on the deterioration of the welfare state. In E.A. Anderson, and R.C. Hula (eds). *The reconstruction of family policy.* New York: Greenwood, 1991, pp 149–163.
45. Danziger, S. Antipoverty policies and child poverty. *Social Work Research and Abstracts.* 1990;26(4):17–24.
46. Moffitt, R., and Wolf, D.A. The effect of the 1981 Omnibus Budget Reconciliation Act on welfare recipients and work incentives. *Social Service Review.* 1987; 61:247–260.
47. Segal, E.A. Welfare reform: Help for poor women and children? *Affilia.* 1989; 4(3):42–50.

48. Stoesz, D. A new paradigm for social welfare. *Journal of Sociology and Social Welfare.* 1989;16(2):127–150.
49. Chilman, C.S. Welfare reform or revision? The Family Support Act of 1988. *Social Service Review.* 1992;66:349–377.
50. Nichols-Casebolt, A.M., and McClure, J. Social work support for welfare reform: The latest surrender in the war on poverty. *Social Work.* 1989;34:77–80.
51. Harris, S. *A social worker's guide to the Family Support Act of 1988: Summary, analysis, and opportunities for implementation.* Silver Spring, MD: NASW Press, 1989.
52. Kamerman, S.B. The new politics of child and family policies. *Social Work.* 1996; 41:453–465.
53. Sidel, R. The enemy within: A commentary on the demonization of difference. *American Journal of Orthopsychiatry.* 1996;66:490–495.
54. Withorn, A. "Why do they hate us so much?" A history of welfare and its abandonment in the United States. *American Journal of Orthopsychiatry.* 1996;66:496–509.
55. National Governors' Association, National Conference of State Legislatures, and American Public Welfare Association. *Analysis of the Personal Responsibility and Work Opportunity Reconciliation Act of 1996 (Conference agreement for H.R. 3734: PL 104–193),* August, 1996. (Available from the National Governors' Association, Hall of States, 444 N. Capitol St., N.W., Suite 267, Washington, DC, 20001)
56. Office of the Assistant Secretary for Planning and Evaluation, U.S. Department of Health and Human Services. *Summary of provisions: Personal Responsibility and Work Opportunity Reconciliation Act of 1996 (H.R. 3734).* Washington, DC: Author, January, 1997.
57. Super, D.A., Parrott, S., Steinmetz, S., and Mann, C. *The new welfare law.* August, 1996. (Available from the Center on Budget and Policy Priorities, 820 First Street, N.E., Suite 510, Washington, DC 20002).
58. DeParle, J. A sharp decrease in welfare cases is gathering speed. *The New York Times.* February 2, 1997; Section 1:1, 12.
59. Edin, K., and Lein, L. *Making ends meet: How single mothers survive welfare and low-wage work.* New York: Russell Sage Foundation, 1997.
60. Poole, D.L. Welfare reform: The bad, the ugly, and the maybe not too awful. *Health and Social Work.* 1996;21:243–246.

10

Potential Effects of the 1996 Welfare Reform Legislation on the Economic Status, Health, and Well-being of Low-income Families

MARY ELIZABETH COLLINS AND LENA LUNDGREN-GAVERAS

Historically, concerns about low-income families and the Aid to Families with Dependent Children (AFDC) program that served them resulted in minor adjustments to the program, but left the basic program framework intact. In recent years, however, there have been growing concerns about welfare resulting in major changes at the federal level. The enactment of the Personal Responsibility and Work Opportunity Reconciliation Act of 1996 (P.L. 104-193) dismantled the previous AFDC program that served poor families with children and has allowed states increased discretion in designing new welfare programs. This chapter focuses on the welfare-to-work aspects of new legislation and examines the potential implications of these changes on the economic status, health, and well-being of adults and children previously served by AFDC and now served by Temporary Assistance for Needy Families (TANF).

WELFARE TO WORK

Prior to the enactment of the Personal Responsibility and Work Opportunity Reconciliation Act of 1996, legislation contained in the 1981 Omnibus Budget Reconciliation Act and the 1988 Family Support Act had already aimed to strengthen the employment component of AFDC. The Job Opportunities and Basic Skills Training (JOBS) program of the Family Support Act required states to place up to 20% of single parents in job activities, after exempting those with child care, health, or family problems. Moreover, since the Family Support Act, states have been allowed increased flexibility to design their own programs, many of which have emphasized work requirements. Yet, although policy developments since the 1980s have encouraged work from AFDC recipients and have allowed increased state experimentation, the most recent legislation intensified both of these policy developments.

Replacing AFDC, the new legislation went into effect October 1, 1996, creating Temporary Assistance for Needy Families (TANF). In this legislation, there are substantial changes in the nature of the relationship between the federal and state governments, the federal commitment to poor families, and the funding mechanism through which aid is provided. Previously the federal government guaranteed matching funds to states to fund the AFDC program and had a defined guarantee of assistance to families who met the eligibility requirements and who complied with the conditions of the program. Under the current legislation, federal funding is fixed and provided to states through a block grant rather than through matched funding. As a consequence of the block grant, funding assistance to families is no longer guaranteed; federal funding is fixed regardless of possible variation in the size of welfare caseloads. Furthermore, the change in the federal-state relationship results in reduced federal oversight of state programs and consequent increased state discretion in designing and implementing programs.

Although states are allowed increased freedom in several areas of program design, there are very specific federal requirements regarding mandatory work and time limits for receipt of aid. With respect to work requirements, the legislation requires states to fulfill specific employment levels in order to receive full federal funding. For example, in 1997, 25% of single parents must work at least 20 hours per week and 75% of parents in two-parent families must work at least 35 hours per week. These numbers rise each year until 2002, when states are required to have 50% of single parents working at least 30 hours per week and 90% of parents in two-parent families working at least 35 hours per week. Failure to meet these standards will result in reduced amounts of funding for states. The legislation also narrowed the definition of work by establishing limits on the percentage of welfare recipients in vocational training and high school education and by placing a greater emphasis on employment, on-the-job training, and community service requirements.

The federal government also instituted a time limit for receiving assistance. There is now a 5-year lifetime limit on receipt of benefits and a provision to allow states to enact shorter time limits. Up to 20% of state caseloads can be exempt from these limits.

State Examples

Prior to the welfare reform legislation, states were allowed to apply for waivers from the federal government requesting exemption from certain rules of the AFDC program in order to experiment with different means of serving the AFDC population. Several waivers were targeted toward establishing various welfare-to-work incentives. Under the new law, states with waivers can continue to implement and monitor their own program for the duration of the waiver, usually 5 years. Examination of state variation gives some indication of the directions likely to be pursued in the future.

Prior to the passage of TANF, 37 states had waivers aimed at encouraging work.[1] Waivers took various forms and included efforts to increase the amount of income recipients could earn without consequent reduction in their AFDC grant (16 states), to increase the resources and assets families could own (27 states), to allow individual savings accounts (9 states), to divert new applicants for assistance into the work force (10 states), to enforce work or training requirements (29 states), and to extend child care and/or Medicaid benefits (12 states). In addition, 27 states have waivers that will permit legal immigrants to apply for aid under the same condition as citizens. As the federal legislation currently is written, states may opt to give welfare block grants to legal immigrants.

State programs have used various combinations of these and other provisions in designing their programs. A few, more detailed state examples are discussed here.

In Massachusetts, welfare reform was signed into law in February 1995, and the Department of Public Welfare was renamed the Department of Transitional Assistance. The primary focus of Massachusetts welfare reform is on work regulations, benefit reductions for those not working, and time limits for assistance. As in the other states that have recently enacted their own welfare program, the Massachusetts welfare program is both more and less restrictive than TANF. For example, fewer work hours are required. Twenty hours per week of work is required from all able-bodied AFDC parents who are non-exempt and whose child of record is of school age. Community service is required from those who cannot find work. Recipients exempt from the work requirements include disabled parents, parents with a disabled child or spouse, parents with a child younger than the age of two at the time they first receive temporary AFDC, women in their third trimester, victims of domestic violence, parents with a child younger than 3 months, parents younger than 20 attending high school, and caretaker relatives. Exempt parents receive a work incentive in the form of increased income disregards (the standard one third disregard is increased to one half); however, for non-exempt parents, there is no change in the disregard. Massachusetts also has expanded the definition of where teen parents may live in order to receive aid to include any supervised setting. Finally, a major difference, compared with federal legislation is that in Massachusetts a recipient may receive assistance only 4 months in a 60-month period.

Since 1993, the state of Wisconsin has had in place a welfare-to work demonstration project in two of its counties, which has been classified by some as having severe sanctions.[2] Under this effort, recipients may be cut off from aid after 2 years whether or not they obtain a job, and recipients are required to spend 40 hours per week in community work efforts or job training.

In contrast to these two states, in Minnesota the emphasis of welfare reform has been on increased economic incentives to engage in work rather than on punitive measures. Minnesota's Family Investment Plan is aimed at increasing the economic status of families who work and receive welfare. Welfare recipients who work receive larger grants than those who do not; an increase of 20% is added to the grants of those who work. Assets and the earnings limits are also increased. In particular, 38% of welfare recipients' earnings are disregarded when calculating the grant (compared with the usual 33% for the first 4 months). Recipients remain eligible for AFDC until their incomes exceed 145% of the federal poverty level.

Hence, these examples suggest that states have a wide latitude in how they develop their welfare-to work programs. Unfortunately, they also suggest, as Handler notes, that "just about any change will be considered welfare reform and justified as an experiment."[2]

EFFECTS ON ECONOMIC STATUS OF FAMILIES

Although families may exit from welfare in several ways, including a change in family status (e.g., remarriage, child reaching age 18), new legislation is most likely to cause recipients to exit welfare as a result of either their reaching the 5-year limit or a change in employment status. Consequently, we now review what is currently known about likely outcomes of the 5-year limit as well as the employment prospects for this population.

For many, AFDC was temporary economic support until their work or family situation changed. Forty-two percent of AFDC recipients collected welfare for less than 2 years,[3] and most exited welfare for work.[4] Hence, it seems unlikely, for this group, that welfare reform will have much impact.

Longer-term recipients have been of greater public concern and policy attention because their prospects for employability are less optimistic. Because they are less likely to find work, they are also most likely to reach the 5-year time limit. Duncan, Harris, and Boisjoly[5] used data from the Panel Study on Income Dynamics to identify those most likely to be affected by time limits. In summary, the recipients who were young, who had never married, had no high school diploma, and had preschool children at the state of their initial receipt on welfare were most likely to remain on welfare for an extended period of time. These researchers estimated that 40% of the current caseload will reach the 5-year time limit. Further, more than half will reach the limit after 60 consecutive months, and the remainder will be cut off from assistance within 8 years because of intermittent spells on and off welfare.

A 1997 study by the U.S. General Accounting Office (GAO)[6] examined termination of benefits within states that had waivers allowing benefit termination prior to the enactment of welfare reform.

Through December 1996, 14 of the 33 states with benefit termination provisions had not terminated any benefits, in part because many states had a gradual phase-in of this provision. In-depth study of three states (Iowa, Massachusetts, and Michigan) found that although AFDC was a significant source of income prior to termination, between 43% and 48% of terminated households had some income from other sources such as wages, pensions, and child support. Also, about 75% had members who received food stamps, Supplemental Security Income (SSI), housing assistance, or Medicaid. The percentage of households receiving food stamps and Medicaid, however, declined significantly in each state (between 23% and 70%) among cases not returning to welfare. Termination of AFDC was not supposed to have affected families' access to these benefits, but the decline was attributed to families' failure to take the necessary action to retain these benefits.

Although the welfare reform legislation implies that those terminated from welfare will be forced to find work, research suggests this may not be the case. Danziger and Danziger[7] examined the effects of the termination of General Assistance benefits in Michigan on the employment of former recipients. Focusing the analysis on former General Assistance recipients most similar to AFDC recipients (younger than 40, with no benefit-qualifying disability), they found that 2 years after termination 46% of those who were high school graduates were employed compared with 28% of those who were high school dropouts. The median monthly earnings of those employed were still below the poverty line. Consequently, they concluded that even with the powerful incentive of benefit termination, large percentages of former recipients, particularly those lacking a high school education, will remain unemployed and that even those successful in gaining employment will remain in poverty.

Hence, employment prospects are dim for many because of limited education and lack of basic job skills. Burtless[8] reports that less than 56% of mothers who received AFDC in 1992 had completed high school and that they also have tended to perform poorly on standardized tests. Many also lack a previous work history. Pavetti[3] reports that half of those who spend longer than 5 years on welfare entered AFDC with no work experience; 42% first received welfare when they were younger than age 25. These limitations can impede employment even when recipients are otherwise able and willing to work. Surveying employers in four large cities, Holzer[9] estimated that only 4% of jobs required no high school diploma, training, experience, or references. Although most employers indicated a willingness to hire welfare recipients, less than half said they would hire a person with only part-time or short-term work experience. Other studies indicate that employers are reluctant to hire welfare recipients and public job training participants even for entry level positions.[10,11]

Because several job training programs existed throughout the 1980s, evaluations of these programs provide some further information about the prospects of employment for those leaving welfare. Summarizing the numerous job training evaluations, Nightingale and Holcomb[12] stated that the demonstration projects involving job search assistance, work experience, training, or a combination of services had positive, but small, effects on employment rates, ranging from 2% to 10%. Programs generally have had more consistent effects on earnings levels than on employment rates, but these too have been small effects, and there have been no consistent effects on the use of welfare. Moreover, gains in earnings were less likely for those most disadvantaged, specifically those who had not completed high school, had no recent work experience, and had received welfare for the last 2 years.[13] For example, in terms of long-term employment rates, a study conducted during the 1980s in Baltimore, San Diego, Virginia, and Arkansas found that in the fifth year after enrollment, the employment rate averaged 38% among those in the programs and 36% among women in the control group.[14] In regard to earnings and welfare receipt, an evaluation of the California JOBS program found that the program raised the earnings of clients an average of 22% over 3 years, with a consequent decrease of 6% in welfare payments.[13] It is likely that the prospects of employment and earnings gains are less optimistic for those who will be forced off welfare because of time limits and who have not had access to job training programs.

In the current strong national economy, low-skilled, low-paying jobs are available in many areas, and, therefore, many with limited job skills are likely to find work. Becoming employed, however, is only the first step to economic stability and long-term self-sufficiency. Additional research suggests that many who leave welfare for work are unable to effectively improve their standard of living for themselves and their families. In general, the wage rates of low-skilled workers have fallen in real dollars over the last few years, making it increasingly difficult to support a family even when working.[15] When women leave welfare for work, they generally find relatively low paying jobs, usually in the range of $5 to $6 per hour.[13] They are also likely to work only part time. One study of women who moved from welfare to work found that on average they worked just 20 hours per week and earned from $203 to $387 monthly.[16]

Perhaps of greater concern, these initial work experiences generally do not lead to higher paying and more secure jobs. Burtless[17] found that although many women who earn low wages in their twenties eventually work in moderately well paying jobs in their thirties, such advancement is less likely for women who did poorly in high school or who dropped out. Women who did not complete high school experienced an average yearly increase of just seven cents per hour.[17] Pavetti[18] found similar results; women had difficulty moving from bad jobs to good jobs if they lacked education or had young children.

Returns to welfare after the initial work experience are also common. Analysis of the National Longitudinal Survey of Youths (NLSY) found that 39% of those leaving work returned to welfare within a year,[19] and analysis of the Panel Study on Income Dynamics (PSID) found that 22% returned within a year.[20] Even with the support of a job training program, stable employment is difficult to attain. In a study of the Massachusetts Employment and Training (ET) Choices Program, 62% participants lost their first jobs within 12 to 16 months.[21] The reasons for returning to welfare are highly individualized, but they often include the low return of working when considering the loss of benefits and out-of-pocket costs; instability of the jobs themselves or the workers' ability to succeed in the jobs; and problems with child care, health, transportation, or personal family troubles (e.g., family violence.)[22] Because of their substantial impact on the probability of initial and continued employment, child care and access to health care are discussed further.

Child Care

Finding satisfactory child care arrangements is essential to the financial reward of working, success in obtaining and keeping a job, and child safety and optimal development. Given the increased work requirements in federal legislation, more people are likely to enter the work force, resulting in an increased need for child care. The welfare reform legislation has combined the four federal child care programs into the Child Care and Development Block Grant, which will provide $15 billion over 7 years to states for use in helping poor families pay for child care. The child care block grant, like the TANF block grant, eliminates the entitlement to assistance, and, therefore, access to affordable child care may be limited by available funding.

Several analyses have demonstrated that child care is a substantial cost to families and that low-income families, in particular, spend a large part of their income on child care. For example, Kisker and Ross[23] calculate that in 1995 a single mother of one child who is earning minimum wage in a full-time job will make only $8,840, of which 38% will be spent on child care. The cost of child care can effectively prohibit a parent from working. A GAO study on child care estimated the effect of a full child care subsidy on the labor force participation of mothers at different income levels. The study estimates that poor mothers would increase their labor force participation from 29% to 44%, that near-poor mothers would increase their participation from 43% to 57%, and that non-poor mothers would increase their participation from 55% to 65% if they were to receive full child care subsidy.[24]

Although the cost of child care is clearly a key issue in determining whether a mother can or should work, there are further considerations beyond cost. Accessibility and reliability of child care are also important. Because many low-income workers are in part-time, service occupations, their work schedules tend to be at non-regular hours that may not coincide with the operating hours of child care centers. Moreover, the reliability of child care is particularly important for such workers because their jobs frequently lack the paid vacation or sick time that allow other parents the flexibility to meet child care crises.

A study by the GAO[6] estimated the impact of the reform legislation on the supply and demand of available child care. Collecting data at four sites, the study found potential problems in terms of supply, cost, and access. For example, the study estimated that in Chicago, without any increase in care by 2002, the child care supply will be able to meet only 12% of demand. Echoing earlier research, the study found that poor families spend high proportions of their income on child care. For example, in Benton County, Oregon, infant care at a child care center consumes 20% of median household income for a poor family. Centers also were found to lack the flexible hours needed to coordinate with the types of jobs that are often available to low-income workers; the number of centers providing care outside of non-standard work hours was only 12% to 35%.

Quality of child care, aside from its impact on child safety and development, also may directly impinge on parents' ability to work. One study found that a parent's perception of the safety of her child care arrangement and the trustworthiness of her child care provider were important in predicting whether she was still active in employment or job preparation 1 year after enrolling in the JOBS program.[25]

Hence, this review of research indicates that lack of access to child care, lack of quality child care, and lack of federal funding for child care all are likely to negatively affect a low-income parent's ability to adhere to new work requirements. It is interesting that the new welfare legislation both addresses and ignores the consequences of this child care dilemma. Specifically, the new legislation does not allow for states to sanction parents who cannot find child care, but it nonetheless requires states to count such parents in work participation rates. Also, parents with children younger than the age of 1 are exempted, but only once (the exemption cannot be used for subsequent children). Despite any difficulties finding and arranging child care, families still may be cut off from assistance if they reach the 5-year time limit.

Access to Health Care Medical Insurance Coverage

The move from welfare to work has often been complicated by the role that medical insurance coverage may play in individual decision-making about the relative benefit of work versus welfare. Families receiving AFDC have automatically qualified for Medicaid since the program began in 1965, and, consequently, concern about the loss of Medicaid coverage has been a disincentive for adults to leave AFDC as well as an incentive to return to welfare when family health concerns arise.

Although Medicaid has gradually been extended in the late 1980s and early 1990s, and its tie to AFDC has been loosened, many children have continued to lack health insurance. In response to this problem, new federal legislation to expand health insurance coverage to children was passed in September 1997. In the Balanced Budget Act of 1997 (P.L. 105-33), the Social Security Act was amended to add a new title—Title XXI, the State Children's Health Insurance Program (CHIP). Although this effort is a step forward with respect to expanding health insurance coverage for medically indigent populations, it still excludes major groups (e.g., immigrant children, medically indigent adults). Consequently, health care coverage may remain an important influence on decisions to leave welfare, at least for some families, and although the welfare reform law did not affect Medicaid coverage, it is not yet clear how welfare will interface with CHIP.

Further Effects on Health and Well-being

Employment of mothers can have some positive effects on children's development; however, these positive effects have been found in families where mothers voluntarily enter the job market, earn above minimum wage, and have challenging work. For example, Moore and Driscoll[26] found better cognitive functioning and fewer behavioral problems among children whose mothers worked than those whose mothers did not, but the mothers were making at least $7 per hour and engaged in work voluntarily. Others have also found positive effects when mothers work full-time compared with part-time[27] and at more demanding rather than less demanding jobs.[28]

These positive developments are unlikely for most families affected by welfare reform. Families in which parents are unable to work but terminated from assistance will become more impoverished. Those able to find work and remain employed are likely to have better outcomes but unlikely to rise above poverty, at least in the short term. The continued struggles with poverty for both types of families suggest additional, negative effects on family health and well-being. Substantial developmental research has found child poverty to be a risk factor for several negative outcomes. Summarizing numerous studies in this area, Brooks-Gunn and Duncan[29] identified higher incidences of a variety of poor outcomes for children in poverty in the areas of physical health (low birthweight, growth stunting, lead poisoning), cognitive ability (intelligence, verbal ability, achievement scores), school achievement (years of schooling, high school completion), and emotional and behavior outcomes. As one example, a study using data from the National Longitudinal Survey of Youth (NLSY) and the Infant Health and Development Program (IHDP) comparing children in families with incomes less than half of the poverty threshold to those with incomes between 1.5 and 2 times the poverty threshold found the poorer children to score between 6 and 13 points lower on various standardized tests of IQ, verbal ability, and achievement.[30] Poverty also has a strong link to child maltreatment. Data from the National Incidence Study of Child Abuse and Neglect[31] showed that children from families with annual incomes below $15,000 as compared with children from families with annual incomes above $30,000 were more than 22 times more likely to experience some form of maltreatment.

CONCLUSION

This chapter has examined some of the key provisions of the welfare reform legislation and the implications of the legislation for the economic status, health, and well-being of welfare recipients and their children. To summarize, the legislation changed the nature of the federal government's role in providing economic assistance by altering its funding mechanism to states (by providing capped block grants rather than matching funds) and by removing the entitlement status of assistance (that ensured aid to individuals provided they met the program requirements). Additionally, the new legislation institutes two major requirements: families are denied assistance after 5 years and individuals must meet certain work and community service requirements to receive aid. Child care legislation also has been changed to consolidate four previous child care programs into one block grant. Child care, also, is no longer an entitlement and may not be available to many former welfare recipients attempting to enter the labor force.

Medicaid coverage was not directly affected by the changes in the welfare law. Most poor children will continue to be eligible regardless of their family's receipt of welfare benefits. In addition, new legislation (CHIP) that provides added funding to states that either develop or expand low-income children's health insurance is likely to decrease the number of children who lack access to health care. However, this expanded coverage does not include adults. Low-income parents are covered by Medicaid while receiving welfare but will lose Medicaid coverage when they lose cash assistance.

The effects of these changes can be estimated based on earlier research on AFDC recipients and the recent experience of states that used waivers to make changes in their previous AFDC programs. Most AFDC recipients received assistance for a relatively short time period and generally left AFDC when they were able to find work. Long-term recipients generally have been found to have less education and fewer skills and so have required greater supports to enter the job market. In the current economy, low-skilled jobs are often available, so that many of those voluntarily leaving, or being forced off, welfare will be able to find work. Nonetheless, the type of work available usually is not sufficient to lift a family out of poverty. Limitations on access to child care and health insurance coverage aggravate a family's ability to get and maintain work. Therefore, unless long-term job training, access to child care, and health insurance coverage are expanded, the prospects for economic well-being are poor. Given the well-known relationship between poverty and numerous negative life outcomes, the prospects for more general health and well-being are also poor.

These conclusions lead to some specific recommendations. First, given the widespread changes and the potential for negative outcomes, systems for monitoring the effects of welfare reform are imperative. The potential implications outlined in this chapter are based on research examining previous AFDC populations. It is unknown exactly what the effects will be and whether positive and negative unanticipated effects will occur. Such important policy changes require careful monitoring and research as well as early dissemination regarding successful and unsuccessful results. Second, the role of job training and access to educational opportunities in assisting people in both exiting and avoiding welfare needs to be re-emphasized. Because the profile of those at risk for long-term dependency is fairly clear, early intervention efforts with adolescent mothers to assist them in completing high school and continuing on to higher education or vocational training have the potential for achieving the greatest long-term benefits. High-quality educational and training experiences are needed to address the educational deficits of this population. Third, high-quality and accessible child care is a national concern for parents at all income levels who want to be part of the work force. Addressing the problem will require strategies that increase the aggregate supply of child care, provide child care options, enhance and monitor the quality of care, and prioritize child care slots for low-income individuals who are likely to have fewer options. These and other strategies for assisting low-income populations will benefit from solutions that are focused toward the long term. A short-term view, aimed primarily at reducing the welfare rolls is likely to do little to relieve poverty and, in the long run, will create further problems requiring policy interventions.

References

1. Behrman, R.E. *The future of children*. Center for the Future of Children, Los Altos, CA. 1997;7(1):1.
2. Handler, J. *The poverty of welfare reform*. New Haven: Yale University Press, 1995.
3. Pavetti, L. Who is affected by time limits? In I. Sawhill (ed). *Welfare reform: An analysis of the issues*. Washington DC: Urban Institute, 1995.
4. Harris, K.M. Work and welfare among single mothers in poverty. *American Journal of Sociology*. 1993;99(2):317–352.
5. Duncan, G.J., Harris, K.M., and Boisjoly, J. *Time limits and welfare reform: New estimates of the number and characteristics of affected families*. Chicago: Northwestern University/University of Chicago Joint Center for Poverty Research; 1997. Available online at www.spc.uchicago.edu/PovertyCenter/limit/21.html.
6. U.S. General Accounting Office. *Welfare reform: States' early experiences with benefit termination*. GAO/HEHS-97-74. Washington, DC: U.S. General Accounting Office, 1997.
7. Danziger, S.K., and Danziger, S. Will welfare recipients find work when welfare ends? In I. Sawhill (ed). *Welfare reform: An analysis of the issues*. Washington, DC: Urban Institute, 1995. Available online at http://www.urban.org/welfare/overview.htm.
8. Burtless, G. Welfare recipients job skills and employment prospects. *The Future of Children*. 1997;7(1):39–51.
9. Holzer, H. *What employers want: Job prospects for less-educated workers*. New York: Russell Sage Foundation, 1996.
10. Kirshenmann, J., and Neckerman, K. We'd love to hire them but. . . . In C. Jencks, and P. Peterson (eds). Washington, DC: The Brookings Institute, 1991.
11. Lundgren-Gaveras, L., and Cohen, I. The new skills mismatch: An examination of urban employers' perceptions about public job training participants as prospective employees. *Journal of Social Services Research*. 1999.
12. Nightingale, D.S., and Holcomb, P.A. Alternative strategies for increasing employment. *The Future of Children*. 1997;7(1):52–64.
13. Riccio, J., Friedlander, D., and Freedman, S. GAIN: Benefits, costs, and three-year impacts of a welfare-to-work program. New York: Manpower Demonstration Research Corporation, 1994.
14. Friedlander, D., and Burtless, G. *Five years after: The long-term effects of welfare-to-work programs*. New York: Russell Sage Foundation, 1995.
15. Danziger, S., and Gottschalk, P. *America unequal*. Cambridge, MA: Harvard University Press, 1996.
16. Brandon, P. What happens to single mothers after AFDC? *Focus*. 1995;17(2):13–15.
17. Burtless, G. Employment prospects of welfare recipients. In D.S. Nightingale, and R.H. Haveman (eds). *The work alternative: Welfare reform and the realities of the job market*. Washington, DC: The Urban Institute, 1994.

18. Pavetti, L. *Moving up, moving out or going nowhere?: A study of the employment patterns of young women.* Washington, DC: The Urban Institute, 1997. Available online at http://www.urban.org/welfare/jobtr.htm.

19. Pavetti, L. The dynamics of welfare and work: Exploring the process by which young women work their way off welfare. Cambridge, MA.: Malcolm Wiener Center for Social Policy, Harvard University, 1993.

20. Harris, K.M. Life after welfare: Women, work, and repeat dependency. *American Sociological Review.* 1996;61(3): 407-426.

21. Nightingale, D.S., Wissoker, D., Burbridge, L.C., Bawden, D.L., and Jeffries, N. *Evaluation of the Massachusetts Employment and Training (ET) Choices Program.* Washington, DC: Urban Institute Press, 1991.

22. Hershey, A.M., and Pavetti, L.A. Turning job finders into job keepers. *The Future of Children.* 1997;7(1):74–86.

23. Kisker, E.E., and Ross, C.M. Arranging child care. *The Future of Children.* 1997;7(1):99–109.

24. U.S. General Accounting Office. Child care subsidies increase likelihood that low income mothers will work. GAO. Washington, DC: GAO, 1994.

25. Meyers, M.K. Child care in a JOBS employment and training program: What difference does quality make? *Journal of Marriage and the Family.* 1993;55(3):767–783.

26. Moore, K.A., and Driscoll, A.K. *The Future of Children.* 1997;7(1):122–127.

27. Woods, M.B. The unsupervised child of the working mother. *Developmental Psychology.* 1972;6(1):14–25.

28. Piotrkowski, C.S., and Katz, M.H. Indirect socialization of children: The effects of mothers' jobs on academic behaviors. Child Development. 1982;53(6):1520–29.

29. Brooks-Gunn, J., and Duncan, G.J. The effects of poverty on children. *The Future of Children.* 1997;7(2):55–71.

30. Smith, J.R., Brooks-Gunn, J., and Klebanov, P. The consequences of living in poverty for young children's cognitive and verbal ability and early school achievement. In G.J. Duncan, and J. Brooks-Gunn (eds). Consequences of growing up poor. New York: Russell Sage Foundation, 1997.

31. Sedlak, A.J., and Broadhurst, D.D. The third national incidence study of child abuse and neglect. Washington DC: U.S. Department of Health and Human Services, 1996.

11

Child Care

Robert C. Fellmeth

Demand for Child Care in the 21st Century

In 1995, of the nation's 21 million children younger than 6 years of age, 13 million were in child care. Among children younger than the age of 1, 45% received regular child care.[1]

Current Demand: Working Mothers

Child care demand has been driven traditionally by the number of women in the work force. Even the parents of young children are increasingly working. By 1995, almost 60% of women in the United States with children younger than age 3 were working.[2] The trend is expected to continue. In 1992, 75% of all women between the ages of 25 and 54 were working; and the Bureau of Labor Statistics projects that proportion to increase to 83% by 2005.[3]

Full-time child care for preschoolers is divided into two submarkets: full-day infant care and full-day toddler care. Both are included in the numbers previously cited. In addition, demand for a third submarket, part-time day care for those in school, is also increasing as more women work.

Surveys of the important preschool (full-day) submarket indicate who are the identities of current providers. Where mothers are employed, almost 39% of children younger than the age of 5 are now cared for in another's home, and 25.8% are cared for in organized child care facilities. A 1996 Census Bureau population report found 30% of preschoolers in organized child care facilities (centers), 21% with non-relative child care providers (family day care or in-home babysitters), 17% with grandparents, 16% with their fathers, 9% with other relatives, and 7% whose mother worked at home or in other miscellaneous arrangements.[4] The incidence of care by relatives is substantially higher where family income is below the poverty line, with 60% placed with relatives, compared with 46% of children in higher income families.[4]

New Demand: Single-Parent Families and the Effect of Welfare Reform

In addition to the current child care demand created by households in which both parents work outside the home, additional demand comes from unemployed parents who live below the poverty line and who would require child care in order to work. Welfare reform implemented in 1998 requires employment of a large number of parents now receiving Temporary Aid for Needy Families (TANF) assistance (formerly Aid to Families with Dependent Children [AFDC]) (see later discussion of the Personal Responsibility and Work Opportunity Reconciliation Act of 1996).

Impoverished families are a critical new source of demand for child care, because work is required to avoid TANF safety net cut-offs for affected children. As cut-offs begin, there is much concern over the impact on children among those working with the poor. Legal immigrants (non-refugees) arriving after August 1996 now face denial of most safety net help for their children if they experience financial hardship. Parents unable to find jobs over the next 5 years face draconian cuts that would make housing and proper nutrition problematical for many. Mitigation of increasing child harm is impeded by a media which "averts its face" to the impact of welfare reform on children. The media have been preoccupied with celebrities and tabloid trivia, and when welfare reform has received attention, children have been substantially excluded. The rationale behind AFDC was the safety net protection of children, but a major survey found that only 6% of media coverage of the radical alteration of welfare (welfare reform) focused on children. More than two thirds of the articles surveyed did not mention children in their coverage.[5]

Another impediment to mitigation is the public's picture of welfare families, demonized by opportunistic politicians and colored by a parade of afternoon talk show misfits—the welfare queen, a minority, unmarried teen, demanding a right to motherhood at public expense, producing fatherless children who perpetuate the dependency pattern in ever larger numbers and who constitute gangs, increase crime, and incur imprisonment expense.

A subset of TANF families corresponds to this stark picture, but a study of California's recipients reveals the remarkable error in its generalization; the AFDC parent's average age is 31, unmarried mothers younger than 19 make up only 2% of families receiving aid; the average number of children among single-parent recipients is 1.9, and the average child support received from absent fathers is $28 per child per month (much of which goes to recompense public agencies for TANF grants).[6] Fewer of the poor were receiving AFDC, and at substantially reduced grant levels, in 1996 than in the 1970s or 1980s. The TANF account makes up less than 1.5% of the federal budget; 70% of the recipients are children.[6]

Although a large number of recipients have married and have responsibly planned their children, intending to provide for their care, those representing irresponsible decisions by females, or predatory behavior by males, have clearly increased. The growth in the number of single-parent births—not just by teens, but also by older women—forms a substantial portion of the new child care potential demand population.

The employment mandate of the Personal Responsibility and Work Opportunity Reconciliation Act (PRA) brings the single-parent dilemma—child care costs versus work—front and center. The single-parent population's poverty level and incidence increase combine to add appreciably to child poverty. Single-parent families with children live below the poverty line at about five times the rate of married couples with children.[6]

Table 11.1 presents census data detailing the disparity between children who live in married versus single-parent households. Single persons living alone (without children) have a median income of $27,495. Households with one child younger than 6 years old living with a female single parent have a median family income of $11,243, and two persons to clothe, house, and feed. Single-parent households with two or more children younger than 6 years old have a median annual income of $6,948, and must provide for three or more persons. Low income to the degree indicated by these numbers correlates with deficient nutritional intake, IQ diminution, and child disability, which may be particularly critical during brain development from birth to age 6.[7]

Children living in two-parent families consistently have median household incomes three to five times the amount in single-parent households. The disparity holds for all ethnic groups. For example, the median income of the African American two-parent household with multiple children, some younger than 6 and some older than 6, is $34,690; where there is one child older than 6, it is $42,370.[8] Because

TABLE 11.1

U.S. Income of Families with Children: Married vs. Single Parents

All Races	Median Income	
	Married Parents	Female Single Parent
1 child, younger than 6	$40,938	$11,243
1 child, 6–17	$48,869	$18,050
2 or more children, all younger than 6	$40,952	$6,948
2 or more children, some younger than 6, some 6–17	$40,815	$9,742
2 or more children, all 6–17	$47,429	$16,330
No children	$39,766	$27,495

TABLE 11.2

U.S. *Number and Income Trends by Types of Families with Children*

	Single Female Parent		**Single Male Parent**		**Married Couple Parents**	
	No.*	Median Income	No.*	Median Income	No.*	Median Income
1974	4,400	$14,103	424	$28,906	25,236	$40,298
1980	5,634	$14,429	NA	NA	24,927	$41,435
1986	6,297	$13,007	NA	NA	24,645	$43,955
1992	8,230	$13,445	1,549	$22,366	25,714	$44,483

*No. is in 1,000s of households.
 NA, not available.

married couples generally have children a number of years after marriage and as incomes begin to rise, they have a higher median income than do childless couples.*

As Table 11.2 indicates, the overall median income of single females with children is $13,445, as reported in 1992 census data. The overall median income for two-parent households with children is $44,483. The trend in adjusted income is down for single-female or single-male households and up slightly in real spending power for two-parent families with children. Notwithstanding this stark disparity and trend, the number of parents choosing to have children without a second parent, divorcing, or parenting alone for other reasons has doubled from 4.8 million in 1974 to 9.8 million in 1992 and has increased further during the 1990s.

The number of children in single-parent households reached 18.9 million by 1995, according to the most recent (1996) census data. The 5.9 million of these who live with mothers who never married have a median family income of $9,989 per year; 62% of this group lives below the poverty line. The 48.3 million children who live with both parents enjoy a median family income of $46,195 per year, and 10.9% live below the poverty line.[9]

The PRA includes a list of new requirements for those receiving TANF aid. Most germane to child care is the work requirement. The PRA imposes a statutory 60-month absolute limit on TANF grant assis-

---

*This is partly a reflection of length of time working, since younger couples who have not yet had children are closer statistically to initial entry into the work force. It also suggests enhanced resources for children where there is such a delay.

tance; increasing percentages of those receiving aid must be employed full time to avoid federal funding penalties; and states may require employment of TANF parents at earlier intervals. Many jurisdictions are implementing cut-offs of TANF at the 2-year mark for those who have not obtained employment.

The federal statute does require states to provide those who must work with "adequate child care." Child advocates have demanded compliance with this requirement at state and local levels. State governors and the President have announced what appear to be large financial commitments for its provision. All proposed amounts, when combined with what has already been appropriated, would fund child care for a very small proportion of those who must obtain work or suffer TANF cut-offs. However, there is unlikely to be a child care funding shortfall for this particular group because there are not jobs available in the private sector for the vast majority of those receiving TANF assistance.* And although the original Republican Wisconsin model promised a public service job where private employment was unavailable, the PRA and implementing states have opted to abandon this option or to use it only marginally.

One alleged theory behind the PRA is a desire by some to "stop feeding the pigeons." If procreation decisions are monetarily or maternally motivated, it is reasoned, making parents work (at jobs likely not of their choice) and inhibiting "maternal" time by child care substitution could discourage single and impoverished parent birth rates. But the provision of such public service employment and child care would cost substantially more than the rejected AFDC system.

Instead, the mix of incentives adopted is the worst possible alternative for children. TANF grant assistance is assured for 2 years, through early infancy without work requirements. Unless procreation decisions by the poor are made with planning horizons of more than 2 years in the future, the basic economic incentive to eschew abstinence and ignore family planning remains in place. Instead, the PRA format maintains the allegedly perverse incentive decried by PRA sponsors until the child bonds and is too old to be easily adoptable. *Then* the cut-off is imposed.

State and federal officials count on the lack of jobs to save child care costs. Without even greater expenditures for public service jobs (not a likely prospect), the large child care sums ostentatiously and

---

*See detailed discussion of numbers in the expanding job market of California in reference 6: 700,000 TANF parents must compete for a record 400,000 to 600,000 new jobs with 1 million non-TANF candidates for full-time work and another 600,000 for part-time employment. The non-TANF competition is generally more educated, qualified, experienced, and healthy.

proudly announced by public officials for this population are irrelevant. Public officials know that child care is not needed unless jobs exist, and the promised funds will not be spent given the lack of that condition precedent. TANF cuts, however, can proceed. The consequences are dire for millions of children from the mix of employment, child care, and cut-off policy choices made through the PRA.

Notwithstanding this predicted tragedy, child care provision remains important in three respects: (1) To provide an opportunity for as many TANF recipients as possible to meet work requirements and escape cut-offs; some additional TANF parents will obtain jobs and need the "adequate child care" that federal law requires. (2) To allow large numbers of working poor parents to rise above the poverty line toward self-sufficiency in the lower middle class (and to prevent them from falling back into poverty). (3) To improve the quality of care, so the additional time children spend in such care is enriching and educational, rather than a form of warehousing to accommodate adult needs.

Child Care Costs in Relation to Family Income

Two studies have found that child care costs account for 24% to 31% of the budget of the working poor, but only 6% of the budget of upper middle class taxpayers.[9]

For the impoverished, child care costs can preclude meaningful reward for work without subsidy. Table 11.3 presents the average monthly cost of child care in California for 1994. The precise charge varies by facility, but the averages and price ranges represented apply

TABLE 11.3

1994 California Average Monthly Child Care Costs

	Family Day Care	Day Care Center
Infant	$500	$600
Preschooler (2–5)	$400	$400
School-Age	$150 to $216	$190 to $240

These figures are based on surveys in separate counties involving a sample of 13,305 interviews by the Field Research Corporation. Variations in cost by location are substantial, reflecting varying real estate values and costs of living. The rural county figures are generally lower than the averages cited. The specific monthly means for child care centers within the three highest population counties are as follows: infants—Los Angeles $591, San Diego $485, San Francisco $704; preschoolers—Los Angeles $388, San Diego $357, San Francisco $495. The monthly means for family day care centers are as follows: infants—Los Angeles $480, San Diego $425, San Francisco $541; preschoolers—Los Angeles $300, San Diego $265, San Francisco $543.

to the vast majority of families. In 1995, the average cost of full-time child care in a licensed child care center was $7,020 per year for a child younger than 2 years old, and $4,888 per year for a child aged 2 to 5.[11] The 1994 annual rate for after-school care at a child care center was $1,800 to $2,900 per child.[12]

A single mother working full-time at minimum wage with two children younger than 5 (infants or preschool) will earn—after Social Security and other deductions—about the same amount as her child care will cost. One infant will cost 75% of the mother's take-home pay; two children older than 6 will leave her with $3,000 per year in net earned income.

Current Child Care Supply and Assistance

The number of licensed child care centers has responded partially to increased demand, growing almost 300% between 1975 and 1990, with the number of children in child care increasing fourfold.[13] In addition, the number of organized preschool programs for 3- to 5-year-olds has grown in many states to satisfy some of the demand for toddler care. However, these programs, such as federal Head Start and state counterparts, are often structured for half-day duration or for 4 days per week and must be supplemented with additional care where parents must work full-time.

Notwithstanding substantial increases in spaces and subsidies, child care supply remains inadequate and too expensive for much of the demand. Subsidies meet only a fraction of the need, leading to long waiting lists for assistance throughout the nation, large numbers of latchkey children, and substantial reliance on sometimes problematical relative or sibling care, particularly among the impoverished. Measuring this shortfall in light of the additional needs of TANF parents required to work, a General Accounting Office study of four cities and counties concluded that "the current supply of known child care [is] inadequate for meeting even the demand they currently face for children in certain age groups, particularly for low-income populations . . . for example, we estimated that the supply of known child care in Chicago would be sufficient to meet just 14 percent of the demand for infant care that will probably exist by the end of fiscal year 1997."[14]*

---

*The study examined infant, preschool (toddler), and school-age child care in Baltimore, Chicago, and in Benton and Linn Counties in Oregon. The survey found only the supply for preschool children in Baltimore meeting even pre–welfare reform demand. As to the other jurisdictions and groups, supply met from 16% of demand in Chicago for infants to 92% for Benton County preschoolers, with the average approximating 50%.

Consistent with rapid growth in demand and supply, public subsidies for special populations needing assistance have increased as well. The General Accounting Office has identified more than 90 federal funding programs for child care, administered by 11 agencies. Most are specialized programs serving circumscribed populations such as the military, disabled respite care, and college students. Child care complexity is further exacerbated by state programs supplementing their federal counterparts, particularly state-funded preschool programs, or general child care subsidies separate and apart from federal funding streams.

Federally originated programs, which contribute federal funds to state agencies for state administration, have traditionally focused on the AFDC (TANF) program and are largely intended to facilitate the employment of parents on welfare. Historically, these programs have included child care under the federal Job Opportunities and Basic Skills (JOBS) program—combining job training, placement, and child care for TANF parents. Realizing that when these parents obtain jobs, they are unable to continue if child care support is lacking, the federal government advanced "transitional child care" for up to 1 year to those who were newly employed (now extending to two years in some states). Then the federal government, eventually acceding to the obvious, developed "at-risk" child care directed at those who are working but are likely to regress into welfare dependency without child care assistance. Unfortunately, each of these programs (and others) has separate rules, application procedures, and administrative costs—with many parents forced out of employment as they fall between or outside the discrete and separate programs. And they have historically been administered by state departments of social services, separately from the extensive state child care programs often run by state departments of education.

Many of the federal and state programs became indirectly coordinated through the evolution of "resource and referral" (R&R) agencies in most states. These agencies have served very successfully as a "marketplace" for child care—both privately paid and publicly subsidized. Very simply, family child care providers and child care centers notify their local R&R agency when they have slots available and provide information to the R&R about their facilities. The R&R agency also helps on the supply side by assisting new providers with state licensure. Each R&R agency has a widely publicized local hotline number. When a parent needs child care, the line is called and an expert discusses available slots, their location and features. Importantly, the R&R agency also has expertise in available subsidies and can determine whether a parent may qualify and help with the paperwork.

Head Start programs are structurally distinct. Unlike most other federally mandated programs, Head Start is not funded through state agencies but is operated directly by the federal government.

In addition to federal assistance to state programs, separate state programs, and the stand-alone Head Start program, both federal and state jurisdictions sometimes enact tax expenditures. These are usually tax credits to pick up part of child care expenses through tax forbearance, or to businesses who provide child care facilities or services. The major existing subsidy is a federal child care credit. A family whose income is less than $10,000 annually may claim 30% of its child care costs as a tax credit; a family whose income is more than $28,000 annually may claim 20%. The maximum cost for which a credit may be claimed is $2,400 for one child and $4,800 for two or more children.* Studies of the federal system indicate that the credit benefits some poor families, but also tends to extend to the middle class more than do the direct subsidy programs.[15][†]

The Goal of Self-Sufficiency

In addition to child care demand and supply vis-a-vis the private sector, and the issue of subsidies for the impoverished to remove them from welfare dependency, there is a third area of important subsidy demand: the working poor, who are unable to rise above the poverty line and into self-sufficiency without a sliding scale of child care assistance to ease the way.

The scheduled minimum wage increases and the existing federal Earned Income Tax Credit (EITC) will put full-time workers heading the benchmark family of three just above the poverty line if earning the enhanced minimum wage.[‡] A family of four (a parent and three children)

---

*A separate federal "Wee Tot" Earned Income Tax Credit (EITC) Supplement allowed a credit of 5% of earned income up to $388 for a parent who stays home to care for a newborn and in so doing loses eligibility for straight earned income tax credit benefits. That credit was repealed in 1994.

†A study by Harvard University's Professor Bruce Fuller surveyed 1,800 child care centers in 36 states and concluded that families with annual incomes of more than $50,000 pay just 6% of their incomes for child care, whereas families earning less than $15,000 devote 23% of their income for child care. The tax credits provide a tax expenditure of $4 billion annually. One third of the credit goes to families with incomes above $50,000 per year.

‡For example, a full-time worker earning $5.75 per hour will receive $11,960 per year in gross income. After Social Security, Medicare, and state SDI deductions, maximum take-home pay would be $10,991. The maximum EITC credit for a worker with two dependent children is $3,556 and does not provide a credit for additional children. Adding the maximum EITC credit equals $14,547 for full-time work, about 6% more than the $13,655 poverty line for a family of three for 1998.

TABLE 11.4

Wages Necessary to Achieve Self-Sufficiency

For Family with 1 Adult, 1 Infant, 1 Preschooler	Los Angeles–Long Beach, CA	Tulare County, CA
Housing	$855.00	$480.00
Child care	$759.75	$571.45
Food	$281.40	$281.40
Transportation	$117.81	$117.81
Medical care	$176.79	$176.79
Miscellaneous	$219.07	$162.74
Total Taxes (minus EITC and CCTC)	$448.62	$268.77
Earned Income Tax Credit (EITC) (−)	$0.00	($108.75)
Child Care Tax Credit (CCTC) (−)	($80.00)	($92.00)
Self-sufficiency wage (monthly)	$2,858.44	$1,858.56
Self-sufficiency wage (hourly)	$16.24	$10.56

The standard is calculated using U.S. Department of Housing and Urban Development annual Fair Market Rents; State Market Surveys of Child Care, U.S. Department of Agriculture, Low-Cost Food Plan; average costs of commuting using public transportation if available or ownership of 6-year-old car where public transportation is not available; medical costs based on full-time work with employer-provided health coverage, estimated costs from Families USA, National Medical Expenditure Survey; miscellaneous expenses of 10% of all other costs; taxes include sales tax, state income tax, payroll tax, and federal income tax.

would have an income just over 80% of the poverty level at the enhanced minimum wage, and including the maximum EITC benefit.[6,16]*

Apart from the minimum wage, average hourly wages of females from 15 to 24 years of age who have not completed high school or who have only a high school diploma have dropped 16% between 1979 and 1993 in constant dollars. In 1979, 18.5% of all households headed by females from 15 to 24 years old lived below the poverty line; by 1993, the proportion climbed to 38.1% for all races, and to 63% for young African American women.[17]†

Table 11.4 indicates the income needed by a single-parent family with two children (one infant and one preschool child) to be economically self-sufficient in Los Angeles and Tulare counties in California, representing high-cost urban and moderate-cost rural settings, respectively. The amounts shown, based on a series of economic studies, assume minimum housing/nutrition needs and no subsidies.[18]

Under the Bureau of the Census' official poverty thresholds, the study's urban family requiring $34,296 annually or the rural

---

*The estimated poverty line for a family of four is $16,968 for 1998 in this calculation.
†Note that over the same 1979–1993 period, the top 5% of all income earners increased their income 35% in constant dollars, from $89,000 to $121,000.

family needing $22,296 would not be considered poor unless income for a parent and two children is below $1,049 per month, or $12,588 annually.[1]

For those who are able to obtain work, the EITC and higher minimum wage promise to move large numbers of parents and families to the area of $1,000 to $1,400 per month in take-home income. But the various subsidies for impoverished parents (some designed to protect children) here interact to create a difficult barrier to income from the poverty line to this "liveable wage," which would allow modest shelter, adequate nutrition, and child care without public subsidy.

As a single mother of two passes $1,000 per month, she sequentially loses AFDC (now TANF), begins to acquire federal (and some state) tax liability, loses food stamps, progressively loses the EITC, loses eligibility for subsidized school lunches, loses priority for subsidized child care, and loses Medicaid.* Private sector child care and medical coverage for dependents are increasingly rare.[6] The rate of fall-off of this assistance places many parents in a quandary—additional earnings can reduce net benefits available for the family.

The two major costs impeding self-sufficiency as subsidies drop off at the poverty line are housing and child care. Child care costs are critical; it is the single largest expense for working parents with more than two children, or with two children younger than 5, or with two children outside high-rent urban settings.

Quality

A four-state study of quality in child care centers found that only 14% could be rated as high in quality.[19] The Packard Foundation's Center for the Future of Children concluded that "(1) the quality of services is mediocre, on average; (2) the cost of full-time care is high; (3) at the present time, the cost of increasing quality from mediocre to good is not great, about 10%; and (4) good child care is dependent on professionally approved staffing ratios, well educated staff, [and] low staff turnover.[20] One of the leading authorities in the field concludes that the state of child care "reflect(s) the low priority given to children's care and women's work in American society."[20]

---

*1997 federal legislation allocates new tobacco tax funds for child health, allowing Medicaid expansion to 200% or more of the poverty line. Many states are using these funds for private medical care add-on programs, which require substantial co-payments, both per visit and on a monthly basis. Parents are not covered for their own expenses. The new funding may allow a reduction of up to $80 per month in the projected $176 per month medical costs listed in Table 11.4.

CHILD CARE CHANGES AS THE 20TH CENTURY ENDS

Child Care Provisions in the Personal Responsibility and Work Opportunity Reconciliation Act

The 1996 enactment of the PRA led to the creation of a new Child Care and Development Fund (CCDF). This fund absorbed both the "transitional" and the "at-risk" programs described earlier and included as well the old Child Care and Development Block Grant (CCDBG), creating a single "super child care block grant." Under this new "capped entitlement" funding scheme, states receive a mandatory base amount at the level each received previously under Title IV-A in 1992–1994, 1994 alone, or 1995 alone, whichever is highest. These funds are sent as a block grant without any required state match, unlike the previous programs they absorbed. The Congress then appropriated $7.2 billion in total for the grant over 6 years.

A state may obtain additional funds beyond this block grant on a matching basis if the state (1) obligates all of the block grant money allocated to it for the fiscal year it seeks new money, and (2) spends at least as much as it has been spending from its own resources in matching federal funds or in providing its own child care. In other words, more money is available beyond the block grant on a matching basis, so long as the state is spending above and beyond what it previously spent on child care and is not diverting previous state commitment so it can be "supplanted" with federal funds.* If the state complies, it can get its share (based on its percentage of the nation's children younger than 13 years of age) of another $3.5 billion in federal capped entitlement funds at fiscal year 1995 rates. The state must match this funding on a 50/50 basis.

States must spend at least 70% of all of these funds on TANF recipients, those leaving TANF, or those in danger of falling back onto TANF (see the three federal programs described previously and now within the block grant).

As noted, this Child Care and Development Fund also includes the previous Child Care and Development Block Grant (CCDBG),

---

*Such a supplantation danger is an endemic problem in federal-state and state-county relations; the larger jurisdiction wishes to subsidize an increase in resources in an area, which is frustrated when the new money is taken, and an equivalent amount previously spent by the receiving jurisdiction for the subsidized purpose is then subtracted and diverted elsewhere or "supplanted." To discourage these diversions, the donor jurisdiction often requires that there be a "maintenance of effort" (MOE) by agencies receiving funds—to ensure that it maintains the same spending it had been committing and treats new money as a genuine "add-on."

which had financed the resource and referral agencies described earlier, given grants for quality improvement (monitoring, training, technical assistance), and expended 78% of its funds on direct services to purchase child care with certificates, contracts, grants, or as part of before- and after-school care—mostly for the working poor.* This CCDBG continues within the Fund at $6 billion nationally over the next 6 years but is subject to annual appropriations approval. Money not obligated by the state by the end of the fiscal year reverts to the federal government for redistribution to other states.

Although these are substantial increases, the Congressional Budget Office has estimated that if states simply maintain current spending for the working poor so they can remain on the job and meet the minimum work requirements of TANF recipients, the spending is $1.4 billion short over its 6-year period.[21]

Whatever the prospects of meeting these counts through job production, increases are necessarily limited by child care availability. Further, child care aid withdrawal from the currently working poor will stimulate their job losses and add to the recipient population—cancelling the gain made from a newly employed TANF parent taking that child care aid.

The Child Care and Development Fund combines three existing Title IV-A programs, including the at-risk category of working poor, resource and referral provision, and spending for child care quality enhancement. It feeds some of the other substantive programs previously listed.

The President's 1998 Proposal for Child Care

The President's 1998 proposal involves an increase in public funding and tax credits of $21.3 billion over 5 years. Over this timeline, the proposal would

- Add $7.5 billion to the Child Care and Development Fund, doubling the number of potential recipients (from 1 million to 2 million). A state match is required.

- Add $3.4 billion for Head Start and for Early Head Start, bringing the total number of children in the former to 1 million and in the latter to 40,000.

---

*Most of its clients were the working poor—with 67% earning below the poverty line, and 90% below 150% of the line. Essentially, it funded parents who were at risk of falling back onto AFDC (TANF) but had not been on AFDC previously and therefore would not be eligible for the at-risk program.

- Add $800 million to a currently small ($200 million) before/after-school program for school-age children. The 21st Century Community Learning Center Program requires local matches to create school- or locally based child care.

- Add $3 billion in challenge grants to local communities (administered by states) to improve learning quality and safety in facilities serving preschool children. Funds may be used for training, licensing and accreditation, linking child care to health services, reducing child-caregiver ratios, providing home visits, and parent/consumer education.

- Allocate $250 million for student child care accreditation scholarships, to provide 50,000 scholarships per year over the 5-year timeline.

- Add $500 million to fund state enforcement of minimum safety and health standards.

- Increase tax expenditures by $5.2 billion in the form of credits for families who use the Dependent Care Tax Credit. The additional credit will provide an additional average tax cut of $358 for families whose income is below $60,000.

- Provide $500 million in new tax credits to businesses that provide child care facilities for their employees, expand existing facilities, train child care workers, or provide resource and referral help to employees. The credit covers 25% of qualified expenses with a per business cap of $150,000 per year.

The President proposes substantial additional investment in the supply and quality of child care. His proposal does not address some important problems. It does not resolve the balkanized fragmentation of agencies, programs, requirements, and subsidies. This failure is particularly important to those who suffer TANF cuts. Along with those cut-offs comes the loss of the social worker who has previously coordinated child care (and Medicaid) subsidies, to make participation where needed more likely.

The proposed program does not address the paramount question of TANF cut-offs. How much of the proposed additions to the Child Care and Development Fund (the largest new commitment) will be needed given limited private employment vis-a-vis those required to work? Why does a proposal not calculate how many will be cut off not because they have refused a job, but because none is offered or available? How much would be required to provide public service employment for this group whose children face cut-offs unprecedented over the last two generations? After the requisite need is determined, how much is required for child care subsidy? The amount will be many times the figure proposed.

Finally, the program does not consider the working poor. The single parent attempting to work her way into self-sufficiency is not appreciably assisted by the mix of new programs offered. The tax credits are not expected to be "refundable"—a critical error that allows them to disproportionately benefit the middle class not requiring this help and to abandon the impoverished and working poor.* The existing Fund increases will only be relevant to the extent that new jobs are won by generally less qualified TANF parents, as discussed earlier. The working poor population is not given the critical child care bridge into self-sufficiency.

A Vision for Child Care in the New Millennium

Adequate Supply

The first requirement must be an adequate supply of spaces where acceptable relative care is unavailable and an adequate subsidy to allow parents to work. This requirement is essential where parents suffer TANF cut-offs if not employed.

If the national policy to restrict the safety net protection of children continues, adults and not children must face the consequences. The current paradigm is a game of musical chairs for millions of children, with the TANF parents of more than 3 million children certain to be left standing when the music stops and unemployment continues. Those children are then in a catch-22 no civilized society can countenance: parents are cut off from basic safety net support and their children must either go without essentials or suffer surrender by otherwise loving and competent parents to whom they have bonded into state foster care (at a public cost substantially more than that of TANF). If we have decided to inhibit decisions to have children without ability to provide for them privately, required public service work provides such a disincentive. It, or some other alternative, is ethically compelled short of the current disincentive—reliance on the misery of children.

---

*The Earned Income Tax Credit (EITC) is an example of a refundable credit that benefits the poor. Those who qualify receive a reward regardless of their tax liability. However, the educational and child care credits proposed by the President have been not refundable; they only offset tax liability. Because the working poor are on the edge of tax liability (e.g., annual income in the $10,000 to $14,000 range), they do not owe enough in taxes to use the credit. Those who pay taxes above the level of the credit can take advantage of it.

Where public service employment is provided (or if the PRA sponsors' unrealistic projections of full employment were to prove accurate), child care supply will have to be increased many times the proposed funding in the President's plan, in addition to the costs of public service employment itself. For a somewhat different alternative, see the section on Prevention.

Rational, Efficient, and Comprehensible Child Care

The historical pattern of child care subsidies is a patchwork of federal and state programs to meet the needs of narrow populations or to facilitate removal of parents from welfare rolls. The predictable result has been fragmentation, confusion, inefficiency, barriers to care, and high administrative costs. These problems are exacerbated for parents cut off from TANF. Such a cut-off deprives parents of the single social worker who historically arranges for child care (and Medicaid) options.

It is part of the holy grail of child advocates that children need a seamless system of child care, based on the needs of the children involved. Creating a universal sliding scale of child care subsidy, based on income, is advisable. In the alternative, those needing government services should be able to avail themselves of the same technologic advances used in the private sector to rationalize confusing alternatives. A "social service" card could be issued to all impoverished or otherwise eligible parents, with a magnetic coded strip updated periodically for income, family size, child disabilities, and other qualifying facts. Swiping such a card through a machine could array all available programs, giving a parent the efficiency of a shopper's choice, and the same card would qualify for services chosen without endless forms, trips across town, lines, and interviews for each service each eligible child needs. Either a child needs and deserves a public investment for the benefit of all of us, or not. If so, barriers to its provision should be bureaucratically minimal and technologically facilitated.

Safe and Enriching Child Care

In addition to adequate child care supply, quality is important. Recent research indicates that child care and preschool programs can contribute meaningfully to the cognitive development of a child and assist in his or her socialization. Parental roles remain primary, but attentive and stimulating child care can be a benefit. Unfortunately, the child care industry pays those to whom our children are entrusted low wages, among the lowest in the nation. As discussed previously, the political trend remains focused on warehousing children in the lowest-cost arrangement so parents can work and move off welfare.

In the 21st century, four areas of improvement can lead to fruitful investment in the future of children. First, control over child care should pass from departments of social services concerned about adult welfare accounts to state departments of education concerned about child development.

Second, child care must be intelligently regulated through a licensing system specifying the number and qualifications of providers, ensuring "Trustline" clearance of providers and employees from sex offender lists, subject to facility spot inspections, and subject to a flexible system of civil penalties for violations—high and certain enough to get the attention of providers, yet low enough to maintain the incentive to provide adequate supply.

Third, the increased number of impoverished children in child care gives us the chance to ensure immunization coverage, health checks, and adequate nutrition. The last is currently addressed through the Child and Adult Care Food Program (CACFP), and those young children in child care with parents hovering near the poverty line are especially vulnerable to nutritional shortfall, particularly given food stamp benefit reductions. Moreover, infant and preschool settings reach children during the 0 to 5 years of age period, when brain development makes adequate nutrition a particularly important investment.

Finally, the 21st century should yield creative use of public and marketplace-based incentives to upgrade educational quality, such as scholarships; certification standards; tax credits for computer, educational telecommunications, and other capital enhancements; and higher recompense (including public subsidy premiums) for enhanced quality. A variety of marketplace strategies and rewards, together with public subsidies, can be designed to direct care providers toward further enrichment of the children in their charge, rather than toward higher volume and minimum interaction.

Financing

Public subsidies required may be financed from a wide variety of possible sources. The Ewing Marion Kauffman Foundation and the Pew Charitable Trusts have published a compendium of current financial sources.[22] Current sources of child care financing include children's services special (property) taxing districts (Florida), a special Families and Education Levy (Washington); allocation of a minimum percentage of the budget for children's education or services (California's Proposition 98, San Francisco's Proposition J), a dedicated sales tax (Aspen, CO), a local option sales tax (Ames, IA), a voluntary income tax check-off for child care (Colorado), various state child care and employer tax credits (22 states), enterprise zone tax credits (Colorado), property tax abatement for child care facilities (Travis County, TX), child care licensing fees, vanity license plate revenues (Kids' Plates in California and Massachusetts), lottery revenue (Georgia and Florida), tax exempt bonds (Illinois), state loan guarantees (Maryland), public grants (New York), and others.

The 1980s and 1990s have been a period of "looking out for number one." A long-standing national tradition of sacrifice and investment in our children, to give them more than we had, has been violated. A study of California public spending on children since 1989 created private and public adult "selfishness indices." The former measured maternal unwed birth rates and paternal child support contribution rates, adjusted for inflation. The latter measured almost all public spending for children per child in poverty, as a percentage of adult personal income. Both indices have fallen markedly since 1989, with 1998 representing record levels of adult private and public commitment to themselves over their children.[6] This self-destructive trend is reflected in the disproportionate political power of the elderly, now with a poverty rate one third the level for their grandchildren. Senior citizens, deserving of respect and assistance, receive publicly arranged financial and medical security substantially beyond either provided for the nation's children.

A Path to Self-Sufficiency

Child care is the doorway out of welfare and poverty for the children of single parents. Even with one young child, blue-collar single parents cannot work and surmount the poverty line without child care help. It makes little sense to responsible parents to work full-time to pay someone else to care for their children, and take home virtually no net pay to house and feed them. The result of insufficient assistance is TANF dependency. With TANF timelines, cut-downs to token TANF grants, and reduced food stamps will come increased homelessness and undernutrition.

The plight of single-parent households is particularly stark. Successful child care can do more than provide a safety net stopgap to allow initial employment. In combination with an enhanced Earned Income Tax Credit, it can bridge the gap from the $1,000 to $1,400 per month barrier to eventual self-sufficiency. Without sliding scale assistance well beyond that currently provided, millions of parents are vulnerable to a slide back well below the poverty line, often without a TANF safety net for their children where their previous allocation or state policies preclude it. The goal of a safety net should be a hand up toward self-sufficiency, with the incentive from work always present in the form of incremental financial gain.

Given the dominant role of child care costs in the personal budgets of working parents, it is the critical mechanism (in combination with the EITC) to provide a bridge. Income qualification for child care subsidies should remain 100% up to 125% of the poverty line, and then decline gradually and incrementally as family income increases above that level.

Prevention of Unintended and Unwed Pregnancies

Underlying all recommendations for child care for the 21st century is a new contract for our children. Currently, children are most often an unintended byproduct of adult sex. Many adults treat conception as a form of divine intervention. Intellectually, we all know that it is substantially controllable and that control must be discussed as mature adults.

A covenant can be agreed on, and made a part of our education and culture, that children deserve a bona fide attempt by two married parents to prepare for them and to provide for their needs. If such an ethic were to take hold, much would follow. One consequence would be increased political backing for strong safety net support. Where the cause of child poverty is lay-off, illness, divorce, or trauma affecting parents, public support for child safety net support would be strong and reliable. That support would allow much more to be expended on enriched child care for the smaller number of children then in need. And substantial resources would remain to begin the important work of improving child care quality for all children.

References

1. National Center for Education Statistics, U.S. Department of Education. Quoted in the White House Virtual Library Database, http://www.whitehouse.gov/cgi.
2. Bureau of Labor Statistics. *Employment status of the civilian noninstitutional population by sex, age, presence and age of youngest child, marital status, race, and Hispanic origin.* Washington, DC, U.S. Department of Labor, March, 1995.
3. Bureau of Labor Statistics. Bulletin 2452. Washington, DC, U.S. Department of Labor, April, 1994.
4. Casper, L.M. *Who's minding our preschoolers?* (Current Population Reports). Washington, DC: Bureau of the Census, U.S. Department of Commerce, March, 1996.

5. Children Now. *Children and welfare reform: High stakes, low coverage.* Oakland, CA, January 15, 1998.
6. Fellmeth, R.C. *California Children's Budget 1998–99.* San Diego, CA, Children's Advocacy Institute, 1998.
7. Fellmeth, R.C., Kalemkiarian, S., and Reiter, R. *California children's budget 1995–96.* San Diego, CA, Children's Advocacy Institute, 1995, pp 1–46 and 1–47.
8. Bureau of the Census, U.S. Department of Commerce. *Money income of households, families, and persons in the United States: 1992.* (Current Population Reports, Consumer Income, Series P60-184). Washington, DC, 1993, pp 68–76.
9. Saluter, A. Martial status and living arrangements, Current Population Reports, Washington, DC, Bureau of the Census, U.S. Department of Commerce, 1998, 36.
10. Phillips, D.A. (ed). *Child care of low-income families: Summary of two workshops.* Washington, DC: National Academy Press, 1995.
11. California Child Care Resource and Referral Network. *The California Child Care Portfolio 1997.* San Francisco, 1997.
12. California Child Care Resource and Referral Network. *Regional market rate survey of California child care providers.* San Francisco, 1994, pp 16–17.
13. Willer, B., Hofferth, S., and Kisker, E.E. *The demand and supply of child care in 1990.* Washington, DC: National Association for the Education of Young Children, 1991.
14. U.S. General Accounting Office. *Welfare reform: Implications of increased work participation for child care.* Washington, DC, U.S. Government Printing Office, May, 1997.
15. Ribadeneira, D. Day care credits said to favor well off. *Boston Globe,* September 18, 1992, p 3.
16. Center on Budget and Policy Priorities. *The 1995 Earned Income Credit campaign, EITC participation for tax year 1995, by state.* Washington, DC, 1994.
17. May, R. *1993 poverty and income trends.* Washington, DC, Center on Budget and Policy Priorities. March, 1993, pp 19–20, 61.
18. Pearce, D. Wider Opportunities for Women. *The self sufficiency standard for California.* Washington, DC, 1996, p 5.
19. Helburn, S. (ed). *Cost, quality, and child outcomes in child care centers: Technical report.* Denver, CO: Department of Economics, Center for Research in Economic and Social Policy, University of Colorado, 1995.
20. Helburn, S., and Howes, C. Child care cost and quality. *Financing Child Care.* The Future of Children, Summer/Fall 1996;6(2):79–80.
21. Smith, S., Fairchild, M., and Groginsky, S. National Conference of State Legislatures. *Early childhood care and education: An investment that works.* Washington, DC, January, 1997, p 68. (citing an August 14, 1996 Congressional Budget Office memorandum)
22. *Financing child care in the United States: An illustrative catalog of current strategies.* Ewing Marion Kauffman Foundation and Pew Charitable Trusts, January 13, 1998. See http://www.pewtrusts.com/docs/childcare/index.htm.

12

Child Abuse and Neglect

PATTI R. ROSQUIST AND RICHARD D. KRUGMAN

Whether one approaches family health from a medical, legal, mental health, or social perspective, child abuse and neglect is an enormous and complicated problem. The incidence of child maltreatment is increasing despite recognition of the problem in medical literature for over a century. Recent federal legislation affecting health, welfare and parental visits may exacerbate our ability to deal with the problem. Keys to prevention are being slowly elucidated; however, much research remains to be done. The large task of addressing this issue begins with the willingness to acknowledge that child abuse and neglect exists and that its solution will require a public health approach.

INCIDENCE AND PREVALENCE

The precise incidence and prevalence of child abuse and neglect is difficult to determine. Nonetheless, recent studies are providing more reliable estimates. Despite a decrease in the incidence of unintentional trauma, there continues to be an increase in intentional injury.[1,2] Three million cases are reported to child protective services in the United States each year. More than 1 million of these are confirmed as child abuse or neglect. According to 1993 case-level data on substantiated or indicated victims, 52% suffered from neglect, 20% were victims of physical abuse, 12% were victims of sexual abuse, 4% were victims of emotional maltreatment, and 4% suffered medical neglect.

Almost 30% of victims of child maltreatment were younger than 4 years of age, 25% were from 4 to 7 years old, 21% were 8 to 11, and 26% were 12 to 17. The gender of maltreated children was roughly evenly split between males and females. Forty-three percent of victims of fatal child abuse were younger than 1 year of age. Women were counted as perpetrators 1.6 times as often as men, and perpetrators are five times more likely to be relatives than nonrelatives. More than half of the victims suffered from neglect.[3,4]

When following the incidence of child abuse and neglect over time, the National Incidence Study revealed that there have been significant increases in the incidence of child abuse. The number of abused and neglected children nearly doubled from 1986 to 1993. Girls were sexually abused three times more often than boys; boys had a greater risk of serious injury. Children are consistently vulnerable to sexual abuse from at least as early as the age of 3 years. Family risk factors include single-parent families and poverty. Children in larger families were at greatest risk for neglect.[5]

The rate of victimization of children is approximately 15 per 1,000. About 80% of perpetrators were parents of the victims. Depending on the source, it is reported that between 1,000 and 2,000 children die from severe child abuse each year.[5,6] Some researchers suggest that there is an 85% underestimation because of the way death certificates are recorded, incomplete investigations, and inaccurate medical diagnoses.[6]

In a recent survey about the incidence of physical abuse or sexual abuse in childhood, it was found that childhood maltreatment was common: 30.2% of males and 21.1% of females reported a history of physical abuse; 12.8% of females and 4.3% of males reported a history of sexual abuse.[7]

These incidence and prevalence data tell only part of the story. In addition to the immediate suffering and cost, child maltreatment affects the mental and physical health and development of children for decades. For example, victims have increased rates of adolescent suicide, alcoholism and drug abuse, anxiety and depression, criminality and violence, and learning problems. Melton suggests that although the acute and chronic problems of child maltreatment are great, a broader and equally concerning perspective is that child abuse may reflect the decline of a society.[8] Although knowledge about the incidence, etiology, treatment, and prevention of abuse has increased in recent years, more information is needed.

HISTORICAL PERSPECTIVE

In the United States childrearing practices were traditionally viewed as personal and largely private responsibilities, and therefore the government has been reluctant to legislate in this area. Although the first formal legal response to child abuse and neglect in the United States was documented in 1874, it was not until the early part of the 20th century that organizations were established to address the welfare of children. These Societies for the Prevention of Cruelty to Children were organized by philanthropic organizations primarily in major cities and for the most part addressed the plight of dependent, neglected and abandoned children, as well as those children exploited in the child labor system. Federal legislation regulating child labor, the creation of the Children's Bureau (1912), and the Social Security Act of 1935 all were major events which provided an infrastructure for dealing with the exploitation of children. None of this legislation, however, directly addressed physical exploitation of children and overt child abuse in a meaningful way. Even though evidence of abuse was regularly reported and documented in medical circles, little was done from a public policy perspective, and the problem remained out of the public eye.[9,10] It was not until the early 1960s when C. Henry Kempe's work was published, that major public recognition of the problem began to occur. Considerable attention was paid to the problem in the 1960s: the Children' Bureau developed a model child abuse reporting law, federal regulation required child welfare systems to develop child protection programs, and states improved their legal, detection, enforcement, and service systems. In 1974, the National Center on Child Abuse and Neglect (NCCAN) was created in the U.S. Department of Health and Human Services as an effort to coordinate a national program for improving knowledge, promoting prevention strategies, and improving service systems. Although considerable progress has been made, child abuse continues to be a significant problem. Our understanding of the factors which lead to child abuse, and our knowledge of the best methods to prevent and treat the problem demand continuing improvement.

ETIOLOGY

With respect to one set of societal problems, it has been shown that alcohol and drug use is associated with an increased risk of homicide of other family members.[1] In another study, children born to women who used cocaine during pregnancy were at increased risk for maltreatment. The authors concluded that a mother's cocaine use is a marker of increased risk.[11]

Discipline and parenting is a controversial subject. Corporal punishment of children is actively debated by professionals dealing with children. As more information is gathered, the relationship between spanking and antisocial behavior may be established.[12] Yet the effects of corporal punishment are difficult to separate from the family and social context.[13] Smith found that harsh discipline was associated with lower IQ in children and that harsh discipline plus low maternal warmth was associated with an even greater decline in intelligence.[14] Bross notes that "most child maltreatment is not the product of insanity but rather an exaggeration of accepted practices."[15]

The effects of recent federal legislation may exacerbate some of the complex causes of child maltreatment. Specifically, welfare reform bill H.R. 3734, the Personal Responsibility and Work Opportunity Reconciliation Act of 1996, eliminates Emergency Assistance to Families with Children and Aid to Families with Dependent Children (AFDC) and allows for Temporary Assistance for Needy Families block grants of federal funds to the states. However, the act stipulates that states must have 25% of their welfare recipients engaged in work and that recipients must begin working within 2 years and are limited to 5 years of benefits for a lifetime. Some experts in child abuse and neglect have expressed concerns that these changes may increase the risk for child abuse and neglect. The incidence and severity of child abuse and neglect will need to be monitored as these legislative changes are implemented.

PREVENTION AND INTERVENTION STRATEGIES

The spectrum of etiology, severity, and consequences of child maltreatment is very broad—from relatively subtle effects such as decreases in cognitive function to fatal child abuse, in which context is not relevant. With child maltreatment manifesting in so many ways, it is not surprising that opportunities for intervention, treatment, and prevention are many as well.

There is little agreement on what defines adequate care for our children—whether as parents, citizens, or legislators. The standard of care may be set at various points, from preventing additional harm after a crisis to affirmatively advocating for prevention of abuse. Some professionals attempt to address preventing additional harm, whereas others seek to prevent maltreatment from occurring.

Prevention strategies include both general and specific approaches. Examples of general approaches include community programs that address poverty and violence. Specific strategies include targeted interventions such as a violence prevention curriculum for children[16] or prenatal and early childhood home visits. Such visits have been shown to reduce the number of subsequent pregnancies, use of welfare, child abuse and neglect, and criminal behavior. The effect is greater for women who are unmarried and from low socioeconomic background.[17] Clearly, specific interventions have been shown to modify behavior.[16,17] Unfortunately, a systematic approach to the prevention of child abuse and neglect has not yet been studied.

Consequently, child abuse and neglect prevention research needs to be a funding priority. Regardless of one's role in child protection, decisions must frequently be made based on common sense, experience, and personal beliefs because scientific studies may not have been done to provide a sound, literature-based decision-making process. These gaps in knowledge need to be filled by child protection research. There are many risk factors for abuse. Each of them represents an opportunity for a separate prevention strategy. Successful unintentional injury prevention strategies might be adapted to slow the increase in intentional injuries.[1] Specific needed areas of inquiry include evaluation of current prevention, intervention, and treatment programs, the perception of children of the current child protection system, and the relationship between domestic violence and child maltreatment.[8]

A coordinated, systematic curriculum using existing resources could possibly change attitudes and behavior in a cumulative way. In the meantime, the costs and benefits of many specific interventions remain to be tested. Perhaps children can learn skills that could enhance future parenting effectiveness and promote optimal child development of the next generation.

Beginning with primary and secondary education, some existing curricula teach conflict resolution skills based on the premise that violence is not an acceptable response to conflict. Secondary school students could be targeted for parenting education before they become parents. In early adulthood, susceptible individuals need access to drug, alcohol, and smoking cessation treatment prior to becoming parents. In addition to targeted home visits, prenatal care addressing new parent coping skills might prove helpful in decreasing the incidence of shaken baby syndrome.

Several general parenting issues can be addressed throughout childhood. At pediatric health supervision and immunization visits, health care providers can elicit concerns about behavior and offer age-appropriate anticipatory guidance. Parents need to know about community resources before abuse occurs.

When family dysfunction becomes apparent, early therapeutic intervention may be more effective than later intervention during adolescence. At times, hospitalization of the child becomes necessary. A broader view of child protection to include identifying and building on family strengths may ameliorate the need for foster care in some instances. In the event of fatal child abuse, state fatality review teams can assist communities in identifying specific needs. In other words, many preventive and therapeutic interventions need to be explored in order to find the most cost-effective and humane strategy to approach the problem of child abuse and neglect. The results of such a strategy can only be evaluated by providing long-term follow-up for families.

Cost is an important factor. In 1992, more than $2 billion was spent on foster care alone.[6] We also know that children identified as being at high risk for child abuse or neglect have significantly more hospitalizations.[18] But while the cost of protecting children must be monitored, so ought the cost of not protecting children.

But what if child abuse and neglect were a genetic problem? Whether genetically determined or genetically influenced, the possibility that abusive or neglectful behavior is not merely a social problem could transform how society and health professionals deal with it.

This intriguing possibility should keep anyone from being certain that they know what needs to be done in an area so understudied.[19,20]

CONCLUSION

From this review of incidence, federal legislation, causes, and potential preventive strategies for child maltreatment, the need for a clear statement on child protection policy and focused child protection programs is clear. Such a policy must stem from informed public discussion, acknowledgment of the severity of the problem, and the need to support research. Each individual needs to know more about child abuse. For maternal and child health professionals, this means remaining up to date on current literature. For society, it means investment in research, both biomedical and biosocial, as well as a commitment to outcomes research on programs in place to help children. A comprehensive public policy should be based on known effective strategies and support research to uncover additional approaches. These will likely focus on strengthening neighborhoods and improving parental competence. A system is needed that responds to parents' needs so they can get assistance prior to abuse. The task is large but necessary. After all, the prevention and treatment of child abuse is basic to the preservation of our communities.[19]

References

1. Rivara, F.P., and Grossman, D.C. Prevention of traumatic deaths to children in the United States: How far have we come and where do we need to go? *Pediatrics.* 1997;97:791–797.
2. Rivara, F.P., Mueller, B.A., Somes, G., Mendoza, C.T., Rushforth, N.B., and Kellerman, A.L. Alcohol and illicit drug abuse and the risk of violent death in the home. *JAMA.* 1997;278:(7):569–575.
3. U.S. Department of Health and Human Services, National Center on Child Abuse and Neglect. *Child abuse and neglect case-level data 1993: Working paper 1.* Washington, DC: U.S. Government Printing Office, 1996.
4. U.S. Department of Health and Human Services, National Center on Child Abuse and Neglect. *Child maltreatment 1995: Reports from the states to the National Child Abuse and Neglect Data System.* Washington DC: U.S. Government Printing Office, 1997.
5. Sedlak, A.J., and Broadhurst, D.D. *Executive Summary of the Third National Incidence Study of Child Abuse and Neglect.* Washington, DC: U.S. Department of Health and Human Services, National Center on Child Abuse and Neglect, 1996.
6. U.S. Advisory Board on Child Abuse and Neglect. *A nation's shame: Fatal child abuse and neglect in the United States.* Washington, DC: U.S. Government Printing Office, 1995.
7. MacMillan, H.L., Fleming, J.E., Trocme, N., Boyle, M.H., Wong, M., Racine, Y.A., Beardslee, W.R., and Offord, D.R. Prevalence of child physical and sexual abuse in the community. *JAMA.* 1997;278(2):131–135.

8. Melton, G.B., and Flood, M.F. Research policy and child maltreatment: Developing the scientific foundation for effective protection of children. *Child Abuse and Neglect.* 1994;18(supplement):1–28.

9. Caffey, J. Multiple fractures in the long bones of infants suffering from chronic subdural hematoma. *AJR.* 1946;56:163.

10. Silverman, F.N. The Roentgen manifestations of unrecognized skeletal trauma in infants. *AJR.* 1953;69:413.

11. Leventhal, J.M., Forsyth, B.W.C., Qi, K., Johnson, L., Schroeder, D., and Votto, N. Maltreatment of children born to women who used cocaine during pregnancy: A population based study. *Pediatrics.* 1997;100(2):258.

12. Straus, M.A., Sugarman, D.B., and Giles-Sims, J. Spanking by parents and subsequent antisocial behavior of children. *Archives of Pediatric and Adolescent Medicine.* 1997;151:761–767.

13. Lindner Gunnoe, M., and Mariner, C.L. Toward a developmental-contextual model of the effects of parental spanking on children's aggression. *Archives of Pediatric and Adolescent Medicine.* 1997;151:768–775.

14. Smith, J.R., and Brooks-Gunn, J. Correlates and consequences of harsh discipline for young children. *Archives of Pediatrics and Adolescent Medicine.* 1997;151: 777–786.

15. Bross, D. Law and the abuse of children. *Currents in Modern Thought: Child Abuse and Society's Response.* 1990;473–487.

16. Grossman, D.C., Neckerman, H.J., Koepsell, T.D., Liu, P., Asher, K.N., Beland, K., Frey, K., and Rivara, P. Effectiveness of a violence prevention curriculum among children in elementary school: A randomized controlled trial. *JAMA.* 1997;277 (20):1605–1611.

17. Olds, D.L., Eckenrode, J., Henderson, C.R., Kitzman, H., Powers, J., Cole, R., Sidora, K., Morris, P., Pettit, L.M., and Luckey, D. Long-term effects of home visitation on maternal life course and child abuse and neglect: Fifteen year follow-up of a randomized trial. *JAMA.* 1997;278(8):637–643.

18. Leventhal, J.M., Pew, M.C., Berg, A.T., and Garber, R.B. Use of health services by children who were identified during the postpartum period as being at high risk of child abuse or neglect. *Pediatrics.* 1996;97:331–335.

19. Krugman, R.D. Editorial. *Child Abuse and Neglect.* 1997;21(3):245–46.

20. Krugman, R.D. Future directions in preventing child abuse. *Child Abuse and Neglect.* 1995;19:273–279.

13

Health Care Issues of Children in Placement: The Example of Foster Care

MARY CARRASCO

Although in recent years both legislation and policy have emphasized family preservation and the maintenance of children with their natural families, the number of children in foster care and other out-of-home placements has continued to increase. On any given day there are approximately 500,000 children in foster care. These children are typically placed because of abuse or neglect, but there are also significant proportions of children in foster care as a result of delinquency, mental health problems, or physical or development disability. As a result, the supervision and coordination of services may involve child protective agencies, juvenile justice systems, mental health/mental retardation programs, or a combination of these and other social service and educational programs. These children are certainly not a homogeneous population, and they often have very complex and varied physical and mental health problems. In spite of the fact that children in foster care and other out-of-home placements often have regular, extensive, court-mandated contact with health and social service agencies, they remain one of the neediest groups in terms of health status. This point has been demonstrated by the fact that inadequacy of health care services has been a major factor in class action suits that have been filed to improve the child welfare system. Although this chapter focuses primarily on children in foster care, the issues identified are often similar for homeless children and for children in group home or residential placement arrangements.

Poor Health Status of Children in Placement

Numerous studies have documented the high frequency of chronic physical conditions, physical and developmental delays, and mental health problems among this population.[1–6] The early studies of the health of foster children helped promote the development of recommendations by the Child Welfare League of America and by the American Academy of Pediatrics that all children entering foster care receive a full health assessment. Although one might expect that children would be in poor health status on entry into placement, there are indications that these health problems persist during the time of placement as well.[7] The persistence of these problems is of particular concern because children entering foster care are fully covered by medical insurance (usually Medicaid) and typically have been under supervision by some type of social service agency.

Studies involving carefully done health assessments of children entering foster placement report that anywhere from 70% to more than 90% of the children studied had an abnormality in at least one body system.[1,5] These results are very similar to the author's own recent experiences in a clinic that serves large numbers of dependent and neglected children at a major children's hospital medical center. Halfon[3] reported growth failure in 43% at entry into care, and many of these children are at further risk for growth and eating disorders while in foster placement. He reported infections/parasites in 17%, hematologic abnormalities in 21%, nervous system abnormalities in 30%, respiratory abnormalities in 18%, gastroesophageal abnormalities in 15%, genitourinary abnormalities in 10%, skin abnormalities in 23%, and congenital abnormalities in 8%. Chernoff and colleagues[1] reported that 25% failed the vision screen and 15% failed the hearing screen at initial examination. In addition to acute health problems, about 80% have at least one chronic health problem and 25% have three or more chronic problems.

Approximately 60% of preschool children in foster care have a developmental disability, and 35% to 85% have severe mental health disturbances.[8] Diamond[5] and Schor[4] both found that 70% of foster children are inadequately immunized, and there are no indications that the situation has changed much since the time of their studies. Hochsteadt[6] found that "at the time of placement, most of these children have had inadequate physical and emotional nourishment and poor medical and psychosocial care."

Additionally, after entry into the system, despite numerous mandated examinations, Halfon and Klee[2] found that "delivery of health services to foster children is fragmented and often uncoordinated." Much of this may result because of poor communication and follow-up with foster parents. In one study, it was reported that only 27% of foster parents were aware of the need for follow-up care of problems identified in pre-placement physical examinations.[5]

REASONS FOR POOR HEALTH STATUS

There are many reasons for the poor health status of these children. The overwhelming majority come from a poverty background, which places them at higher risk. In addition, they often have been living in unstable homes where proper health care and preventive behaviors were not emphasized, particularly during the period immediately prior to removal from the home. Given that across the country serious neglect is the most common reason for placement outside the home, it is easy to understand that medical needs would not have been attended to. Moreover, some children have experienced active physical, sexual, and emotional abuse, resulting in increased need in terms of both physical and mental health issues. What is of major concern is the fact that the health problems are often not appropriately recognized and assessed, and even when identified, the health status of these children may not improve during the foster care experience.

Major issues related to the high level of unrecognized and untreated health problems in these children can generally be classified into two broad categories: (1) the lack of an initial comprehensive health assessment (many of these examinations are done in the emergency room setting or in part-time clinics), and lack of follow-up on this examination; and (2) the lack of regular, continuous, comprehensive primary health care and a related lack of focus on secondary and tertiary health care needs. These factors are now complicated by mandated entry into the managed care system for most Medicaid recipients. Although managed care may hold promise for better case management, care coordination, and prevention efforts, issues regarding fiscal responsibility, accountability, and adequate financial reimbursement to providers may be further complicated.

LIMITATIONS OF PRESENT SYSTEM FOR HEALTH ASSESSMENTS

In most situations, a physical examination is required immediately prior to, or within 24 to 48 hours of, actual placement. This examination generally serves to meet medical and legal requirements rather than serving a health status enhancement function. The examination serves to ensure either that there are no prior injuries that personnel at the new placement would be "accused" of causing or that there is documentation of these injuries or prior conditions. Some significant physical and mental health problems in children may not be identified during the physical examination. In addition, important information about prior conditions, immunizations, behavioral problems, and the like may not be obtained—factors that are essential in determining the health needs of children. In spite of the fact that this initial examination is often cursory, and because other medical information is not available, the fact that the examination has occurred serves to inappropriately convince foster parents, case workers, and others that the child's health needs are being adequately addressed. As a result, caregivers may not think that the child requires any additional assessments or services.

During most mandated physical examinations that occur close to the time of placement, an accurate medical history is rarely available and no mechanism exists for the recommendations of the physician to be communicated to, interpreted for, or acted on by child welfare caseworkers, foster care staff, or family members. When a foster parent may be aware of a specific health need, care is often postponed because of the expected temporary nature of the placement. When medical records are available, they are often incomplete, and there is no centralized responsibility for coordinating the flow of information.

The examinations are most often conducted by rotating staff in the acute care facilities, who although clinically competent, are often unaware of the underlying purpose of the appraisal or the nature of the Children and Youth Services (CYS) system. In many cases the examinations may not be carried out by clinicians trained in pediatrics. Because many different physicians are involved, liaison with CYS and its caseworkers is difficult and usually non-existent. The American Academy of Pediatrics Committee on Community Health Services[9] reported that "hospital emergency rooms, visiting public health nurses and clinics usually provide episodic and fragmented care. Continuity is nonexistent and care is rarely comprehensive."

LACK OF COORDINATION

A major limitation of the current system concerns implementation of recommendations for care that are made by the examining physician. In some instances, these recommendations are not recorded or if recorded are not in sufficient detail for implementation. Even when follow-up recommendations are adequate, information usually is entered into the child's medical facility record, which does not accompany the child. In those cases where a medical record and/or recommendations for follow-up care do accompany the child, problems can still occur. As previously mentioned, in many cases there is no systematic communication of physician recommendations to the appropriate caregivers or caseworkers. In addition, CYS caseworkers are not trained to interpret medical findings, and no single individual or program has responsibility for communication and interpretation.

In addition to the obstacles to follow-up care of problems revealed by pre-placement health examinations, there is typically no system or mechanism to monitor the immunization and preventive health status of these foster children or to place these children in appropriate, community-based "medical homes" that will provide continuity of care. Most service agencies such as CYS have limited funds or other resources to provide for or coordinate health care for these children, other than those resources available through Medicaid, which has routinely reimbursed these labor-intensive examinations at the routine office visit level.

Currently, in most communities foster children are assigned to the Medicaid system starting the day they are placed. Sometimes, however, they do not have an assigned Medicaid number at the time of placement. This makes it more difficult for the provider to obtain the limited reimbursement provided through Medicaid. Most physicians who are willing to consider providing care to children in foster care may be reluctant to provide care, not because of the very limited reimbursement, but because they find it difficult to negotiate the foster care system to obtain the necessary social and medical information on the child. When providers do take the time to work with the system, the child is often moved to another placement and the time spent in developing the carefully mapped out health plan appears to be wasted.

Additional problems are encountered because natural parents maintain legal guardianship of their children residing in foster care, making consent for non-emergent care problematic at times. In some jurisdictions, the courts routinely provide a permission to obtain medical records and to provide routine health care services for these children. When this is not done, problems may be encountered in the administration of immunizations even when prior immunization status is known. There are also significant and related communication gaps between health care providers, agency caseworkers, and the parents or caregivers. This situation is aggravated by the fact that children may frequently move between caregivers (one third moving more than three times while in care) and by the high turnover rate among caseworkers in the social agencies responsible for coordinating service. In addition, there is often no formal mechanism for providing for the education of parents, foster parents, and caseworkers about health care needs, and of physicians about the foster care system and the special health care needs of foster children. As a result, even when health problems are identified, there may be inadequate follow-up.

The delivery of mental health services is often complicated further by the fact that many areas deliver these services in "catchment areas," each of which requires the completion of an intake process at their particular site. As children in foster care move frequently, the actual delivery of services is problematic. The delivery of services in the context of the family (with the goal of reunification) is almost never addressed appropriately. The solution to this particular challenge would result in a marked improvement in successful return of children to their natural homes and greatly decreased cost to the entire welfare system.

As indicated earlier, the move toward managed care for Medicaid recipients will certainly have a significant impact on health care services for children in foster care as well as other vulnerable populations. Within the framework of managed care, many jurisdictions, however, have chosen to include children in foster care as part of the required "carve out" (i.e., they could not be placed in managed care). This move represents a recognition that this is a group of "special needs children" who are at risk for poor health status. The carve out strategy has been adopted to ensure that these children are guaranteed quality care; however, such a move also will remove this group from any potentially positive benefits of managed care (e.g., aggressive case management services). In any case, whether under managed care or traditional indemnity coverage, more aggressive measures are required to ensure appropriate health care.

STRATEGIES FOR SYSTEM IMPROVEMENT: THE POTENTIAL OF CASE MANAGEMENT

Recommendations to improve health status of children in foster care typically are in the general areas of coordinating the timing and increasing the depth of the initial health assessment; improving data collection and record keeping; coordinating and tracking services; and providing training for physicians, caseworkers, legal and advocacy personnel, and for foster parents. A variety of specific approaches are presented in the literature.[2,7] There is, however, little indication that many of the recommended strategies have been implemented, and in cases where implemented, the results have not been documented. These recommendations and policy and program strategies should continue to be actively pursued. Within the changing health care environment, however, the use of aggressive case management for children in out-of-home placements is a strategy that also shows considerable promise.

Case management (service coordination) is a term that was regularly used to describe the function of arranging and coordinating services for clients and patients—a function closely akin to that of social casework. The operational definition of this term has changed in recent years, however, and is now more commonly associated with provider-focused case management—typically part of a managed care health coverage plan. In spite of the fact that case management now may include a strong emphasis on efficiency and cost containment, it still emphasizes coordination, communication, and comprehensiveness of services, all important factors in assuring quality health care. It also promotes the establishment and maintenance of a consistent primary care arrangement, or "medical home" for each child, no matter what their living arrangement.

A positive impact of case management was dramatically demonstrated in a recent study at our Children's Hospital. Aggressive case management was provided to a randomly selected group of children followed up for 1 year. There was a marked improvement in immunization status at the 1 year follow-up (97% completely immunized) as compared with the control group (immunization status actually declined to only 57% completely immunized). These results are consistent with those emerging from other case management efforts with high-risk populations. It is anticipated that a formalized case management program for children in foster care, whether under the umbrella of managed care or through traditional coverage, can considerably improve the overall health status of children in foster care. Decision makers in both the child welfare and the health care systems should work toward the implementation of these systems improvements.

References

1. Chernoff, R., Combs-Orme, T., Risley-Curtiss, C., and Heisler, A. Assessing the health status of children entering foster care. *Pediatrics*. April, 1994;93(4):594–601.
2. Halfon, N. and Klee, L. Health services for California's foster children: Current practices and policy recommendations. *Pediatrics*. August, 1987;80(2):183–191.
3. Halfon, N. Mendonca, A., and Berkowitz, G. Health status of children in foster care: The experience of the center for the vulnerable child. *Archives of Pediatric and Adolescent Medicine*. 1995;149:386–392.
4. Schor, E. The foster care and health status of foster children. *Pediatrics*. 1982; 69:521–528.
5. Diamond, P. Care of children in foster care. Presented at Conference on Child Abuse: Challenges and Controversies. New York, March 10, 1988.
6. Hochsteadt, N.J., Jaudes, P.K., Zimo, D.A., and Schachter, J. The medical and psychosocial needs of children entering foster care. *Child Abuse and Neglect*. 1987; 11(1):53–62.
7. Simms, M. and Halfon, N. The health care needs of children in foster care: A research agenda. *Child Welfare*. September–October, 1994;73(5):505–24.
8. Szilagyi, M. The pediatrician and the child in foster care. *Pediatrics in Review*. February, 1998;19(2):39–50.
9. American Academy of Pediatrics, Committee on Community Health Services. Health needs of homeless children. *Pediatrics*. 1990;82:938–940.

14

Homeless Women and Their Children

PETER SHERMAN AND IRWIN REDLENER

Although homelessness brings to mind the stereotype of a man panhandling on a street corner, in fact, single women and their children now make up a significant and increasing proportion of this population. At the same time that the demographics of homelessness are changing, this country is profoundly transforming the nature of the programs that traditionally have provided shelter, food and other services for the nation's poor. This alteration in the safety net is likely to have serious implications for the welfare of homeless women and their children. In order to predict the impact that these changes will have on this population, it is important to have an understanding of the forces that create and maintain the condition of homelessness in families.

NUMBERS OF HOMELESS

Although it is well substantiated that homelessness is a major problem for many communities, it is not how many individuals are homeless in the United States. Estimates are in the range of 1.7 to 3 million per year, with the number varying according to the definition of homelessness and the methodology used to tabulate individuals.[1]

The most common method of counting the number of homeless individuals, point-in-time estimation, tends to underestimate the number of homeless persons because it focuses on the chronically homeless and misses many of those who are homeless for a short period of time. Many surveys do not count people who are homeless because they are doubled-up with other families or are living in hidden areas, such as cars, tunnels, or parks.

Retrospective studies provide a different picture. Link, in 1990, randomly surveyed a cross-section of people living in the United States, via telephone, to ask whether they had ever experienced homelessness. Literal homelessness was defined as living in a park, abandoned building, street, train or bus station, shelter, or another temporary residence. Even though this methodology is likely to underestimate homelessness by missing those who do not have telephones and those who are currently homeless, the proportion reporting a history of homelessness was striking. Lifetime prevalence was 7.4% for literal homelessness and 14% if those living doubled-up with others were included.[2] These were not just brief episodes of homelessness. Forty-six percent reported their length of homelessness to be between 1 month and 1 year, and 13% were homeless for more than a year. This translates to more than 13 million adult Americans reporting literal homelessness at some point in their lives. If one includes doubling-up, the number increases to 26 million. This figure includes large numbers of single mothers and their children.

There are several estimates of the number of homeless children and adolescents. The Federal General Accounting Office in 1989 reported that there are 68,000 to 100,000 homeless children on any given night residing in the United States.[3] According to the U.S. Conference of Mayors, in the 29 cities it surveyed in 1996, families with children made up 38% of the homeless population.[4] In the same year, in New York City one half of the homeless population consisted of families and 1 of 10 children younger than 5 years old lived in a homeless shelter.[5]

CAUSES OF HOMELESSNESS

When single-parent families were queried about why they were homeless, 28% related it to housing problems, 20% to economic hardship, 31% to family and/or relationship problems, and 14% to drug use or violence.[6] However, to understand system-wide causes of homelessness, it is necessary to examine its roots in poverty, housing shortages, and the current labor market.

There are differing schools of thought concerning the causes of homelessness. One view is that it is caused by the combination of low wages and a shortage of affordable housing. Another view is that homeless families have certain psychosocial characteristics that make them vulnerable to housing loss. Both viewpoints are applicable depending on the type of population that is being studied. It is important to understand the difference between direct causes of homelessness, such as a deficiency of affordable housing, and characteristics that make people more vulnerable to homelessness, such as domestic violence.

In cities where the housing market is very tight and there is a paucity of low-income housing, one will find more families that are homeless as a result of economic factors. This is due to the fact that a relatively small loss of income can leave a person in the situation of not having access to affordable housing because such housing is exceedingly scarce. Cities that have a better supply of affordable housing will find more homelessness caused by psychosocial factors, because it is not the lack of affordable housing per se that causes homelessness, but rather the inability of the person to access housing because of individual dysfunction. The interaction of these different factors may help explain the disparate findings reported in studies of homelessness. Cognizance of these factors is also important in designing programs that are responsive to an individual community's needs.

A clear and direct correlation exists between poverty and homelessness. The U.S. Department of Housing and Urban Development (HUD) classifies those families who have incomes that are less than 50% of the median family income in their community, are renters, and do not receive federal housing assistance in the category of "worst case housing needs."[7]. Since the early 1980s, there has been a large increase in the number of people falling into this category. Between 1979 and 1990 the number of people living below the federal poverty level increased by 41%. Families with children accounted for more than half of that increase.[8] By 1995, 21% of children in the United States lived in poverty, compared with 14% of children in 1969. Children of color are the most vulnerable, with 66% of Hispanic and 62% of African-American children living in female-headed households falling into this category.[9] The proportion and numbers of homeless families mirror these trends.

For those who are working, poverty is fueled by a service economy that pays low wages and often provides only part-time work with few or no benefits. Underemployment (unemployed or those working part-time because they cannot find a full-time job) increased from 8.2% in 1973 to 12.6% in 1993. Those earning wages below the poverty line went from 12.6% of workers in 1973 to 23.9% in 1993. The percentage of workers earning less than 75% of the poverty line doubled during this same period.[10] Even though the minimum wage was raised to $5.15/hour in 1997, full-time employment at that rate puts a worker at only 83% of the poverty line for a family of three.[5] In 1995, the share of poor children living in a household headed by a full-time year-round worker was 21%, the highest level since these data were first collected in 1975.[5] HUD reports that of those families with children who fall into the category of "worst case housing needs" more than four out of five have earnings that exceed the equivalent of full-time work at minimum wage.[7]

Low wages are exacerbated by a lack of affordable housing. Between 1973 and 1993, 2.2 million low-rent units were lost. At the same time, those requiring low-rent housing increased by 4.7 million. This has resulted in the largest shortage of low-rent housing on record.[11] The Section 8 Housing program, a federal program that subsidizes rental costs for poor families, is unable to address this housing gap, owing to insufficient funding. Since 1988 federal spending for housing assistance has decreased 78%.[12] Between 1977 and 1980, HUD was able to provide rental assistance to an average of 290,000 low-income households per year. Between 1981 and 1993 this number dropped to an average of 74,000 per year.[11] The average wait for Section 8 Housing assistance is about 32 months. Some cities have had to stop accepting applicants for some of their assisted housing programs.[4]

Despite this, no new vouchers or certificates were issued in 1996 or 1997.[7] Thus, it is no surprise that only 26% of those eligible for assisted housing receive it.[13]

Most importantly the number of families headed by single women, the population most vulnerable to becoming homeless, has soared. In 1996, 68% of children lived with two parents, compared with 85% in 1976. In that same year, 24% of children lived only with their mother. This trend has been fueled by rising divorce rates, out-of-wedlock births, and a growing number of mothers who never marry.[9]

Poverty in families headed by single women has been aggravated by a decrease in the value of Aid to Families with Dependent Children (AFDC). Providing AFDC and food stamps still places a family below the poverty line in every state except Alaska, and below 75% of the poverty line in 39 states.[14] The median AFDC grant for a family of three declined from $671 per month in 1970 to $367 in 1992.[1] This is a 45% decline, adjusting for inflation.

This overall combination of decreasing income, coupled with an increase in the number of families headed by single women and a scarcity of affordable housing, is working to produce an epidemic of homeless families in the United States.

FACTORS PUTTING FAMILIES AT RISK FOR HOMELESSNESS

Numerous studies have examined homeless families headed by single mothers in an attempt to create a profile of the mother at risk for becoming homeless. By predicting which families are at risk for homelessness, it would be possible to effectively target homeless prevention programs. Unfortunately, results are conflicting, principally because homeless families are not a homogeneous population. As previously indicated, there is a great deal of geographic variation in the root causes of homelessness, given that the housing and economic status of one locale may be very different from that of another. Another reason is that admission criteria for shelters vary considerably from one area to another. There is also a large variation in the allowable and actual length of stay among shelters. The profile of a family and the effects of homelessness may be very different in a family that stays in a shelter for a few days as compared with a family that is in residence for several months.

Another important reason for conflicting findings pertaining to the profile of homeless families is the variation in study designs. Few studies actually compare homeless subjects with matched poor housed subjects. Without a comparison group, it is not possible to separate out predisposing factors that are unique to homelessness. Even when control groups are used, they are often not well matched, making comparison difficult. Another methodological issue is that the number of families studied tends to be small, which decreases the ability of the study to statistically differentiate between the two populations.

In spite of these variations, research studies have uncovered important information about risk factors. One study that examined a large number of homeless families, and used a case-control design to compare them with housed families who were receiving AFDC, found several interesting results. Predictors of homelessness were foster care placement as a child and drug use by a respondent's primary female caretaker. Additional factors associated with homelessness were fewer social supports, frequent heroin or alcohol use, and mental health hospitalization within the past 2 years.[6] Other investigators have also found that these factors identify homeless women.[12,15] Although they are powerful predictors, they still identify only a small subset of homeless women. Protective factors included being the lease holder of an apartment, receiving AFDC and/or a housing subsidy in the prior year, graduating from high school, and having a large nonprofessional support network.[16]

Numerous studies have found a correlation between homelessness and having a history of being abused as an adult or a child. Shinn found that 11.4% of homeless women had a history of being physically abused as a child as compared with 6.5% of housed poor women. Twenty-seven percent of the homeless women had been abused or threatened as adults as compared with 16.6% of housed women.[17] Several studies found higher rates of battering among homeless women when compared with housed women.[6,18,19]

Other investigators were unable to confirm these findings. Goodman found no difference in both childhood and adult episodes of both physical and sexual abuse in comparing the two groups.[20] Both groups had experienced strikingly high rates of abuse at some point during their lifetime, with approximately 90% of both populations reporting some form of physical or sexual abuse during their lifetimes. The investigator hypothesized that their study failed to find a difference between the populations because of the changing nature of the homeless population. Because housing had become scarcer since the previous studies were carried out, a greater number of higher functioning families were homeless. This tended to diminish the potential differences between housed and homeless poor families. The investigator also felt that the high rate found in their study was due to the use of a more sensitive instrument to measure abuse. The overall picture does suggest that a history of abuse is a common experience among homeless women.

Investigators have found significant differences between housed and homeless mothers regarding a history of living in foster care or a group home as a child, with homeless mothers reporting higher rates of both experiences.[15] Shinn found that 21.6% of homeless mothers reported running away as minors, compared with only 6.5% of housed mothers. In addition, a higher percentage of homeless mothers reported the experience, as children, of living on the street.[17]

These findings suggest that experiences interfering with a person's ability to form supportive relationships places a mother from an economically impoverished background at increased risk for homelessness, and in fact, other investigators have found the absence of a supportive network to be an important risk factor for homelessness. In Shinn's study, families were contacted at their point of entry into the homeless shelter system to gather information about support networks. Thus, the study was able to capture the support system that existed for a person just prior to entering the homeless system. Homeless families were compared with families on welfare. The percentage of those with supportive family contacts were similar between the two groups. What was interesting was that the homeless families had "used up" resources on which they could depend for housing in an emergency. Of the housed families, 18.4% had at least one contact where they could reside in an emergency, whereas only 4.4% of the homeless families had such a contact. For those younger than 30 years of age the difference was even more striking, being 27% and 4%, respectively.[17] Thus, one can conjecture that it is not the direct lack of social support, but rather the lack of a socially supportive network that can provide housing in an emergency, that puts a family at risk for homelessness.

Bassuk found that homeless families moved much more frequently and had a much higher rate of living doubled-up just prior to being homeless. In addition, homeless mothers demonstrated a paucity of social supports. Twenty-two percent of homeless women were unable to name any individuals whom they could turn to for support, as compared with 2% of housed women. Only 26% of the homeless women could name three adult supports, as compared with 74% of the housed women.[16] Wood found other differences with, for example, 37% of the homeless mothers naming a child younger than 18 years old as a support, whereas only 13% of the housed mothers did so.[6]

Economic supports were also found to be lacking in homeless mothers. Bassuk found that housed mothers received more entitlements such as AFDC, food stamps, housing subsidies, and Supplemental Security Income (SSI). She found that 24% of homeless women had not been granted AFDC in the previous year as compared with 7% of housed mothers.[15] It is possible that mothers who later became homeless were less effective in obtaining benefits than those who were able to maintain their housing. Whether this explains the correlation found between homelessness and specific individual characteristics, such as history of abuse, lack of education, and substance abuse, remains to be clarified.

IMPACT OF HOMELESSNESS ON CHILDREN'S HEALTH AND DEVELOPMENT

Few studies compare the health of homeless children with poor housed children. Therefore, it is not clear whether there is a significant difference in the health of the two populations. When parents were asked to rate the health of their children, 13% of homeless children were reported to be in fair or poor health, compared with 3.2% of the general pediatric population and 6.5% of those living in poverty. However, 44% of the problems were clustered in 15% of the children.[21] Another investigator did not find any difference in the general health of homeless children compared with poor children.[22]

In addition, children who present to clinical services with complaints of an acute nature, such as an upper respiratory infection, are frequently found to have serious problems of a more chronic nature. For example, while the typical rate for a subspecialty referral in a general pediatric practice is 1 of every 55 to 60 patient encounters, the New York City Children's Health Project, which serves homeless children, reports that approximately 1 of every 14 patient encounters results in a referral.[23]

Alperstein found several areas of significant difference when comparing housed and homeless children. Of homeless children, 3.8% had an elevated serum lead level above 30 μg/dl, whereas this occurred in only 1.7% of housed poor children. Inpatient pediatric admission rates were 11.6/1,000 for homeless children and 7.5/1,000 for poor housed children. Twenty-seven percent of homeless children had delayed immunization as compared with 15% of housed children.[24] Wood also found high rates of underimmunization, with 27% of children younger than 5 years old not immunized against diphtheria, pertussis, tetanus (DPT), 33% not immunized against polio, and 28% having never received a measles-mumps-rubella (MMR) vaccine.[22]

Of particular concern is the nutritional status of homeless children. When parents were asked whether their children got enough food, 21% of the homeless families replied that there had been insufficient food 4 days or more in the preceding month because of lack of money, compared with 7% of housed poor families. Twenty-three percent of the homeless families reported hunger in their children secondary to insufficient food resources, compared with 4% of the housed poor. Fourteen percent of the homeless families stated that they ate in a fast food restaurant or convenience store at least four times per week, compared with 4% of housed families. Nine percent of the girls in homeless families were at less than fifth percentile for weight for height, which is indicative of failure to thrive, and 12% of the children had weight for height greater than 95%, indicative of obesity.[24] Given the importance of adequate nutrition for development in the infant and young child and the risk factors associated with obesity in later life, these are disturbing findings.

Developmental, educational, and psychological outcomes in homeless children are equally worrisome. Homeless children have a higher rate of developmental delay when compared with housed poor children. Fifty-four percent of homeless children had at least one area of delay, compared with only 16% of housed children in one study.[26] The greatest differences were found in the language and personal/social subscales. Rescorla and colleagues found significant differences between homeless and housed poor preschoolers on receptive vocabulary and visual motor development. Yet only 35% of the homeless children were enrolled in an early intervention program, compared with 85% of the housed children.[27] A recent report found that 180,000 homeless preschool children do not attend school because of inadequate funding, lack of transportation to school, state non-compliance with federal law regarding barriers to school enrollment, and long waiting list for preschool spaces.[28]

The situation of school-age children also causes concern. Rubin and co-workers found that homeless children scored significantly lower on the Wechsler Intelligence Scale for Children-Revised (WRAT-R), a measure of academic achievement.[29] Another investigator found lower scores on the Wide Range Achievement Test-Revised (WISC-R), which reflects knowledge gained as the result of experience.[27] In another study, 41% of homeless mothers reported that their children were failing or doing below-average schoolwork in comparison with 23% of housed mothers.[19] Because the differences found are related to a lack of knowledge rather than innate intelligence, these studies suggest that poor school performance may be due to a disruption in schooling secondary to homelessness rather than innate differences in intelligence. The exact cause of this—whether increased prevalence of illness, depression, or school absence—remains to be determined.

The Department of Education reported in 1989 that 30% of homeless children did not attend school.[30] The National Coalition for the Homeless in 1991 estimated this to be as high as 50%.[31] On a positive note, a 1995 national study found that only 14% of homeless children were not attending school.[32] This improvement may be attributable to decreased barriers to school enrollment resulting from enforcement of the educational provisions of the McKinney Act. Congress enacted the McKinney Act in 1987 to provide funds for shelter, food, and health care of homeless people. Subtitle VII-B of the Act, as amended in 1990, requires that states receiving McKinney funding eliminate barriers to education for homeless children. Specifically, it is stated that homeless children have the same right to a free and appropriate education as housed children. States are required to revise any laws or regulations that might act as a barrier to education, and children are not to be separated from the mainstream school environment because they are homeless. Although many such barriers have been eliminated, a 1995 survey found four states with residency requirements, five requiring prior school records, 15 with immunization requirements, 15 with legal guardianship requirements, and 30 with transportation requirements that hinder school enrollment for homeless children. On a cautionary note, the budget for the educational portion of the McKinney Act remains at the 1992 level of funding, even though the number of homeless school-age children has doubled.[30]

Evidence that homeless children may suffer from behavioral and psychological problems is persuasive. Using the Children's Depression Inventory, one study found the mean score of homeless children to be 10.3, while that of housed children was 8.3. A score of 9 indicates the need for psychiatric evaluation. Thirty-one percent of a group of homeless children, compared with 9% of housed children, scored at a level indicating the need for further evaluation when tested with the Children's Manifest Anxiety Scale.[19] Homeless preschoolers scored significantly higher on the Child Behavior Checklist when compared with a group of housed children.[27] This test reflects anxiety, depression, and acting-out behavior.

LONG-TERM OUTCOME OF HOMELESSNESS ON WOMEN AND CHILDREN

Current research demonstrates that homeless families are not a homogeneous population. Some families are homeless due solely to economic circumstances, such as loss of a job or onset of an illness that overwhelms a person's financial resources. However, some homeless families fit more of a psychological profile, suggesting that factors such as mental illness, substance abuse, or lack of education are involved in the etiology of homelessness.

Less clear is whether the experience of homelessness, in itself, adversely affects a person's ability to function. Although differences in the psychological and developmental characteristics of homeless children compared with poor housed children have been identified, it is not clear whether this is the result of processes that occurred prior to homelessness or were precipitated by homelessness. Regardless of their cause, these factors may continue to hamper the child's functioning even after the period of homelessness has ended.

It is also possible that homelessness adversely affects parents, therefore making future episodes of homelessness more likely. Some adults may become "institutionalized" once they enter the homeless system and lose skills needed to function autonomously. Clarification of these issues will be central to designing future homeless prevention programs.

THE IMPACT OF WELFARE REFORM ON HOMELESS FAMILIES

Changes that have been made to the welfare laws can have an impact on homelessness in two ways: They can affect those who are currently homeless, and they can increase or decrease the overall number of homeless families. The central tenet of the Personal Responsibility and Work Opportunity Reconciliation Act of 1996 (P.L. 104-193) is that economic assistance to needy individuals is time-limited. Most recipients will have a lifetime limit of 5 years for receiving financial subsidies.

Given what is known about the economic and psychosocial causes of homelessness and their relationship to affordable housing, preventing further increases in the number of homeless families will demand intensive efforts to implement the transition of those receiving welfare to other means of economic support. For a large proportion of this population, entering the job market and becoming economically self-sufficient may be extremely difficult.

Twenty-five percent of the single-parent families receiving welfare or Temporary Aid to Needy Families (formerly AFDC) must be working and/or in training currently. This number rises to 50% by 2002. Because most of these families are headed by single women who have young children, lack adequate education, and possess few job skills, this mandate presents a particularly problematic set of challenges. Adequate education, job training, and child care is central to enabling these women to afford housing without the safety net of welfare.

Although the block grants to states provide some of these items, they are inadequate for meeting current needs. The Congressional Budget Office estimates that P.L. 104-193 falls $12 billion short of providing the funding needed to enable states to provide transition services required to meet job training requirements. It is estimated that $1 billion in additional monies would be needed to provide adequate child care provisions.[33]

Even when successful, welfare-to-work programs have typically increased employment rates among welfare recipients only 5% to 10%. For those who find employment, wages are typically around $6.00 per hour, which is insufficient to afford the typical child care cost of $1.60 per hour per child.[34]

Using computer simulation to gauge the impact of welfare reform on poverty, one study estimated that the percentage of families with children who live below 75% of the poverty line in New York City will increase from 10% to 17% of the total population. This means that 16,000 families will be pushed below the poverty line and 110,000 families will be pushed below 75% of the poverty line.[35]

Although the changes in welfare laws focus on the economic issues, studies show that many homeless parents also present with psychological issues. It is necessary to address problems of child abuse, domestic violence, substance abuse, as well as psychiatric and medical illness that lead to homelessness. Some parents will need to receive economic support from Supplemental Security Income (SSI) because of disabling conditions that prevent them from holding full-time jobs. Families will need access to medical, psychological, and educational services to help them become more self-sufficient and free from dependency on the welfare and homeless shelter system.

Although the long-term effects of homelessness on children are not established, it is prudent to provide needed educational, medical, and psychological services to prevent the entry of children into the ranks of homelessness as adults. Under the new legislation, Temporary Aid to Needy Families and Medicaid eligibility are determined separately and individuals who do not qualify for welfare will be able to remain on Medicaid. The decoupling of Medicaid from Temporary Aid to Needy Families may result in individuals not realizing that they may still qualify for Medicaid even though they have lost their eligibility to receive welfare benefits, unless an effort is made to publicize Medicaid eligibility criteria.[36] Comprehensive health care is an important component in the services needed to limit the damaging effects of homelessness on children.

References

1. Children's Defense Fund. *The state of America's children yearbook.* Washington, DC: Children's Defense Fund, 1994, pp 37–44.
2. Link, B.G., Susser, E., Stueve, A., Phelan, J., Moore, R.E., and Stuening, E. Lifetime and five-year prevalence of homelessness in the United States. *American Journal of Public Health.* 1994;84:1907–1912.
3. Committee on Community Health Services. Health needs of homeless children and their families. *Pediatrics.* 1996;98:789–791.

4. Waxman, L., and Hinderliter, S. *A status report on hunger and homelessness in America's cities:* 1996. Washington, DC.
5. Children's Defense Fund. *The state of America's children: Yearbook 1997.* Washington, DC: Children's Defense Fund, 1997.
6. Wood, D., Valdez, R.B., Hayshi, T., and Shen, A. Homeless and housed families in Los Angeles: A study comparing demographic, economic, and family function characteristics. *American Journal of Public Health.* 1990;80:1049–1052.
7. U.S. Department of Housing and Urban Development, Office of Policy Development and Research. *Rental housing assistance at a crossroads: A report to Congress on worst case housing needs.* U.S. Dept. of Housing and Urban Development, 1996.
8. National Coalition for the Homeless. *Homeless families with children, NCH fact sheet #7.* National Coalition for the Homeless, March, 1977.
9. Federal Interagency Forum on Child and Family Statistics. *America's children: Key national indicators of well-being.* Office of Juvenile Justice and Delinquency Prevention. 1997.
10. Hardin, B. Why the road off the street is not paved with jobs. In J. Baumohl (ed). *Homelessness in America.* Phoenix, AZ: Oryx Press, 1996.
11. Lazere, E. *In short supply: The growing affordable housing gap.* Washington, DC: Center on Budget Policy and Priorities; 1995.
12. Nunez, R. *Hopes dreams and promises: The future of homeless children in America.* New York Institute for Children and Poverty, 1994.
13. Dolbeare, C. Housing policy: A general consideration. In J. Baumohl (ed). *Homelessness in America.* Phoenix, AZ: Oryx Press, 1996.
14. Parrott, S. *The Cato Institute Report on Welfare Benefits: Do Cato's numbers add up?* Washington, DC: Center on Budget and Policy Priorities, 1996.
15. Bassuk, E.L., Weinreb, L.F., Buckner, J.C., Browne, A., Salomon, A., and Bassuk, S.S. The characteristics and needs of sheltered homeless and low-income housed mothers. *JAMA.* 1996;276:640–646.
16. Bassuk, E.L., Buckner, J.C., Weinreb, L.F., Browne, A., Bassuk, S.S., Dawson, R., and Perloff, J.N. Homelessness in female-headed families: Childhood and adult risk and protective factors. *American Journal of Public Health.* 1997;87:241–247.
17. Shinn, M.B., Knickman, J.R., and Weitzman, B.C. Social relationships and vulnerability to becoming homeless among poor families. *American Psychologist.* 1991; 46:1180–1187.
18. Weitzman, B.C., Knickman, J.R., and Shinn, M. Predictors of shelter use among low-income families: Psychiatric history, substance abuse, and victimization. *American Journal of Public Health.* 1992;82:1547–1550.
19. Bassuk, E.L., and Rosenberg, L. Why does family homelessness occur? A case-control study. *American Journal of Public Health.* 1988;78:783–788.
20. Goodman, L.A. The prevalence of abuse among homeless and housed poor mothers: A comparison study. *American Journal of Orthopsychiatry.* 1991;61:489–500.
21. Miller, D.S., Lin, E. Children in sheltered homeless families: Reported health status and use of health services. *Pediatrics.* 1988;81:668–673.
22. Wood, D.L., Valdez, R.B., Hayshi, T., and Shen, A. Health of homeless children and housed, poor children. *Pediatrics.* 1990;86:858–866.
23. Redlener, I. Overcoming barriers to health care access for medically underserved children. *Journal of Ambulatory Care Management.* 1993;16:21–28.
24. Alperstein, G., Rappaport, C., and Flanigan, J.M. Health problems of homeless children in New York City. *American Journal of Public Health.* 1988;78:1232–1233.
25. Eddins, E. Characteristics, health status and service needs of sheltered homeless families. *The ABNF Journal.* Spring, 1993;4(2):40–44.
26. Bassuk, E.L., and Rosenberg, L. Psychosocial characteristics of homeless children and children with homes. *Pediatrics.* 1990;85:257–261.
27. Rescorla, L., Parker, R., and Stolley, P. Ability, achievement, and adjustment in homeless children. *American Journal of Orthopsychiatry.* 1991;61:210–220.
28. National Law Center on Homelessness and Poverty. *Blocks to their Future: A report on the barriers to preschool education for homeless children.* Washington, DC: National Law Center.

29. Rubin, D.H., Erickson, C.J., San Augustin, M., Cleary, S.D., Allen, J.K., and Cohen, P. Cognitive and academic functioning of homeless children compared with housed children. *Pediatrics.* 1996;97:289–294.
30. Bassuk, E.L. Homeless families. *Scientific American.* 1991;265:66–72.
31. National Coalition for the Homeless. *Education of homeless children and youth.* National Coalition for the Homeless, Washington, February, 1997.
32. Anderson, L.M., Janger, M.I., and Panton, K.L. *An evaluation of state and local efforts to serve the educational needs of homeless children and youth.* Washington, DC: U.S. Department of Education. 1995.
33. Edelman, P. The worst thing Bill Clinton has done. *The Atlantic Monthly.* March, 1997;43–58.
34. Center for the Future of Children. Welfare to Work Executive Summary. *The Future of Children.* 1997;7:2–7.
35. Waldfogel, J., Villeneuve, P., and Garfinkel, I. *The impact of welfare reform for families with children in New York.* Paper prepared for presentation at Impact 97 Conference, January 14, 1997 (revised May 19, 1997).
36. Ku, L., and Coughlin, T. How the new Welfare Reform Law affects Medicaid. *New Federalism: Issues and Options for States.* Urban Institute, 1997;A-5.

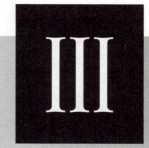

III

Health
Expenditures
and Insurance

15

Overview of Health Insurance for Children and Youth

HELEN M. WALLACE

Health insurance is a major factor in making basic quality medical and health care easily, readily, and quickly available. For children and youth, health insurance is essential for well-child care and preventive health services, maintenance of well-child status, early identification of health problems, and access for those with health problems to a source of early counseling and treatment. Health insurance must be accompanied by health protection, health promotion, and health education.

THE POLITICS OF CHILDREN'S HEALTH

Interest in expanding health coverage for children through new policies is high. Several factors underlie this growing interest:

- Children continue to be the largest group of Americans without health insurance, accounting for one of every four uninsured persons in 1995.
- The number of uninsured children remains high despite expansion of Medicaid, in substantial part because of a decline in employer-based coverage.
- Public opinion polls show widespread support for the enactment of children's health insurance reform.
- In addition to Medicaid, more than 30 states offer some type of children's health insurance program financed through a combination of public and private funding as well as in individual payments.

The joint efforts of such groups as children's advocates and consumer advocates along with support by providers have produced a commitment to promote and expand access to children's health care.

THE CONSEQUENCES OF LACK OF INSURANCE FOR CHILDREN AND YOUTH

Children are particularly vulnerable to the lack of health insurance because they need preventive and acute care for their optimum growth and development. If they do not receive care when they need it, their health can be affected for the rest of their lives.

Without health insurance, many families face difficulties securing preventive and basic health care for their children. Consequently, uninsured children and youth are less likely than insured children to secure needed health and preventive care. Children without health insurance or with gaps in coverage are less likely to have routine physician visits or have a regular source of medical care. They are less likely to have seen a physician in the past year and have fewer physician visits. When they do seek care, they more often do so at a clinic rather than through a private physician or health maintenance organization. They are also less likely to receive care for injuries, see a physician if chronically ill, or secure dental care.

In addition, these children may not be appropriately immunized to prevent childhood illnesses. Kogan and colleagues[1] have pointed out that children without health insurance have fewer immunizations and are at increased risk for delaying early treatment of health problems that may lead to complications requiring hospitalization. Lack of health care coverage for children has been cited as an important factor in delaying access to both acute and preventive care.

In a nationally representative study of U.S. preschool-age children, nearly one quarter (22.6%) had a period when they were without health insurance. Further, 60% of these children had a gap in health insurance coverage for more than 6 months. These findings suggest that a sizable number of children in the United States lack continuous health insurance coverage during a critical period of their development. Lack of coverage may be particularly harmful for children with emerging disabilities, chronic illness, or birth defects. Gaps in health insurance coverage may also preclude the receipt of preventive care; hearing, vision, and developmental screening; and early intervention. Children are in particular need of primary health care providers who can track developmental milestones, ensure the maintenance of immunization and other health maintenance schedules, monitor abnormal conditions, and serve as the first contact of care.

PROFILE OF UNINSURED CHILDREN IN THE UNITED STATES

Hall and associates[2] report that there are an estimated 8 million uninsured children in the United States in 1995. An understanding of the characteristics of these children is essential for the design of appropriate outreach and enrollment strategy benefit packages and health care provision arrangements for uninsured children.

Demographic Characteristics

Uninsured children are more likely to live in the South and the West (Fig. 15.1, Table 15.1); however, they are not disproportionately con-

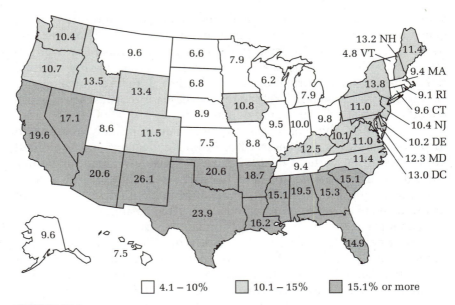

FIGURE 15.1

Percentage of uninsured children, by state, 1994. *Source:* GAO

TABLE 15.1

Child Health Coverage: Best and Worst States (Percentage of Children Without Health Insurance)

	Best States			Worst States	
Rank		Percent	Rank		Percent
1.	Minnesota	6.7%	51.	New Mexico	24.7%
2.	Wisconsin	6.8	50.	Texas	22.7
3.	Vermont	7.5	49.	Oklahoma	22.6
4.	Hawaii	8.0	48.	Arizona	20.2
5.	Michigan	8.3	47.	Louisiana	19.0
6.	North Dakota	8.7	47.	Arkansas	19.0
7.	Massachusetts	9.0	46.	Nevada	18.7
8.	Nebraska	9.1	45.	California	18.3
9.	Washington	9.3	44.	Mississippi	17.7
10.	Ohio	9.4	43.	Florida	17.1
10.	South Dakota	9.4			
10.	Alaska	9.4			

Source: U.S. Census Bureau. Current Population Survey, March 1994 through March 1996. Calculations by Children's Defense Fund. *CDF Reports.* March, 1997;18:6.

centrated in either urban or rural areas. Uninsured children are more likely to live in a household whose head has not completed high school, and their families are more likely to be poor or nearly poor.

Sources of Medical Care and Health Care Utilization

There are substantial differences in sources of care and utilization of medical services between uninsured and insured children. Among subgroups of children such as those with special health care needs, access to routine medical care varies substantially, and health insurance has been found to be an important predictor of utilization of medical care. Uninsured children who have a chronic disease, such as asthma, face difficulties of access to care and utilize substantially fewer outpatient and inpatient services. Generally speaking, uninsured children are 3–4 times likely to receive medical care from a physician when it seems reasonably indicated.

Uninsured children are three to four times more likely to lack a usual source of routine care and sick care. The majority of insured children receive their medical care, both routine and sick, in physicians' offices, whereas uninsured children are more likely to receive their medical care in publicly supported outpatient clinics and health centers. Similar proportions of uninsured and insured children are reported as using emergency departments as a usual place of care.

Uninsured children are more likely not to have had any routine care visits at all or are more likely to have an interval of 3 years or more between routine care visits. Thirty percent (30%) of uninsured children are not up-to-date with well-child care visits as recommended by the American Academy of Pediatrics, as compared with 22% of insured children.

There is a lack of primary care physicians in many areas of concentrated poverty. It is necessary to ensure that primary care practitioners are available to provide care to this population. Comprehensive and continuous care, attributes of the concept of a "medical home," are associated with significant beneficial effects.

Health Status

The link between health insurance coverage and individual health status is a major topic of debate in the current discussion of health care reform. However, results of various studies demonstrate evidence to support the connection. An eight-county study in California showed that lack of health insurance was associated with adverse health outcome. Data from the 1984 National Health Immunization Survey showed that adolescents in fair or poor health were more than twice as likely to be uninsured as those described as being in excellent health. A nine-county survey in Washington found that more members of uninsured families reported poorer health status than those from insured families.

Factors Independently Associated with Being Uninsured[3]

Factors associated with being uninsured include being of Mexican ethnic background, living in southern or western regions of the United States, living with a head of household whose education level is less than the 12th grade, and being in a family that is poor or nearly poor (see Figure 15.2).

Health-related outcomes associated with lack of insurance include the following:

- Having different sources for routine and sick care
- Never having had routine care
- No physician visit in last 12 months
- Not up-to-date with well-child care

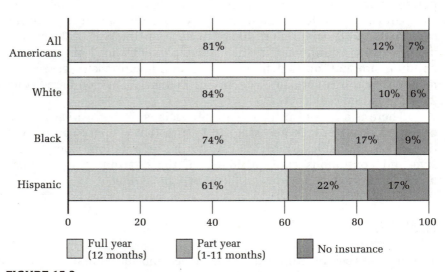

FIGURE 15.2

Health insurance coverage, by race. *Source:* Population Reference Bureau. *Population Today.* November, 1994;22(11):6. (Data from U.S. Bureau of the Census, Survey of Income and Program Participation [SIPP] 1990–1992.)

- Low income
- More likely to lack a usual source of medical care
- Low rate of utilization of health services

Characteristics of Uninsured Children and Youth[4]

1. One of three children were uninsured for a month or more during 1995 and 1996. Nearly half are uninsured for at least 12 months, and many are uninsured for 2 full years.

2. Almost half of uninsured children (49%) had uninsured periods of 12 months or longer.

3. Most children without insurance are from working families. The overwhelming majority of those uninsured for a month or more are from families where the head of household works, and a large proportion of them work full-time. More than half of all uninsured children are from families with moderate incomes.

4. Uninsured children are two times more likely to live with a married (69%) than a single parent (31%).

5. Four of five uninsured children (80%) lived in families where neither parent was covered by an employer-provided health insurance plan at the time the children were uninsured.

6. Non-Hispanic white children made up a majority (55%) of children without health insurance for 1 month or longer. Hispanic children made up 22%; blacks, 19%; and all others, 4%.

7. Most uninsured children's parents were also uninsured.

8. Lack of insurance coverage limits children's access to health care.

9. Uninsured children often do not see doctors for conditions that require treatment and that could require long-term care.

10. Uninsured children were three to four times more likely to lack a usual source of care.

11. Children without health insurance were nearly four times as likely to go without at least one needed service—medical care, dental care, prescriptions, eyeglasses, or mental health care.

SOURCE OF HEALTH INSURANCE FOR CHILDREN YOUNGER THAN AGE 18[5]

Even though lack of health insurance is a barrier to obtaining basic primary and preventive care services that are crucial to a child's development, many children in the United States remain uninsured. In 1994, the

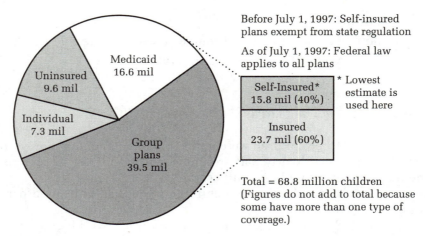

Before July 1, 1997: Self-insured plans exempt from state regulation

As of July 1, 1997: Federal law applies to all plans

Self-Insured*
15.8 mil (40%)

Insured
23.7 mil (60%)

* Lowest estimate is used here

Total = 68.8 million children (Figures do not add to total because some have more than one type of coverage.)

FIGURE 15.3

Children younger than age 18 with selected sources of health insurance coverage (1993, millions). *Source:* EBRI, 1996.

number of uninsured children younger than age 18 reached 10 million, or 14.2% of all children, according to the General Accounting Office.

Private coverage (employer-based) and individually purchased insurance for children declined steadily between 1987 and 1993, from 73% to 67.4% of all children (see Figure 15.3).

While private coverage was losing ground, Medicaid picked up the poorest of the uninsured as a result of expansions mandated by Congress beginning in 1986. These expansions, however, were not sufficient to offset completely the loss in private insurance.

RECENT EVENTS IN CHILDREN'S HEALTH INSURANCE

In August 1997, a new $24 billion initiative to expand health coverage to some of the estimated 10 million children who lack medical/health insurance was passed. The program is the largest federal investment in children's health care since Congress created Medicaid in 1965. This new initiative is financed largely by a tax increase of $0.15 per pack in the federal levy on cigarettes. At the time of this writing, the final details were still being worked out, including:

- The number of children and youth to be covered;
- what will be covered, e.g., basic health care, mental health, vision, hearing, drugs;

- how to spend the money—the degree of flexibility in deciding how to spend the money.

At the time of this writing (October 1997), the details of the new State Children's Health Insurance Program are not publicly known. Such major aspects as how many children will be covered, what services will be covered (e.g., basic health care, mental health, vision, hearing, drugs), and how the funds will be spent are still to be determined. In fact, initial decisions about some of these issues may shift as experience is gained with this significant and important program—both for the new group of children to be included as well as the remaining millions of children yet to be covered by health insurance.

It is likely that there may be flexibility in the use of funds in the states. It is recommended that both national and state plans be established to evaluate methodology and outcome, to establish pilot demonstration programs, and to permit rapid sharing of information about such demonstration and evaluation efforts.

References

1. Kogan, M.D., Alexander, G.R., Tertelbaum, M.A., Jack, B.W., Kotelchuck, M., and Pappas, G. The effect of gaps in health insurance on continuity of a regular source of care among preschool aged children in the United States. *JAMA.* 1995;274: 1429–1435.
2. Hall, J.L., Szilagi, P.G., Rodewald, L.E., Byrd, R.S., and Weitzman, M.L. Profile of uninsured children in the United States. *Archives of Pediatrics and Adolescent Medicine.* April, 1995;149:398–406.
3. Families USA. *One out of three: Kids without health insurance, 1995–1996.* Washington, DC: March, 1997.
4. Rosenbaum, S. Reforming child health care. In S.B. Kamerman, and A.J. Kahn (eds). *Child health, Medicaid, and welfare reform.* Pages 1–22. New York: Columbia University School of Social Work, 1996, pp 1–22.
5. Greenberg, J., and Zuckerman, B. State health care in Massachusetts. *Health Affairs.* July–August, 1997;16:188–193.

APPENDIX: AMCHP SUMMARY

State Children's Health Insurance Program   (P.L. 105-33 *enacted* August 5, 1997)

A.   EFFECTIVE DATES

The State Children's Health Insurance Program (SCHIP) is effective Federal Fiscal Year 1998 through Federal Fiscal Year 2007. States become eligible for payments beginning October 1, 1997.

B.   PURPOSES

The law establishes the State Child Health Insurance Program under a new Title XXI of the Social Security Act. Under the law, states are

- able to expand Medicaid, create their own children's health program or implement a combination of the two;
- eligible for payment once they have submitted their state plans to the Secretary of Health and Human Services (HHS) and have received approval;
- permitted to use 10% of these funds for noncoverage purposes defined as administration, outreach, and other child health assistance.

C.   FUNDS

The law appropriates $24 billion over the first five years and approximately $50 billion over ten years. Of the $24 billion, $8 billion will be raised through an increase in the cigarette tax effective 2000.

- For Fiscal Years 1998–2001, the law annually appropriates $4.275 billion.
- For Fiscal Years 2002 and 2004, the law annually appropriates $3.15 billion.

This Summary of the State Children's Health Insurance Program (P.L. 105-33 enacted August 5, 1997) was produced by AMCHP and is reproduced here with their permission.

- For Fiscal Years 2005 and 2006, the law annually appropriates $4.05 billion.
- For Fiscal Year 2007, the law appropriates $5.0 billion.

Before funds are allocated to the states and the District of Columbia, total amounts will be reduced by .25% for allocations to the territories and commonwealth. Of this .25%,

- Puerto Rico would receive 91.6%,
- Guam would receive 3.5%,
- Virgin Islands would receive 2.6%,
- American Samoa would receive 1.2%, and
- Northern Mariana Islands would receive 1.1%.

Funds will initially be allocated to the states based on each state's percentage of uninsured children adjusted for a state cost factor. Over time, that formula will change to include both the percentage of uninsured children plus the percentage of low-income children in families below 200% poverty.

- For Fiscal Years 1998–2000, states will receive federal allocations totally based on the number of uninsured children in families below 200% of poverty. Census Bureau data from the March *Current Population Surveys* will be used to determine the three year average for low-income uninsured children.
- For Fiscal Years 2001, the formula will change and will be based on 75% of a state's uninsured children plus 25% of a state's population of low-income children.
- For Fiscal Years 2002–2007, the formula will change again and be based on 50% of a state's uninsured children plus 50% of low-income children. The state cost factor is based on a state's average annual wage per employee compared to the national average. States have three years to spend their allotments.

D. ELIGIBILITY

States have to develop their children's health plans targeting low-income children. Low-income children are defined as those who satisfy all of the following criteria:

- meet the eligibility standards determined by the state;
- live in families with income below 200% of the poverty level (In states that have Medicaid levels above 150% of poverty on

the date of enactment, August 5, 1997, they can expand coverage to low-income children beyond the 200% cap, up to 50% higher than the state's previous Medicaid eligibility level.);

- are not eligible for Medicaid and not covered under another health plan; and
- are covered under a health insurance program which has been in operation before July 2, 1997 and which receives no federal funds.

In addition, eligibility standards

- can include geography, age, income, and resources, residency, disability status, access to other health insurance and/or duration of eligibility;
- within any defined class or group must serve children in lower income families first rather than children from families with higher incomes; and
- cannot prohibit children with pre-existing conditions from receiving coverage.

E. BENEFITS

States have four options in the area of benefits. Coverage of benefits must be governed by one of the following rules.

- It can be equivalent to those provided in a benchmark benefit package (listed below);
- It can have the same actuarial value as one of the benchmark benefit packages. States that choose the actuarial value of a benchmark plan must provide benefits in the basic benefits category listed below;
- Florida, Pennsylvania and New York have their state benefits packages "grand fathered" under this legislation; or
- A state can develop its own benefit plan. In this case, the Secretary of HHS will have to determine, upon application by a state, that the benefits provide appropriate coverage.

The Benchmark Benefit package includes one of the following:

- the standard Blue Cross/Blue Shield preferred provider option service benefit plan offered under the Federal Employees Health Benefits Plan,

- the health coverage that is offered and generally available to state employees, or
- the health coverage that is offered by an HMO and has the largest commercial enrollment in the state.

States are required to cover basic benefits which include inpatient and outpatient hospital services, physicians' surgical and medical services, lab and x-ray services and well-baby and well-child care, including age-appropriate immunizations.

States also have to cover 75% of the actuarial value of additional benefits if they are included in the benefit package selected by the state. If these additional benefits are not included in that benefit package, the state does not have to cover them. Additional benefits include prescription drugs, mental health, vision and hearing.

F. Cost Sharing

States must describe in their state plans the amount, if any, of premiums, deductibles, coinsurance and other cost sharing imposed. Cost sharing

- is permitted on premiums, deductibles, and coinsurance based on family income that would not favor children from higher-income families over those from lower income families;
- is prohibited on preventive services or benefits;
- must be imposed pursuant to a public schedule;
- must be nominal and may be based on a sliding scale for children in families below 150% of poverty so long as costs do not exceed 5% of a family's income.

G. Payments to States

The Secretary of HHS will make quarterly payments to states with an approved child health assistance plan.

A state would receive its federal allotment, or enhanced FMAP, based on its current Medicaid FMAP. The enhanced FMAP = the FMAP + (30% × 100 − FMAP). The enhanced FMAP can be no higher than 85%.

The allotments will be reduced by the cost of the state's presumptive eligibility program under Medicaid and costs of covering targeted low-income uninsured children under Medicaid.

The 10% limit on payments for administration, outreach and other child health services can be waived if a state establishes, to the satisfaction of the Secretary, that

- the coverage provided meets the benefits and cost sharing requirements of Title XXI,
- the cost of such coverage is no more than it would be otherwise, and
- such coverage is provided through the use of a community-based health delivery system.

A state may use Title XXI funds to purchase family coverage for families that include targeted low-income children. The state must establish, to the satisfaction of the Secretary, that cost of such family coverage is more cost-effective when compared with the cost of covering only children, and does not substitute for other health insurance coverage.

Funds may not be used to pay for

- children eligible for Medicaid using standards in effect April 15, 1997;
- services that a private insurer would be obligated to cover;
- services for which payment can reasonably be expected to be made under any other federally operated or financed health insurance program or the Indian Health Service; or
- abortion services or for health benefits coverage that includes coverage of abortion except in cases of rape, incest, or when necessary to save a woman's life.

Federal funds or program spending that is largely subsidized by federal funds may not be claimed as the required non-federal share of costs.

The Secretary may make payments to states on the basis of advance spending estimates made by the state, and may adjust payments to account for overpayment or underpayment in prior quarters.

H.   STATE MATCHING REQUIREMENTS

For the new children's health funds, a state will have to match 70% of its Medicaid matching rate. For example, a state that pays 50% of Medicaid costs would pay 35% of costs for new children. This matching rate applies to either Medicaid expansions or a new child health insurance program. Each state must pay at least 15% of such costs.

I.   MAINTENANCE OF EFFORT

Medicaid eligibility must be maintained using income and resource standards in place in the state on June 1, 1997.

States that choose to expand Medicaid cannot use income and resource standards that are more restrictive than those used as of June 1, 1997.

Spending on state-only child health initiatives, in effect on April 15, 1997, must be maintained.

J.   STATE CHILD HEALTH PLANS

States have to submit to the Secretary a plan identifying how they intend to use the federal funds. Plans will have to describe

- the current insurance status of children, including targeted low-income children;
- current state efforts to provide or obtain coverage for uninsured children;
- how the plan is designed to coordinate with current state efforts to increase coverage of children;
- the methods of establishing and continuing eligibility and enrollment (see below), including a methodology for computing family income that is consistent with the method used for Medicaid beneficiaries;
- cost-sharing requirements, the health care delivery method (e.g. managed care, fee-for-service, direct provision of services, or vouchers) and utilization control systems;
- the procedures used to accomplish outreach and enrollment assistance to families of eligible children and to coordinate with other public and private health insurance programs;
- the methods of establishing and continuing eligibility and enrollment; and
- the provision of child health assistance to targeted low-income children in the state who are Indians.

Procedures established for eligibility have to ensure that

- only targeted low-income children receive assistance,
- children found through screening to be eligible for Medicaid are enrolled in Medicaid,
- the new insurance does not substitute for coverage under group health plans, and
- there is coordination with other public and private programs providing coverage.

K. PROCESS FOR SUBMISSION, APPROVAL AND AMENDMENT OF PLANS

A state plan would become effective in a specified calendar quarter that is at least 60 days after the plan is submitted.

All state child health plans would be required to identify

- specific strategic objectives aimed at increasing health coverage,
- performance goals for each strategic objective identified, and
- performance measures that are objective and verifiable so that when compared with the performance goals, indicate the state's performance.

Plans must include

- assurances that the state will collect data, maintain records, and furnish reports as required by the Secretary as well as provide the required annual assessments and evaluations; and
- a description of the process for obtaining ongoing public involvement in the design and implementation of the plan.
- A state may amend its child health plan at any time with a plan amendment. Plan amendments must be approved for the purposes in the legislation and would take effect on dates specified in the amendment.
- Amendments restricting or limiting eligibility require prior public notice of the change before taking effect.
- Unless the state is notified in writing within 90 days that a plan or amendment was disapproved, the plan or amendment would be approved.
- In the case of a disapproval, the Secretary would provide a state with a reasonable opportunity for correction.

L. ANNUAL REPORTS AND EVALUATIONS

States are required to provide an annual report to the Secretary by January 1 following the end of each fiscal year assessing the operation of the plan and the progress made in reducing the number of uninsured children during the prior fiscal year.

States are also required to provide an evaluation by March 31, 2000 assessing

- the effectiveness of the state plan in increasing the number of children with health coverage;
- the effectiveness of specific elements of the plan, such as characteristics of families and children assisted and quality of coverage provided;
- the effectiveness of other public and private programs in the state in increasing health coverage for children;
- state activities to coordinate the plan with other public and private programs providing health care and financing, including MCH services and Medicaid;
- trends in the state affecting the provision of health care to children; and
- plans for improving the availability of health insurance and health care for children.

Also due by March 31, 2000 are recommendations for improving the program.

The Secretary would be required to submit to Congress a report based on the state evaluations by December 31, 2001.

M. OTHER

States have the option of providing for a presumptive eligibility period for children under the age of 19 using Medicaid providers and qualified Head Start, child care, and WIC agencies.

The legislation requires states to continue Medicaid coverage for disabled children who were receiving SSI on the date of enactment of the welfare law (August 22, 1996) even if they lose SSI because of the new definition of disability.

16

Title XXI—The State Children's Health Insurance Program: What the New Authority Means for States

SHELLY GEHSHAN

In August 1997, President Clinton signed into law Title XXI of the Social Security Act, called the State Children's Health Insurance Program, which provides a framework for expanding state children's health insurance programs and $24 billion over 5 years to fund them. This is the largest federal investment in insurance coverage for uninsured Americans since passage of the Social Security Act in 1965.

States were already moving forward to fill gaps in coverage for children. Twenty-nine states have expanded Medicaid to cover more children than mandated by federal law, 7 states have established separate programs, and 24 states have developed private, charitable programs. Dozens of bills were introduced in the 1997 legislative sessions. However, the passage of Title XXI means that states that were heretofore unable to expand health insurance for children now have a new funding source available to support their efforts. This chapter describes the problem of uninsured children, outlines the options available to states under the new law, and describes current state activities to provide health insurance for children.

THE PROBLEM OF UNINSURED CHILDREN

Approximately one of seven children younger than the age of 19 (approximately 10 million) are without any form of health insurance. Of the 71 million children in the United States in 1995, 59% had employer-based health insurance, 23% had Medicaid, and 14% had no insurance. A majority of children without health insurance live in two-parent families where at least one parent works full time. Even so, most are low-income families; nearly 60% of uninsured children live in families with incomes below 150% of the federal poverty line, or $24,075 per year for a family of four.[1] The two most common reasons children are without employer-based health insurance are that the parent who worked has lost a job or the dependent coverage available is simply too expensive to buy.[2]

Insurance for children has been affected by trends in insurance for adults. Employer-sponsored insurance for adults is shrinking as more companies trim their work forces and use more temporary, part-time, and contract employees. The growth of the service sector of the economy has meant that many new jobs do not have benefits. Insurance costs are also a significant factor. The rising cost of health care during the 1980s and 1990s has driven up the cost of health insurance. As a result, many employers are not offering dependent coverage. If they do, they are paying for a smaller portion of the cost of the family policy, making it unaffordable for some lower-income workers. The decline in private health coverage is primarily due to the fact that fewer adults and children are being covered as dependents of employees. Some analysts believe that, given current trends, in 20 years, employer-sponsored dependent coverage will be a thing of the past.

Despite the increasing number of uninsured adults, changes in Medicaid eligibility have held the number of uninsured children relatively stable during the 1990s. In the late 1980s, Congress moved to "de-link" Medicaid and Aid to Families with Dependent Children (AFDC) in an effort to expand Medicaid for pregnant women and children. As a result, nearly 5 million more children were brought into the program between 1989 and 1993. Approximately half of the 34.2 million people now enrolled in Medicaid nationwide (17 million) are children. Although policymakers feared that expanding Medicaid coverage for women and children would displace private insurance, the data suggest that the effect has been very small. Although the data are far from conclusive, by one estimate, only 15% of the overall decline in private insurance is attributable to increases in Medicaid rolls.[3] Employers' decisions to decrease coverage is influenced by many factors, principally the cost of premiums.

Adding to the problem is the fact that nearly one third of the 10 million uninsured children (2.9 million) are eligible for but not enrolled in Medicaid. There are many likely explanations. Families may not know their children are eligible and do not apply for Medicaid benefits. The stigma of being on public assistance, along with the complex application process, may cause some families to delay applying for Medicaid until they are driven to do so by a child's specific medical problem. Finally, about half of those who are denied benefits are actually eligible but cannot supply the documentation needed to complete the process.[4]

Although some believe that people without insurance somehow get the health care they need, that is often not true, particularly for children. One study showed that, among uninsured adults, nearly half had problems getting the care they needed in the previous year.[5] For children, the failure to get care is even more serious because much of what they need is preventive, behavioral, developmental, or related to learning problems. Among young children, for example, 4% have a developmental problem, 7% have a learning disability, and 13% have an emotional or behavioral problem.[6] Uninsured children are less likely than other children to receive care from a doctor as opposed to a clinic or hospital, get routine check-ups, be properly immunized, and get dental care. If problems are not identified early, they can lead to serious difficulties. For example, undiagnosed and untreated learning disabilities or vision problems can lead to poor literacy skills and school performance. Untreated ear infections can lead to permanent hearing loss. The price of delaying care or getting no care at all can be life-long difficulties for a child.

OPTIONS FOR CHILDREN'S HEALTH COVERAGE UNDER TITLE XXI

Title XXI, the new State Children's Health Insurance Program, is, like Medicaid, an optional program that requires states to supply matching funds and comply with requirements related to eligibility and benefits. States must initially submit a plan for approval by the Secretary of Health and Human Services. The plans must describe the extent of the problem, current efforts to solve it, plans for the use of funds, eligibility standards and outreach activities for the new program, quality assurance mechanisms, coordination with other state programs, and the proposed system of service delivery. Although funds are available October 1, 1997, states have 3 years to spend them. Given the speed with which the bill was enacted and the complexity of the new program, implementation is likely to be an incremental process that takes years.

There are two basic options under Title XXI: expanding Medicaid or establishing a new program. States can utilize a combination of the two, and many are likely to. Because development of the state plan will require a detailed examination of the state health system, many states may take the opportunity to craft a plan that fills a number of gaps. The target population for the new program is children younger than age 19 in families with incomes less than 200% of the federal poverty line who are not covered by any other insurance program. The six states that now cover children above the 200% level (Hawaii, Minnesota, Rhode Island, Tennessee, Vermont, and Washington) are allowed to expand up to 50% above their current level.

States have substantial flexibility under the new law in crafting their plan. States can determine eligibility for the program based on age, geography, income, residency, disability, and access to other insurance. This means that states could target the program to disabled children, children residing in medically underserved areas, children older than age 14, and those under 200% of the federal poverty level (the so-called "OBRA" children who are currently being phased in 1 year at a time). States can also consider offering family coverage if they can prove that it is cost effective.

Two other provisions can also be used to increase access to the state's current Medicaid program, even if the state chooses to develop another program separate from Medicaid.

1. The law allows states to use "presumptive eligibility" for children, which means providers can begin to serve children who appear to be under the income limit until their application is completed.

2. The law also allows states to provide 1 year of continuous eligibility for children, even if their family income changes.

Implementing these two provisions would assist states in servicing hard-to-reach children by enrolling them when they present for care and maintaining their enrollment for a year.

States are allowed to spend up to 10% of their total federal and state program funds on administration, outreach, and contracting directly with providers for health services. States can request a waiver of this limit and fund more services directly if they can prove that the benefits provided are those required under the law, that the cost of care is not more expensive than other care rendered under the program, and that the care is delivered by community-based agencies such as federally qualified health centers or disproportionate share hospitals. This provision is controversial because 10% is a relatively small amount for administration and outreach, particularly in light of the millions of children who are eligible for but not enrolled in Medicaid. Critics also fear that a waiver of this ceiling could potentially allow states to divert money from children's health coverage and use it to compensate providers who have sustained cuts in other federal payments.

At this point, state officials, the policy community, health care providers, and advocates all are examining the new law and beginning discussions about how their states will implement Title XXI. How quickly states respond will depend on many factors, including whether they have a program in place, whether their legislature has a special session scheduled that can be used to appropriate the funds needed for the state match, the quality and tenor of the working relationship in the state between the legislative and executive branches, and the clarity of the guidance issued by the Department of Health and Human Services. The seven states that have a program already in place (Colorado, Florida, Massachusetts, New Jersey, New York, Pennsylvania, and Washington) will be able to build on them, but they still face many decisions about how to redesign and expand their programs. Many other states who have expanded Medicaid beyond mandated levels may examine further expansions in lieu of or in addition to establishing a new program. The 16 states that have neither expanded Medicaid nor developed a separate program will have fewer coordination problems but more basic groundwork to lay.

The alternatives of expanding Medicaid or establishing a new program are basically the same ones that states have had. A key question is how states will evaluate the pros and cons of these two approaches as they design their programs. There are a number of advantages to using Medicaid as a basis for Title XXI expansions. Medicaid provides a comprehensive benefit package, which is particularly good for children with special needs or those who have been uninsured and poorly served before enrollment. Medicaid also has an existing administrative and reimbursement system and a network of providers. Under traditional Medicaid programs, states are required to provide inpatient care; services provided by a physician, nurse practitioner, or nurse midwife; skilled nursing care; home health care for people in nursing facilities; family planning; laboratory and x-ray services; and screening for children younger than age 21.* In addition, states can add a number of optional services. Those most relevant for children include emergency medical services, clinic services, eyeglasses, dental services, and prescription drugs.

Using Medicaid as the vehicle for Title XXI is no guarantee that needy children will enroll and receive services, however. Even special Medicaid waiver programs targeted at children, such as those in Maryland and Rhode Island, have had lower enrollments than expected. Most states have found that designing effective outreach, simple enrollment processes and forms, and efficient administrative systems is essential in working with families to get their children enrolled in Medicaid.

The main advantage of establishing or expanding a program separate from Medicaid is that states can use a more limited benefit package which costs less and allows them to insure more children. Before Title XXI, states used programs separate from Medicaid so they could cover children who were not eligible for Medicaid, require co-payments and premiums from families, and pay providers less. These things are all allowable under Title XXI. State programs have allowed them to circumvent other requirements in the Medicaid program, such as ensuring that benefits be made available to everyone who is eligible or that recipients be able to use any provider they choose. However, there are a whole new set of requirements under Title XXI which will govern the design and implementation of non-Medicaid programs.

CURRENT STATE ACTIVITIES

Expanding Medicaid Eligibility

Because all states receive federal funds to match their share of the costs, most have relied on Medicaid expansions to increase the avail-

---

*Screening refers to early and periodic screening, diagnosis, and treatment (EPSDT). States are required to provide EPSDT and to pay for services needed for conditions detected during EPSDT visits, even if they are not ordinarily covered under the state Medicaid plan.

ability of health insurance. In addition to expansions under the new Title XXI, there are two ways that states can expand eligibility for Medicaid. Under Section 1902(r)(2) of the Social Security Act, states can use income and asset guidelines that are more liberal than those applied to recipients of cash assistance programs for special populations such as children. Most states have used this provision to increase eligibility in small increments, such as including older children or children at higher income levels.

The other way to offer Medicaid eligibility to needy children and adults who otherwise would not be eligible is to apply for a research and demonstration waiver (1115). Hawaii, Minnesota, Tennessee, and Vermont, for example, have implemented large-scale managed care programs under 1115 waiver authority that allow them to cover more children. In Minnesota and Vermont, the states first expanded coverage using 1902(r)(2) authority, then included those children into the waiver program once it was approved and implemented. Both 1115 waivers and 1915(b) waivers allow states to circumvent many requirements that have made Medicaid expansions too expensive or difficult for states to administer. Waivers are required if states wish to provide fewer or different services to segments of the eligible population, to restrict recipients' choice of providers and enroll them in managed care, to require co-payments and premiums for families based on their income, to establish a program in only part of a state, or to establish reimbursement rates that are not consistent among providers. The following three states have used very different approaches to expanding Medicaid.

Rhode Island. RIteCare is an 1115 research and demonstration waiver program that was developed to target low-income women and children and enroll them in managed care. The program originally expanded coverage for pregnant women and children younger than age 6 with family incomes to 250% of the federal poverty line. RIteCare has a very comprehensive benefit package that includes primary care, inpatient care, dental care, home health and skilled nursing care, substance abuse treatment, prescriptions, and free bus passes. In April 1996, the program was expanded to include children up to age 8 and now enrolls more than 44,000 children.* In May 1997, Rhode Island allowed children up to age 18 to enroll, largely because the expected number of younger children did not enroll. Many of the families who apply for insurance for their children under the new program would have been eligible previously.

---

*This figure represents children up to age 14. Figures for children over 14 are not broken out from adults.

Minnesota. In 1987, Minnesota established a limited children-only health program. The program, originally funded by a cigarette tax, used Medicaid providers and paid them Medicaid rate to provide outpatient services. Children ages 1 to 8 who were below 185% of the federal poverty line were eligible. In 1992, the state embarked on an ambitious health care reform effort that established a new program called MinnesotaCare, which included adults, provided more services, and covered more children. Children younger than age 21 with family incomes of up to 275% of the federal poverty line are eligible. The state later obtained an 1115 waiver to enable it to limit patients' choice of providers, using managed care, and require family co-payments. To qualify for MinnesotaCare, families must have been without employer-supported coverage for 18 months and uninsured for 4 months. This provision was added to ensure that employers did not cancel their coverage to take advantage of the availability of a state-funded program. There are no co-payments required for preventive care and no limits on inpatient care for children.

MinnesotaCare is paid for with Medicaid funds, premiums (families contribute small payments based on a sliding scale), and a 2% tax on health care providers that is passed on to all insurers, including companies that self-insure and are thus exempt from state regulation under the Employee Retirement Income Security Act. There is also a 1% tax on Blue Cross/Blue Shield. These funds provide coverage for 95,000 people, including approximately half of the state's 100,000 uninsured children.

Washington. In 1988, Washington established its Basic Health Care Plan to provide low-cost insurance to uninsured adults in some counties. In 1994, the pilot program was expanded statewide, and a new companion program, called Basic Health Care Plus, was established. The Plus program provides coverage for children younger than age 19 with family incomes of up to 200% of the federal poverty line who are not in families receiving cash assistance. Plus is a Medicaid program that offers the same benefit package as traditional Medicaid through a choice of managed care plans. About 60,000 children are covered. What is unique about this program is the fact that, although it is a Medicaid program, it is coupled with a program for uninsured adults so whole families can receive coverage. In addition, although the program uses managed care plans, the state did not implement the program under a waiver because families have a choice of plans for their children.

Programs Using State Funds

A number of states have designed programs using their own funds to provide health insurance for children. The programs, generally for children who are not eligible for Medicaid either because of age or income, vary considerably, although almost all use contracts with managed care providers to deliver services and hold down costs. Most also use an existing administrative system, such as the State Health Department, the Medicaid agency, or schools, to distribute information, verify eligibility, enroll children, and contract with providers. To save money, most programs offer a limited benefit package and require co-payments and premiums from families, generally on a sliding scale. Even though health insurance coverage for children is relatively cheap, the need for these programs is great; most of them cover a relatively small portion of the state's uninsured children. Program size has been limited by state appropriations, and states often restrict new enrollment until more funding is available. New York, Florida, and Pennsylvania have been granted special attention in the State Children's Health Insurance Program to continue to use their current benefit package. Other states with programs will have the option to expand them using Title XXI funds if they comply with the requirements of the law. They can also change their programs and use the new funds to serve new groups of children.

Florida Healthy Kids. This innovative program uses schools as the administrative base for the program, as well as to advertise the availability of benefits and establish eligibility. School-age children and their 3- and 4-year-old siblings are eligible if they are uninsured, in school, and not enrolled in Medicaid. The program offers a full range of services and some special services, including physical therapy, speech and occupational therapy, and substance abuse treatment for pregnant teenagers. Children's premiums are subsidized if they participate in the school lunch program. Uninsured children whose family incomes are above 185% of the federal poverty line pay premiums based on a sliding scale that differs by county. Health services in each county are provided by one health maintenance organization that receives a fixed payment for enrolled children. Florida Healthy Kids is funded by state general revenue funds, county property and other taxes, health district taxes, school board funds, and family premium payments. The program, operating in nine counties, covers approximately 47,000 children. It is being expanded to include as many as half of the uninsured children in the state by the end of 1997.

New York. Created in 1990, the statewide Child Health Plus program now provides health insurance for 110,000 predominantly low-income children in New York. The State Department of Health contracts with private insurers that have in place networks of providers. Insurers process one-page applications that can include a variety of documents as proof of income; no resource or assets limits are imposed.

Uninsured children younger than age 13 who live in the state (even if they are not legal residents) and whose family incomes are under 222% of the federal poverty line are eligible. Families with incomes below 160% of the federal poverty line do not pay a premium; those between 160% and 225% of the federal poverty line pay $25 per child per year, up to a maximum of $100 per family. The program is financed from the Bad Debt and Charity Pool (funded by taxes on providers) as well as premiums and co-payments from families. Designed to offer primary care, Child Health Plus covers preventive services, emergency care, outpatient surgery and diagnostic tests, outpatient substance abuse treatment, short-term physical and occupational therapy, chemotherapy, and dialysis. A recent expansion added inpatient care. However, the plan does not cover dental care or speech therapy.

Private Programs and Partnerships

Some states have chosen to provide start-up funds or contribute funds to private programs, rather than establish a new state program or expand Medicaid. The most extensive private efforts are the Caring Programs for Children, which are charitable foundations set up by Blue Cross/Blue Shield organizations in 24 states to provide an insurance package for uninsured children who are not eligible for Medicaid. Each program is run separately and collects private and corporate donations to purchase insurance for needy children. Most Blue Cross/Blue Shield plans provide matching funds for other private donations, and all plans loan the program office space and supply staff and administrative support. Currently, four states contribute their own funds into Caring Programs to purchase insurance for children: Kansas, Michigan, Montana, and Pennsylvania. States could consider using Caring Programs as a vehicle for providing insurance coverage to children under Title XXI.

In Pennsylvania, the Caring Program is used as a model for a large-scale health insurance program for children called the State Children's Health Insurance Program (CHIP). Separate public-private plans are operating in three different regions of the state, with privately funded insurance plans augmenting coverage in two of the three. The public-private programs together provide health insurance for nearly 50,000 children. Coverage is "layered," so that the fully subsidized BlueCHIP program covers children in families with incomes up to 185% of the federal poverty line, and two sliding scale programs cover children whose family income falls between 185% and 235% of the federal poverty line.

CONCLUSION

The State Children's Health Insurance Program will significantly change the structure and availability of insurance for children. It is unclear at the outset how many of the nation's uninsured children will be able to receive coverage through the new programs, but states will be responsible for crafting and implementing programs to provide the best coverage possible for the greatest number of low-income children.

References

1. U.S. General Accounting Office. *Health insurance for children, many remain uninsured despite Medicaid expansion.* GAO/HEHS-95-175. Washington, DC: GAO, July, 1995.
2. Sheils, J., and Aleczih, L. *Recent trends in employer health insurance coverage and benefits.* Washington, DC. The Lewin Group, September 3, 1996.
3. Cutler, D., and Gruber, J. Medicaid and private insurance: Evidence and implications. *Health Affairs.* 1997;16(1):194.
4. Shuptrine, S. *Southern regional project on infant mortality.* Washington, DC: Southern Governors' Association, 1986.
5. Donelan, K., Blendon, R.J., Hill, C.A., Hoffman, C., Rowland, D., Frankel, M., and Altman, D. Whatever happened to the health insurance crisis in the United States? *JAMA.* 1996;276(16):1346.
6. Evans, A. *Financing and delivery of health care for children.* Washington, DC: National Academy of Social Insurance, May, 1994.

17

A View from the Field: Lessons Learned From More Than Twelve Years of Providing Health Care Coverage for Uninsured Children

Charles P. LaVallee and Kevin D. Sunderman

WESTERN PENNSYLVANIA CARING FOUNDATION FOR CHILDREN

Beginnings

In 1985, uninsured children were not an issue. Millions of children went without needed health care because they did not have health insurance; families worried every day about the one accident or sickness that could bankrupt them—but not many people noticed it, and even fewer tried to do anything about it. It took an economic disaster and the consequent swelling of the ranks of the uninsured in one region of the United States for one innovative solution to this problem to come about.

The Western Pennsylvania Caring Foundation for Children (Caring Foundation) began in 1985 to respond to the needs of uninsured children falling through the cracks of the health care system. The Caring Foundation emerged out of the massive dislocation resulting from the collapse of the steel industry in western Pennsylvania. In the early 1980s, the Pittsburgh area lost 140,000 manufacturing jobs, affecting hundreds of thousands of family members directly. Many neighborhood businesses, from barber shops to grocery stores, also failed as the money dried up in these old steel communities. This was a major crisis for the region, both economic and emotional.

Thousands of workers had lost their jobs, and along with them, their health care benefits. As these families struggled to get back on their feet, they carried the extra burden of anxiety for their children, the worry that their families were now exposed to sickness or accident with no health insurance. As one displaced steelworker, himself the son of a retired steelworker, put it, "You can pay for rent, groceries or health care. You can't get all three. This is not a choice anyone should have to make for their children." This father was not even considering the purchase of health care *coverage*; taking his children for medical care when they were sick or hurt was always an agonizing decision when the cost could mean going without food or falling behind in rent.

The Western Pennsylvania Caring Foundation for Children was born out of listening to the needs of these parents. Two ministers, John T. Galloway, Jr., and William F. Ewart, from Fox Chapel Presbyterian Church in a suburb of Pittsburgh, listened to the anguish of these families who had nowhere to turn. The parents asked for help for their children—they would forgo health care coverage for themselves, but they wanted their children to be cared for. Time and again the ministers heard the typical parental response: "Don't worry about me, but please do something for my kids." The ministers met with the late Eugene J. Barone, then President and CEO of Blue Cross of Western Pennsylvania, to share the problems of uninsured children.

Lesson 1

....

Listen to those who are to be the beneficiaries of any program that will be developed.

- Programs cannot be effectively developed and structured without being connected to needs of those who are to be served.

In response to these inquiries, and as an expression of its mission, Highmark Blue Cross/Blue Shield (formerly Blue Cross of Western Pennsylvania and Pennsylvania Blue Shield) launched the Caring Program for Children. The Western Pennsylvania Caring Foundation for Children implemented outreach and fundraising initiatives and provided administrative services for the Caring Program for Children.

The first program of its kind in the nation, the Caring Program offered primary and preventive health care coverage to uninsured children from low-income families. The Caring Program's initial benefits package was designed to offer basic services to the greatest number of children. This package was made up of five core benefits: doctor office visits for sick and well-child care, immunizations, diagnostic testing, emergency care, and outpatient surgery. No child was then or has ever been excluded because of a pre-existing condition.

Initially, the children served were from families who earned less than 100% of the federal poverty level (FPL), yet were ineligible for medical assistance (approximately 50% FPL in Pennsylvania in 1985) (Fig. 17.1).

The program was financed through community contributions (Fig. 17.2) either donated at-large for any child who was uninsured in western Pennsylvania or targeted to children from a specific geographic area. The community contributions were matched by Highmark, both to inspire the community and to reach more children. Highmark also donated the administrative costs of the program. Thus,

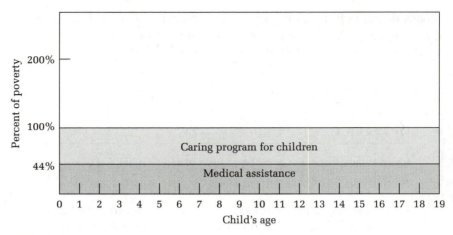

FIGURE 17.1

....

Caring Program for Children eligibility, 1985.

every dollar received from the community was doubled and went to health care costs of the children. In 1985, the cost to sponsor a child in the program was $156 per child per year. The Caring Program began with an enrollment of 200 children.

Lesson **2**

....

Start—no matter how small the beginning steps are.

- There is no need to have a "perfect" program.
- Begin—meet the needs that can be met.
- Success cannot be built on until a program has begun.
- Leadership means both action and risk: no program like this had been created before.

The health care delivery system for the enrolled children was the Blue Cross/Blue Shield (BCBS) network of 12,000 physicians and all the hospitals in western Pennsylvania. These children received the same care from the same providers that any other private BCBS

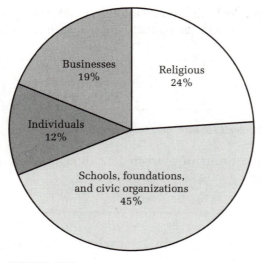

FIGURE 17.2

Community donations to Caring Program, 1985–1997.

customers received. The Caring Program administration used the strengths of private sector systems and experience.

Lesson **3**

Use the strength of the private sector.

- No one needs to reinvent the wheel.
- Take advantage of existing administrative efficiency, out-reach expertise, and strong networks of physicians who can serve children in both rural and urban settings.

The Caring Program children were mainstreamed—not set apart in their own "special" program. All enrolled children received a standard Blue Cross/Blue Shield card, identical to those used by any other BCBS members. From the beginning, one of the guiding principles has been to uphold the dignity of all participating families by not setting them apart or making them feel different. Families overwhelmingly respond in favor of this inclusion in the mainstream of health care coverage.

Lesson 4

Maintain the dignity of enrolled families.

- No family wants to be treated, or thought of, as a second-class family

---

The goal of the Western Pennsylvania Caring Foundation for Children was to create a model that could

- Demonstrate that it was possible to provide coverage
- Be replicated
- Be driven up to scale
- Inspire the nation

Building a Model

Philanthropy alone could not solve the problem of the uninsured. The ultimate goal was to establish a model that could be built on and greatly expanded, to serve children until the need was met in other ways and philanthropy was no longer necessary to finance the coverage.

The response to providing the coverage was extremely positive from both the enrolled families and the western Pennsylvania community. The families were very grateful, not only for the coverage, but also for the relief from the burden of worry they had for their children. The community embraced the program as well. From its inception, more than 30,000 community partners have worked to identify eligible children and raise funds.

The Western Pennsylvania Caring Foundation for Children was a catalyst, empowering communities to help their own. Applications were primarily distributed to community partners, who then distributed them to potential families. The number one source of referrals to the program came from friends or relatives—a finding that shows the importance of grassroots knowledge of the program and the necessity of getting the word out about the program throughout the region in order to make possible word-of-mouth referrals.

Collaborative efforts exist with groups such as schools, religious groups, civic organizations, minority advocacy groups, county assistance offices, local stores and restaurants, physicians and hospitals, hundreds of local programs, local government officials, majors, supervisors, WIC (Special Supplemental Food Program for Women, Infants and Children), unions, hospitals, job centers, businesses and corporations, as well as individuals. Parents of enrolled children have also participated in community efforts and in mobilizing their schools to find eligible children. The Caring Foundation has also aired television public service announcements featuring Fred Rogers of the television program *Mister Rogers' Neighborhood*, worked with the Pittsburgh Steelers football team and area schools, and built grassroots efforts in every county in western Pennsylvania.

When the 10 million uninsured children in America are looked at as a whole, many might feel overwhelmed at attempting to find a solution to so large a problem. But when people can feel the problem closer to their own level—300 uninsured children in their school district; 500 uninsured children in their county—then the problem becomes manageable. Communities want to help their own children.

L e s s o n 5
....

Commitment and participation of the community at the grassroots level are essential.

- Communities *want* the opportunity to respond to their own uninsured children—they need a vehicle for doing so.
- The spirit of "neighbor helping neighbor" is a powerful instrument for change.

The Caring Foundation's outreach staff makes an average of 600 presentations per year; approximately 350,000 fliers and 50,000 applications are distributed yearly, and every year more than 10,000 new children are enrolled, while 3,000 to 4,000 children are referred to Medical Assistance.

The power of committed individuals joined together and focused on helping children is very effective in getting things done. The partnerships formed in western Pennsylvania represented a broad spectrum of the community:

- 170 western Pennsylvania schools, a dozen corporations, and the Pittsburgh Steelers have worked in partnership with the

Caring Foundation since 1989 to find uninsured children and raise more than $2 million for other children in need.

- In one rural mountainous county, a group of coal miners banded together to find uninsured children and to raise funds for the Caring Foundation.

- Thousands of churches have taken leadership roles in reaching children, from entire denominational bodies and dioceses to individual community churches at the local level.

- In a rural northern Pennsylvania county, one family foundation undertakes to pay for the cost of every enrolled child in the county with the goal that no child in the county should be without health care coverage solely through a lack of finances.

- In another county, area businesses through the Chamber of Commerce passed out program information to their customers, and all the churches included information in their bulletins every Sunday for a month.

- Three hospital CEOs and a community leader from a semi-rural western county brought together 100 of the most influential people from their county and pledged that no child in their county would go without health care coverage. They have been true to their word since 1987.

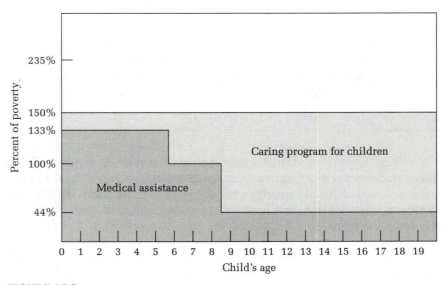

FIGURE 17.3

Caring Program for Children eligibility, 1989–1992.

Caring Program eligibility guidelines first changed as Medical Assistance guidelines expanded under the Omnibus Reconciliation Acts of 1986–1990 (Fig. 17.3).

EXPANDING THE MODEL

National Caring Programs for Children

The model that had been established in western Pennsylvania was receiving significant attention and interest throughout the country. The Western Pennsylvania Caring Foundation for Children worked closely

TABLE 17.1

Caring Programs Starting Dates

Western Pennsylvania	May 1985
Missouri, St. Louis	January 1987
North Carolina	November 1987
Alabama	March 1988
Maryland	March 1988
North Dakota	January 1989
Kansas	February 1989
Ohio	March 1989
New York*	September 1989
Iowa	October 1989
Wyoming	August 1990
Southeastern Pennsylvania	September 1990
Michigan	November 1991
Texas	January 1992
Utah	April 1992
California	July 1992
Mississippi	July 1992
Missouri, Kansas City	August 1992
Massachusetts*	November 1992
Virginia*	December 1992
Montana	January 1993
Georgia	April 1993
Louisiana	July 1993
South Dakota	December 1993
Idaho	January 1994
Oklahoma	August 1995
West Virginia	October 1996

*As other health care initiatives were launched, Caring Programs were no longer needed in these states.

(Author's note: With the implementation of Title XXI, the role of the philanthropically based Caring Program will be evaluated, and many will be completely absorbed through this implementation. See later discussion of Title XXI.)

with the Maternal and Child Health Bureau of the U.S. Department of Health and Human Services. Through SPRANS (Special Projects of Regional and National Significance) grants, the Caring Foundation was able to replicate its innovative model throughout the United States (Table 17.1). Blue Cross/Blue Shield Plans launched programs in their own regions.

The Children's Health Insurance Program of Pennsylvania

In 1992, a long-standing dream of the Western Pennsylvania Caring Foundation for Children came true. In December of that year, the Children's Health Insurance Program of Pennsylvania was signed into law by then-Governor Robert F. Casey. Pennsylvania State Representative (now Pennsylvania State Senator) Allen G. Kukovich was the primary sponsor of the legislation, funding for which came from two cents per pack of the state's cigarette tax (each penny generates approximately $10.5 million annually).

When it came time to design the details of the legislation, Kukovich looked to a program that was already covering children right in his own home district. "My initial strategy of modeling the Children's Health Insurance Program after the Caring Program for Children," he explained, "was that the Caring Program was a program that worked, it was cost-effective, and it had a good image in the state."

The Caring Foundation administers the Caring Program for Children, as well as the Children's Health Insurance Program in western Pennsylvania (where it is known as BlueCHIP). This public-private partnership was based on a private model supported by philanthropy, demonstrating a program that worked. The infusion of public dollars dramatically expanded the number of children who could be reached—the Caring Foundation receives more money from the state in a month than it does through an entire year of fundraising.

The benefits provided through BlueCHIP were comprehensive. The Caring Program's benefits were then adjusted to match those of BlueCHIP (Table 17.2). The expansion of benefits was made possible by a substantial increase in support by Highmark Blue Cross/Blue Shield. The cost of these benefits for enrolled children is approximately $850 per child per year.

The initial eligibility for BlueCHIP targeted specific groups of children. The Caring Program modified its eligibility requirements to create a seamless system of health care coverage for children in western Pennsylvania (Fig. 17.4). This was to ensure that there would be no overlap or duplication of services on the one hand, while leaving no gaps in coverage on the other.

TABLE 17.2

Caring Program for Children and BlueCHIP Benefits, 1985–1998

Caring Program	Benefit	BlueCHIP
1985	Doctor office visits	1993
1985	Immunizations	1993
1985	Diagnostic testing	1993
1985	Emergency care	1993
1985	Outpatient surgery	1993
1993	Dental	1993
1993	Vision	1993
1993	Hearing	1993
1993	Prescription drugs	1993
1994	Hospitalization	1993
1994	Mental health	1994

From the families' standpoint, the Caring Program/BlueCHIP could have been a single program, covering all their children. In other words, a single application received from a family in need of health care coverage enrolls children in BlueCHIP or the Caring Program. Whichever program the child is eligible for, he or she receives the same benefits, the same care, provided by the same physicians.

To increase the number of children served, BlueCHIP expanded its eligibility guidelines. BlueCHIP also covers children from birth to age 6

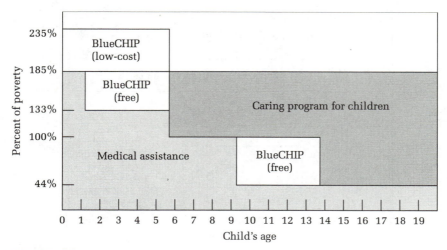

FIGURE 17.4

Caring Program for Children and BlueCHIP eligibility, 1993.

in families earning more than the eligibility limit for free coverage. These families pay a portion of the cost of their premiums. The Caring Program has also matched this subsidized coverage, offering the same benefits to older children in this same group of families. The families share in covering their children, paying $20 per month per child, with a family cap of $50 per month regardless of the number of children enrolled.

The goal of this low-cost coverage is to enable families to move forward without sacrificing their children's health care. The low cost a family pays for this coverage serves as a bridge to obtaining employer-provided coverage or to buying their own insurance.

More than 100,000 western Pennsylvania children have received health care coverage since 1985 through this model public-private partnership, the most comprehensive such partnership in the nation, empowering parents to care for all the children in their families.

So that all uninsured children, regardless of their families' income, would have an option to obtain health care coverage, families earning above 235% FPL—the fastest growing segment of the uninsured population in Pennsylvania—were able in 1997 to purchase Caring Program coverage for their children at cost.

Eligibility for the programs now is much wider than the initial guidelines between 50% and 100% of the federal poverty level. At this point, children from families up to 235% FPL and beyond can be covered (Fig. 17.5).

In 1997, Pennsylvania's Governor Tom Ridge and the state legislature increased the funding to the Children's Health Insurance Program

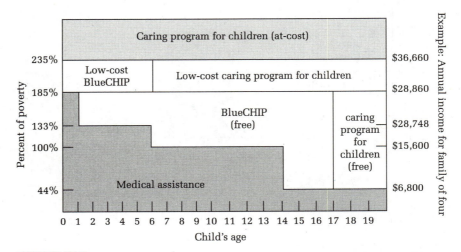

FIGURE 17.5

Caring Program for Children and BlueCHIP eligibility, 1998.

from two to three cents per pack of the cigarette tax, which increased enrollment in the Commonwealth to approximately 54,000 children.

The Western Pennsylvania Caring Foundation for Children began in 1985 by providing approximately 200 children with a basic package of primary and preventive benefits. By the end of 1997, more than 100,000 western Pennsylvania children had received health care coverage through the Caring Program for Children and the state-sponsored Children's Health Insurance Program, 97% of whom were in managed care. In addition, several hundred thousand more children had been covered through some two dozen variations on the Caring Program for Children throughout the nation and through state programs like Pennsylvania's Children's Health Insurance Program.

IMPACT OF THE PROGRAMS

The impact of living without health insurance is great, as is the impact of opening the doors to the health care system—on the children, their families, and the community as a whole.

Even with comprehensive coverage available to, and used by, enrolled children, the top three utilized services are primary care services:

- Physician office visits for illness
- Physician office visits for preventive care
- Immunizations

Studies of Caring Foundation participants by the University of Pittsburgh Graduate School of Public Health show the impact of the Caring Foundation on the families:

- Decrease in unmet medical care, vision care, dental care
- Increase in children having primary care physician
- Increase in children having dentist
- Decrease in limitation of activity due to lack of health insurance
- 97% of the parents were satisfied or very satisfied with the Caring Program
- 91% of the parents responded that it was easy or very easy to obtain health care services
- 77% of the parents thought the application was easy to fill out
- 93% of the parents felt that it was important to be able to complete the application at home

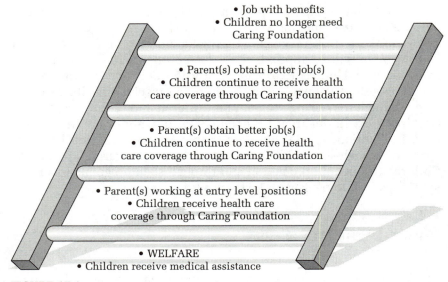

FIGURE 17.6

Climbing the ladder of self-sufficiency.

Additional data show the impact on the community of having children enrolled in BlueCHIP or the Caring Program:

- Through these two programs alone, the total number of uninsured residents of western Pennsylvania has been reduced by 5%.
- Total health care costs to the private sector in western Pennsylvania are estimated to have decreased by 1% as a result of these two programs, presenting $60 million in savings by the community (1985–1997).

A significant number of children no longer need the program every year because their parents gain employment with dependent coverage (Fig. 17.6). It is critical to note that the average length of stay in these programs is only 19 months. The Caring Foundation offers families a change to climb the ladder of self-sufficiency without sacrificing the health of their children.

The Western Pennsylvania Caring Foundation for Children provides the following:

- Coverage for children
- Improved health status for children
- Reduced cost shifting
- Lowered rate of uninsured

- Dignity of families
- Chance for families to climb the ladder of self-sufficiency

TITLE XXI: ANOTHER DREAM COME TRUE

A further step to provide America's children with health care coverage, the State Children's Health Insurance Program was enacted as part of the Balanced Budget Act of 1997. This new program, Title XXI of the Social Security Act, entitles participating states to annual federal allotments that must be used for low-income uninsured children. Providing $20.3 billion over the next 5 years to expand children's health coverage, Title XXI was based in part on the success of states like Pennsylvania in providing health care coverage to uninsured children. In fact, Pennsylvania was one of only three states with existing children's health insurance programs that were "grandfathered" into Title XXI.

The Western Pennsylvania Caring Foundation for Children and its public-private partnership, with its history of serving the needs of uninsured children, was closely examined in the crafting of this legislation. The Administration, members of Congress, and their staffs sought input from the Caring Foundation.

In his budget address on February 3, 1998, Pennsylvania Governor Ridge proposed a $15 million expansion for the Children's Health Insurance Program. This additional $15 million, added to existing state resources, is expected to draw down $80.3 million of federal funding for the first 12 months of the expanded program. "With these state dollars, and the expected new federal funding, we will be able to enroll approximately 122,000 new children in the program," said Ridge.

MEANS TO AN END

Creating legislation and providing funds for uninsured children are not enough. Nor is it enough to create or expand a program and simply announce the changes. If uninsured children cannot be found, they cannot be enrolled. In the experience of the Caring Foundation, parents of uninsured children had to have been provided with solid information about the program (for example, through schools, churches or synagogues, television advertisements) an average of at least three times before they would respond. Many had the "it's-too-good-to-be-true" syndrome—they simply did not believe that their children were eligible for comprehensive health care coverage.

It is imperative to remain focused on the goals for our children. Providing health care coverage is the first step. The next is that children receive appropriate and quality health care. Finally, our focus must remain on the health of our children. In order to ensure the care and the health of our children, as well as to successfully implement Title XXI, a key area of concern is outreach to eligible families.

Partnership with the community is needed; dollars must be invested in outreach. Although Title XXI provides $20.3 billion over 5 years for uninsured children, results are not automatic. Up to 10% of the total funding can be earmarked for outreach. This amount must be used, and used well. If we fail here, the whole program may fail. We will have wasted a great opportunity, perhaps the opportunity of a lifetime—our own lifetime and our children's lifetime.

The Western Pennsylvania Caring Foundation for Children's experience in Pennsylvania, a large and diverse state, demonstrates that providing health care coverage to America's children is within our reach.

Sidebar: *One Family's Story*

Joyce Oliverio is a bright talkative parent of three who has walked a long road the past few years.

"We were uninsured for over a year," she remembers. Joyce has a college degree in education, but because teaching jobs are hard to get, when her husband got laid off, the family had nothing to fall back on.

"The scariest part," she says, "is that you never know when something is going to happen. You worry that one of the kids is going to do something that will get them hurt.

"You worry, knowing that one emergency room visit will cost two paychecks, knowing that with one big accident we could lose our house."

Bobby, who is now 10 years old and going to Beechview Elementary School, got bitten by a dog during this time. His arm healed quickly, but, says Joyce, "it took us over a year to pay off the doctor bills from that accident.

"The worry is always there. You're always thinking, What if . . . ? What if . . . ?"

"What if they get hurt? What if they get sick? What if you have to take them to the doctor and then lose everything you have?"

"What if you don't take them to the doctor and then it turns into something worse?"

Joyce had that worry with Anthony, who is in eighth grade at West Liberty Academy. For years Anthony had to live with sore throats every couple weeks, missing a few days of school every time.

Finally, after enrolling in the Caring Program, Anthony had his tonsils removed and he hasn't had a sore throat in more than 2 years.

"It was scary at the time, not being able to do anything about it," says Joyce.

"You feel like a bad parent, not taking them to the doctor or the dentist. But you have to put things off."

"You don't want to mess up their lives just because of something you don't do. But you end up having to gamble with things you don't want to gamble with—your kids' health."

Finally, with nowhere else to turn, Joyce heard about the Caring Program and signed her family up.

"The Caring Program helped us get through years where we wouldn't have had anything else," Joyce says.

All three kids went to the dentist and the eye doctor, got regular check-ups, and had all the normal problems taken care of.

Anthony got glasses, which he badly needed, while Shannon, a sophomore at Pittsburgh's High School for the Creative and Performing Arts, got help of another kind.

Ever since fifth grade Shannon's feet had hurt, rubbing on her shoes. The pads or slightly larger shoes she got never really helped because the bones of her feet were shaped a little wider than usual. Shannon just learned to live with sore feet.

Until the Caring Program anyway. Once a part of the program, Shannon had an operation for her feet, and now sore feet are just a memory.

There are other benefits to the Caring Program as well. "It gives you peace of mind," says Joyce. "It takes that worry off your shoulders.

"It's also nice that you get a card that looks like anyone else's. No one, including doctors and nurses, knows you're any different than anyone else. No one treats you any differently."

Today, Joyce and her family are no longer with the Caring Program. Joyce now has a job with benefits, while her husband continues to build up his own repair business. They've moved ahead, allowing another family to benefit from the Program.

"The Caring Program was great," says Joyce. It gave us a cushion, the security to go out there and find a good job and not worry that our children's health was at risk."

General References

1. Lave, J.R., Keane, C.R., Lin, C.J., Ricci, E.M., Amersbach, G., and LaVallee, C.P. Impact of a children's health insurance program on newly enrolled children. *JAMA.* 1998;279(6):1820–1825.
2. Lave, J.R., Keane, C.R., Lin, C.J., Ricci, E.M., Amersbach, G., and LaVallee, C.P. The impact of lack of health insurance on children. *Journal of Health and Social Policy.* 1998;10:57–73.

18

Managed Care and Children

Dana Hughes

Since the early 1980s, the health care system in this country has been radically transformed from one dominated by fee-for-service arrangements to one increasingly dominated by managed care. Within this short period of time, the number of Americans enrolled in some form of managed care rose 14-fold.[1] The largest increases in managed care enrollment have occurred in the private market; however, managed care also has swept government insurers such as Medicaid. After federal restrictions on managed care enrollment were significantly relaxed, the number of Medicaid beneficiaries enrolled in managed care rose from 750,000 in 1983 to nearly 12 million in 1995.[2] An estimated 16.7 million children, or 22% of all children younger than age 20, were enrolled in managed care plans in 1994.[3]

The significance of this change is only partially understood today. Managed care, in a variety of forms and names, has been a means of financing and delivering health care for more than 50 years. The number of persons enrolled in managed care plans was, however, relatively low until recently. Thus, the extent to which past experience can help predict future effects is limited. However, research on managed care does suggest that this move is likely to at least partially achieve its intended objectives of helping contain costs and improving access to care for some of those enrolled. It may also have some unintended consequences, such as reducing access to needed care for other populations. Managed care may also improve the quality of care for some people, while making it worse for others.

This chapter provides an overview of managed care and examines the implications that its widespread adoption has for children. In particular, this chapter examines managed care for children enrolled in Medicaid, because of the extraordinary rate at which state Medicaid programs are converting to managed care. The sheer magnitude and speed of this move demand special analysis and scrutiny if lessons are to be learned from this experience. Moreover, because children who are Medicaid beneficiaries are generally from low-income families or are disabled, they may be more vulnerable to changes in how health care is delivered and financed.

What Is Managed Care?

The term *managed care* refers to a variety of financing and delivery arrangements. The single unifying characteristic of these various approaches is that enrollees are encouraged or required to obtain care through a network of participating providers who are selected by the managed care organization and agree to abide by the rules of that organization.[4] This is in contrast to fee-for-service arrangements, in which patients typically may seek care from any licensed health care professional or organization and providers may perform services based on their individual judgments about what is appropriate or needed. Within this general approach are a vast number of managed care models, which are derived from three major models:

- *Fee-for-service case management*, in which beneficiaries are assigned to a primary care case manager (generally a physician or clinic) that furnishes or arranges primary care services, authorizes use of specialty services, and coordinates such care. Sometimes referred to as managed indemnity plans or MIP, these arrangements place providers at no financial risk; instead, they are paid on a fee-for-service basis and receive a monthly case management fee. This lack of financial risk would lead many not to characterize MIPs as true managed care. However, they are commonly considered as such in the context of Medicaid.

- *Partially capitated arrangements*, in which plans or providers are placed at risk for only certain services. Each month, the plan or provider is paid a capitated fee covering those specified services for which it is responsible and at financial risk. Other services are reimbursed on a fee-for-service basis as they are rendered.

- *Fully capitated arrangements*, in which plans are at full financial risk for all or nearly all services to which the patient is entitled. Plans may provide services within the plan or arrange for them out of plan; they are paid on a capitated basis reflecting the range of covered services and the patient's risk.

Managed Care and Health Care Delivery for Children

How do these various models influence the delivery of health care for children? Perhaps the easiest way to understand managed care's effect on service delivery is to contrast managed care with fee-for-service. As Table 18–1 demonstrates, managed care differs from fee-for-service in a number of significant ways. One of the primary distinctions between these two methods of financing and delivering care is the requirement that patients select providers from a pool prescribed by the plan. Generally, patients select a primary care provider who provides the bulk

TABLE 18.1

A Taxonomy for Categorizing Health Insurance Plans

	Type of Plan				
	FFS	FFS CM	PPO	POS	HMO
Sponsor assumes financial risk*	−/+	−/+	−/+	−	−
Intermediary assumes financial risk*	+/−	+/−	+/−	+	+
Physicians assume financial risk[†]	−	−	−	+	+
Restriction on consumer's choice of provider[‡]	−	−/+	−/+	−/+	+
Significant utilization controls placed on provider's practice[§]	−	+	+	+	+

FFS, traditional fee-for-service indemnity plan; FFS CM, fee-for-service case management; PPO, preferred provider organization; POS, point of service or open-ended health maintenance organization; HMO, health maintenance organization (including independent practice association). − = absent; + = present

Sponsor is an employer or government. *Intermediary* is usually a health plan or other entity that serves as an administrative conduit. The left side of the slash reflects a plan where an employer purchases a full-premium benefit from the insurer. The right side reflects a self-insured (or minimally insured) private plan or government plan where risk resides with the sponsor.

[†]Primary care physicians at a minimum, but may also involve other providers.

[‡]In FFS CM, PPOs and PSOs, consumers' choice is limited through incentives and disincentives rather than mandatory restrictions. They have the option to seek covered care from outside the plan. The right side of the slash reflects care when this "out of plan" option is exercised.

[§]Usually defined as mandated prior authorization for non-emergency hospitalization.

Adapted from Weiner, J.P., and de Lizzovoy, G. Razing a tower of Babel: A taxonomy for managed care and health insurance plans. *Journal of Health Politics, Policy and Law.* 1993;18(1):75–103.

of care and approves referrals to specialists as he or she deems appropriate. This approach limits the patients' choice of primary care providers and eliminates their ability to "self-refer" to care.

In some instances, the list of available providers is quite extensive; in others, it may be quite limited. There is, however, an expectation that listed providers are truly available, unless their practice is listed as being closed. This is in contrast to the situation in which all licensed physicians are listed as "available," but in fact accept few Medicaid patients.

This approach also can serve to ensure linkage to a "medical home" in the form of a primary care provider who is chiefly responsible for a patient's care, which is considered advantageous, if not essential, for children.

Managed care also generally shifts financial risk from the sponsor of coverage—government or employer—to another payer or to providers. For example, under Medicaid managed care, the payer (the federal and state governments) shifts its financial risk to participating health plans. Although the payer is still responsible for the premium, financial risk for costs beyond the premium rests with the plan or is passed on in part or in full to providers. From the perspective of the payer, the principal advantage of this approach is that it introduces limits and predictability in expenditures. Although costs may rise from year to year based on re-negotiated contracts with plans, the payer knows with some certainty how much will be expended within the time frame of a given contract. This is in stark contrast to fee-for-service arrangements in which the payer is largely unable to either control or predict spending, because retrospective payments are made as services are rendered.

CHALLENGES AND OPPORTUNITIES

Most observers would agree that the transition from fee-for-service arrangements to managed care presents both challenges and opportunities in the provision of services to children, at least in theory. Managed care has the potential to affect access to health care, the quality of care received, and health care costs in countless ways. Proponents of managed care argue that it can result in improvements over fee-for-service through enhanced coordination and convenience of health services, emphasis on prevention, and flexible benefits.[5] Unlike fee-for-service, which merely promises to reimburse patients for the care they obtain, managed care plans have an obligation to provide services to the people enrolled in the plan. This means that the plan has to know who is enrolled and should keep track of the services they receive. A conventional fee-for-service insurer may not even know how many children are covered in a family, let alone whether they have received their immunizations, especially if such services are excluded from the benefit package. A managed care plan should know exactly which children are enrolled and whether their immunizations are up-to-date, thus providing mechanisms to improve access to and coordination of care. Opponents of managed care argue the opposite, citing the potential to create barriers for children through financial disincentives to provide quality care, risk selection, limitations on providers and services, and other system-related obstacles to care, especially specialty and sub-specialty care. Which of these perspectives is correct, if either, remains an unresolved question.

Indeed, in the absence of clear empirical evidence, any resolution to this debate is necessarily based on conjecture and speculation. Few data with respect to managed care and children exist to prove one view or the other. Although numerous studies have been conducted on the effect of managed care in general,[6] few studies have been conducted specifically on the impact for children. It is questionable, moreover, whether findings from studies pertaining to adults can be applied to children given how different children's needs for health services are from those of adults.

MANAGED CARE, ACCESS, QUALITY, AND COSTS

As previously stated, few studies have been conducted that examine the impact of managed care on children. What data are available are derived largely from Medicaid demonstration projects conducted in the early and mid-1980s as well as a few more recent studies of Medicaid managed care. It remains instructive, however, to outline what is known from these limited studies. After a comprehensive review of the literature that was published in *The Future of Children* in 1993, Freund and Lewit concluded that

> *It is difficult to document that managed care consistently results in decreases in hospital use for children or that it uniformly increases access to physicians, especially primary care providers, as claimed.[7]*

Similarly, they found little evidence that the health status of children or the quality of care they receive is any better under managed care than under traditional fee-for-service plans, and they concluded that "it is difficult to prove that managed care reduces the total societal costs of health care for children ... or slows the growth of these costs." They write:

> *About the only consistent finding is that managed care reduces emergency room use by children enrolled in Medicaid and tends to concentrate their care among a smaller number of primary care providers.*

Another comprehensive review of the literature studied the same work as well as research published since the Freund and Lewit article.[8] In addition, the authors included reports and other materials not found in the peer review literature. They, too, found mixed results in terms of access, quality, and costs. They concluded that, because of the different circumstances and conditions under which managed care is operating for Medicaid beneficiaries in the 1990s, it is uncertain whether either the positive or negative findings hold lessons for today.

MANAGED CARE FOR LOW-INCOME CHILDREN

Currently, most states have implemented managed care programs for Medicaid beneficiaries, principally those who are enrolled through TANF.[8] Because children constitute the majority of the AFDC populations, this conversion to managed care represents a marked change in children's health care. Examination of managed care's impact on children is important because children's health care needs are so different from those of adults, and as such, they require special consideration in the design and organization of health services.[9,10]

Yet, little is known about the impact of managed care on children, as indicated earlier. What little is known suggests that managed care, if not properly designed, may not necessarily produce the desired results. Because virtually no research has been conducted on non-poor children, the information from existing studies provides little guidance about those needed design elements. However, available information related to Medicaid managed care, as well as data that describe the needs of Medicaid beneficiaries, does suggest the following considerations for the design of Medicaid managed care.

Different Health Care Needs of Medicaid Beneficiaries

As a group, children are especially vulnerable to the health risks associated with poverty, such as poor housing and sanitation, inadequate diet, general family stress, and hardship.[11] These threats, as well as the social isolation and environmental hazards that accompany poverty, are associated with increased health problems.[11,12] For example, low-income children are more likely to have a learning disability and to have a long-term emotional or behavioral problem.[13]

Because of their more stressful living circumstances, Medicaid beneficiaries often have a greater need than the general population for services that affect health status but are not considered "medical care," such as psychosocial support and care coordination. As a result, low-income children often require access to a broad array of providers, such as social workers, counselors, and health educators, as well as effective linkages to public health programs and "non-health" public programs, such as housing and food assistance. However, many of these services are often not covered by traditional managed care plans.

Pent-up Demand

Research shows that low-income children receive less health care than the general population despite a higher level of need.[14-16] As a group, poor children are less likely to have a regular source of care. Poor children also use fewer physician visits after adjustment for need.[11,14,15] Taking into account greater likelihood of health problems, coupled with historical underuse of services, utilization may be higher among Medicaid covered children, at least initially. Managed care plans may expect to initially lose money on this population as "catch up" occurs.

Eligible for More Benefits

Non-Medicaid beneficiaries in managed care generally sign up for a set of benefits that are negotiated with the employer and the plan, based on a notion of what the plan can reasonably provide and on the premium paid. In the case of Medicaid, the benefits to which beneficiaries are entitled are set by federal law and go beyond what is generally covered in typical managed care plans. Indeed, under the Early Periodic Screening and Diagnosis Treatment (EPSDT) program, children are entitled to the full range of federally allowed Medicaid services, even if those services are not contained in the state plan.[17] Under shared risk arrangements, the financial incentives can restrict availability of these extended services. In fact, a 1990 survey of Medicaid directors found that only half of the states that enroll children in managed care planned to revise their contracts to ensure compliance with the EPSDT mandates.[18]

Fluctuating Eligibility

In theory, shared risk arrangements encourage provision of preventive health care to achieve future savings by preventing expensive hospitalization and treatment. Without assurances that patients will be enrolled in the future, there is little incentive to provide preventive health care to either public or privately insured patients. Yet, it is estimated that 40% of Medicaid AFDC enrollees go on and off Medicaid during the course of a year.

Low Rates of Payment

Typically, managed care rates are set at a discounted amount of annual fee-for-service expenditures for each eligibility category. Medicaid rates, however, are already typically well below market fees, particularly in pediatrics. For example, the average Medicaid fee paid to a pediatrician in 1989 for an established patient was nearly half the market fee.[19] In states where fee-for-service rates for pediatric care are especially low, the customary managed care rate-setting methodology could reinforce the incentive to underserve.

To ensure that managed care addresses the needs of low-income children, the design of Medicaid managed care programs should take into account the special circumstances and characteristics of this population.

WHY WE DON'T KNOW MORE

Why don't we know more about the impact of managed care on children and how to design optimal programs for them? Although there is a large and growing body of literature based on the Medicaid managed care demonstrations of the 1980s, the applicability of these data are limited. Indeed, most of the current knowledge available regarding managed care and children is derived from studies of Medicaid recipients.[20] The limitations of this research are based, in part, on the fact that these studies assessed Medicaid managed care programs operating before 1990, when the nature of managed care was dramatically different. Most of the Medicaid managed care demonstration programs were largely voluntary for Medicaid beneficiaries compared with today, when virtually all Medicaid families, especially those on AFDC, are required to enroll in managed care plans. This has implications both for the kinds of individuals who are enrolled in managed care (and their health care needs) and for the scope of the transformation to managed care, and hence the ability to make adjustments to address problems that arise. In addition, many of these studies lacked control groups in fee-for-service delivery systems. Consequently, the findings of studies from the mid-1980s may not be relevant to the current managed care environment. Moreover, virtually no studies have been conducted on non-poor children in managed care settings. Although conventional Medicaid programs have many of the aspects of fee-for-service from the perspective of the providers, they actually routinely incorporate two important aspects of managed care—enrollment and limited co-payments. State Medicaid agencies usually know exactly for whom they are responsible, thus mimicking the responsibility of the managed care plan and the ability to focus on enrolled populations rather than just "users." Reflecting the low-income status of its enrollees, the Medicaid law precludes use of co-payments and deductibles for children and mandates a broad benefit package. Thus, although managed care may offer important "denominator responsibility" and low financial barriers to comprehensive benefits in contrast to coverage for employed populations, this may not be a particular advantage for Medicaid recipients. Similarly, children with special needs covered by targeted programs may find little in the way of additional benefits and coverage under managed care, and in fact, may find that some needed services, particularly specialty care, may be obtained only out-of-plan. For these reasons, as well as the different health care needs of poor and non-poor children, it is not clear that the results related to children enrolled in Medicaid apply to privately insured children.

The diversity of approaches to managed care further complicates efforts to understand its impact, because different models are likely to have different impact on access and costs.[8] For example, the ability of sponsors, intermediaries, and physicians to absorb risk is so variable that utilization may be more tightly controlled in models in which physicians hold the risk as compared with large employers or large health plans. Care must be taken, therefore, to distinguish between the various approaches when analyzing the impact of managed care on children and designing programs for them.

Lack of strong evidence about the impact of managed care on children is also a function of fundamental problems with the current state of knowledge about measuring the impact of health services in general, which prohibit a fuller understanding of managed care. There is little agreement about which outcomes to monitor, measurements of outcomes, and appropriate comparison groups, particularly with respect to children. After years of effort, researchers have managed to produce a handful of basic quality of care measures. The measures that do exist tend to be applicable to high-prevalence health conditions experienced by large numbers of individuals (such as prenatal care and immunization rates) rather than low-prevalence conditions that affect relatively few individuals with high health needs but that may constitute a better test of quality in the case of a prepaid health care system that has a built-in incentive to underspend on its enrollees.

SUMMARY AND RECOMMENDATIONS

The adoption of managed care in place of fee-for-service health care is rapid and widespread. Between 1975 and 1994, the number of Americans who received care in health maintenance organizations alone rose by more than sevenfold, from 6 million to 51.1 million.[21] As of 1994, nearly one fourth of all children were enrolled in managed care plans. Among low-income children, the managed care penetration is higher. As of June 1996, 40% of Medicaid beneficiaries, the majority of whom are children, were enrolled in managed care plans.[22] Given current trends, the proportion of Medicaid-covered children enrolled in managed care is likely to continue to rise. Between 1983 and 1995, the number of Medicaid beneficiaries enrolled in managed care rose 15-fold.[2]

This dramatic shift to managed care has significant implications for children. Most observers agree that, if well designed and executed, managed care may have the potential to reproduce for children the cost savings, improved quality, and greater access that it has for middle-class adults. However, the evidence in support of managed care, although convincing for middle-class adult populations, is inconclusive and sometimes contradictory when considering children. As already mentioned, information derived from the managed care experiences undertaken thus far offer little guidance about what constitutes optimal design and implementation for children, with the exception of Medicaid managed care.

Policymakers and program planners concerned about children currently face a significant dilemma. The movement toward managed care has developed an undeniable momentum. At the same time, there is very little empirical evidence to demonstrate that this is an appropriate direction or to indicate ways to maximize the potential benefits and minimize the potential harm. At a minimum, this lack of conclusive data suggests the need to slow the conversion momentum until information can be gleaned from the current experiences about the impact on children, and modifications made, as needed. In particular, there is a need for research on the impact of managed care on non-poor children, for whom there is virtually no reliable information available. A commitment to and investment in research and monitoring by the federal and state governments, philanthropic organizations, and health plans are key to this.

We do have enough information to suggest the need for explicit steps to ensure that managed care plans address the needs of children and, as appropriate, the needs of poor children. At the very least, this means that plans must have available providers who are trained in pediatrics, particularly for children with special health care needs. In addition, health plans for Medicaid-enrolled populations must adapt their plans to this group's unique needs and circumstances. The principal distinctions between Medicaid-enrolled children and other children can provide guidance as to some of the aspects of plans that should be examined and possibly altered.

References

1. Freudenheim, M. Health care in the era of capitalism. *New York Times.* April 7, 1996, Section 4, page 6.
2. Roland, D., and Hanson, K. Medicaid: Moving to managed care. *Health Affairs.* 1996;15(3):150–152.
3. Leatherman, S., and McCarthy, D. Opportunities and challenges for promoting children's health in managed care organizations. In R.E. Stein (ed), *Health care for children: What's right, what's wrong, what's next?* New York: United Hospital Fund, 1997.
4. Rosenbaum, S., Serrano, R., Magar, M., and Stern, G. Civil rights in a changing health care system. *Health Affairs.* 1997;16(1):90–105.
5. Saucier, P. *Public managed care for older persons and persons with disabilities: Major issues and selected initiatives.* Waltham, MA: The Center for Vulnerable Populations, 1995.
6. Miller, R.H., and Luft, H.S. Managed care: Past evidence and potential trends. *Frontiers of Health Services Management.* 1993;9(3):3–37.
7. Freund, D.A., and Lewit, E.M. Managed care for children and pregnant women: Promises and pitfalls. *The Future of Children.* 1993;3(2):92–122.
8. Rowland, D., Rosenbaum, R., Simon, L., and Chait, E. *Medicaid managed care: Lessons from the literature.* Washington, DC: Kaiser Commission on the Future of Medicaid, 1995.
9. Halfon, N., Inkelas, M., and Wood, D. Nonfinancial barriers to care for children and youth. *Annual Review of Public Health.* 1995;16:447–472.
10. Wehr, E., and Jameson, W.J. Beyond benefits: The importance of a pediatric standard in private insurance contracts to ensuring health care access for children. *The Future of Children.* 1994;4(3):115–133.
11. Wise, P., and Meyers, A. Poverty and child health. *Pediatric Clinics of North America.* 1988;35:1169–1186.
12. Egbuonu, L., and Starfield, B. Child health and social status. *Pediatrics.* 1982;69:550–557.
13. Zill, N., and Schoenborn, C.A. Developmental, learning, and emotional problems: Health of our nation's children, United States, 1988. *Advance Data from Vital and Health Statistics,* No. 190. Hyattsville, MD: National Center for Health Statistics, 1990.
14. St. Peter, R.F., Newacheck, P.W., and Halfon, N. Access to care for children: Separate and unequal? *JAMA.* 1992;267:2760–2764.
15. Newacheck, P.W. Access to ambulatory care for poor persons. *Health Services Review.* 1988;23(3):401–419.
16. Newacheck, P.W., and Halfon, N. Access to ambulatory care for economically disadvantaged children. *Pediatrics.* 1986;78:813–819.
17. United States Congress. *Budget Reconciliation Act of 1989.* P.L. 101–329.
18. Fox, H.B., Wicks, L.B., and Newacheck, P.W. State Medicaid health maintenance organization policies and special-needs children. *Health Care Financing Review.* 1993;15(1):25–37.
19. McManus, M., Flint, S., and Kelly, R. The adequacy of physician reimbursement for pediatric care under Medicaid. *Pediatrics.* 1991;87:909–920.
20. Health Management and Gini Associates. *Evaluation of the Michigan Medicaid program's physician sponsor plan, 1989–1990, Part I. Analysis of cost effectiveness issues in the AFCD population.* Lansing, MI: Health Management Associates and Gini Associates, 1991.
21. Troy, T.N. Does managed care work? *Managed Healthcare.* July, 1996;6(7):20–41.
22. Health Care Financing Administration Web Page. [Internet web page] http://hcfa.gov/medicaid/pntrtn3.tmt. April 29, 1997.

19

The Supplemental Security Income Program for Children

JOHN REISS, HELEN M. WALLACE, AND MERLE McPHERSON

Program Background

The Supplemental Security Income (SSI) program has been an important part of the federal government's social benefits safety net for low-income children with special needs for almost a quarter of a century. SSI is a nation-wide program, administered by the Social Security Administration (SSA), that provides monthly cash payments based on the income of the child's family. As stated in the 1971 House Report on SSI, "disabled children who live in low-income households are certainly among the most disadvantaged of all Americans and . . . are [therefore] deserving of special assistance in order to help them become self-supporting members of our society."[1] In most states, children who are SSI beneficiaries also qualify for health care services through the Medicaid program.

In 1975, Congress assessed the impact of the SSI program on disabled children and concluded that, in the absence of a formal referral procedure for rehabilitative services, children receiving SSI had only a "haphazard" chance of coming in contact with an agency providing services to disabled children.[2] To address this problem, Congress amended the SSI program and created the Supplemental Security Income–Disabled Children's Program (SSI-DCP), which was administered in most states by the Title V Maternal and Child Health/Children with Special Health Care Needs (CSHCN) agency. This program was an innovative effort to ensure that children receiving SSI benefits had the comprehensive care and services they required. Individual service plans, written under the authority of the state Title V agency, were a hallmark of this program. In 1981 the SSI-DCP was integrated into the new Maternal and Child Health Services Block Grant, and subsequently most states discontinued a distinct SSI-DCP. However, today, state Title V CSHCN programs remain actively involved with many children receiving SSI benefits. As mandated in the provisions of the Omnibus Budget Reconciliation Act (OBRA) of 1989 (P.L. 99-272), state Title V CSHCN programs (1) receive referrals of SSI beneficiaries who are younger than the age of 16 years, and (2) provide rehabilitation services to these children to the extent these are not provided through Medicaid (Title XIX) [Section 501(a)(1)(C) of Title V].

In the 1990s, the SSI program underwent two major changes. The first of these changes was mandated in February 1990 through the Sullivan v. Zebley U.S. Supreme Court decision. This Supreme Court decision brought about a liberalization of the SSI childhood disability criteria that allowed an estimated 300,000 additional children to qualify for SSI benefits during the period 1990–1996. The second change was mandated by Congress in 1996, as part of the Personal Responsibility and Work Opportunity Reconciliation Act (P.L. 104-193). This Congressional reform of the SSI program tightened the SSI childhood disability criteria and will result in the loss of SSI benefits for an estimated 180,000 SSI current child beneficiaries.

In the Zebley decision, the Supreme Court found that the SSA was not implementing the SSI program as intended by Congress. Because the SSI legislation did not make a distinction between child and adult applicants, the Court found that the procedures used by SSA to determine the SSI eligibility of children, which were not comparable to those used with adults, were unconstitutional. For adults, the SSI disability determination process included an assessment of the adult's "functional status"; SSA did not use a comparable assessment of functioning for child applicants. It was this procedure of not assessing a child's functional status that the Supreme Court determined to be unconstitutional because it discriminated against children; i.e., children had to meet a stricter standard to qualify for SSI than did adults who applied for SSI.

As a result of this ruling, SSA

- Contacted the 452,000 children who had been denied benefits between January 1, 1980, and February 11, 1991, based on medical evidence only (termed the "Zebley class"); reevaluated the 339,000 who responded to SSA; and found approximately 135,000 of these eligible for SSI.

- Developed methods for assessing the functional status of children, known as the Individualized Functional Assessment (IFA).

- Developed improved methods for working with other public and private agencies that work with disabled children, to gather better information about the medical condition and functional status of child applicants.

- Implemented an active outreach program and worked to improve the ways in which parents get information about the program and apply for benefits.

Also, in December 1990, SSA issued regulations revising and expanding its medical standards for assessing mental impairments in children by incorporating functional criteria into the standards and adding such impairments as attention deficit hyperactivity disorder (ADHD), mood disorder, and personality disorder. This revision was undertaken in response to the Social Security Disability Benefits Reform Act of 1984 (P.L. 98-460) and was under way prior to the Zebley decision.

As is discussed in detail later, Congress closely followed the rapid growth in the number of SSI child beneficiaries after the Zebley decision and the growth in the total cost of the program. In 1996, more than $5 billion was paid in SSI benefits to children. Much attention was given to the number of SSI child beneficiaries with mental impairments, especially those eligible because of attention deficit hyperactivity disorder and other disorders that have been broadly characterized as behavior problems.

PROGRAM DESCRIPTION

The SSI program provides an income supplement to low-income disabled adults and children. Eligibility for the program is based both on financial status (income and assets) and on disability status.

Benefits

The maximum federal SSI monthly payment for a child was $484 in 1997 and was increased to $494 in 1998. The amount a given SSI beneficiary receives is based on income, the SSI cash benefit being reduced as income increases. For children younger than 18 who are living with their parents, the parents' income is considered when calculating the benefit amount. In most cases, for children 18 and older, family income is not considered.

In addition to the federal payment, states have the option of providing a supplemental cash benefit in order to address the special needs of selected SSI beneficiaries in the state and/or in recognition of the variations in the cost of living from one state to another. All but seven states and the Northern Mariana Islands provide supplement to some SSI beneficiaries. Fifteen states and the District of Columbia have chosen to have SSA administer the supplemental payments on the state's behalf. The other 28 states administer supplemental payments themselves. The amount of supplemental payment ranges from a few dollars up to $156 and averages about $80 per month.

In addition, most children who are eligible for SSI are also eligible for Medicaid. In 32 states and the District of Columbia, a child who is found eligible for SSI is automatically enrolled in Medicaid. Seven other states provide Medicaid to all SSI beneficiaries, but a separate Medicaid application must be completed. The remaining 11 states do not use SSI status as a criteria for qualifying for their Medicaid program, but rather use more restrictive income, resource, or disabilities standards. These states are often referred to as "209(b)" states; the name comes from the section of the law that authorizes states to use the more restrictive guidelines.[3]

Because the income eligibility requirements for SSI are, in general, more liberal than those for Medicaid, the SSI Program provides disabled children in 39 states and the District of Columbia access to the health care services through the state Medicaid program for which they may not otherwise qualify. In addition, SSI child beneficiaries are referred to the Title V CSHCN program in their state, which, in turn, assists many SSI child beneficiaries to access health and other needed supportive services that may be available through public and private programs.

Extent of Coverage of Disabled Children by SSI

In December 1989, immediately prior to the Zebley decision, approximately 296,000 children were receiving SSI benefits. In 1992, this number had more than doubled, to 623,845. In December 1995, there were 974,189 children receiving SSI, more than three times the number of beneficiaries in 1989. As of June 1997, the number of SSI child beneficiaries had increased to 1,022,028.

In September 1994, the General Accounting Office (GAO) issued a report on the rapid rise of children on the SSI disability roles, comparing the impact of the new Mental Impairments Listings (issued in 1990) with that of the Individualized Functional Assessment (IFA), which was implemented as a result of Zebley. GAO reported that approximately 60% of the growth in child beneficiaries during 1991 and 1992 was attributable to the mental impairments listing, and 40% was due to the IFA. The SSA Office of Disability attributes 69% of the growth in the SSI rolls to the revised listings. The diagnostic categories of blind and disabled children, ages 0 to 17 years, receiving SSI benefits in December 1988 and June 1997 are shown in Table 19.1. Mental retardation is, by far, the largest diagnostic group, both in 1988 and in 1997 (approximately 41%). The next most frequently diagnostic group in 1997 was mental disorders (other than mental retardation) at 25.4%. This diagnostic category constituted only 6.2% of SSI child recipients in 1988.

Eligibility for SSI: Citizenship, Residency, and Financial Status

Eligibility for the SSI program is based on citizenship, residency, financial status (income and assets), and disability status. With certain

TABLE 19.1

Diagnostic Categories of Blind and Disabled Children, Ages 0–17 Years,
Receiving Supplemental Security Benefits (December 1988 and June 1997)

Category	1988		1997	
	Number	%	Number	%
Mental Retardation	108,600	41.9	346,770	40.6
Diseases of nervous system/sense organs	66,100	25.5	97,200	11.4
Mental disorder (other than mental retardation)	16,000	6.2	217,420	25.4
Neoplasms	6,900	2.7	13,680	1.6
All other (e.g., endocrine or blood disorders; conditions of circulatory, respiratory, gastrointestinal, genitourinary, or musculoskeletal system; congenital anomalies; injury; infectious diseases)	37,300	14.4	178,620	21.0

exceptions, in order to be eligible for SSI a child must be a U.S. citizen or national and reside in one of the 50 states, Washington, DC, or the Northern Mariana Islands. Certain children of U.S. Armed Forces personnel stationed abroad are exempt from the residency requirement.

To determine the financial eligibility of a child younger than 18 years old, SSA evaluates the child's and the families' income and resources. For a child to qualify for SSI, the monthly income and resources that are available to the child must be less than dollar limits specified in the SSI regulations. The month after the child's 18th birthday, parental income and resources are not counted in the young adult's financial eligibility. Thus, a child who did not qualify financially before his or her 18th birthday may qualify when the parent's income is no longer considered.

The rules and procedures for determining financial eligibility are complicated, so the following example provides only a general idea of the family income criteria. In 1997, a disabled child in a family with two working parents and two children, one who has a disability and another who does not, could have a family income of up to $33,444 and still qualify. The maximum income level is higher in those states that provide supplements.

After SSA determines that the child meets the citizenship and residence requirements and appears to qualify financially, information about the child's disability and a list of additional sources of information are sent to a state Disability Determination Services (DDS) agency. SSA does not make disability determinations directly, but contracts with a state DDS agency to carry out this determination. State DDSs operate under federal regulations and instructions issued by SSA. It is the responsibility of the DDS to decide whether the child has any medically determinable condition and whether that condition produces a disability severe enough to make the child eligible for SSI benefits.

Eligibility for SSI: Disability Status

The rules and procedures for determining disability eligibility are also complicated. State DDSs use a team made up of a disability examiner and a medical or psychological professional to decide whether, based on the written information that is available to them, the child meets SSI disability criteria. As part of the disability determination process, a disability examiner develops a complete medical and functional history for at least the 12 months preceding the child's application for SSI. Staff of the DDS never examine the child, nor do they meet with the child/family face-to-face. In determining SSI eligibility, the DDS uses the following sequential process.

In Step 1, the examiner determines whether the child is engaged in substantial gainful activity (SGA) (i.e., is working). If the applicant does engage in SGA, then the claim is rejected. If the applicant child does not engage in SGA, the examiner proceeds to Step 2. In Step 2, based on the available documentation, the examiner determines whether the child applicant has a medically determinable impairment or combination of impairments that is severe.

In Step 3, the examiner determines whether the child's impairment(s) meets the definition of disability. As specified in P.L. 104-193, for individuals younger than the age of 18, a child is considered disabled if "that individual has a medically determinable physical or mental impairment which results in marked and severe functional limitations, and which can be expected to result in death or which has lasted or can be expected to last for a continuous period of not less than 12 months." In applying this definition, the examiner refers to SSA's Listing of Impairments and decides whether the child's impairment or combinations of impairments meet or medically equal the requirements of a listing, or whether the functional limitations caused by the impairment(s) are the same as the disabling functional limitations of any listing and, therefore, are functionally equivalent to that listing. The Listing of Impairments identifies for each of the major body systems impairments that, for a child, cause marked and severe functional limitations. Most of the listed impairments are permanent or are expected to result in death, or include a specific statement of duration.

Prior to the passage of the Personal Responsibility and Work Opportunity Reconciliation Act of 1996 (P.L. 104-193), a child was considered disabled for purposes of eligibility for SSI if he or she "... suffer[ed] from any medically determinable physical or mental impairment of comparable severity" to an impairment(s) that would make an adult disabled.[4] Following the Zebley decision, "comparable severity" for children was determined through an Individualized Functional Assessment (IFA).

However, P.L. 104-193 repealed the comparable severity criterion in the Act, directed SSA to discontinue the use of the IFA in evaluating a child's disability, and directed SSA to eliminate references to maladaptive behavior in the domain of personal/behavioral function in the Listing of Impairments for children. Thus, under the new law, a child's impairment or combination of impairments must cause more serious impairment-related limitations than were required under the old law and prior SSI regulations.

The IFA generated much of the controversy about the SSI program because critics alleged that parents coached their children to fake mental and behavioral disorders. These allegations prompted several examinations of the program by SSA, the Health and Human Services Office of Inspector General, and the General Accounting Office. Although these reviews did criticize some aspects of the program, none of these investigations substantiated allegations of widespread fraud. (For a discussion of the role that the media played in focusing public and Congressional attention on alleged fraud in the SSI program, see "A Media Crusade Gone Haywire," Forbes MediaCritic, September, 1995.)

While the IFA has been eliminated, the new SSI disability determination process does take into consideration the impact of an impairment on a child's functioning. Four methods are used in determining whether a child's impairment has the same disabling functional consequences as a listed impairment: (1) limitations of specific functions (i.e., walking, talking); (2) limitations resulting from chronic illness that are characterized by frequent illnesses or attacks or by exacerbations and remissions; (3) limitations resulting from the nature of the treatments required or the effects of medication; and (4) broad functional limitations.

In evaluating broad functional limitations, the following six areas of functioning may be considered: (1) cognition/communication; (2) motor; (3) social; (4) responsiveness to stimuli; (5) personal; and (6) concentration, persistence, or pace. The first three areas are taken into consideration in evaluating the broad functional limitations of all child applicants (birth to age 18). Responsiveness to stimuli is applied only to applicants from birth to age 1. The areas of "personal" and "concentration, persistence, or pace" apply to children from ages 3 to 18.

A finding of "functional equivalence" is made when a child has an *extreme limitation* in one area of functioning or *marked limitations* in two areas of functioning. For the purposes of the SSI program, a child is considered to have a marked limitation if the child scores between 2 and 3 standard deviations below the mean on a standardized measure of functional abilities; for children from birth to age 3, the child is functioning at more than one half but no more than two thirds of chronological age; or, for children from ages 3 to 18, the degree of limitation interferes seriously with the child's ability to function. A child is considered to have an extreme limitation if the child scores 3 standard deviations or more below the mean on a standardized measure of functional abilities; for children from birth to age 3, the child is functioning at one half of chronological age or less; or, for children from ages 3 to 18, there is no meaningful functioning in a given area.

Appeals

SSI child applicants whose disability claim is denied have the right to appeal. There are three levels of administrative appeal: reconsideration, hearing before an administrative law judge, and Appeals Council review. If a child's claim is denied at each of these three steps, then the case can be reviewed in federal court. Historically, approximately one half of those cases that have gone through the appeals process have ultimately been approved.

Summary

The SSI program for children serves as a critical component of the nation's social service system for low-income children with special needs. Because SSI is a cash assistance program, parents have the flexibility to decide how to best use the SSI benefits to meet the needs of their child and family, such as special food, clothing, equipment, transportation, unreimbursed medical expenses, increased cost of utilities, and child care, including care by a parent who cuts back on work in order to provide such care.

In addition, in many states, SSI-eligible children are also eligible for needed health care services through the state Medicaid program. Further, because new beneficiaries are referred to state Title V CSHCN programs, the SSI program can serve as a mechanism for linking children with special needs and their families to the family-centered, community-based services that they need.

In the following section, additional recent changes to the SSI program are identified, and the implications of these changes on children with special needs are discussed.

IMPACT OF WELFARE REFORM ON
CHILDREN WITH SPECIAL NEEDS

The Welfare Reform Act of 1996 brought about marked changes in the SSI program that will significantly affect current SSI beneficiaries and future SSI applicants. As part of the background and descriptive information on the SSI program, changes to the SSI disability criteria and disability determination process were described. In this section, changes to the SSI Program and other benefits program, as mandated by the Welfare Reform Act of 1996, are summarized, potential impacts on children with disabilities and their families are identified, and the implications for programs serving this population are defined.

Children will have to quality for SSI benefits on the basis of a more narrow definition of childhood disability.

On February 11, 1997, the SSA published new rules for determining SSI eligibility for children. As already detailed, these rules specify that, in order for a child to qualify for SSI, he or she must have a medically determinable physical or mental impairment of substantial duration that results in marked and severe functional limitations. These rules eliminate the "comparable severity" standard, and remove the Individualized Functional Assessment (IFA) step from the disability determination process for children. (The IFA step had been added in response to the Zebley decision.) In addition, in keeping with the welfare reform legislation, the medical listings were modified to eliminate references to "maladaptive behavior" when evaluating personal/behavioral functioning for children with mental impairment.

In addition, SSA was required to redetermine the SSI eligibility of approximately 288,000 children who had been deemed eligible through the IFA process or due to functional limitations associated with maladaptive behavior. The August 22, 1997, deadline for SSA to complete these redeterminations was extended to February 22, 1998 (or "as soon thereafter as practical") under a provision of the Balanced Budget Act of 1997. Although the redetermination process was initiated soon after the regulations were issued, the welfare reform legislation stated that no children were to lose their SSI benefits until July 1, 1997, or the date of their redetermination (whichever was later).

Impact

Following the publication of the new SSI eligibility rules, the Administration estimated that approximately 50% of the redetermined cases would be terminated. Through an initial screening process, SSA determined that more than 28,000 of the 288,000 "redetermination cases" should remain on the SSI roles. Of the remaining 260,000 cases, a redetermination had been completed on 227,000 cases by October 4, 1997. Of these, 91,216 (40.2%) had been "continued" (redetermined as eligible for SSI) and 135,841 (58.8%) had been "ceased" (redetermined as not eligible, based on the new criteria). Of those children who have lost benefits, more than 80% have mental disorders or mental retardation.

Slightly less than one half of those that were determined to be ineligible filed a request for reconsideration within the 60-day deadline for appeals. As of October, a review had been completed for 5,683 (8.5%) of the appealed cases. After reconsideration, 3,276 (58%) of the terminations were reversed, and 2,407 (42%) of these terminations were upheld. (Historically, the reversal rate at this stage of appeals is about 10%.) The 2,407 children whose terminations were upheld have the right to appeal through another three levels of review. Thus, about 123,000 (43%) of the 288,000 redetermination cases were found eligible under the new criteria. About 130,000 ceased cases were awaiting a redetermination at the reconsideration level, and 70,000 had been dropped from the SSI roles because they were redetermined as no longer eligible and did not file an appeal. The remaining 33,000 cases were awaiting the outcome of the initial redetermination.

Projection from interim data must be viewed as tentative; however, child advocates estimated that up to 160,000 children would lose their SSI benefits as a result of the reevaluation process. Further, it was anticipated that the vast majority of these children would have mental disorders or mental retardation. Advocates also voiced concern that SSI child beneficiaries who have a combination of impairments would have more difficulty qualifying under the new rules if none of their medical conditions matched one of the medical impairments on the Listing of Impairments.

In addition, the Congressional Budget Office estimated that between 1996 to 2002 about 267,000 new SSI child applicants who would have qualified for SSI under the old eligibility rules will be found not eligible under the new statute. However, this estimate may be low. Approximately 48,000 of these denials will be as a result of eliminating reference to "maladaptive behavior" in the mental impairment listings.

Starting in August 1996, the national allowance rate for new SSI applicants (whose claims were evaluated using the new definition of disability) was about 32%. This compares with an SSI allowance rate of about 43% in 1989, prior to the Zebley decision, when the eligibility standard was more restrictive. Thus, the number of new applicants who do not qualify for SSI because of the change in eligibility criteria may exceed the 276,000 CBO estimate.

In October 1997, in response to concerns and criticisms, the new Social Security Commissioner, Kenneth Apfel, ordered a comprehensive review of SSA's implementation of legislative changes to the SSI program. The findings of this review were made public in December 1997, identifying three areas of concern: (1) the status of children classified as having mental retardation; (2) the actual case processing in some areas; and (3) confusion regarding appeal rights. In response to these areas of concern, SSA will review the cases of some 45,000 children who were found not eligible for SSI through the redetermination process. In addition, the families of children who lost benefits and who did not appeal that decision will be given a second opportunity to do so. As a result of this re-review of selected cases and the second opportunity to appeal, SSA estimated in December 1997 that only 100,000 children will lose SSI as a result of the changes in the eligibility criteria.

Medicaid benefits will be retained by children who lose SSI.

Under the provisions of the Welfare Reform Act, SSI and associated benefits (i.e., Medicaid) for those recipients who did not meet the new eligibility criteria would have been terminated beginning in July 1, 1997, or the date of the redetermination, whichever came later.

However, under the State Children's Health Insurance Program (SCHIP) provisions of the Omnibus Budget Reconciliation Act of 1997 (Section 4913), states were required to continue Medicaid eligibility for disabled children who lost SSI benefits because of the changes in the definition of childhood disability until the child's 18th birthday. Prior to the passage of SCHIP, it was estimated that 50,000 of the 135,000 who would lose SSI as a result of redetermination would also lose Medicaid, with the other 85,000 qualifying for Medicaid under other eligibility criteria, such as age and family income.

Impact

The intent of Section 4913 was to ensure that those children who are terminated from SSI through the reevaluation process continue to be covered under the Medicaid program. However, although this provision appears to be straightforward, a number of complex issues must be addressed. In November 1997, the Health Care and Financing Administration (HCFA) issued directions to state Medicaid programs regarding implementation of this provision. Although these instructions addressed some issues of concern, many operational issues remain unanswered.

For example, in some states, SSI beneficiaries are automatically eligible for and are automatically enrolled in Medicaid. In other states,

SSI beneficiaries are automatically eligible for Medicaid but must submit a separate application for that benefit. In those states where an SSI beneficiary must submit a separate application, there were children (on August 22, 1996) who, because of their SSI status, were eligible for Medicaid but had not applied for that benefit. If such children are terminated from SSI under the reevaluation process and apply for Medicaid following SSI termination, it is not clear whether they would be "grandfathered" in as SSI beneficiaries. Further, if a child who is terminated from SSI moves across state lines, it is not clear how continuing eligibility for Medicaid is to be handled. The child may move from a state with more restrictive Medicaid/SSI eligibility to a state with more liberal Medicaid/SSI eligibility, or vice versa.

If the income or assets of the family of an SSI child beneficiary exceed the SSI financial limits, the child loses SSI and associated Medicaid benefits. As specified in the November 1997 HCFA instructions, those children who are terminated from SSI but continue to receive Medicaid as a result of SCHIP will be required to continue to meet SSI financial eligibility, and the state Medicaid agency has responsibility for monitoring and redetermining financial eligibility status. However, as previously noted, determining financial eligibility for SSI is a complex process, requiring significant staff training. The issue of training of Medicaid agency personnel to apply SSI financial eligibility criteria has not been addressed.

The November 1997 HCFA instructions also specify that those children who are terminated from SSI but continue to receive Medicaid as a result of SCHIP will be required to continue to meet the SSI disability criteria that were in effect prior to the passage of the Personal Responsibility and Work Opportunity Reconciliation Act of 1996. As with financial eligibility, the state Medicaid agency will have responsibility for monitoring and redetermining disability status. The determination of disability, based on SSI criteria and procedures, is a complex and highly specialized task, which is carried out by state DDSs under contract from SSA.

Although the Title XXI/SCHIP legislation ensures continuing Medicaid benefits to those who lose SSI, this legislation does not extend Medicaid coverage to the estimated 267,000 children who would have qualified for SSI between 1996 and 2002 if the SSI eligibility criteria had not been changed. There are no provisions within the SCHIP legislation that helps ensure that these children are given priority for coverage under Title XXI.

SSI *continuing disability reviews.*

The Welfare Reform Act requires SSA to conduct a continuing disability review (CDR) once every 3 years for recipients younger than age 18 with non-permanent impairments and not later than 12 months after birth for low-birthweight babies. The SSI-related provisions of the Budget Reconciliation Act of 1997 permits SSA to schedule a continuing disability review of low-birthweight babies after the child's first birthday if the SSA Commissioner determines that a given child's impairment is not expected to improve within 12 months of the child's birth. CDRs are conducted to ensure that SSI beneficiaries whose medical and functional status improves significantly are not maintained on the disability roles.

Impact

This provision will mean that some children will lose SSI and associated Medicaid benefits; however, no data are currently available on the proportion of current SSI beneficiaries whose medical and functional status improve to the degree that they no longer qualify for SSI benefits.

Requirement that child beneficiaries access necessary and available services.

As part of the CDR, the representative payee (in most cases the parent) of an SSI child beneficiary is required to present evidence that the child is receiving treatment that is considered medically necessary and available (unless SSA determines that such treatment would be inappropriate or unnecessary). If the representative payee (parent) refuses without good cause to cooperate, SSA may change the payee. The child will continue to receive SSI benefits, however.

Impact

This provision may help promote improved coordination and collaboration between SSA, families, and other state programs serving children with special needs, such as the state Title V CSHCN program.

However, there are no provisions within this (or other) SSI legislation that ensure that all SSI beneficiaries have a comprehensive plan of care that identifies medically necessary treatments and available sources of those treatments. Thus, parents will be held accountable for accessing services, without benefit of direction from a plan of care.

Under the Title V legislation, state CSHCN programs are to receive the names of SSI child beneficiaries from SSA/DDS and are to use MCH Block Grant Program funds to, in part, "provide rehabilitative services to SSI beneficiaries (under the age of 16) to the extent that these services are not available through the Medicaid Program (Title XIX)."

Included in the new Title V Block Grant Guidance is a performance measure that specifically addresses state Title V CSHCN program responsibilities for SSI beneficiaries. The measure, as stated in the draft guidance, is "the percent of state SSI beneficiaries less than 16 years old who are receiving rehabilitative services from the state CSHCN program." Further, Title V responsibility for providing and promoting family-centered, community-based care serves as a basis for states to establish a policy whereby all SSI disabled children are eligible to participate in or benefit from the state Title V CSHCN program. Thus, state Title V CSHCN programs could participate in the development and monitoring of comprehensive care plans for all CSHCN and SSI child beneficiaries.

It is important to note, however, that Title V is not an entitlement program. State CSHCN programs have limited funding and personnel, can set eligibility criteria that are different from the SSI-eligibility criteria, and can limit the scope of services provided or funded. It is also important to note that other federally based, state-operated programs (i.e., developmental disabilities, child mental health, Part H/early intervention, vocational rehabilitation) are not required by statute to collaborate with the state Title V CSHCN agency in addressing the needs of SSI child beneficiaries.

This provision appears to require that SSA, as part of the periodic CDR for each SSI beneficiary, determine what services and treatments are considered "medically necessary" or "inappropriate or unnecessary" and are available. SSA would need to do this in order to have a point of reference against which to judge if a given child's representative payee has presented evidence that "the child is receiving treatment which is considered medically necessary and available, unless SSA determines that such treatment would be inappropriate or unnecessary."

This provision appears to raise several significant issues. First, in most states, SSI child beneficiaries are eligible for Medicaid. Under Medicaid's EPSDT program, eligible children, birth to age 21, are to receive early and periodic screening, evaluation, and diagnosis and treatment (EPSDT) services. As specified in the Omnibus Budget Reconciliation Act (OBRA) of 1989, each state Medicaid Program is required to provide any medically necessary follow-up or treatment service that is reimbursable under Medicaid, whether or not the service is included in its Medicaid plan. Currently, many states are enrolling Medicaid beneficiaries, including those who are SSI beneficiaries, in Medicaid managed care plans. Under such plans, a primary care provider, or designated individual, serves as a gatekeeper and must preauthorize delivery of specialty treatment services.

In carrying out this mandate, will SSA develop its own criteria for medically necessary (including intensity and duration of services) or will SSA defer to the judgment of others regarding the medical necessity of a given treatment for a given child? How will SSA handle those cases in which there are differing judgments among providers, payers, and parents regarding medical necessity. Professionals from different disciplines may have different judgments regarding the necessity of a given service. Gatekeepers, employed by managed care organizations and other third party payers, may be restrictive in approving services, because their interest may be in minimizing costs rather than maximizing the functioning of a child. This issue of the medical necessity of service is one which is currently being addressed in early intervention and school-based special education programs. As is evidenced by these programs, the issue of medical necessity is very complex and not easily resolved.

Second, SSA will be required to determine whether a given treatment or service is, in fact, available to a given child. Maintaining an up-to-date database of sources of services needed by children with special needs and their families is a daunting task. There are numerous state and local initiatives (many of which are maintained by Title V CSHCN programs and Part H programs) to develop and maintain information and referral (I&R) databases and services. If SSA is to carry out this mandate in a cost-effective manner, functional linkages to existing I&R databases must be developed. Further, this may serve as an opportunity to document gaps in the service system and needs of children and families that are not currently met by the existing system of care.

SUMMARY

The Supplemental Security Income (SSI) program for children has recently undergone significant changes that will reduce the number of children who receive cash benefits through this program. However, the SSI program, along with state Title V CSHCN programs, state Title XVI Medicaid programs, and the new Title XXI Child Health Insurance Program (three other programs authorized under the Social Security Act), continues to provide low-income children with special needs supports they need to become self-supporting members of our society.

References

1. House Report No. 92-231 (Ways and Means Committee), May 26, 1971, reprinted at 1972 U.S.C.C. & A.N. 4989, 5133–5134.
2. Senate Report No. 94-1265 (Finance Committee), December 16, 1975, reprinted at 1976 U.S.C.C. & A.N. 6019, 5133–5134.

3. P.L. 92-603, §209(b), 86 Stat. 1329, 1465 (1973).
4. Social Security Act, Section 1614(a)(3)(A).

Additional References

Perrin, J.M., and Stein, R.E.K. Reinterpreting disability: Changes in Supplementary Social Security Income for children. *Pediatrics.* 1991;88:1047–1051.

Crocker, A.C. Improved support for children with disabilities. *Pediatrics.* 1991;88:1057–1059.

Social Security Administration, U.S. Department of Health and Human Services. *Social Security and SS benefits for children with disabilities.* SSA Publication No. 05-10026. January, 1992.

Schulzinger, R. *The impact of children's SSI program changes in welfare reform.* Washington, DC: The Bazelon Center for Mental Health Law; August 7, 1996.

20

The Health Insurance Portability and Accountability Act of 1996 (Kassebaum-Kennedy Act): Preliminary Phase

HELEN M. WALLACE

The Health Insurance Portability and Accountability Act of 1996 (HR3103), sponsored by Senators Kassebaum and Kennedy, guarantees the right to purchase health coverage for an estimated 25 to 30 million workers who lose or leave their jobs, even if they are sick.[1] The bill, however, does nothing about the 45 million Americans, including approximately 10 million children, without health insurance.

This new legislation was passed by the House of Representatives on August 1, 1996,[2] and by the U.S. Senate on August 2, 1996.[3] It was signed into law by President Clinton on August 21, 1996. The provisions of the legislation became generally effective July 1, 1997.

PURPOSE OF ACT

The Act was designed to improve portability and continuity of health insurance coverage in the group and individual markets; to combat waste, fraud, and abuse in health insurance and health care delivery; to promote the use of medical savings accounts; to improve access to long-term care services and coverage; and to simplify the administration of health insurance.

DESCRIPTION OF THE LEGISLATION

The legislation is divided into five Titles. Four Titles are explained briefly.

Title I: *Improved Availability and Portability of Health Insurance Coverage*

- The legislation limits exclusions for pre-existing conditions. It prohibits health insurers from limiting or denying coverage to individuals covered under a group health plan for more than 12 months for a medical condition that was diagnosed or treated during the previous 6 months.
- The legislation ends "jobs lock" by making health coverage portable. Because the bill limits pre-existing exclusions and provides credit for prior continuous coverage, workers will no longer be locked into jobs or prevented from starting their own businesses for fear of losing health insurance coverage.
- The legislation guarantees availability of health coverage for small employers.

- The legislation prohibits discrimination against employees and dependents based on health status, medical condition, claims experience, receipt of health care, medical history, genetic information, evidence of insurability (including domestic violence), or disability.

- The legislation guarantees reviewability of health coverage to employers and individuals. The legislation requires health insurers to review coverage to all employers as long as premiums are paid.

- The legislation helps individuals leaving or losing their job to maintain health coverage.

Title II: Preventing Health Care Fraud and Administrative Simplification; Duplication and Coordination of Medicare Benefits

The legislation creates a new coordinated program to combat health care fraud and abuse, including a program to coordinate federal, state, and local law enforcement efforts. This will involve Medicare payment and utilization audits. Education on health care provider efforts on quality of care and payment rules will be provided, as well as guidance regarding penalties and sanctions. A new health care fraud and abuse data collection program will be created.

Title III: Tax-Related Health Care Provisions[4]

The legislation includes a demonstration project to test the impact of Medical Savings Accounts (MSAs), a 4-year pilot project. It also increases the deduction for health insurance expenses of self-employed individuals. Long-term care expenses are deductible as medical expenses beginning 1997.

Title IV: Application and Enforcement of Group Health Plan Requirements

The legislation provides for enforcement of group health insurance requirements.

This new federal legislation requires insurance companies to cover people for health care for existing medical problems and to enable workers to keep health insurance when they leave their jobs. The law prohibits insurers from denying health insurance to people with pre-existing conditions. The bill requires employers to sell health insurance to all employees who want it, and prohibits excluding any workers from coverage, as sick employees sometimes are. It bans employers from cancelling coverage when employees get sick.[5]

SPECIAL COVERAGE RULES FOR DEPENDENTS[6]

If a group health plan or issuer of group health plans makes coverage available to a dependent of an individual, that person is a participant under the plan. A person becomes a dependent through marriage, birth, adoption, or placement for adoption. The plan would have to provide for a special dependent enrollment period during which an individual would be enrolled under the plan as a dependent and, in the case of the birth or adoption of a child, the spouse of the individual could be enrolled as a dependent of the spouse. The dependent enrollment period would have to be at least 30 days, beginning on the date dependent coverage is made available or on the date of the marriage, birth, adoption, or placement for adoption.

HEALTH INSURANCE REFORM[6]

Virtually every state will need to adopt legislation ensuring that its standards for the individual and small-group market reflect the new federal law. If states do not enforce the law, the federal government may step in. States may want to take actions so that they can keep their traditional role of insurance regulator. States must enforce the federal law's standards at the minimum, but can go further. The amount of work each state needs to do depends on the level of reform already in place.

The law is intended to provide a safe harbor for a specified payment practice, resulting in the following:

1. An increase in access to health care
2. An increase in the quality of health care services
3. An increase in patient freedom of choice among health care providers
4. An increase in competition among health care providers
5. An increase in the ability of health care facilities to provide services in medically underserved areas or to medically underserved populations

6. A decrease in the cost to federal health care programs, with particular reference to practitioner or provider

7. Any other factors the Secretary of Health and Human Services deems appropriate in the interest of preventing fraud and abuse in federal health care programs

SYNOPSIS OF THE HEALTH INSURANCE REFORM ACT (S10280)[7]

What the Bill Does (The Good News)

1. Limits (but does not eliminate) pre-existing conditions exclusions.

2. Ensures availability of individual policies for those who leave jobs voluntarily, for themselves and their dependents.

3. Prohibits insurers from charging more or denying coverage to individuals in poor health in group plans.

4. Makes long-term care expenses deductible from federal income tax.

5. Increases the deductibility of premiums for the self-employed.

What the Bill Does (The Bad News)

1. Allows the creation of 750,000 medical savings accounts (MSAs), a compromise provision reconciling the views of Republicans, who did not want any, fearing they would benefit the healthy and the wealthy.

2. Criminalizes transfer of assets to qualify for Medicaid.

3. Lets insurers sell policies duplicating benefits.

What the Bill Does Not Do

1. Does not address the cost of individual policies.

2. Does not extend limits on pre-existing condition exclusions and individuals holding individual policies.

3. Does not provide protection for mental health conditions.

4. Does not help the insured at all.

POTENTIAL SIGNIFICANCE OF THE NEW LEGISLATION[8]

The potential significance of this new federal legislation is considerable. It should provide health insurance coverage for the previously employed person who has lost his or her job and for the family—that is, continuity of coverage with health insurance. It may raise or protect quality of health care. It may reduce the cost of health insurance and health care in the long run. It should provide coverage for human reproductive care, for the preventive care of well children and youth, and for the care of sick children and youth.

CHILDREN'S CONTINUITY OF COVERAGE
UNDER THE KASSEBAUM-KENNEDY BILL

This Act is expected to increase the availability of private health insurance coverage for certain children.

A special report by Markus[9] makes an effort to clarify the eligibility for selected children under the new Kassebaum-Kennedy legislation. Further experience is needed to clarify this basic issue. Health and Social Welfare personnel working with families and children with chronic conditions are advised to analyze and test this issue, as further experience is gained.

References

1. *ATMCH Newsletter.* Fall 1996; p 3.
2. *Health Insurance Portability and Accountability Act of 1996.* 104th Congress, House of Representatives, 2nd Session, Report 104-736.
3. *Health Insurance Portability and Accountability Act of 1996.* P.L. 104-191. August 21, 1996. pp 1936–2103.
4. *Summary. The Health Insurance Portability and Accountability Act. HR3103.* Prepared by Staff of the Senate Labor and Human Resources Committee and the Senate Finance Committee, 1997.
5. *Conference Report* as passed by the House of Representatives on August 1, 1996, and by the U.S. Senate on August 2, 1996. Signed into law by the President on August 21, 1996.
6. Aston, G. Insurance reform moves to the states. *American Medical News.* February 3, 1997, pp 3 and 22.
7. Kirk, M.A. *Medical savings plans: The experiment begins. The New York Times.* February 16, 1997, p 9.
8. Families USA. Quoted in *ATMCH Newsletter.* Fall, 1996, p 5.
9. Markus, A.R. Children's continuity of coverage under the Kassebaum/Kennedy Bill. *Health Policy and Child Health.* Special Report. George Washington University Center on Health Policy Research, Fall, 1996.

21

National Health Expenditures

KATHARINE R. LEVIT, HELEN C. LAZENBY, BRADLEY R. BRADEN,
CATHY A. COWAN, PATRICIA A. McDONNELL, LEKHA SIVARAJAN,
JEAN M. STILLER, DARLEEN K. WON, CAROLYN S. DONHAM,
ANNA M. LONG, AND MADIE W. STEWART

This chapter was adapted from the original article "National Health Expenditures,
1995," by Katharine R. Levit, Helen C. Lazenby, Bradley R. Braden, Cathy A. Cowan, Patricia A. McDonnell, Lekha Sivarajan, Jean M. Stiller, Darleen K. Won, Carolyn S. Donham, Anna M. Long, and Madie W. Stewart, published in *Health Care Financing
Review*, Fall 1996, Volume 16, Number 1, pages 175–199.

There are no comparable data for children and youth published since 1987.

Reprint Requests: Anna Long, Office of National Health Statistics, Health Care Financing
Administration, 7500 Security Boulevard, N3-002-02, Baltimore, Maryland 21244-1850.
E-mail: along1@hcfa.gov.

This chapter presents data on health care spending in the United States for various types of medical services and products and their sources of funding from 1960 to 1995. In 1995, $988.5 billion was spent to purchase health care in the United States, up 5.5% from 1994. Growth in spending between 1993 and 1995 was the slowest in more than three decades, primarily because of slow growth in private health insurance and out-of-pocket spending. As a result, the share of health spending funded by private sources fell, reflecting the influence of increased enrollment in managed care plans.

GENERAL TRENDS IN NATIONAL HEALTH EXPENDITURES

In today's health care system, providers and third-party payers face intense pressures. Increases in health care spending during the late 1980s and early 1990s in relation to overall economy-wide growth focused the attention of purchasers on the problems of rising costs. As the federal government attempted to control cost increases associated with Medicare and Medicaid, employers sponsoring health insurance for their workers evaluated alternatives to conventional private health insurance (PHI) plans more intensely. Both private and public sectors reacted with increased enrollment in managed care plans. Under heightened pressure from managed care plans to reduce cost growth, health care providers were transformed from "revenue generators" who individually orchestrated activity within the health care system to "cost centers" within a larger, managed care system.[1] Faced with competition for patients, an increased proportion of providers are responding to incentives to minimize costs. Managed care plans negotiated rate discounts with providers in return for provider access to large groups of patients; these plans also altered patterns of care through an emphasis on preventive services and elimination of unnecessary care and demanded cost-conscious decision-making by providers in delivery of health care. Faced with lower expected revenue growth, providers were forced to find ways to reduce expense growth to remain financially viable and competitive.

Health system changes are reflected in the matrix of spending trends recorded in national health expenditures (NHE). Most prominently, growth in health spending in 1994 and 1995 reached its lowest points in more than three decades of measuring health care spending (Fig. 21.1). Nominal expenditures grew 5.1% in 1994 and 5.5% in 1995; real (inflation-adjusted) growth measured 2.7% in 1994 and 2.8% in 1995. Decelerating growth reflects changes occurring within the provider and PHI components of the health care industry during the 1990s.

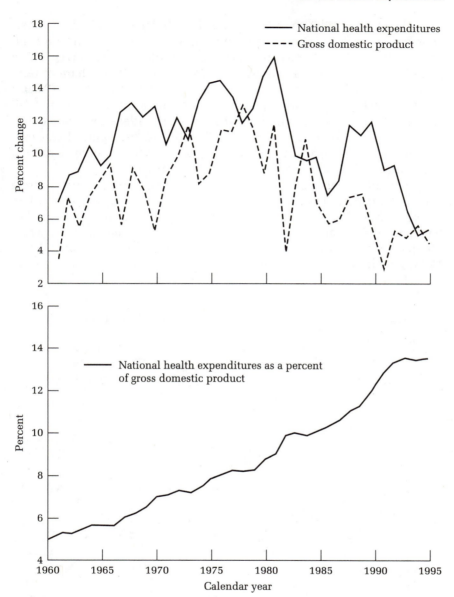

FIGURE 21.1
....

Percentage growth in national health expenditures and gross domestic product, and national health expenditures as a percentage of gross domestic product for calendar years 1960 to 1995. *Source:* Health Care Financing Administration, Office of the Actuary (data from the Office of National Health Statistics).

During the 1993 to 1995 period, health care spending as a percentage of gross domestic product (GDP) exhibited virtually no change: It stabilized between 13.5% and 13.6% (see Fig. 21.1). There were three additional periods since 1960 when the NHE share of GDP remained stable for 3-year periods: 1964 to 1966, 1977 to 1979, and 1982 to 1984. Each of these periods was characterized by strong GDP growth. For the first time in more than three decades, however, stability in NHE as a percentage of GDP in the 1993 to 1995 period was precipitated by a slowdown in the rate of growth of health care spending, rather than an upswing in overall economic growth.

The effects of health system changes are evident in the contrast between private and public sector financing. From 1960 to 1990, growth in spending by both the private and public sectors was similar, with only two notable exceptions: the period of 1966 to 1967, when Medicare and Medicaid were introduced, and the period of 1974 to 1975, which recorded the effects of the 1973 expansion of Medicare to

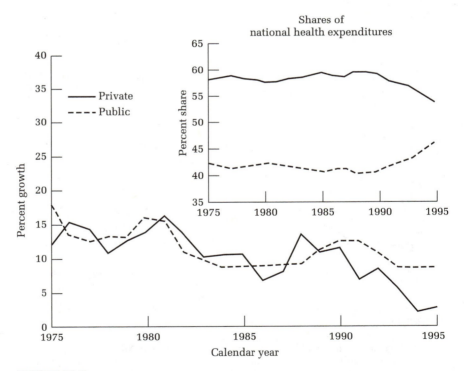

FIGURE 21.2

Percentage growth and percentage share of public and private national health expenditures for calendar years 1975 to 1995. *Source:* Health Care Financing Administration, Office of the Actuary (data from the Office of National Health Statistics).

cover the disabled population. Each of these major expansions in public program coverages produced offsetting, step-wise shifts in public and private financing responsibilities, with the share shouldered by the public sector increasing. The unique feature of the shift toward a larger public share beginning in 1990 is that it was not driven by public sector initiatives to add new populations or expand services, although the number of people covered by the Medicaid program did increase. In fact, public sector expenditure growth has continued at approximately the same average annual rate since 1990 (9.9%) as between 1980 and 1990 (10.5%). At the same time, average annual growth in private spending decelerated markedly between 1990 and 1995, to 5.2%, from the 11.2% average annual growth experienced during the 1980 to 1990 period (Fig. 21.2).

PERSONAL HEALTH CARE EXPENDITURES BY CATEGORY

The disparity in growth among different types of personal health care (PHC) services narrowed in 1995. For all services except other personal health care, spending growth ranged from a low of 4.5% (for hospital services) to a high of 8.9% (for dental services). The one exception, other personal health care services, which accounts for 2.8% of PHC, is dominated by Medicaid home- and community-based waivers and miscellaneous services that are provided by non-health care establishments. Spending for this sector grew 14.9% in 1995, faster than all other PHC sectors, but slower than it did in 1994 (Table 21.1).

The changing distribution of health care spending mirrors the impact of managed care and, to a lesser extent, changes in Medicare payment policies. The share of PHC expenditures spent on hospital and physician services has declined over the past 5 years, while spending on home health services, nursing home care, and other personal health care services has increased (Fig. 21.3). These increases have paralleled increases in Medicare spending for home health and skilled nursing facility services.

Hospital Care

Hospital care expenditures, the single largest component of personal health spending at 39.8% amounted to $350.1 billion in 1995. Registering growth of less than 5% in the last 2 years, spending for hospital services was among the slowest growing of any PHC services.

The American Hospital Association's panel survey of community hospitals[2] reports that overall admissions per 1,000 population in-

TABLE 21.1

Personal Health Care Expenditure Aggregate Amounts, Percentage Distribution, and Average Annual Percentage Change, by Type of Expenditure: Selected Calendar Years 1960–1995

Type of Expenditure	1960	1970	1980	1985	1990	1991	1992	1993	1994	1995
	Amount in Billions									
Personal Health Care	$23.6	$63.8	$217.0	$376.4	$614.7	$676.6	$740.5	$786.9	$827.9	$878.8
Hospital Care	9.3	28.0	102.7	168.3	256.4	282.3	305.4	323.3	335.0	350.1
Physician Services	5.3	13.6	45.2	83.6	146.3	159.2	175.7	182.7	190.6	201.6
Dental Services	2.0	4.7	13.3	21.7	31.6	33.3	37.0	39.2	42.1	45.8
Other Professional Services	0.6	1.4	6.4	16.6	34.7	38.3	42.1	46.3	49.1	52.6
Home Health Care	0.1	0.2	2.4	5.6	13.1	16.1	19.6	23.0	26.3	26.6
Drugs and Other Medical Non-Durables	4.2	8.8	21.6	37.1	59.9	65.6	71.2	75.0	77.7	83.4
Prescription Drugs	2.7	5.5	12.0	21.2	37.7	42.1	46.6	49.4	51.3	55.5
Vision Products and Other Medical Durables	0.5	1.6	3.8	6.7	10.5	11.2	11.9	12.5	12.9	13.8
Nursing Home Care	0.8	4.2	17.6	30.7	50.9	57.2	62.3	67.0	72.4	77.9
Other Personal Health Care	0.7	1.3	4.0	6.1	11.2	13.6	15.4	17.9	21.7	25.0
	Percentage Distribution									
Personal Health Care	100.0	100.0	100.0	100.0	100.0	100.0	100.0	100.0	100.0	100.0
Hospital Care	39.3	43.9	47.3	44.7	41.7	41.7	41.2	41.1	40.5	39.8
Physician Services	22.4	21.3	20.8	22.2	23.8	23.5	23.7	23.2	23.0	22.9
Dental Services	8.3	7.3	6.1	5.8	5.1	4.9	5.0	5.0	5.1	5.2
Other Professional Services	2.6	2.2	2.9	4.4	5.6	5.7	5.7	5.9	5.9	6.0
Home Health Care	0.2	0.3	1.1	1.5	2.1	2.4	2.6	2.9	3.2	3.3
Drugs and Other Medical Non-Durables	18.0	13.8	10.0	9.8	9.7	9.7	9.6	9.5	9.4	9.5
Prescription Drugs	11.3	8.6	5.6	5.6	6.1	6.2	6.3	6.3	6.2	6.3
Vision Products and Other Medical Durables	2.7	2.5	1.7	1.8	1.7	1.7	1.6	1.6	1.6	1.6
Nursing Home Care	3.6	6.6	8.1	8.1	8.3	8.4	8.4	8.5	8.8	8.9
Other Personal Health Care	2.9	2.0	1.9	1.6	1.8	2.0	2.1	2.3	2.6	2.8

Average Annual Percentage Change from Previous Year Shown

Personal Health Care	—	10.5	13.0	11.6	10.3	10.1	9.5	6.3	5.2	6.1
Hospital Care	—	11.7	13.9	10.4	8.8	10.1	8.2	5.9	3.6	4.5
Physician Services	—	9.9	12.8	13.1	11.8	8.8	10.4	4.0	4.4	5.8
Dental Services	—	9.1	11.1	10.2	7.8	5.6	11.0	6.0	7.3	8.9
Other Professional Services	—	8.8	16.3	21.2	15.8	10.4	10.0	10.0	6.1	7.0
Home Health Care	—	14.5	26.9	18.9	18.4	22.4	22.3	17.1	14.4	8.6
Drugs and Other Medical Non-Durables	—	7.6	9.4	11.4	10.1	9.4	8.6	5.4	3.6	7.3
Prescription Drugs	—	7.5	8.2	11.9	12.2	11.9	10.6	6.1	3.8	8.1
Vision Products and Other Medical Durables	—	9.6	8.8	12.4	9.2	7.0	6.3	5.1	2.8	7.2
Nursing Home Care	—	17.4	15.4	11.7	10.7	12.2	9.0	7.6	8.1	7.5
Other Personal Health Care	—	6.5	12.0	8.8	12.9	20.7	13.3	16.4	21.6	14.9

NOTE: Numbers may not add to totals because of rounding.
Source: Health Care Financing Administration, Office of the Actuary (data from the Office of National Health Statistics).

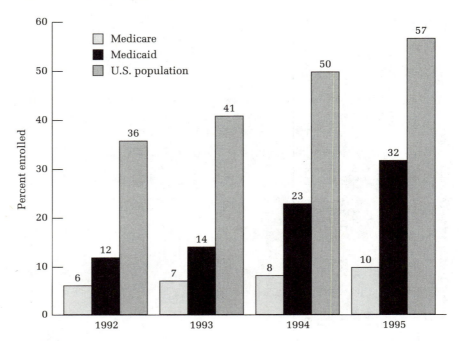

NOTE: Figures given for U.S. resident population enrollment in managed care for 1992 and 1993 exclude dependents and are therefore not strictly comparable to later years.

FIGURE 21.3
....

The nation's health dollar for calendar year 1995. *Source:* Health Care Financing Administration, Office of the Actuary (data from the Office of National Health Statistics).

creased in 1995 by 0.4%, the first such increase in more than a decade. Growth in admissions per 1,000 population in 1995 comes from admissions for the population age 65 and older; meanwhile, admissions per 1,000 for the population younger than age 65 continued to decline but at a slower rate. Despite the slight increase in admissions per 1,000 population, inpatient days in community hospitals continued to fall by almost 3% overall, indicating declining overall length of stay. When the number of beds is not reduced to match the decline in days, occupancy rates fall and excess capital grows. In 1995, overall occupancy rates in community hospitals fell to less than 60%,[3] the lowest rate in history. Such rates put renewed pressure on hospitals to develop new sources of revenues, to negotiate with managed care plans for access to patients, and to integrate both with other local and national hospital organizations and with physicians and other health care providers and insurers.[1]

An increasing number of hospitals are expanding their lines of business to provide more than just inpatient and outpatient hospital care. In addition to fitness facilities and home health care agencies, they are using excess bed capacity to add rehabilitation and skilled nursing or sub-acute care facilities to broaden their revenue base.[4] Creating sub-acute care facility units from underused inpatient units enables hospitals to compete for the follow-up institutional care that discharged patients often need for full recovery. Incentives exist for hospitals to discharge patients as soon as possible. Medicare's inpatient hospital payment is diagnosis-based and prospectively determined, regardless of length of hospital stay. Managed care plans, which often pay for hospitalization on a daily rate, also encourage fewer inpatient days. But community nursing homes, traditionally providing custodial services and limited medical care, are frequently not staffed and equipped to handle patients discharged from hospitals "quicker and sicker." Hospitals with a sub-acute care unit can discharge patients from their hospital stays quickly and admit them to the skilled nursing or sub-acute care unit for their follow-up care, maximizing their revenue from the overall stay.

With the rise of enrollment in managed care plans and falling occupancy rates, hospitals have been forced to consider the benefits of mergers and alliances with local and national hospital organizations. Squeezed by high operating expenses, competition from market-area providers, and the prices managed care organizations were willing to pay providers for services, hospitals have sought alliances with similar community facilities or with national chains. Some alliances have been based on geographic location and others on religious affiliation. Most have been aimed at integrating services, reducing competition, and increasing cooperation in order to compete effectively for managed care business.[1] Increasingly, largely consolidated for-profit hospital organizations are buying nonprofit facilities facing difficulties in the highly competitive hospital marketplace. For-profit chains strengthen the market positions of acquired facilities by cutting costs. Communities worry, however, that takeovers of their local facilities will threaten the existence of hospital-provided charity and preventive services and cost jobs in their community.[5,6]

Expenditures for inpatient services in community hospitals accounted for 62% of all hospital revenues in 1995. Growth in inpatient expenditures has slowed since 1990, paralleling decreases in inpatient day and length of stay. Some of this deceleration can be attributed to the rise of managed care. According to the *HMO and PPO Industry Profile*, health maintenance organizations (HMOs), the most restrictive type of managed care plan, cover about 20% of the resident population. "HMO members experience fewer total hospital days per thousand, fewer admissions per thousand, and shorter average lengths of stay than the population at large . . . HMO members were hospitalized about two-thirds as often as the population as a whole in 1993 [and] . . .

spent about half as many days in the hospital. Growth in other types of managed care organizations (especially PPOs) and the increasing use of utilization review by indemnity health insurance plans" may also have contributed to this trend.[7]

Nearly all hospital care was financed by third parties in 1995, with only 3.3% paid by consumers in out-of-pocket expenditures. PHI accounted for a 32.3% share. Total public funding accounted for a 61.2% share; Medicare and Medicaid, the primary subset of public payers, financed 47% of hospital care. The remaining 3.2% of hospital revenues came from philanthropic and nonpatient sources such as hospital gift shops, parking facilities, and cafeterias.

Physician Services

Expenditures for physician services reached $201.6 billion in 1995, an increase of 5.8% from the previous year. Spending for services in this sector accounted for 22.9% of PHC (see Table 21.1). For the last 3 years, growth in spending for physician services has been lower than the growth in overall PHC expenditures. This slow growth is linked to the expansion of managed care.

The health care system in the United States has historically been controlled by providers, with physicians typically deciding type and place of treatment. In recent years, the growth of managed care has caused the locus of control to shift from provider to insurer,[8] with the insurer having more input into treatment plans. This fundamental change in the health care delivery system has been precipitating changes in the organization of physician practices, demand for types of physician specialties, utilization of physician services, and income of physicians. In 1993 and 1994, these changes contributed to the slow-down of growth in expenditures for physician services. By 1995, physician expenditures showed a slight upturn in growth rate, although growth was still lower than the growth in PHC spending. There is anecdotal evidence to suggest that increased utilization and referral to specialists may be part of the reason for the slight acceleration in growth.[9,10]

The share of physician expenditures funded by PHI rose between 1990 and 1995, consistent with managed care's emphasis on services provided by primary care physicians. Meanwhile, the share funded by Medicare remained unchanged as a result of the implementation of the Medicare Fee Schedule (MFS) to pay physicians for services and volume performance standards (VPS) to limit the effect of induced utilization increases. Payment mechanisms used by both managed care and Medicare put pressure on physicians to curb expenditure growth. There is no evidence to suggest that physicians shifted costs to private insurers with the advent of the MFS, because physicians were restrained by market forces from raising prices. Managed care and MFS caused spending growth to drop to 5.8% in 1995 from 11.8% in 1990.

Changes in the way physicians deliver services are evident in U.S. Bureau of the Census[11] data on revenue sources of physician offices. From 1992 to 1994, the percentage of revenues earned from the delivery of inpatient hospital services fell, while those earned through the delivery of services in doctors' offices and hospital outpatient settings rose. Part of the decline in percentage of revenues from hospital services may be associated with falling number of inpatient days.

Growth in managed care enrollment had a direct impact on physician organizations. The number of physicians signing contracts with managed care organizations is on the rise. In 1990, 61% of physicians had a managed care contract; by 1995 that proportion had grown to 83%. Although physician participation in managed care had grown substantially, the percentage of revenues received through managed care contracts grew more slowly—from 28% in 1990 to 33% in 1995.[12]

As the number of managed care contracts has increased, the structure of physician practices has changed. Group practices have become more prevalent. Physicians have joined together in larger group practices to offer the breadth of services necessary to attract managed care contracts and to consolidate expenses. Groups can also absorb some of the risk associated with managed care contracts. Within physician practices, the proportion of physicians who are employed has increased, while the proportion of physicians in solo practices or self-employed in group practices has declined.[13] Employed physicians tend to work fewer hours, see fewer patients, and earn lower income than physicians who own a practice.[14] As the number of employed physicians increases, earnings of physicians on average could fall.

In 1994, physicians' income decreased for the first time in recent history. This may be a result of the growth in managed care contracts. The decline was more pronounced for the high earners, whereas the income of low earners continued to rise.[15] The decline also affected primary care physicians and procedure-oriented physicians differently. Primary care physicians' income increased faster than average, while the income of procedure-oriented physicians declined or increased at a slower-than-average rate.[16]

As the impact of managed care on the health industry has increased, there has been more emphasis on primary and preventive care and less on the services of specialists. Since 1990, the demand for specialists has dropped, as measured by physician recruitment advertising, and the demand for generalists has been rising.[17] This change in type of physician will also affect the future of medical schools and the

TABLE 21.2

Physician Contacts[1] per Person, by Age: Calendar Years 1987–1994

Age Group	1987	1988	1989	1990	1991	1992	1993	1994
Total[2]	5.4	5.3	5.3	5.5	5.6	5.9	6.0	6.0
Under 15 Years	4.5	4.6	4.6	4.5	4.7	4.6	4.9	4.6
15–44 Years	4.6	4.7	4.6	4.8	4.7	5.0	5.0	5.0
45–64 Years	6.4	6.1	6.1	6.4	6.6	7.2	7.1	7.3
65 Years or Over	8.9	8.7	8.9	9.2	10.4	10.6	10.9	11.3

[1]A consultation with a physician (or another person working under a physician's supervision) in person or by telephone, for examination, diagnosis, treatment, or advice. Place of contact includes office, hospital outpatient clinic, emergency room, telephone, home, clinic, health maintenance organization, and other places located outside a hospital.
[2]Age-adjusted.
Source: National Center for Health Statistics, 1995.

type of training available to incoming students. As an indication of this trend, the percentage of recently graduated residents unable to find full-time jobs in their specialties amounted to more than 6% in two hospital-based specialties (anesthesiology and pathology) and one surgical specialty (plastic surgery). Similar rates for various primary care specialists were 2.1% or less.[18]

Utilization of physician services remained stable over the 1993 to 1994 period at approximately 6 contacts per person per year, after rising steadily from 5.3 contacts per year in 1989.[19] The contribution to the increase in number of physician contacts per person differed by age group. For the population age 65 years or older, the number of physician contacts per person grew consistently between 1989 and 1994 but experienced a particularly large increase between 1990 and 1991. For the population age 15 to 64, utilization increased between 1989 and 1992 but has remained fairly constant since (Table 21.2), possibly a response to increased enrollment in managed care.

Prescription Drugs

Americans purchased $55.5 billion worth of prescription drugs in 1995. Prescription drug spending growth has been slower than that of PHC in 1993 and 1994 (6.1% and 3.8%, respectively) but jumped to 2 percentage points faster than PHC in 1995 (8.1%). Surveys show that about two thirds of the accelerated 1995 growth comes from an increase in the number of prescriptions sold. Depending on the survey used, this increase ranged from 5.7%[20] to 7.8%.[21]

Long-Term Care

Long-term care (LTC) includes spending for care received through free-standing nursing homes and home health agencies. This sector accounted for almost one eighth of PHC expenditures in 1995, or $106.5 billion, with public programs (mainly Medicaid and Medicare) financing 57.4%.

Nursing Home Care

In 1995, spending for nursing home care climbed to $77.9 billion and accounted for 8.9% of total spending for PHC. Growth in nursing home care expenditures decelerated from 8.1% in 1994 to 7.5% in 1995. The nursing home expenditure estimate for 1995 implies a $127 average charge per day for care in free-standing nursing facilities. At that rate, a 1-year stay would cost more than $46,000 in 1995.

Home Health Care

Expenditures for free-standing private and public home health agencies amounted to $28.6 billion in 1995. Expenditures for the services and products provided by these agencies were 3.3% of PHC expenditures in 1995, a small but increasing share.

Public sources, predominantly Medicare and Medicaid, financed 55.3% of home health care spending in 1995. Out-of-pocket payments by patients or their families funded one half of all private spending. PHI and non-patient revenue equally funded the remaining portion of private spending.

Home health agencies seeking to maintain or boost revenue levels are also developing sub-acute care expertise.[4] As with nursing homes, more highly trained staff are designed to better serve patients discharged from hospitals but still in need of substantial home care for full recovery from their illnesses.

MANAGED CARE

In recent years, enrollment in employer-sponsored PHI has shifted dramatically away from conventional fee-for-service insurance into managed care plans. Such plans typically charge lower average premiums than traditional indemnity plans[22,23] by controlling provider costs

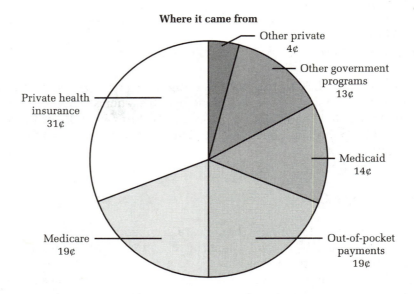

Where it came from

- Other private 4¢
- Other government programs 13¢
- Medicaid 14¢
- Out-of-pocket payments 19¢
- Medicare 19¢
- Private health insurance 31¢

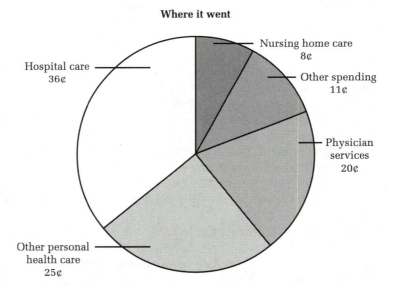

Where it went

- Nursing home care 8¢
- Other spending 11¢
- Physician services 20¢
- Other personal health care 25¢
- Hospital care 36¢

NOTES: Other private includes industrial inplant health services, non-patient revenues, and privately financed construction. Other personal health care includes dental services, other professional services, home health care, drugs and other non-durable medical products, vision products and other durable medical products, and other miscellaneous health care services. Other spending covers program administration and the net cost of private health insurance, government public health, and research and construction.

FIGURE 21.4
....

Percentage of Medicare enrollees, Medicaid recipients, and U.S. population enrolled in managed health care plans for 1992 to 1995. *Sources:* Health Care Financing Administration, Office of Managed Care; Dial, T.H., Pan, L., Bergsten, C., et al. *HMO and PPO industry profile: 1995–96 edition.* Washington, DC: American Association of Health Plans, May, 1996.

and utilization of services. In 1986, almost 90% of health plan participants in medium and large firms enrolled in traditional fee-for-service plans; however, by 1993 the number of participants had dropped to 50%.[24] Enrollment in HMOs, typically the most restrictive of the managed care plans, grew from 13% to about 23% of all employer-plan participants between 1986 and 1993.

The fastest growing type of managed care plan was the preferred provider organization (PPO). These plans grew from 1% of health plan participants in 1986 to 26% in 1993.[24] PPOs attempt to lower costs by establishing networks of providers who are paid according to negotiated fee schedules. Many traditional fee-for-service plans now also generate a list of preferred providers for participants. The advantage to the participant for using the preferred provider is lower out-of-pocket costs.

Survey data from KPMG Peat Marwick[23] indicate that employees continue to migrate away from conventional fee-for-service plans and into managed care plans. In 1995, HMO enrollment in employer-sponsored plans nearly equaled the enrollment in conventional plans; it was predicted to edge ahead in 1996.[23] Almost one half of the U.S. resident population was covered by an HMO or PPO plan in 1994[7] (Fig. 21.4).

COVERED SERVICES

Throughout the late 1980s and early 1990s, the breadth of services covered by employer-sponsored PHI greatly expanded. For example, an increasing number of insurance plans began offering home health and hospice care coverage as less expensive alternatives to hospital stays. Much of this expansion was driven by cost-containment strategies aimed at substituting lower cost services for more expensive care and by the desire to attract healthier participants.

The rise in the availability of covered services was accelerated by the migration of employers and employees toward managed care health plans including HMO, PPO, and point-of-service (POS) plans. Managed care health plans, particularly HMOs, were much more likely to provide their members with coverage for many basic preventive services, such as routine physical examinations, well-baby care, well-child care, and immunizations and inoculations. For example, data from KPMG Peat Marwick[23] indicate that in 1995 HMO enrollees were almost twice as likely to be covered for adult physicals as enrollees in conventional plans.

Although conventional plans have been slow to catch up, many have greatly expanded their coverage during the first half of the 1990s into areas such as adult physicals and well-baby and well-child care. However, despite such increases, these conventional plans still lag behind most managed care plans, particularly HMOs, in the overall level of preventive services coverage.

Expansions in covered services continued in 1996. More recent survey data from KPMG Peat Marwick indicate that the biggest increases for preventive services were in POS plans. POS plan offerings for both adult physicals and well-child care coverage increased, and HMO plans were increasingly likely to cover chiropractic care. Although just over one half the HMO plans are now offering such coverage, they still remain far behind non-HMO plans, which almost universally cover chiropractic services.

MEDICARE

Medicare's Hospital Insurance and Supplementary Medical Insurance programs funded $187 billion of spending for health services and supplies in 1995, an 11.6% increase over 1994 spending. Ninety-eight percent of these expenditures were for PHC services for the 37.5 million aged and disabled Medicare beneficiaries enrolled on July 1, 1995.

Medicare is the largest public payer for PHC expenditures and for each of the service components covered by the program except nursing home care. Over time, with few exceptions, Medicare has financed increasingly larger shares of spending for each service component. In 1995, Medicare funded 20.9% of spending for PHC, a full percentage point more than it funded in 1994. One third of all spending for hospital care and one fifth of expenditures for physician services are funded by Medicare. Faster growth in the Medicare population, compared with the general population, and the aging of frail elderly Medicare enrollees are contributing factors to these increasing funding shares.

Medicare expenditures for hospital care totaled $112.6 billion in 1995, 10.5% higher than in 1994. Expenditures for hospital care services cover inpatient, outpatient, and hospital-based home health agency and skilled nursing facility services. Relatively high growth in Medicare hospital expenditures that has continued in recent years may be, in part, the result of expansions of hospital-based, sub-acute units that allow Medicare patients to be discharged quickly from hospitalization and admitted into the same facility's sub-acute care unit. This permits hospitals to limit expenses incurred for Medicare hospitalizations, which are compensated at a fixed amount regardless of length of stay, and continue treating the patient under Medicare's cost-based reimbursement policies for skilled nursing home care.[25]

MEDICAID

Combined Federal and State Medicaid spending for PHC accounted for 15.1% of total PHC in 1995, or $133.1 billion. Medicaid largely funds institutional services. In 1995, hospital care and nursing home care accounted for two thirds (36.9% and 25.7%, respectively) of combined federal and state Medicaid spending. The program is the largest third-party payer of nursing home care, financing 46.5% in 1995.

In fiscal year 1995, there were 36.3 million persons who received some type of Medicaid benefit. The groups of children and adults in families with dependent children represented 68.3% of all Medicaid recipients in 1995, yet consumed only 26.2% of program benefits. Nearly one half of all Medicaid recipients were children (17.2 million), who consumed only 15% of all Medicaid benefits. These children also accounted for more than two thirds of all family-based criteria recipients but consumed only a little more than one half of the benefits to families. Conversely, the aged, blind, and disabled represented just over one quarter of all recipients but consumed nearly three quarters of program benefits (Table 21.3).

Medicaid is funded jointly by federal and by state and local governments. For a state to receive federal matching funds, it must adhere to minimum requirements for eligibility and services set by the federal government. Within this broad framework, state governments are afforded considerable flexibility in designing the total scope of the program within the constraints of the state budgetary process. One way

---

TABLE 21.3

Medicaid Recipients and Expenditures by Eligibility Category: Fiscal Year 1995

Category	Recipients (Thousands)	Expenditures (Billions)	Percent Distribution	
			Recipients	Expenditures
All Eligibility Categories[1]	36,282	$120.1	100.0	100.0
Aged, Blind, and Disabled	9,977	85.9	27.5	71.5
Families	24,767	31.5	68.3	26.2
Children	17,164	18.0	47.3	15.0
Adults[2]	7,604	13.5	21.0	11.2

[1]Includes children and aged and non-aged adults categorized as "other" or unknown not shown separately.
[2]Adults in families with dependent children.
NOTE: Data reported on Health Care Financing Administration Form 2082.
Source: Health Care Financing Administration, Bureau of Data Management and Strategy, 1995.

states use this flexibility is through Medicaid waivers. There are two types of Medicaid waivers: program waivers (including home- and community-based service waivers and freedom-of-choice waivers) and research and demonstration waivers. Home- and community-based waivers allow states to place Medicaid-eligible persons into alternative, non-institutional settings for certain types of medical and personal care. Freedom-of-choice waivers allow states to place Medicaid beneficiaries into mandatory managed care plans (where beneficiaries have a choice of a minimum of two providers). Research and demonstration waivers (section 1115 of the Social Security Act) allow federal Medicaid requirements to be waived in order to conduct experimental, pilot, or demonstration projects.

The recent slowdown in Medicaid expenditure growth from 1993 to 1994 (from 12.6% to 8.5%), which continued in 1995 (8.4%), was partially driven by a slowdown in the growth of overall program recipients (7.3% in 1993 to 4.8% in 1994 and 3.5% in 1995). In addition, the change in the proportion of the Medicaid population enrolled in managed care rather than fee-for-service may also have contributed to the overall expenditure slowdown. State Medicaid programs view managed care as a way to constrain cost growth. In shifting recipients to managed care plans, states also shift the risk for health care costs to the plans. As an increasing number of states used this cost-containment option, managed care enrollment grew quite rapidly. The Medicaid managed care population represented only 9.5% of all Medicaid recipients in fiscal year 1991, but by fiscal year 1995 tripled in share to 32.1%. In 1995, HMOs represented 62% of all Medicaid managed care programs; prepaid health plans, 25%; primary care case management programs, 12%; and health insuring organizations, 1%.[26]

The slowdown in Medicaid expenditure growth between 1993 and 1994 was also marked by a sharp deceleration in federal Medicaid spending. (The state share of Medicaid expenditures, however, grew at a steady rate.) There was a marked increase from 1993 to 1994 in the percentage of states with higher-than-average federal matching rates who also showed lower-than-average expenditure growth. In other words, the poorest states showed the slowest growth in Medicaid spending during this period, which slowed the growth in overall federal matching contributions. This composition change caused the federal percentage contribution to Medicaid spending to fall.

CONCLUSION

This chapter describes the latest shifts that have occurred within the health care system. Growth in private sector spending fell to low rates between 1993 and 1995, contributing heavily to the slow overall spending growth in those years. National health expenditures as a share of the nation's output of goods and services were stable for 3 years, breaking the trend of rapid annual increases registered in the late 1980s and early 1990s. Questions about whether these trends will continue and how the federal sector (primarily Medicare) will react to current changes in the health care marketplace continue to be asked. How will physicians react to slow or negative income growth? How will managed care plans respond to rapid increases in prescription drug use? How will issues of quality and bias selection be addressed by managed care plans? What will happen to managed care premium increases once the transition of privately insured persons to these plans has stabilized? The answers are not yet clear.

References

1. Duke, K.S. Hospitals in a changing health care system. *Health Affairs.* Summer 1996;15(2):49–61.
2. American Hospital Association. National Hospital Panel Survey. Chicago, 1995 (Unpublished).
3. Heffler, S.K., Donham, C.S., Won, D.K., and Sensening, A.L. Health care indicators: Hospital, employment, and price indicators for the health care industry: Fourth quarter 1995 and annual data for 1987–95. *Health Care Financing Review.* Summer 1996;17(4):217–256.
4. Lewin-VHI, Inc. *Subacute care: Policy synthesis and market area analysis.* Available on the Internet at: http://aspe.os.dhhs.gov/daltcp/home.htm. Contract number HHS-100-93-0012. Prepared for the Office of the Assistant Secretary for Planning and Evaluation, U.S. Department of Health and Human Services, Washington, DC, 1995.
5. Langley, M., and Sharp, A. As big hospital chains take over nonprofits, a backlash is growing. *The Wall Street Journal.* October 18, 1996, A1.
6. Rundle, R.L. Tenet Healthcare's bid to buy OrNda signals it means to stay independent. *The Wall Street Journal.* October 18, 1996; B3.
7. Dial, T.H., Pan, L. Bergsten, C., Hobart, J., Whitmore, H., Musker, J., and Gabel, J.R. *HMO and PPO industry profile: 1995–96 Edition.* Washington, DC: American Association of Health Plans, May, 1996.
8. Zwanziger, J., and Melnick, G.A. Can managed care plans control health care costs? *Health Affairs.* Summer 1996;15(2):185–199.
9. Wooton, S. Physicians are ordered to limit referrals. *Baltimore Sun.* August 3, 1996; C3.
10. Rice, T., Stearns, S., DesHarnais, S., Pathman, D., Tai-Seale, M., and Brasure, M. Do physicians cost shift? *Health Affairs.* Fall 1996;15(3):215–225.
11. U.S. Bureau of the Census. *Service annual survey: 1994.* Washington, DC: U.S. Department of Commerce, August, 1996.
12. Emmons, D.W., and Simon, C.J. Managed care evolving contractual arrangements. In *Socioeconomic Characteristics of Medical Practice, 1996.* Chicago: American Medical Association, April, 1996.
13. Kletke, P.R., Emmons, D.W., and Gillis, K.D. Current trends in physicians practice arrangement from owners to employees. *JAMA.* 1996;276(7):555–560.
14. American Medical Association. *Socioeconomic characteristics of medical practice, 1996.* Chicago: American Medical Association, April, 1996.
15. Simon, C.J., and Born, P.H. Physician earnings in a changing managed care environment. *Health Affairs.* Fall, 1996;15(3):124–133.

16. Moser, J.W. Trends and patterns in physician income. In *Socioeconomic Characteristics of Medical Practice, 1996*. Chicago: American Medical Association, April, 1996.

17. Seifer, S.D., Troupin, B., and Rubenfeld, G.D.: Changes in marketplace demand for physicians. *JAMA*. 1996;276(9):695–699.

18. Miller, R.S., Jonas, H.S., and Whitcomb, M.E. The initial employment status of physicians completing training in 1994. *JAMA*. 1996;275(9):708–712.

19. National Center for Health Statistics. *Health United States, 1995*. U.S. Department of Health and Human Services, Public Health Service. Washington, DC: U.S. Government Printing Office, June, 1996.

20. IMS America. Data from the U.S. Hospital Audit. Plymouth Meeting, PA, 1996.

21. Schondelmeyer, S., and Seoane-Vazquez, E. Prescription trends: 1996 survey. *American Druggist*. June, 1996;213(6):25.

22. Foster Higgins. *National survey of employer-sponsored health plans, 1994*. Report. New York: Foster Higgins Survey and Research Services, 1994.

23. KPMG Peat Marwick. *Health benefits in 1996*. (Also yearly editions for 1991–1995.) Newark, NJ: KPMG Peat Marwick, 1991–1996.

24. U.S. Bureau of Labor Statistics. *Employee benefits in medium and large firms, 1993*. Bulletin 2456. U.S. Department of Labor. Washington, DC: U.S. Government Printing Office, November, 1994.

25. Anders, G. Pricey operation: A plan to cut back on Medicare expenses goes awry; costs soar. *The Wall Street Journal*. October 3, 1996;A1.

26. Health Care Financing Administration. *Medicaid managed care enrollment report*. Summary Statistics as of June 30, 1995. Baltimore, MD: 1996.

22

Quality Health Insurance for All Our Children

Donald Schiff

The crisis in providing quality health care for all children in the United States will clearly be a major issue as we move into the new millennium. The persistent opposition that influential sectors of our society (business, state governments, and special interest groups) have demonstrated toward declaring that health care is a "right" for all of our children is a painful reminder that the achievement of this goal remains in the future.

Because our nation draws its strength at every level—from President to factory worker to artisan—from a population that is ethnically and economically diverse, we cannot allow any potential contributor to our society to fail to maximize her ability because of a lack of adequate health care. In the latter years of the 20th century, quality comprehensive health insurance[1] is the best available vehicle for ensuring a healthy citizenry. (See Appendix at end of chapter.)

ISSUES OF CHILD HEALTH CARE

Multiple studies have provided clear evidence that children who do not have health insurance are not perceived by their parents to be in as good health as those who do. They do not visit doctors as often, nor do they receive regular care for a variety of important acute health problems (pharyngitis, urinary tract infections, injuries) or chronic ones (asthma, obesity, developmental delays).

There have been advances producing declining infant mortality rates (we remain 25th among industrialized nations)[2] and increasing immunization levels in children at 2 years of age.[3] (The recommended immunization schedule is shown in Table 22.1.) However, major areas of morbidity and mortality, including non-intentional injury, poisoning, child abuse, murder, suicide, mental illness, and human immunodeficiency virus (HIV) infection, are some of the child health areas that continue to demand our ongoing intervention.

A further consideration of the current status of child health care reveals a widespread lack of awareness and understanding of the availability and importance of preventive care for this specific age group. The widespread screening of newborns for common metabolic diseases (e.g., phenylketonuria, hypothyroidism) during the 1990s has prevented disastrous complications for thousands. Introduction of new vaccines protecting against potentially deadly *Haemophilus influenzae* B and chickenpox has saved additional thousands from illness and death. New vaccines currently being tested against rotavirus (the cause of common, severe diarrhea) will, when put into general use, help contain another international disease. But less well known preventive measures—such as the early detection of anatomic defects

TABLE 22.1

*Recommended Childhood Immunization Schedule United States,
January–December 1998*

Vaccines[1] are listed under the routinely recommended ages. [Bars] indicate range of acceptable ages for vaccination. Catch-up immunization should be done during any visit when feasible. Broken border ovals indicate vaccines to be assessed and given if necessary during the early adolescent visit.

Vaccine ▼ / Age ►	Birth	1 Month	2 Months	4 Months	6 Months	12 Months	15 Months	18 Months	4-6 Years	11-12 Years	14-16 Years
V Hepatitis B[2,3]	Hep B-1	Hep B-2			Hep B-3					Hep B[3]	
A / **C** Diphtheria, Tetanus, Pertussis[4]			DTaP or DTP	DTaP or DTP	DTaP or DTP		DTaP or DTP[4]		DTaP or DTP	Td	
C H. influenzae type b[5]			Hib	Hib	Hib[5]	Hib[5]					
I Polio[6]			Polio[6]	Polio	Polio[6]				Polio		
N Measles, Mumps, Rubella[7]						MMR			MMR[7]	MMR[7]	
E Varicella[8]						Var				Var[8]	

Accelerated Schedule For Infants And Children Under 7 Years Old Who Start The Series Late*

Visit	Vaccine doses
1st visit (at least 4 months of age)	DTaP/DTP #1, Polio #1, Hib[a], MMR (as soon as child is 12 months), HB #1
4-8 weeks after 1st visit	DTaP/DTP #2, Polio #2, Hib[a], HB #2
4-8 weeks after 2nd visit	DTaP/DTP #3, Polio #3, Hib[a]
6 months after 3rd visit	DTaP/DTP #4, Hib[a], HB #3
Age 4-6 years (before school entry)	DTaP/DTP #5[b], Polio #4[b], MMR #2 (at least 1 month after MMR #1)
Age 11-16 years	Td

a. Immunologically normal children age 5 years and older do not need Hib vaccine. If Infant starts series at age 7-11 months, give 2 doses 2 months apart and booster dose at 12-15 months. If Infant starts at age 12-14 months, give 1st dose. Give 2nd (and last) dose at least 2 months later. If child starts at age 15 months to 4 years, give just one dose.

b. The USPHS and the AAP consider DTaP/DTP #5 and Polio #4 necessary unless the DTaP/DTP #4 and Polio #3 were given after the 4th birthday.

* If child was born on or after 11-22-91, initiate the hepatitis B vaccine series.

Children Beginning Immunization At Age 7 Years Or Older

Visit	Vaccine doses
1st visit	Td #1, Polio #1, MMR #1, HB #1
4-8 weeks after 1st visit	Td #2, Polio #2, HB #2
6 months after 2nd visit	Td #3, Polio #3, HB #3
10 years after 3rd Td	Td
At age 11-12 years	MMR #2 (at least 1 month after MMR #1)

Minimum Intervals Between Vaccine Doses

Vaccine	Dose 1-2	Dose 2-3	Dose 3-4
DTP/DTaP (DT)	4 Weeks	4 Weeks	6 Months
Comb. DTP-Hib	1 Month	1 Month	6 Months
Hib			
HbOC	1 Month	1 Month	•
PRP-T	1 Month	1 Month	•
PRP-OMP	1 Month	1 Month	*

* Hib booster dose should be administered no earlier than 12 months of age and at least 2 months after the previous dose of Hib vaccine.

Vaccine	Dose 1-2	Dose 2-3	Dose 3-4
Polio*	4 Weeks	4 Weeks	4 Weeks
MMR	1 Month		
Hepatitis B	1 Month	2 Months**	
Varicella	4 Weeks		

* Sequential IPV/OPV, all-OPV, or all-IPV.

** This final dose is recommended at least 4 months after the first dose and no earlier than 6 months of age.

The above table shows the minimum intervals acceptable between doses of vaccine. All vaccines should be administered as close to the recommended schedule as possible in order to maximize the protection from vaccine. It is not necessary to restart the series of any vaccine due to extended intervals between doses.

TABLE 22.2

Recommendations for Preventive Pediatric Health Care

Each child and family is unique; therefore, these **Recommendations for Preventive Pediatric Health Care** are designed for the care of children who are receiving competent parenting, have no manifestations of any important health problems, and are growing and developing in satisfactory fashion. **Additional visits may become necessary if circumstances suggest variations from normal.**

Committee on Practice and Ambulatory Medicine (RE 9535)

These guidelines represent a consensus by the Committee on Practice and Ambulatory Medicine in consultation with national committees and sections of the American Academy of Pediatrics. The Committee emphasizes the great importance of **continuity** of care in comprehensive health supervision and the need to avoid **fragmentation** of care.

A prenatal visit is recommended for parents who are at high risk, for first-time parents, and for those who request a conference. The prenatal visit should include anticipatory guidance and pertinent medical history. Every infant should have a newborn evaluation after birth.

AGE[4]	INFANCY[3]									EARLY CHILDHOOD[3]				MIDDLE CHILDHOOD[3]				ADOLESCENCE[3]										
	NEWBORN	2-4d[2]	By 1mo	2mo	4mo	6mo	9mo	12mo	15mo	18mo	24mo	3y	4y	5y	6y	8y	10y	11y	12y	13y	14y	15y	16y	17y	18y	19y	20y	21y
HISTORY Initial/Interval	•	•	•	•	•	•	•	•	•	•	•	•	•	•	•	•	•	•	•	•	•	•	•	•	•	•	•	•
MEASUREMENTS Height and Weight	•	•	•	•	•	•	•	•	•	•	•	•	•	•	•	•	•	•	•	•	•	•	•	•	•	•	•	•
Head Circumference	•	•	•	•	•	•	•	•	•	•																		
Blood Pressure												•	•	•	•	•	•	•	•	•	•	•	•	•	•	•	•	•
SENSORY SCREENING Vision	S	S	S	S	S	S	S	S	S	S	S	O[5]	O	O	O	O	O	S	O	S	O	S	O	S	O	S	O	S
Hearing[6]	S/O	S	S	S	S	S	S	S	S	S	S	O	O	O	O	O	O	S	S	S	S	S	S	S	S	S	S	S
DEVELOPMENTAL/BEHAVIORAL ASSESSMENT[7]	•	•	•	•	•	•	•	•	•	•	•	•	•	•	•	•	•	•	•	•	•	•	•	•	•	•	•	•
PHYSICAL EXAMINATION[8]	•	•	•	•	•	•	•	•	•	•	•	•	•	•	•	•	•	•	•	•	•	•	•	•	•	•	•	•
PROCEDURES – GENERAL[9] Hereditary/Metabolic Screening[10]		•																										
Immunization[11]	•		•	•	•	•		•	•	•			•		•			•	•		•		•		•			
Lead Screening[12]							←	•			•																	
Hematocrit or Hemoglobin					↔																							
Urinalysis														•														
PROCEDURES – PATIENTS AT RISK Tuberculin Test[15]									←—————————————————————→																			
Cholesterol Screening[16]														←——————————————————————————————————————→														
STD Screening[17]																		←———→										
Pelvic Exam[18]																		←———————————————————————————————→							•	•	•	•
ANTICIPATORY GUIDANCE[19]	•	•	•	•	•	•	•	•	•	•	•	•	•	•	•	•	•	•	•	•	•	•	•	•	•	•	•	•
Injury Prevention[20]	•	•	•	•	•	•	•	•	•	•	•	•	•	•	•	•	•	•	•	•	•	•	•	•	•	•	•	•
INITIAL DENTAL REFERRAL[21]												•																

1. Breastfeeding encouraged and instruction and support offered.
2. For newborns discharged in less than 48 hours after delivery.
3. Developmental, psychosocial, and chronic disease issues for children and adolescents may require frequent counseling and treatment visits separate from preventive care visits.
4. If a child comes under care for the first time at any point on the schedule, or if any items are not accomplished at the suggested age, the schedule should be brought up to date at the earliest possible time.
5. If the patient is uncooperative, rescreen within six months.
6. Some experts recommend objective appraisal of hearing in the newborn period. The Joint Committee on Infant Hearing has identified patients at significant risk for hearing loss. All children meeting these criteria should be objectively screened. See the Joint Committee on Infant Hearing 1994 Position Statement.
7. By history and appropriate physical examination; if suspicious, by specific objective developmental testing.
8. At each visit, a complete physical examination is essential, with infant totally uncothed, older child undressed and suitably draped.
9. These may be modified, depending upon entry point into schedule and individual need.
10. Metabolic screening (eg, thyroid, hemoglobinopathies, PKU, galactosemia) should be done according to state law.
11. Schedule(s) per the Committee on Infectious Diseases, published periodically in *Pediatrics*. Every visit should be an opportunity to update and complete a child's immunizations.
12. Blood lead screen per AAP statement "Lead Poisoning: From Screening to Primary Prevention" (1993).
13. All menstruating adolescents should be screened.
14. Conduct dipstick urinalysis for leukocytes for male and female adolescents.
15. TB testing per AAP statement "Screening for Tuberculosis in Infants and Children" (1994). Testing should be done upon recognition of high risk factors. If results are negative but high risk situation continues, testing should be repeated on an annual basis.
16. Cholesterol screening for high risk patients per AAP "Statement on Cholesterol" (1992). If family history cannot be ascertained and other risk factors are present, screening should be at the discretion of the physician.
17. All sexually active patients should be screened for sexually transmitted diseases (STDs).
18. All sexually active females should have a pelvic examination. A pelvic examination and routine pap smear should be offered as part of preventive health maintenance between the ages of 18 and 21 years.
19. Appropriate discussion and counseling should be an integral part of each visit for care.
20. From birth to age 12, refer to AAP's injury prevention program (TIPP®) as described in "A Guide to Safety Counseling in Office Practice" (1994).
21. Earlier initial dental evaluations may be appropriate for some children. Subsequent examinations as prescribed by dentist.

Key: * • = to be performed for patients at risk   S = subjective, by history   O = objective, by a standard testing method   ↔ = the range during which a service may be provided, with the dot indicating the preferred age.

NB: Special chemical, immunologic, and endocrine testing is usually carried out upon specific indications. Testing other than newborn (eg, inborn errors of metabolism, sickle disease, etc.) is discretionary with the physician.
The recommendations in this publication do not indicate an exclusive course of treatment or serve as a standard of medical care. Variations, taking into account individual circumstances, may be appropriate.

in young children, including those of the heart, hip, eye, and hearing—can, with early recognition and intervention, bring about a positive outcome for an affected child. An evaluation of cognitive and motor development as well as socialization is also part of the health-promoting pediatric visit. Effective treatment plans initiated promptly can be critically important when abnormalities are found. Because injuries are the most common cause of death in children after age 1, considerable time is spent during health promotion visits on a discussion of auto seat restraints, water heater temperature controls, smoke detectors, bicycle helmets, and other safety measures.

The failure of pediatricians and other child advocates to fully inform the policymakers and the public about the importance and success of pediatric prevention methods has resulted in the current lack of a public policy that would ensure quality health care insurance for every U.S. child.

A common misconception suggests that only catastrophic insurance at a low cost is really necessary for family protection. If this view

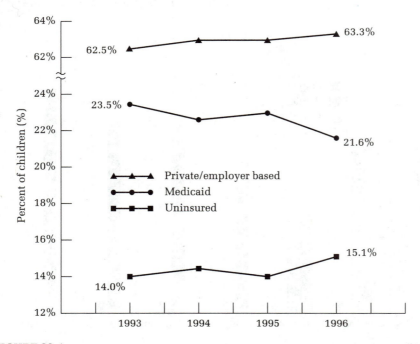

FIGURE 22.1

Health insurance status of U.S. children younger than age 19, 1993–1996. *Source:* From American Academy of Pediatrics, Division of Health Policy Research. *Analysis of 1994–1997 March demographic file of the current population survey.* Elk Grove Village, IL: American Academy of Pediatrics, 1997.

prevails, initial costs would be lower, but the annual toll of disease and injury resulting from the absence of a pediatric prevention program (Table 22.2)[4] would clearly be more expensive in both dollars and the damaged lives of our children.

CURRENT INSURANCE COVERAGE

The percentage of children covered by employer-based insurance was 63% in 1996 (Fig. 22.1), but this varies widely depending on family income (Fig. 22.2).[6] The number covered by Medicaid, 16.2 million (21.6%),[5] has risen slightly because a number of states have raised the percentage of federal poverty level income required for eligibility. In spite of this change, the number of children younger than 19 years of age uninsured in the United States continues to rise (now 11.3 million),[5] and there had been no indication that this would change[7] until the surprising passage of a State Children's Health Insurance Plan as part of the Budget Reconciliation Act of 1997 (Figs. 22.3 and 22.4).

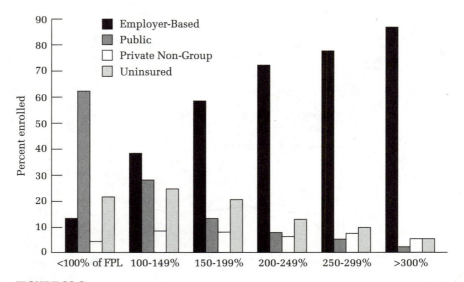

FIGURE 22.2

Primary source of health insurance coverage for children younger than age 18 years, by family income, 1995. (From Merlis, M. *Employer coverage and the Children's Health Insurance Program under the Balanced Budget Act of 1997: Options for states.* Institute for Health Policy Solutions, August/September, 1997.)

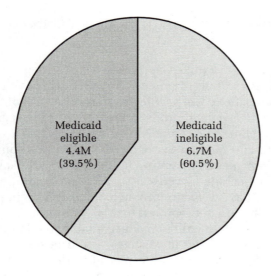

FIGURE 22.3

....

Uninsured children before Title XXI (under age 19 projected at 11.0 million for 1998). (From American Academy of Pediatrics analysis of 1993 to 1997 March Demographic File, Current Population Survey and 1998 State Population Projections by Single Year of Age, Sex, Race and Hispanic Origin (Series A). U.S. Census Bureau, December, 1997.)

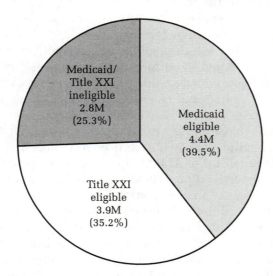

FIGURE 22.4

....

Uninsured children and legislated eligibility per Title XX (under age 19 projected at 11.0 million for 1998). (From American Academy of Pediatrics analysis of 1993 to 1997 March Demographic File, Current Population Survey and 1998 State Population Projections by Single Year of Age, Sex, Race and Hispanic Origin (Series A), U.S. Census Bureau, December, 1997.)

State Children's Health Insurance Program

The new legislation, which was passed by a strong bipartisan vote, will allow millions of children currently without health insurance to acquire this protection. The new legislation (Title XXI of the Social Security Act) provides federal funds in the form of a block grant awarded to states that submit an acceptable plan to the Secretary of the Department of Health and Human Services (HHS). Twenty-four billion dollars derived from general operating funds and a $.15/pack tax on cigarettes will be distributed over a 5-year period beginning October 1, 1997. Each state has 3 years to initiate its plan and begin receiving federal dollars. States are not required to apply for these funds; any dollar not expended by a state will be made available to other states. The allotment formula varies, but most states would receive a match of two federal dollars for each state dollar placed in the program. This is not an entitlement plan, and each eligible family is required to apply for the new option.

Under Title XXI states may expand Medicaid coverage, institute a new subsidized children's insurance plan, or create a combination of the two. The statute makes funds available for targeted low-income children to 200% of the federal poverty level (FPL) and may not be used for children who are eligible for Medicaid or other insurance coverage or who are living in a public institution.

Medicaid, which was designed to be the health care safety net for poor children, has failed to perform that function for up to 4 million at-risk children. Various state policies and dysfunction within families are responsible for the lack of enrollment of millions of Medicaid-eligible children.

Some states have elected to retain an optional family asset test that penalizes families that own a car needed to take them to work but which has a value of up to $2,000. Some states keep the family eligibility based on the federal poverty level at the lowest possible level required by federal law. In many states, for children younger than 6 years, this is 133% of the FPL, for children aged 6 to 15, 100% of the FPL, and between 15 and 19 years of age, less than 100% of the FPL. Some states and counties attempt to reduce Medicaid enrollment by limiting outreach efforts and failing to provide translation services and convenient office hours to facilitate the process. A number of states place physician and dental reimbursement rates so low that it becomes prohibitive for physicians to agree to care for Medicaid patients without limiting their numbers in each practice.

However, states that are instituting Medicaid expansion under Title XXI can have a major impact on the number of uninsured children in the United States. The benefits package for these new enrollees in Medicaid is identical to the current Medicaid benefits. Because more uninsured children (4 million)[5] are eligible for health care coverage under Medicaid than Title XXI, an aggressive outreach program by each state with an emphasis on making enrollment easy is necessary to reach this population.

The Balanced Budget Act also included three new provisions that can increase children's health care coverage through a broadening of the Medicaid program:

1. *Presumptive Eligibility*
   States now have the option of establishing a presumptive Medicaid eligibility procedure to facilitate the enrollment of children. Children may be enrolled in Medicaid on a temporary basis relying on information supplied by families. This is especially useful for children of parents employed at low wage jobs that do not offer health insurance coverage.

2. *Coverage of Supplemental Security Income Children*
   States are now required to continue Medicaid coverage for all disabled children who were receiving Supplemental Security Income (SSI) on August 22, 1996, but who lost their eligibility as a result of the 1996 law that restricted SSI disability standards for children.

3. *Twelve-Month Continuous Eligibility*
   States now have the option to guarantee 12 months of coverage to children enrolled in Medicaid regardless of whether the child experiences a change in family income that would render him or her ineligible for Medicaid during the 12-month period.

Each state will determine the income eligibility in its own program. The maximum allowable limit will be 200% of the FPL or 50 percentage points above the state's Medicaid eligibility level, whichever is higher.

Benefits

If a state chooses to implement a State Children's Health Insurance Program, it can choose the benefits package from among five basic options.

1. Blue Cross/Blue Shield preferred provider option offered to federal employees under the Federal Employees Health Benefits Plan

2. State employee health plan

3. Health maintenance organization (HMO) with the largest insured commercial, non-Medicaid enrollment in the state

4. Coverage that is the actuarial equivalent to one of the first three options

5. Another benefit package approved by the Secretary of HHS

Cost Sharing

- Limited, depending on a family's income, but will vary state by state
- *Below 150% of poverty level*: premiums no greater than those in Medicaid and cost sharing consistent with Medicaid
- *Above 150% of poverty level*: premiums and cost sharing must not exceed 5% of a family's income

Beyond Federal Mandates

Forty-one states had expanded Medicaid eligibility for pregnant women and children beyond federal mandates prior to the implementation of the 1997 Budget Reconciliation Act.

- Thirty-five states exceed the federal mandate for eligibility for pregnant women and infants.
- Thirteen states exceed the minimum income eligibility thresholds for children between 1 and 5.
- Thirty-eight states exceed the income and/or age requirements for children 6 and older.

States have used a variety of mechanisms to expand eligibility for Medicaid beyond federal requirements.[8] Section 1902 and 1115 options were used to gain flexibility and design better programs to meet their policy goals.

Projected Outcomes of Title XXI

The vigorous push by states to expand children's health care through their partnership with the federal government is evidence of the recognition by the general public of the priority that this societal need deserves. Title XXI offers a laboratory and specific period of time (5 to 10 years) during which we will observe and record the progress made toward the goal of improving our children's health by increasing access to health insurance. Our optimism must be tempered by the views of policy analysts who have predicted that only half of the children not currently covered by health insurance will become covered under Title XXI. If this estimate is accurate, between 4 and 6 million children will remain uncovered and at risk.

There are important potential problems associated with Title XXI legislation.

1. It provides no entitlement for children or families. States submit a plan to HHS if they are interested in participating. A number of states have declined to do so at this time. If states do participate and prepare a plan that is approved, parents are also required to apply and enroll their children.

2. Each state has great flexibility in determining the details of the plan, including
   a. Eligibility standards—family income level can vary from 185% to 285% FPL;
   b. Benefit plans; and
   c. Premium and co-pay as family contributions to subsidized insurance programs.

   Although these state plan variations can be productive as a means of broadening our experience in understanding the response of families to multiple options, it is also confusing to many and can lead to a significant migration of families to those states that have more comprehensive benefits in their plans.

3. *Crowd out* is the term used to describe the process of a family dropping employer-based children's health insurance and the substitution of insurance paid for under Title XXI. Measures designed to minimize this effect are limited and their effectiveness unpredictable.

The dizzying array of programs, services, and funding mechanisms currently used in the patchwork quilt of health care for our nation's children has outlived its limited usefulness.

The ineffective approach to closing the huge gaps in the safety net by pursuing the popular political philosophy of devolving increasing power to the states will predictably continue the inequities for millions of children who will have either no health insurance or a less than adequate plan depending on where they live or the choices their parents make. The promotion of self-reliance and independence, which is admirable in so many aspects of our public policy, has had a major role in placing the most vulnerable members of our society, our children, at a significant disadvantage, because their health insurance decisions are made by others (parents, parent's employer, or government).

Managed care was first proposed by Paul Ellwood[9] as a mechanism by which health care costs would be brought under control through a competitive market approach without sacrificing quality care. It has not become sufficiently widespread (70% population covered in some states) so that its impact on U.S. health care can be examined.

Although it is clear that some managed care organizations (MCOs) can provide quality health care at a reasonable cost, there are others that appear to have significant problems. Reports of rationing of care, barriers to consultations by subspecialists, and unexplained refusals to authorize established treatments, including bone marrow transplants, have increased over the past few years. Federal investigation of Columbia HCA for fraud raises additional questions as to whether health care can be considered in the same category as other business ventures.

How the investment world views health care and its management was revealed when it was reported that U.S. Health Care was planning to strengthen its physician network by spending additional money. Wall Street's response was to drop its value by $1 billion.[10]

The move by most states toward mandating that Medicaid recipients receive their care through MCOs may expose this vulnerable population to additional risk.[11]

A PLAN FOR THE FUTURE—"PEDIACARE"

For these reasons, the future of health care for children must be founded on a plan that ensures appropriate health care for *every* American child. It cannot be based on considerations of geography, family income, job status, previous health history, or parental initiative. Children clearly are unable to make the decision to obtain their own health care and should not be subject to societal vagaries that so often negatively affect them.

The goal of a nation devoted to helping all of our children cannot be delayed any longer. The call for quality health insurance for every child is not intended to bring government control into our children's lives. In fact, it must not. Although the plan is designed to be significantly funded at the federal level, it will be administered by the states, with parents making the choices as to when and where care will be received.

The new system would be developed over time. It should be put into place incrementally, recognizing that with experience, ways to improve the plan will become apparent. The experience already gained through the years of Medicaid, Medicare, private insurance, and managed care will be invaluable in the planning.

Uninsured children would gradually be melded into current options, including private insurance, Medicaid, employer-supported plans, the newly designed state children's insurance plans, in the new "Pediacare" plan.

Funding

Funding for Pediacare would come from a private-public partnership based on family contributions on a sliding income scale and the federal and state government general operating funds. Because health care costs will vary somewhat geographically, it will be necessary to vary costs by state or region.

Each family's contribution would be determined by annual income and can be deducted by the payroll deduction method as is now done for Social Security and Medicare.

Employers, who have long complained about being pressured to include health insurance as a fringe benefit, would no longer receive any tax benefit for providing health insurance for children and would be expected to gradually drop their contribution.

Specific Roles and Responsibilities (Table 22.3)

States. States would use their Medicaid contributions to set up and maintain agencies whose purpose would be to administer the plan and provide information about health care organizations to the public, enabling families to select a plan. Additional responsibilities would include oversight of the MCOs, data collection, and evaluation of outcome measures and quality of care.

Managed Care Organizations. MCOs would be certified by the state and would approve claims and reimburse providers according to contracts with hospitals and physicians. They would be viewed as a quasi-public utility with reasonable limits on profit.

Providers. Hospitals and physicians would contract with MCOs and provide services directly to patients. Physicians would continue to be independent practitioners with the same options they now have.

TABLE 22.3

Outline of Roles for Each Participant

Family

- Enrolls in a plan
- Chooses health care provider
- Pays payroll deduction—sliding scale based on income
- May pay co-pay based on income

Physician

- Contracts with MCO
- Provides care
- Submits claims based on capitation or fee for service

Managed Care Organization

- Certified by state
- Quasi-public utility
- Negotiated profit limit
- Contracts with providers
- Contracts with individual families for children's health care coverage
- Claims approval
- Reimburses providers per schedule (capitation, fee for service)
- Collects data
- Responds to complaints

State

- Creates "Pediacare" agency
- Certifies managed care organization
- Provides information to general public concerning physicians, hospitals, managed care organizations
- Receives funds from federal government and disburses to MCOs
- Collects data from MCO
- Monitors costs
- Monitors outcome
- Monitors other quality measures
- Provides outreach
- Promotes enrollment

Federal Government

- Establishes national guidelines for benefits
- Collects payroll taxes
- Major funding source from general operating fund
- Distributes funds to states for Pediacare program
- Collects data
- Publicizes outcome and quality measures

They may practice independently, in small or large groups, or become employees of hospitals or MCOs.

Families. Families would be able to choose any certified state-licensed physician to care for their child—a choice guaranteed by their insurance.

Federal Responsibility. The federal government would approve basic benefit programs that will be comprehensive and uniform across the country, as is currently done in the Medicare and Medicaid plans. General guidelines would incorporate the advice of recognized professional authorities, including the American Academy of Pediatrics and Centers for Disease Control and Prevention.

An additional federal role would be to collect the payroll taxes for the Pediacare program and maintain these funds for disbursement to the states as needed for implementation of the program. Federal general operating funds would provide the other source of funds for the program.

Compilation of data from the states to produce an annual public report on children's health is also a proper task for the federal government.

Political Realities

Objections to this type of plan will come from every direction, but not from the families of those children who are uninsured or underinsured. They have too often experienced the ill effects of the lack of this type of comprehensive program.

The political barriers to obtaining broad acceptance of a new child health plan present themselves at once and are truly formidable. The memory of the Clinton Health Plan of 1993–1994 and its failure to gain acceptance is a major obstacle. A child health plan (Pediacare) would be called the "New Clinton Health Plan" by critics. It would be labeled "socialized medicine" and characterized as the next step toward government control of all health care. In reality, it would and should be viewed as a needed, and far too long delayed, thoughtful approach to protecting our nation's children and thereby our country's future.

Although guidelines and some standards would be put in place at the national level, these would be used only to provide a level playing field of appropriate health care for all children. States would administer the plan, and ultimately each family will make decisions for their own children.

Projected Cost of Pediacare

Costs of medical care continue to rise erratically and somewhat unpredictably. Nevertheless, it should be anticipated that the cost of Pediacare will be influenced by population growth as well as a continuation of the technological revolution and will certainly grow in the future.

Current estimates of the cost of comprehensive care of our child population slightly exceeds $100 billion. With our annual health bill at $1 trillion, it is clear that we can create a more efficient, effective productive system for a "bargain" sum, and we must move forward to accomplish this at the earliest possible opportunity.

References

1. American Academy of Pediatrics, Committee on Child Health Financing. *Scope of health care benefits for newborns, infants, children, adolescents and young adults through age 21 years.* Elk Grove Village, IL: American Academy of Pediatrics, 1997.
2. Population Reference Bureau. *1995 world population data sheet.* Washington, DC: 1995.
3. Advisory Committee on Immunization Practices, U.S. Department of Public Health and American Academy of Pediatrics Committee on Infectious Disease. Recommended childhood immunization schedule, United States, January–December, 1998.
4. American Academy of Pediatrics Committee on Practice and Ambulatory Medicine. Recommendations for preventive health care. 1996.
5. American Academy of Pediatrics, Division of Health Policy Research. *Analysis of 1994–1997 March demographic file of the current population survey.* Elk Grove Village, IL: American Academy of Pediatrics, 1997.
6. Merlis, M. *Employer coverage and the Children's Health Insurance Program under the Balanced Budget Act of 1997: Options for states.* Institute for Health Policy Solutions, August/September, 1997.
7. Himmelstein, D.U., and Woolhandler, S. The Oregon Health Plan. *New England Journal of Medicine.* 1998;338:395.
8. Call, K.T., Lurie, N., Jonk, Y., et al. Who is still uninsured in Minnesota? Lessons for state reform efforts. *JAMA.* 1997;278(14):1127–1208.
9. Ellwood, P.M., and Enthoven, A.C. Responsible choices: The Jackson Hole Group Plan for Health Reform. *Health Aff (Millwood)* 1995;14:24–39.
10. Anders, G. *Health against wealth.* Boston: Houghton-Mifflin, 1996.
11. Ellwood, P., and Lundberg, G. Managed care: A work in progress. *JAMA.* 1996; 276(13):1083–1086.

APPENDIX: AMERICAN ACADEMY OF PEDIATRICS

Scope of Health Care Benefits for Infants, Children, and Adolescents Through Age 21 Years

All newborns, infants, children, adolescents, young adult patients through age 21 years, and pregnant women must have access to comprehensive health care benefits that will ensure their optimal health and well-being. The following services should be included in the health benefit plans offered by all private and public insurers. These services should be delivered by appropriately trained and board eligible/certified pediatric providers, including primary care pediatricians, pediatric medical subspecialists, and pediatric surgical specialists. All providers of prenatal care should be able to identify a full range of medical and psychosocial risks and to refer patients for appropriate care throughout pregnancy. These services should be delivered in a variety of appropriate settings, and coordinated through the child's medical home. They also should be delivered in an efficient manner that does not compromise the quality of care. As these services are physician-directed and prescribed, they should include but are not limited to all of the following:

1. Medical care, including: (a) health supervision with preventive care and immunizations according to the American Academy of Pediatrics' "Recommendations for Preventive Pediatric Health Care," and (b) diagnosis and treatment of acute and chronic illness, developmental disabilities, learning disorders, and behavioral problems.

2. Surgical care.

3. Mental health, substance abuse, and services for other psychosocial problems including therapy, crisis management, day treatment, and residential care. This should also include evaluations and treatment of learning disabilities and related disorders such as attention deficit hyperactivity disorder.

4. Emergency medical and trauma care services for children.

5. Inpatient hospital and critical care services.

6. Pediatric critical care, pediatric medical subspecialty, and pediatric surgical specialty consultations occurring either in the inpatient or outpatient setting.

7. Family planning services.

8. Pregnancy services, including: (a) genetic counseling and related services as needed; (b) prenatal care; (c) prenatal consultation with a pediatrician or board eligible/certified provider of pediatric care; (d) care for all complications; (e) counseling and services for all pregnancy management options; and (f) care for the pregnancy of a dependent of a policyholder.

9. Care of all newborn infants, including: (a) attendance at and management of high-risk deliveries or those mandated by hospital regulations; (b) health supervision; (c) treatment of congenital anomalies and other medical and surgical conditions; (d) newborn intensive care services; and (e) when indicated by the infant's physician, a follow-up visit in the child's home or in the physician's office within 48 hours of discharge.

10. Laboratory and pathology services including screening for metabolic and other congenital disorders.

11. Diagnostic and therapeutic radiology services.

12. Anesthesia services including anesthesia when appropriate for all "covered" procedures.

13. Early intervention services and therapies for developmental, rehabilitative, and habilitative purposes including, but not limited to: (a) physical therapy; (b) speech therapy and language services; (c) occupational therapy; and (d) audiology.

14. Home health care services including, but not limited to, private duty nursing, attendant care, and respite care.

15. Intermediate or skilled nursing facility care in lieu of hospital care.

16. Hospice care.

17. Case management and care coordination integrated with child's primary care provider and family as required by those with special health care needs.

18. Medical and social services required to evaluate and treat suspected child physical and sexual abuse in both inpatient and outpatient settings.

19. Transfer/transport to a hospital or health facility.

20. Preventive and restorative dental care and oral surgery.

21. Nutritional and lactation counseling services.

22. Prescription drugs, medical and surgical supplies, and special nutritional supplements, including, but not limited to, those prescribed under national clinical trials for acquired immunodeficiency syndrome/human immunodeficiency virus and other conditions.

23. Rental or purchase and service of durable medical equipment including, but not limited to, equipment necessary to administer aerosolized medication and to monitor their effects, corrective eyeglasses or lenses, hearing aids, breast pumps, prostheses/braces, electrical and other types of ventilators, cardiorespirator monitors, oxygen concentrators, and customized wheelchairs.

IV

Health Issues
and Policy
Implications

23

Maternal and Infant Health in the United States: Implications for Women's Health

LOIS McCLOSKEY AND PAUL H. WISE

Pregnant women, mothers, infants, and children through adolescence traditionally have been considered the maternal and child health (MCH) population. Likewise, commonly used indicators of the health and welfare of the population have focused on these groups. In this chapter, we address the traditional health status indicators for pregnancy, birth, and infancy (through 1 year of life) and use these data as the basis for a discussion of how health care services and policies should be designed as we approach the 21st century. We point to three imperatives for improving the health of mothers and infants: (1) to expand the MCH population to include women regardless of their reproductive status; (2) to extend the boundaries of the field to encompass the social, economic, cultural, and political contexts in which the health of mothers and children occur; and (3) to design integrated services that recognize the connections between the health of women and infants and the social environments in which they live. This final imperative, of course, lies at the heart of this textbook, with its focus on the significance of social welfare policies for the health of families.

CHANGING DEMOGRAPHICS

The demographics of the MCH population are continually in flux. A few recent trends are important to note as a backdrop for the discussion of the health status of mothers and infants. First, as women in the "baby boom" cohort have begun to age beyond their reproductive years, the number of women giving birth has declined by about 1% per year over the past decade.[1] The fertility rate (number of births/total number of women of reproductive age) also continues to fall in virtually all demographic subgroups.

Second, the demographic profile of the birthing population has changed considerably in recent years, reflecting changes in the society as a whole. Hispanics constitute the fastest growing population group in this country, accounting for 10% of the total U.S. population in 1995 (a 25% increase since 1989).[2] Between 1989 and 1995, births to Hispanic women accounted for a growing proportion of all births in the United States, rising from 14% to 18% between 1989 and 1995.* This is due to the increasing number of Hispanic women (particularly Mexican women) of childbearing age as well as to a higher fertility rate in this group.† The proportion of women giving birth in the major

---

*1989 is the first year for which virtually all states (all but three) reported Hispanic origin on their birth certificates.
†The fertility rate among whites in 1995 was 64.5; for blacks, 71.7; for Asian/Pacific Islanders, 65.6; and for American Indians, 70, compared with 103.7 for Hispanic women.

racial groups as defined on birth certificates (white, black, American Indian, Asian or Pacific Islander) remained relatively stable over these years (white, 80%; black, 15%; American Indian, 0.01%; Asian/Pacific Islander, 4%).[3] By the year 2000, it is expected that close to 40% of births in the United States will be to women of color.

The rise in the proportion of births to unmarried women between 1980 and 1994 (18.4% to 32.6%) has received widespread public attention. It is a trend observed across most demographic groups, although rates vary by age and race/ethnicity. Contributing to the rise are the increase in the proportion of births to Hispanic women (a group with the highest rates of unmarried childbearing), an increase in the number of single women relative to the number of married women in the population, the declining fertility rate among married women, changes in reporting, and larger economic realities, including improved wage opportunities for some women and decreased earnings for men, especially less skilled young men.[1,4] At the same time, it is important to note that the probability of a single woman giving birth has not risen significantly, and for blacks has declined during this time period.[1]

The third trend of great import is the changing face of the poor in this country. Increasing numbers of mothers, namely single mothers, and their children are counted among the country's poor or near poor. Single adult families are the largest group among the poor, constituting almost 43% of poor families. Further differentiated by race, the largest group in real numbers is white single mothers and their children. About 40% of all children younger than age 18 live at or below the poverty level. Almost half of poor families are white (48%), 27% are black, 21% are Hispanic, and 4% are of other racial or ethnic background.[4]

There is no question that members of racial and ethnic minorities shoulder disproportionate amounts of the poverty burden. Almost one third of African American or Hispanic people live in poor families, much higher than the 12% poverty rates among non-Hispanic white persons. Native Americans and recent immigrants, like generations of immigrants before them, are also more likely to be poor. Reasons for high rates of poverty in these groups are deep and enduring. Among the most important are discrimination in housing, particularly among African Americans, discrimination in employment and wages, lack of access to high-quality education, and cultural and language barriers faced by new immigrants.[4]

The combination of the dramatic alterations in the safety net available to poor families and the demographic patterns that have taken root in the 1990s is likely to reinforce this face of the poor well into the first decade of the new millennium. The price of poverty and near poverty in health is high and can be seen as clearly in the indicators of maternal and infant health as in any other health statistics. The impact of inequalities of race/ethnicity, class and gender is powerfully witnessed by disparities in infant mortality, maternal mortality, and the associated morbidities. It is impossible to reflect back or to project forward in the area of maternal and infant health without recognizing the larger contexts of immigration, fertility, discrimination, poverty, health, and social policies.

CHANGING POLICY ENVIRONMENT

Of central importance to maternal and infant health have been changes in policies that shape insurance coverage for health services. Medicaid, the primary publicly funded health insurance program for children and pregnant women in the United States, has undergone incremental expansion over the past decade, such that adolescents and more of the working poor have become eligible. However, these expansions left millions of poor, non-pregnant women without coverage. Medicaid is an entitlement program, meaning that it is offered to all children and pregnant women that meet eligibility criteria, and is jointly funded by federal and state governments. It is a financing program, not a health care delivery program, and relies on local health care systems to provide services. Although the program's general structure is based on federal standards, there remains considerable variation among the states regarding eligibility criteria and covered services.

Traditionally, Medicaid has been closely linked to welfare eligibility. For decades, the Aid to Families with Dependent Children (AFDC) program was the primary cash assistance program for poor families and the principal gateway for poor children and women into the Medicaid program. However, recent federal legislation abolished the AFDC program and replaced it with the Transitional Assistance for Needy Families (TANF), a non-entitlement program with strict eligibility time limits and maternal work requirements. With the introduction of TANF, the linkage between welfare and Medicaid was formally severed, giving states far greater control of their respective welfare programs. It is likely, therefore, that the eligibility criteria and enrollment procedures for the two programs may be quite distinct in many jurisdictions. In addition, the strict requirements regarding maternal work and other behaviors are likely to reduce functional coverage to large groups of reproductive-aged women.[5]

Concern for the impact of these more restrictive welfare policies on children led to the recent passage of the State Children's Health Insurance Program (CHIP), Title XXI of the Social Security Act, which will allow states to provide health insurance to many children who are currently uninsured but do not meet Medicaid eligibility criteria. Although CHIP will expand public insurance for many children, it is important to recognize that the administrative complexity of the state-based programs may mean that only a fraction of the 11 million uninsured children in the United States are likely to benefit. Moreover, although any program that expands health insurance for anyone should be welcomed, one must question whether this program will detract politically from broader efforts to provide health insurance to all American citizens in need.

The implications of these changes on the provision of health services to women and children may be dramatic. Although current policies will allow families to maintain Medicaid coverage based on pre-existing (1996) eligibility criteria, enrolling in Medicaid may require new, more complex procedures in many areas. Further, unless states update their criteria, the proportion of low-income women who can satisfy the 1996 program standards will shrink over time as the cost of living increases.[6] Non-pregnant women remain the most vulnerable group. The emphasis of TANF on maternal employment may mean that parents or other caretakers will be under new pressures to work and may have less time to spend with their children at home and reduced freedom to attend daytime clinical visits. The continued evolution of welfare policy in the United States, therefore, is likely to have a profound impact on the practical guarantee of access to care for poor families.

Beyond health insurance coverage, the growth of managed care systems has also had a major impact on the provision of services to women and children in the United States. These systems generally attempt to control patients' access to services through mandated approval and cost-sharing mechanisms. The challenge of managed care is to ensure that its controlled clinical environment expands access to care rather than restricts it. Particularly for children with considerable health care needs, managed care can enhance the coordination of different levels of care.[7] However, such integrated care for traditionally underserved communities is likely to require policies and programs that specifically facilitate and monitor mechanisms of referral and health service provision and ensure their reach into communities.

Although the profoundly dynamic character of health care policy in the United States cannot be overstated, it is that this evolution is occurring amid unprecedented progress in preventive and therapeutic capability that will define patterns of maternal and infant health outcomes for years to come.[8] Therefore, the greater our capability to improve health, the greater the collective burden on public policy to ensure that this capability is accessible to all those in need.

KEY INDICATORS OF MATERNAL AND INFANT HEALTH: IMPLICATIONS FOR PREVENTION

Infant Mortality—Variations by Race, Ethnicity, and Class

The infant mortality rate* has long been understood to be one of the most vivid indicators of an entire society's health and well-being. Its two components, the neonatal[†] and postneonatal[‡] death rates, reflect different aspects of the dependence of the young on their caretakers and environment. In lesser developed countries (and in developed nations up until the second half of the 20th century), about two thirds of infant deaths occur after the first month of life. These deaths are not closely related to reproduction but primarily are due to enteric and respiratory infections that become fatal in the context of inadequate nutrition. In these countries, pregnancy and lactation shelter the fetus and infant early in life, and as the infant begins to separate from the mother, vulnerability to the larger environment increases. In more developed or industrialized countries, the burden of infant death (about two thirds) shifts to the neonatal period. In large measure, these deaths are related to extreme prematurity and very low birthweight—being born too soon and/or too small.

The overall infant mortality rate in the United States has declined steadily since the early 1930s. However, since the 1960s it has remained consistently higher than the rate in many other industrialized countries. In 1960, the United States ranked 12th internationally and in 1995 our country ranked 21st.[9] In addition to some differences in how live births are defined and reported, this unfavorable standing is rooted in the persistent race- and class-based disparities in the neonatal and postneonatal rates in this country. The U.S. standing on infant mortality also has been disappointing relative to its own national goals. The Healthy People 2000 objective was to reduce the rate to no more than 7.5 among all infants and to no more than 11 for black infants. In 1995, the overall rate was 7.6, the lowest rate ever recorded for the United States.[10] This is the good news. The bad news is that the infant mortality rate for blacks in the United States was 15.1 in 1995, making the Healthy People 2000 goal appear unreachable.[11] The ethnic

---

*The infant mortality rate (IMR) is a period rate measured as the number of infant deaths (deaths to live born infants before 1 year of age) occurring during a year period per 1,000 live births in the same period.
†The neonatal mortality rate (NMR) is defined as the number of deaths to live-born infants age 28 days or less per 1,000 live births in the same period.
‡The postneonatal mortality rate (PNMR) is defined as the number of deaths to live-born infants age 29 days to 1 year per 1,000 live births in the same geographic region and time period.

groups with the lowest infant mortality rates in the United States are the Chinese, Japanese, and Filipinos. U.S.-born blacks, U.S.-born Hispanics, Puerto Ricans, Hawaiians, and Native Americans fare worse.

As shown in Figure 23.1, the chance of survival for white infants has remained close to two times higher than for blacks during the past three decades and reached 2.4 in 1993, 1994, and 1995.[11] The disparity during these years was equal in the neonatal and postneonatal periods. This two-fold difference is projected to prevail throughout the next century.[12]

The racial disparity seen in infant mortality statistics is not explained simply by excess rates of poverty among blacks in the United States. It is present in all groups of women regardless of their level of education or family income, and it is highest among those with a college education or more and among those with an annual income of more than $35,000.[12,13] In addition, the risk of low birthweight and infant mortality among U.S.-born black women is significantly higher than that among foreign-born blacks.[14,15] These findings raise many questions about the realities underlying the statistics and move us away from explanations based solely on differences in poverty and education rates. They push researchers to go beyond existing categories

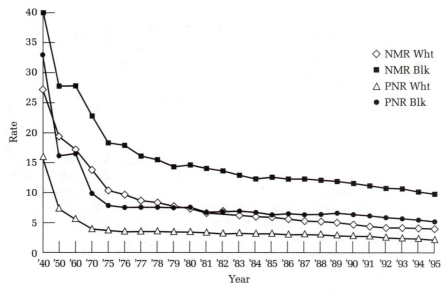

FIGURE 23.1

U.S. neonatal and postneonatal mortality rates by race, 1940 to 1995. *Source:* Report of Final Mortality Statistics, National Center for Health Statistics.

(of race and education) to explore their social meanings for white and black women.[16,17] How does the life experience of stress differ among white and black college-educated women? How does their economic status differ, their assets, their salary, their housing? What discrimination do they face and how do they respond? What are the possible ways that these realities translate into biologic risk? Researchers have begun to examine the impact of long- and short-term discrimination— both individual and structural—on health; however, little attention has been paid to it in maternal and infant health.[18–21]

The same wide gap does not appear between whites and Hispanics overall, despite excess poverty rates among Hispanics in the United States. However, there is great variation within the Hispanic population in the United States. In 1995, although the overall Hispanic infant mortality rate was 6.3, Cubans had the lowest rate (5.1) and Puerto Ricans the highest (8.6).[11]

Similar to findings among blacks, being born outside of the United States is protective for Hispanic families. Foreign-born women do not experience high rates of low birthweight associated with low-income communities, whereas U.S.-born Hispanic women and Puerto Rican women do.[15,22] It is generally accepted that being born in a Latin American country is a marker for the persistence of a Hispanic cultural orientation. This may mean a lifestyle that is healthier (less use of tobacco, alcohol, and illicit drugs and a lower-fat diet), lower stress levels, and stronger family supports and cultural identity—all able to buffer the effects of poverty on the health of women and their infants.[23,24]

The racial disparity in infant mortality mirrors that seen in many child and adult health indicators. Yet infant death is a particularly powerful symbol of the unequal chances of individuals and communities based on their race, ethnicity, and economic status. It is not until the chances for survival improve among infants born to African American, Native American, Puerto Rican, and other U.S.-born Latina women that the health of the entire population will be improved and be favorably reflected in this health indicator.

An examination of the specific components of the infant mortality rate offers insights about how such improvements can be promoted within communities and supported by health and social policy. The process of community-wide fetal and infant mortality reviews (FIMRs) has been disseminated widely in the United States as a result of initiatives of the Maternal and Child Health Bureau (MCHB) and the American College of Obstetrics and Gynecology (ACOG).* The primary ob-

---

*According to an ACOG survey of all state maternal and child health directors in 1995, FIMRs were being conducted in 120 locales (within 35 states), many of them funded by state and local health departments.

jective of FIMRs has been to stimulate community-wide education and action on the problem of infant mortality at the local level. In the process of case review, systems failures are identified and strategies for addressing them are recommended. Findings of select projects are mentioned in the discussion that follows.

Neonatal Mortality. Neonatal mortality is defined as the number of live-born infants who die during the first 28 days of life. It accounts for approximately two thirds of all infant mortality in the United States. The neonatal mortality rate dropped rapidly between 1940 and 1970 as a result of antibiotics and environmental improvements that stemmed the role of infection and malnutrition early in life. The rate continued to decrease at a slower pace until the mid 1980s, largely as a result of neonatal intensive care interventions, followed by a period of stagnation (Figure 23.2). Throughout the entire 50-year period, the two-fold differential between black and white neonatal mortality remained.

Although congenital anomalies continue to account for a large portion of neonatal deaths, prematurity and its associated complica-

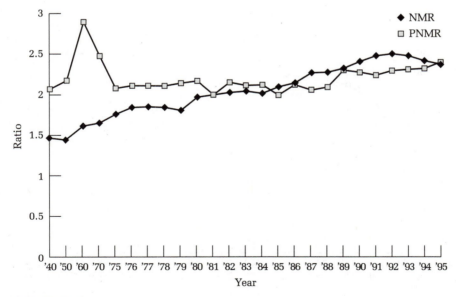

FIGURE 23.2

Black:White ratios of U.S. neonatal and postneonatal mortality rates, 1940 to 1995. *Source:* National Center for Health Statistics.

tions have remained the most important determinant of neonatal mortality patterns in the United States since the 1950s. In recent years, the majority of neonatal mortality has been the result of deaths occurring in neonates born at less than 26 weeks' gestation.[25,26] (Fig. 23.3).

The striking concentration of mortality in the most premature groups is largely the result of the major reductions in the mortality of critically ill newborns born at gestations greater than 28 weeks.[27,28] Important clinical strides in the treatment of respiratory distress syndrome, including surfactant therapy, as well as other related conditions have had a significant impact on neonatal survival.[29] However, although the impact of these technical strides have been well recognized, the policies that have continued to afford access to these advances must also be appreciated. Regionalized systems of referral have been crucial to ensuring that high-risk pregnant women and newborns are treated in clinical facilities with special expertise. In turn, regional policies that support the educational activities, communication, and coordination so essential to regionalized systems of care have been of critical importance to the provision of intensive services. In addition, financial mechanisms, including Medicaid, have also been of major importance in ensuring the provision of complex and often costly health services. The dual impact of technical innovation and facilitative policies has been to reduce dramatically the mortality rates of crit-

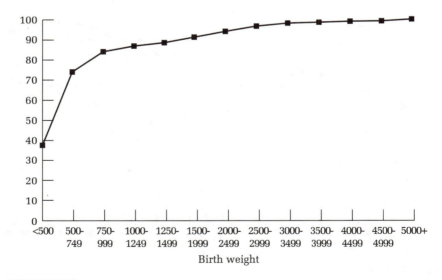

FIGURE 23.3

Cumulative percentage of neonatal mortality by birthweight (United States, 1988).

ically ill newborns and has left that much more glaring persistent elevations in the birth rate of extremely premature newborns.

The concentration of mortality into the most premature newborns has important implications for the traditional strategies to improve birth outcomes through tightly focused prenatal interventions. Given the large portion of neonatal deaths occurring to newborns of 25 weeks of gestation or less, approaches that attempt to identify women in need only after they become pregnant may not provide for a large window of opportunity to prevent extreme prematurity. In addition to the practical difficulties inherent in attempting to intervene early enough in pregnancy to prevent extreme prematurity, the underlying determinants of prematurity and other adverse birth outcomes themselves may require a more comprehensive approach. The clinical epidemiology of prematurity suggests heterogeneous origins.[30] Chronic medical conditions, prior adverse reproductive outcomes, abusive relationships, inadequate social conditions, inadequate nutrition, and behavioral factors such as smoking and drug or alcohol use not only generally predate pregnancy, but also generally require prolonged, continuous interventions. Interventions that act so early in pregnancy that they must be operative prior to conception (e.g., folic acid supplementation to prevent birth defects) are also important.[31] Recent evidence suggests that certain low-grade infectious processes may be an important cause of premature labor and that antimicrobial therapy could reduce a significant portion of the expected premature births.[32,33] However, although the mechanisms of infectious etiologies remain poorly understood, there are some indications that the effectiveness of antimicrobial therapy could possibly be enhanced if the treatment of long-standing infections could be initiated before pregnancy begins.[34] Overall, the reduction of premature births is likely to require comprehensive approaches that integrate specific new clinical interventions to improve birth outcomes within a broader, more comprehensive commitment to the health of women over a lifetime.

Postneonatal Mortality. Deaths that occur between 9 and 364 days after birth account for 38% of all infant deaths.[3] Trends in the postneonatal mortality rate declined steadily from the 1930s until about 1955 as a result of advances in the prevention and treatment of infectious diseases. For the decade that followed, rates in this country stagnated at about 8 per 1,000, dropped to 4.9 by 1970, and have steadily but slowly declined since (see Fig. 23.3). In 1996, 2.5 infants per 1,000 live births died. Historically the rate among blacks has declined more rapidly than that among whites, but in recent years the black : white ratio has remained steady at about 2.5[9,11] (see Fig. 23.2).

Medical factors are more influential in the neonatal period; however, environmental conditions have a profound effect on postneonatal mortality. The biologic vulnerability of infants born at low weight remains a risk for death after 28 days, but the large majority (80%) of infant deaths during the postneonatal period are among infants of normal birth weight.[35] There has been relatively little research attention paid to this category of deaths and how the environment and biology interact (with the exception of research on deaths due to sudden infant death syndrome [SIDS]). This is in part owing to the absence of substantial sociodemographic information on infant death certificates and to the relatively small contribution of postneonatal deaths to overall infant mortality. Sociodemographic correlates include multiple gestation, being male, urban residence, high parity, having an unmarried or adolescent mother, short birth intervals, little prenatal care, lower social class, and being black. In addition, the risk of postneonatal death among infants with the biologic disadvantage of low birthweight is greatly compounded in the presence of these sociodemographic risks.[35,36] Cigarette smoking has been found to exert a stronger influence in the postneonatal than in the neonatal period deaths.[37]

The causes of postneonatal mortality are heterogeneous and difficult to attribute in many instances. The two leading causes are sudden infant death syndrome (SIDS) and congenital anomalies. Accidents and their adverse effects, pneumonia and influenza, homicide, and septicemia are also important causes, although their contribution is quite small in comparison. It is only in the homicide category that a sharp increase (76.3%) occurred between 1979 and 1995. It is not known to what extent this rise is due to changes in the detection and reporting of child abuse during these years.

SIDS, not recognized until the early 1960s, is a diagnosis of exclusion: "the diagnosis given for the sudden death of an infant under one year of age that remains unexplained after a complete investigation, which includes an autopsy, examination of the death scene, and review of the symptoms or illnesses the infant had prior to dying and any other pertinent medical history."[38] In recent years, SIDS has been the subject of intense research and intervention activities. Most striking is the approximately 50% decline in the incidence of SIDS in many countries, including the United Kingdom, New Zealand, Australia, the Netherlands, Norway, Denmark, and Ireland, following the promotion of the supine sleeping position during infancy.[39] Similar reductions in SIDS should be observed in the United States when data from 1996 onward are available.

Males are more likely than females to die of SIDS, as are infants of high birth order. There is an association between lower socioeconomic status and SIDS; however, whether that remains after adjusting for other risk factors such as young maternal age, high parity, bottle feeding, and smoking is not clear.[39] The peak incidence of SIDS is 2 to 4 months of age, suggesting a physiologic vulnerability at the relevant postnatal development phase of the infant. Mounting evidence suggests that this vulnerability is related to brain abnormalities. Specifically, many SIDS infants have had abnormalities in the arcuate nucleus, a portion of the brain that is likely to be involved in controlling breathing and waking during sleep. This helps explain the association between SIDS and the prone sleep position, with the lack of arousal due to airway obstruction or excess carbon dioxide as the probable mechanisms.[38,40]

A number of FIMR projects identified unsafe sleep environment and a lack of understanding about its importance among providers and families as major problems underlying postneonatal deaths in their communities.[41–43] National attention now has been drawn to the issue, and "Back to Sleep Campaigns" have begun to show positive results. Such public education campaigns must be combined with substantial community-based outreach efforts to individual families. Again, in order for improvements to be meaningful they must be equitable. It is crucial that such campaigns and outreach efforts reach all communities in ways that make the information culturally and linguistically accessible.

Congenital anomalies, accounting for more than 17% of postneonatal deaths, require a broad, multi-faceted approach to prevention. Such factors as the aging of the birthing population and environmental and occupational hazards play a large role in maintaining a high prevalence of congenital anomalies. There are also gaps in the health care delivery system. Limited access to genetic counseling and education regarding pregnancy options, even for women with elevated maternal risk for delivering an infant with anomalies, has been documented in several communities by FIMR projects.[41,44] If addressed, such services can lead to reductions in the number of births with lethal congenital anomalies.

The deaths related to being born premature and at low weight are better understood using clinical data. Kempe and colleagues[45] conducted a population-based medical record review of postneonatal deaths in four areas of the United States. They found that 11% were related to prematurity, and in 25% to 44% of these cases, infection was the acute cause of death. However, the large majority (80%) of these infants were never discharged from the hospital. These are postneonatal deaths that represent the success of neonatal technologies in keeping vulnerable infants alive longer. Thus, prevention through follow-up care for high-risk infants is applicable to only a small proportion of these deaths. Such efforts need to be combined with the primary prevention of prematurity through attention to women's primary health care. For those infants who are discharged from the hospital, connection to intensive, family-centered home care is critical. Inadequacies in transition from the hospital to home and community were documented frequently by FIMR projects. The problems relate to both the lack of continuity between community-based providers and hospital care and the absence of resources for intensive early intervention after discharge.

The beneficial effects of home visiting on the long-term outcomes of at-risk infants are well documented.[46–49] Enriched programs, such as those in Elmira, New York, and Memphis, Tennessee, extend from pregnancy through 1 or more years. They focus on the health and well-being of women and their infants and on a broad range of outcomes (e.g., health, child abuse and neglect, encounters with the criminal justice system), and the greatest benefits occur among those deemed at highest risk. Although a large number of postneonatal deaths related to prematurity may not be preventable, the health of those who survive and their families' long-term health can be enhanced.

In summary, understanding postneonatal mortality leads to three major conclusions for health promotion and health care delivery: (1) public information campaigns must be combined with community-based services tailored to individual families; (2) genetic counseling must be accessible to all women, with special attention to cultural and linguistic differences in how congenital anomalies are understood and addressed; and (3) home-based follow-up programs for high-risk infants must be combined with primary prevention aimed at prematurity.

INDICATORS OF MATERNAL HEALTH AND WOMEN'S HEALTH

Maternal Mortality and Morbidity

The maternal mortality ratio* has decreased dramatically in the United States over the last half of the 20th century. At the same time, women continue to experience preventable pregnancy-related deaths, and the race-based disparity characteristic of the earlier part of the century remains in the 1990s. The Centers for Disease Control and Pre-

---

*The maternal mortality ratio is defined as the number of deaths to women during pregnancy or within 42 days (or in some states, 90 days) of termination of pregnancy and result from obstetric causes per 100,000 live births. The pregnancy-related mortality ratio uses the period of 1 year after termination of pregnancy as the parameter.

vention (CDC), in collaboration with the ACOG and state health departments, conducts surveillance of pregnancy-related mortality. The ratio declined from 10.7 in 1979 to 7.1 in 1986, then increased each year from 1987 to 1990 when the ratio reached 10. The ratio for black women in 1990 (the most recent year for which data are available) was four times higher than that for white women (26.7 and 6.5, respectively). The leading causes of pregnancy-related deaths remained hemorrhage, embolism, and pregnancy-induced hypertension for all women, and deaths due to infection and cardiomyopathy increased. The increased risk of death for black women was seen in all causes of pregnancy-related death and was greatest due to complications of anesthesia and cardiomyopathy.[50]

To understand the underlying reasons for the astounding racial disparity in pregnancy-related mortality, it is necessary to consider the content and quality of care, as well as the pre-pregnancy health status and pregnancy-related morbidity of black women.[51] However, such in-depth investigations have not been published. The Year 2000 objective for maternal mortality is to reduce the ratio to no more than 5.0 among black women. If ever to be achieved, this will require a concentration of resources on black women's health and health services.

Maternal mortality is only the tip of the iceberg. It is estimated that for each maternal death, there are 3,100 hospitalizations due to pregnancy-related morbidity.[52] In 1991 to 1992, there were about 17 pregnancy complications requiring hospitalizations for each 100 deliveries, 16 for whites and 26 for blacks, according to data from the National Hospital Discharge Study.[53] Genitourinary tract infections are by far the most frequent reason for obstetric hospitalizations, followed by diabetic conditions, anemia, psychiatric problems, and viruses.[53] As is true for many other maternal and child indicators, women in high-risk sociodemographic groups are those most likely to be hospitalized during pregnancy. The data reflect differences in access to preventive care and the heightened burden of disease carried by these women.

Health of Women

To consider only conventional maternal health indicators, such as pregnancy-related mortality and morbidity, is to miss the significance of women's long-standing health to maternal and infant health. A full discussion of women's health is beyond the scope of this chapter; however, a few major points warrant emphasis.

Lifestyle and access to health information is profoundly important to women, and therefore their families, over a lifetime. McGinnis[54] conducted a detailed analysis of the primary and associated causes of death for women and reported that 19% of all deaths to women (all ages) are tobacco-related; 14% are associated with diet and activity patterns; and an additional 5% are alcohol-related. Addressing these behaviors among individuals requires a model of comprehensive primary care for women, including ongoing risk assessment, counseling and referrals.[55] Addressing them at the societal level requires concentrated public education and information campaigns and local and national policy development, particularly in the area of tobacco and nutrition.

However, women's health is not achieved merely through changes in individual lifestyles and education. The larger contexts in which women live provide the key to understanding patterns in health behavior and health status. As is the case in other areas of maternal and infant health, disparities between women and men and between classes of women point to basic inequities based on gender, race/ethnicity and class.

The case of HIV disease in women provides one of the strongest examples of these connections.[56] Even as the proportion of women among AIDS cases rose from 6%–19% between 1984 and 1995, its case definition, identification, and treatment lagged behind that of men. Further, the vast majority of women with AIDS in the United States are poor women of color, with 75% being classified as non-Hispanic black or Hispanic women. In 1994, the death rate due to HIV among black women was nine times higher than that among white women (5.7 per 100,000 compared to 51.2 deaths per 100,000, respectively).[57] This example clearly points to the necessity of addressing the health of women through multiple approaches, ranging from broad anti-poverty and anti-discrimination policies to a model of health services that incorporates women's biologic, social and economic health.

KEY ISSUES IN HEALTH SERVICES AND HEALTH POLICY FOR MOTHERS AND INFANTS

Health Services

Data on neonatal mortality, postneonatal mortality, and maternal mortality point clearly to the missing link in existing maternal and infant health services and policies: attention to the health of women throughout their reproductive years and beyond. FIMRs, which can examine the match between women's needs and the services available to them, provide further evidence of what is missing. Findings from the Boston Infant Mortality Review were reinforced by projects conducted at many other sites.[58–61] The provider review panels came to the following conclusions:

- Seventy-three percent of infant death cases were preceded by *fragmentation and discontinuity* in the health care of women and infants, including lack of follow-up and linkages across time (preceding pregnancies and between pregnancies) and across systems of care (medical and social).
- Fifty-one percent of women whose infants died had severe *social risk* unrecognized and/or unmatched by needed services in the context of health care. In contrast, 16% were identified as having medical risks that went unrecognized or untreated.
- Forty percent of the women had *repeated unintended pregnancies*, often preceded by a pattern of sexual abuse and/or battering.
- In 38% of the cases, *provider-patient communication issues* were found to be problematic. Interviews with women of color, in particular, emphasized how race, class, and cultural differences between patients and providers often lead to miscommunications that leave women feeling disrespected or not listened to.

Most often the gaps did not consist of inadequate prenatal clinical services. Rather, they consisted of failures to identify and address the links between women's life circumstances and their health behaviors and health status over time. Yet it is on prenatal care that clinical and public policies have focused.

Clinical policies and studies in the 1990s have the definition of prenatal care to include preconception care broadened, consisting of pre-pregnancy risk assessment, ideally done in the context of women's primary care.[62–67] However, preconception care remains an ill-defined and limited concept without a solid home in the health care delivery system and without health policies to support it. In light of the high proportion of all pregnancies that are unintended in the United States, it is a concept that has little meaning unless tied to continuous primary care for women.

Furthermore, public policies devoted to improving birth outcomes have focused primarily on ensuring financial access to prenatal care through the expansion of Medicaid eligibility. Although necessary, these strategies have proven to be insufficient for two main reasons: (1) they address only financial access to care, neglecting the content of care; and (2) they support women only during pregnancy, failing to address access to and quality of primary and preventive care.[58,68–71]

Evaluations of the Medicaid expansions have concluded that "income eligibility expansions must be supplemented by outreach, educational efforts and other means of improving access to prenatal care and improving birth outcomes. Expanded income eligibility under Medicaid can spell the difference between good and bad birth outcomes, but only if the services it finances are enhanced with non-medical supportive services and delivered early enough to make a difference."[72]

Enhanced Models of Prenatal Care and Post-Birth Care

Enhanced models of prenatal care have been tried and evaluated in many communities since the mid-1980's and offer additional lessons. We conducted a review of six studies of community-based models, which had comparison or control groups and research designs deemed adequate to draw conclusions about the program's impact on health status and health care utilization. The programs vary greatly in content and design, but all consisted of home visits, advocacy, education and/or psychosocial support by social workers or community peers. Of the six reviewed, one showed a reduced rate of low birthweight among the intervention group.[73] The program featured indigenous women providing outreach and social support, a feature likely linked to its effectiveness. As a whole, these community-based models are more consistently successful at improving the use of prenatal care.[73–75]

In addition, the randomized clinical trial of a home-visiting model previously mentioned that included prenatal and infancy home visits by nurses for at-risk women and their families for up to two years after birth showed no program effect on preterm delivery or low birthweight.[46,47] However, the model proved effective in improving the health of women during pregnancy (reduced rates of pregnancy-induced hypertension) and the health of children (fewer health care encounters due to injuries or ingestions; fewer hospitalizations for such injuries), and in reducing second pregnancies.[46] In this case, the success of the program was likely rooted in its continuity with families over time.

How enriched services are designed, how continuity can be achieved, and who should be represented on staff are all key issues for the field of maternal and infant health for the next decade. They pose particular challenges in the context of managed care environments. Building partnerships between the insurers and providers of managed care and existing community-based service models must be a high priority. Many such programs have been up and running for several years, supported by a patchwork of federal and state demonstration funds, local health department dollars, and in some cases, infrastructure money for community health centers. They have learned the lessons of cost efficiency even while serving the highest-risk populations. These lessons should be translated into culturally appropriate, cost efficient, and clinically effective services to augment the mainstream approaches to prenatal and primary care for women and infants with complex medical and social risks. This requires some degree of integration with existing clinical services and insurance plans in the managed care environment, but in a way that preserves the autonomy and integrity of community expertise.

Postpartum Care Issues

The importance of care in the postpartum period—long neglected and overshadowed by attention to the antepartum period—has begun to receive attention in this country. The attention has come in the context of the Newborns' and Mothers' Health Protection Act of 1996, prohibiting insurers from restricting the length of hospital stay for a new mother to less than 48 hours. Similar legislation in many states has been accompanied by required benefits for at-home postpartum visits by nurses at intervals during the first 2 weeks after delivery for those with shortened stays. (This legislation and its implications are discussed in Chapter 5.)

Traditionally, postpartum care has been conceived as a series of clinic visits with the maternity provider—6 weeks, 10 weeks, and 18 weeks after birth. Issues covered have been centered on the mother's recovery from childbirth and treatment of any postpartum complications, as well as a vaginal examination and Pap smear, and discussion of contraception. Issues of mental health, lifestyle and health behaviors, social support, attachment, and parenting have not been predominant. Utilization rates have been consistently low, and researchers have paid little attention to the efficacy of this medical and clinic-based model of postpartum care.

Increased awareness about the broad range of health concerns of women during this period, the potential benefits of postpartum home-based services on maternal and child health outcomes, and the trend toward shortened hospital stays has contributed to the emergence of a new model of postpartum care. The new model emphasizes the role of community practitioners (nurse-midwife, family practice physician) in supporting women after childbirth and encourages nursing support through home visits in the immediate post-partum period.[76-77]

A significant additional role for such programs is the potential to assess the need for continued at-home services and follow-up and the linkage to more intensive postpartum/infancy interventions for at-risk families. Such follow-up programs may rely on community-based health workers (sometimes called "doulas" in the partpartum period) to support families with information, emotional and tangible support, and guidance on health and parenting within the context of their own culture.

The postpartum period is an important bridge to all of the issues that are critical to improving women's and infant health: family planning and continuous primary care for women, including monitoring of sexually transmitted infections, cervical cancer screening, nutritional support, and mental health services for women; and strong maternal-infant bonding, good parenting, and good nutrition for infants. In a health care system held together not by planning and continuity but by private enterprise and specialty care, it is difficult to ensure that the bridge is used. Recent policy initiatives that support in-home assessment and support during the immediate postpartum period are a good beginning. The next step is to extend these initiatives into the first 2 years after birth for those who need continued support.

POLICY IMPACT AND FUTURE DIRECTIONS

Despite changes in American society and science, maternal and infant health remains an important reflection of the social and economic well-being of American families. However, although this linkage remains fundamentally intact, the underlying pathways by which social forces shape perinatal health must be seen as inherently dynamic. Increasingly, perinatal indicators will relate to the general health and well-being of women. Accordingly, interventions directed at improving infant health outcomes will have to attend more broadly to the health of women whether they are pregnant or not. In addition, programs essential to the delivery of services to women will have to keep pace with the rapidly changing nature of women's daily lives and strive to integrate traditionally fragmented services and clinical care. Perinatal health will also continue to be highly sensitive to technical innovations in prevention and treatment. Respect for the capacity of technical progress to alter patterns of perinatal health outcomes is essential if policies that afford access to such capacity are to ensure provision to all those in need. These requirements to address more directly the comprehensive health needs of women and the demands of preventive and therapeutic innovation speak strongly for cross-disciplinary interaction and close collaboration between health care and social policy professionals. Such comprehensive strategies to improve maternal and infant health will not only prove more effective but also serve the larger struggle to advance the health and well-being of American families for many years to come.

References

1. Ventura, S.J., Martin, J.A., Curtin, S.C., and Mathews, T.J. Report of Final Natality Statistics, 1995. *Monthly Vital Statistics Report.* National Center for Health Statistics (NCHS). June, 1997;45(11)(suppl).
2. Deardorff, K.E., Montgomery, P., and Hollmann, F.W. *U.S. population estimates by age, sex, race and Hispanic origin: 1990 to 1995.* U.S. Bureau of the Census. Census file RESDO795, PPL-41. Washington, DC: U.S. Department of Commerce, 1996.
3. Ventura, S.J., Peters, K.D., Martin, J.A., and Maurer, J.D. Births and deaths: United States 1996. *Monthly Vital Statistics Report.* National Center for Health Statistics (NCHS). September, 1997;46(1)(suppl 2).
4. Blank, R.M. *It takes a nation: A new agenda for fighting poverty.* New York: Russell Foundation, and Princeton, NJ: Princeton University Press, 1997.
5. Ku, L., and Coughlin, T.A. *How the new Welfare Reform Law affects Medicaid.* Washington, DC: The Urban Institute, 1997.
6. Rosenbaum, S., and Darnell, J. An analysis of the Medicaid and health-related provisions of the Personal Responsibility and Work Opportunity Reconciliation Act of 1996 (P.L. 104-193). Prepared by the Center for Health Policy Research of the George Washington University Medical Center for the Kaiser Commission on the Future of Medicaid, February 1997.
7. Havens, P.L., Cuene, B., Waters, D., Hand, J., and Chusid, M.J. Structure of a primary care support system to coordinate comprehensive care for children and families infected/affected by human immunodeficiency virus in a managed care environment. *Pediatric Infectious Disease Journal.* 1997;16:211–216.
8. Wise, P.H. Confronting racial disparities in infant mortality: Reconciling science and politics. *American Journal of Preventive Medicine.* 1993;9(suppl):7–16.
9. Guyer, B., Martin, J.A., MacDorman, M.F., Anderson, R.N., and Strobino, D.M. Annual summary of vital statistics—1996. *Pediatrics.* 1997;100:905–918.
10. Heck, K.E., and Klein, R.J. Operational definitions for Year 2000 objectives: Priority area 14, maternal and infant health. *Healthy People 2000 Statistical Notes.* December, 1997;14:1–15.
11. Anderson, R.N., Kochanek, K.D., and Murphy, S.L. Report of final mortality statistics, 1995. *Monthly Vital Statistics Report.* National Center for Health Statistics. June 12, 1997;45(11)(suppl 2).
12. Singh, G.K., and Yu, S.M. Infant mortality in the United States: Trends, differentials, and projections, 1950 through 2010. *American Journal of Public Health.* 1995;85:957–964.
13. Schoendorf, K.C., Hogue, C.J., Kleinman, J.C., and Rowley, D. Mortality among infants of black as compared with white college-educated parents. *New England Journal of Medicine.* 1992;326,23:1522–6.
14. David, R.J., and Collins, J.W. Differing birth weight among infants of U.S.-born blacks, African-born blacks, and U.S.-born whites. *New England Journal of Medicine.* 1997;337:1209–1214.
15. Cabral, H., Fried, L., Levenson, S., Amaro, H., and Zuckerman, B. Foreign-born and U.S.-born women: Differences in health behaviors and birth outcomes. *American Journal of Public Health.* 1990;80(1):70–74.
16. David, R.J., and Collins, J.W. Bad outcomes in black babies: Race or racism? *Ethnicity and Disease.* 1991;1:(summer):236–244.
17. Rowley, D., Hogue, C.J.R., Blackmore, C.A., Ferre, C.D., Hatfield-Timajchy, K., Branch, P., and Atrash, H.K. Preterm delivery among African American women: A research strategy. *American Journal of Preventive Health.* 1993;9(6)(suppl):1–5.
18. Krieger, N. Racial and gender discrimination: Risk factors for high blood pressure? *Social Science and Medicine.* 1990;30:1273–1281.

19. Dressler, W.W. Social class, skin color, and arterial blood pressure in two societies. *Ethnicity and Disease.* 1991;1:60–77.

20. Krieger, N., and Sidney, S. Racial discrimination and blood pressure: The CARDIA Study of Young Black and White Adults. *American Journal of Public Health.* 1996;86:1370–1378.

21. Polednak, A.P. Trends in U.S. urban black infant mortality by degree of residential segregation. *American Journal of Public Health.* 1996;86:723–726.

22. Collins, J.W., and Shay, D.K. Prevalence of low birth weight among Hispanic infants with United States-born and foreign-born mothers: The effect of urban poverty. *American Journal of Epidemiology.* 1994;139:184–192.

23. Scribner, R., and Dwyer, J. Acculturation and low birth weight among Latinos in the Hispanic HANES. *American Journal of Public Health.* 1989;79:1263–1267.

24. James, S.A. Racial and ethnic differences in infant mortality and low birth weight: A psychosocial critique. *Annals of Epidemiology.* 1993;3:130–136.

25. Wise, P.H., Wampler, N., and Barfield, W. The importance of extreme prematurity and low birthweight to U.S. neonatal mortality patterns: Implications for prenatal care and women's health. *Journal of the American Medical Womens Association.* 1995;50:152–155.

26. Overpeck, M.D., Hoffman, H.J., and Prager, K. The lowest birth-weight infants and the U.S. infant mortality rate: NCHS 1983 linked birth/infant death data. *American Journal of Public Health.* 1992;82(3):441–443.

27. Paneth, N., Kiely, J.L., Phil, M., Wallenstein, S., Marcus, M., Pakter, J., and Susser, M. Newborn intensive care and neonatal mortality in low-birth-weight infants. *New England Journal of Medicine.* 1982;307(3):149–155.

28. Williams, R.L., and Chen, P.M. Identifying the sources of the recent decline in prenatal mortality rates in California. *New England Journal of Medicine.* 1982;306(4):207–214.

29. Hamvas, A., Wise, P.H., Yang, R.K., Wampler, N.S., et al. The influence of the wider use of surfactant therapy on neonatal mortality among blacks and whites. *New England Journal of Medicine.* 1996;334:1635–1640.

30. Kempe, A., Wise, P.H., Barkan, S.E., et al. Clinical determinants of the racial disparity in very low birth weight. *New England Journal of Medicine.* 1992;327:969–973.

31. Holmes, L., Harris, T., Oakley, G.P. Jr., and Friedman, J.M. Teratology Society Consensus Statement on the use of folic acid to reduce risk of birth defects. *Teratology.* 1997;55:381.

32. Meis, P.J., Gldenberg, R.L., Mercer, B., Moawad, A., Das, A., McNellis, D., et al. The preterm prediction study: Significance of vaginal infections. *American Journal of Obstetrics and Gynecology.* 1995;173:1231–1235.

33. Hillier, S.L., Nugent, R.P., Eschenbach, D.A., et al. Association between bacterial vaginosis and preterm delivery of a low birth-weight infant. *New England Journal of Medicine.* 1995;333:1737–1742.

34. Hauth, J.C., Goldenberg, R.L., Andrews, W.W., DuBard, M.B., and Copper, R.L. Midtrimester treatment with metronidazole plus erythromycin reduces preterm birth only in women with bacterial vaginosis. *New England Journal of Medicine.* 1995; 333:1732–1736.

35. Starfield, B. Postneonatal mortality. *Annual Review of Public Health.* 1985;6:21–40.

36. Bross, D., and Shapiro, S. Direct and indirect associations of five factors with infant mortality. *American Journal of Epidemiology.* 1982;125:78–91.

37. Din-Dzietham, R., and Hertz-Picciotto, I. Relationship of education to the racial gap in neonatal and postneonatal mortality. *Archives of Pediatrics and Adolescent Medicine.* 1997;151:787–792.

38. National Institute of Child Health and Human Development, Public Information and Communications Branch. *Sudden infant death syndrome.* Bethesda, MD, April, 1997.

39. Dwyer, T., and Ponsonby, A.L. SIDS epidemiology and incidence. *Pediatric Annals.* 1995;24(7):350–357.

40. Filiano, J.J., and Kinney, H.C. Sudden infant death syndrome and brainstem research. *Pediatric Annals.* 1995;24(7):379–383.

41. Krieger, J., El-Bastawissi, A., Dickson, A., et al. The Seattle-King County Infant Mortality Review: Modifiable factors contributing to infant deaths (abstract). Annual Meetings of the American Public Health Association, New York, November 17–21, 1996.
42. Lefkow, R.H., Noell, D., and Wright, J. Broward County Fetal and Infant Mortality Review: Final report. Fort Lauderdale, FL: Healthy Mothers–Healthy Babies Coalition of Broward County, 1996.
43. Hauck, F.R., Merrick, C.A., Donovan, M., et al. Risk factors for sudden infant death syndrome: Preliminary results for the Chicago infant mortality study (abstract). Annual Meetings of the American Public Health Association, New York, November 17–21, 1996.
44. McCloskey, L., Plough, A., Power, K., et al. *Case by case: Boston's Infant Mortality Review Project: Report of findings.* Boston: City of Boston, Department of Health and Hospitals, 1993.
45. Kempe, A., Wise, P.H., Wampler, N.S., et al. Risk status at discharge and cause of death for postneonatal infant deaths: A total population study. *Pediatrics.* 1997; 99:3.
46. Kitzman, H., Olds, D.L., Henderson, C.R., et al. Effect of prenatal care and infancy home visitation by nurses on pregnancy outcomes, childhood injuries, and repeated childbearing. *JAMA.* 1997;278:644–652.
47. Olds, D.L., Eckenrode, J., Henderson, C.R., et al. Long-term effects of home visitation on maternal life course and child abuse and neglect. *JAMA.* 1997;278:637–643.
48. Olds, D.L., Henderson, C.R., Kitzman, H., et al. Effects of prenatal and infancy nurse home visitation on surveillance of child maltreatment. *Pediatrics.* 1995;95:365–372.
49. Olds, D.L., Kitzman, H. Review of research on home visiting for pregnant women and parents of young children. *The Future of Children.* 1993;3:53–92.
50. Berg, C.J., Atrash, H.K., Koonin, L.M., and Tucker, M. Pregnancy-related mortality in the United States, 1987–1990. *Obstetrics and Gynecology.* 1996;88:161–167.
51. Atrash, H.K., Alexander, S., and Berg, C.J. Maternal mortality in developed countries: Not just a concern of the past. *Obstetrics and Gynecology.* 1995;86:700–705.
52. Franks, A.L., Kendrick, J.S., Olson, D.R., Atrash, H.K., Saftlas, A.F., and Moien, M. Hospitalizations for pregnancy complications, United States, 1986 and 1987. *American Journal of Obstetrics and Gynecology.* 1992;166:1339–1344.
53. Bennett, T.A., Kotelchuck, M., Cox, C.E., Tucker, M.J., and Nadeau, D.A. Pregnancy-associated hospitalizations in the United States in 1991 and 1992: A comprehensive view of maternal morbidity. *American Journal of Obstetrics and Gynecology* (in press).
54. McGinnis, J.M., and Foege, W.H. Actual cause of death in the United States. *JAMA.* 1993;270:2207–2212.
55. Ruzek, S.B. Towards a more inclusive model of women's health. *American Journal of Public Health.* 1993;83:6–7.
56. Zierler, S., Krieger, N. Reframing women's risk: Social inequalities and HIV Infection. Annual Rev Public Health 1997. 18:401–36.
57. Centers for Disease Control and Prevention 1995. Update: AIDS among women—United States, 1994. MMWR 44:81–84.
58. McCloskey, L., Bigby, J.A., and Brand, A. Beyond prenatal care: Improving birth outcomes in low-income communities through enhancements to clinical services for women. Position Paper of the Working Group on Case Management, Outreach and Community Partnerships of the Infant Mortality Review Project, Boston Healthy Start Initiative, Boston Public Health Commission, April 1997.
59. McCloskey, L., Plough, A.L., Power, K.L., Higgins, C.A., Cruz, A.N., and Brown, E.R. The value of community-wide infant mortality reviews: A case study. *Public Health Reports* (in press). Nov/Dec 1998.
60. Brustman, B., Buckley, K., Cohen, M., and Medvesky, M. *Infant mortality review: Progress report.* New York Sate Department of Health, October, 1993.
61. Casey, S., et al. *Fetal/infant mortality review: Findings and recommendations 1992–1993.* Oakland, CA: Perinatal Network of Alameda/Contra Costa Counties, November, 1994.

62. Public Health Service, Department of Health and Human Services. *Caring for our future: The content of prenatal care.* A Report of the Public Health Service Expert Panel on the Content of Prenatal Care. Washington, DC, 1989.

63. Brown, J.E., Jacobs, D.R., Barosso, G.M., et al. Recruitment, retention and characteristics of women in a prospective study of preconceptional risks to reproductive outcomes: Experience of the Diana Project. *Pediatric and Perinatal Epidemiology.* 1997;11(3):345–358.

64. Moos, M.K., Bangdiwala, S.I., Meibohm, A.R., and Cefalo, R.C. The impact of a preconceptional health promotion program on intendedness of pregnancy. *American Journal of Perinatology.* 1996;13(2):103–108.

65. Cefalo, R.C., Bowes, W.A., and Moos, M.K. Preconception care: A means of prevention. *Baillieres Clinical Obstetrics and Gynecology.* 1995;9(3):403–416.

66. Jack, B. Preconception care (or how all family physicians can 'do' OB) (editorial). *American Family Physician.* 1995;51:1888–1890.

67. Jack, B.W., Campanile, C., McQuade, W., and Kogan, M.D. The negative pregnancy test: An opportunity for preconception care. *Archives of Family Medicine.* 1995; 4:340–345.

68. Guyer, B. Medicaid and prenatal care: Necessary but not sufficient. *JAMA.* 1990;264:2264–2265.

69. Piper, J.M., Mitchel, E.F., and Ray. W, A. Evaluation of a program for prenatal care case management. *Family Planning Perspectives.* 1996;28:65–68.

70. Schlesinger, M., and Kronebusch, K. The failure of prenatal care policy for the poor. *Health Affairs.* 1990;4:91–111.

71. Braveman, P., Bennett, T., Lewis, C., et al. Access to prenatal care following major Medicaid eligibility expansions. *JAMA.* 1993;269:285–289.

72. Lipson, D., and Loranger, L. *The Medicaid expansions for pregnant women and children.* Princeton, NJ: The Robert Wood Johnson Foundation's Changes in Health Care Financing and Organization Program, 1995.

73. Heins, H.C., Nance, N.W., and Ferguson, J.E. Social support in improving perinatal outcome: The Resource Mothers Program. *Obstetrics and Gynecology.* 1987;70: 263–266.

74. Graham, A.V., Frank, S.H., Zyzanski, S.J., et al. A clinical trial to reduce the rate of low birth weight in an inner-city black population. *Family Medicine.* 1992;24: 439–446.

75. Poland, M.L., Giblin, P.T., Waller, J.B., and Hankin, J. Effects of a home visiting program on prenatal care and birth weight: A case comparison study. *Journal of Community Health.* 1992;17:221–229.

76. Williams, L.R., and Cooper, M.K. A new paradigm for postpartum care. *Journal of Obstetric, Gynecologic, and Neonatal Nursing.* 1996;25:745–749.

77. Gagnon, A.J., Edgar, L., Kramer, M.S., Papageorgiou, A., Waghorn, K., and Klein, M.C. A randomized trial of a program of early postpartum discharge with nurse visitation. *American Journal of Obstetrics and Gynecology.* 1997;176:205–211.

On the Horizon: Women's Health as a Family Health Imperative

LISA PAINE

An understanding of women's health and its impact on contemporary American Society as a whole is long overdue. Deficiencies in the current U.S. health care system notwithstanding (most specifically the lack of universal health care), no longer is women's health framed solely within the context of reproductive function. Although maternity care is still often the first entry into primary care, recent changes through policy initiatives that address the specific health needs of midlife women have begun to focus more careful attention on the basic health care needs of women of all ages.

Within these changing women's health perspectives lies a broader focus on what constitutes women's health, a focus that extends well beyond that of reproductive health.[1] Three key concepts lead to the "new" focus on the health of women: (1) health includes social and contextual issues that interact with physical and emotional development; (2) health is best understood from a life span and multi-role perspective; and (3) health is not the absence of disease, but rather the result of a woman's lifelong maintenance of health promotion and disease prevention strategies.[1,2] These concepts reinforce our understanding of the central role women play in maintaining and promoting the health of their families and communities throughout their lives.[3]

In Chapter 23; McCloskey and Wise purport that attempts to improve the health of mothers and infants must include focused attention on the following imperatives: (1) expansion of the maternal and child health (MCH) population to include women regardless of their reproductive status; (2) extension of the boundaries of the field to encompass the social, economic, cultural, and political context in which maternal and infant health occur; and (3) the design of integrated services that recognize connections between the health of women and infants and the social environments in which they live. These imperatives are in concert with recent literature about the changing definitions of women's health and the resulting health policy implications.

Legislative and policy issues resulting from welfare reform and immigration policies may also heighten attention to women's health care issues, including limitations in women's access to comprehensive primary care and fragmentation of clinical service delivery.[4] Equally well established is the uncertainty as to whether new policies, however well intentioned, will lead to an enhancement of the health and welfare conditions of American women[4] (see Chapters 5 and 23). Health care will most likely remain unaffordable as a result of low-wage jobs that are less likely to cover comprehensive services, or unavailable because of the day-to-day demands on the time of working women, especially those in single-parent households with low-paying jobs.[5] In fact, the impending crisis in child care, which is being fueled by welfare to work policies, virtually guarantees that the health care situation for low-income women and their families will reach a critical state in the near future (see Chapters 10, 11, and 23). None of these emerging consequences of welfare reform are surprising, because few welfare reform monitoring efforts deal with the impact on women's lives and their health.[4]

There is no doubt that in the coming years women's health issues will become first and foremost in the minds of clinicians, social welfare and maternal and child health professionals, and health policy leaders. Likewise, services designed to promote the health and welfare of children *must* keep pace with the rapidly changing nature of women's daily lives. Indeed, in pointing out that attention to women's health issues is long overdue, Hutchins advocates a *proactive stance* to the health of women as a family health imperative (see Chapter 40).

Future editions of this book and others regarding the health and welfare of women, children, and families must address in greater detail health care services and welfare policies, immigration policies, and the expansion of managed care systems. Moreover, as noted by Chavkin and

Wise, changes in the structures of welfare and health care "strike directly at the relationship between women's and children's interests,"[4] and children's health cannot be adequately addressed without attention to the broader policy debates focused on the welfare of women. In addition, if women's health—the family health imperative of the future—is to be sufficiently addressed, integration of traditionally fragmented clinical and social welfare services must be made a priority (see Chapter 23).

References

1. Weisman, C.S. Changing definitions of women's health: Implications for health care and policy. *Maternal and Child Health Journal* 1997; 1:179–189.
2. Walker, D.K. Where is women's health in maternal and child health? *Maternal and Child Health Journal* 1997; 1:191–193.
3. Bernstein, J., and Lewis, J.L. The modern health care system and gender bias: The historical and ideological context. In J.A. Lewis and J. Bernstein (eds). *Women's health: A relational perspective across the life cycle.* Boston: Jones and Bartlett Publishers, 1996, pp 3–17.
4. Chavkin, W., Wise, P.H., and Elman, D. Topics for our times: Welfare reform and women's health. *American Journal of Public Health* 1998; 88:1017–1018.
5. Albelda, R., and Tilly, C. *Glass ceilings and bottomless pits: Women's work, women's poverty.* Boston: South End Press, 1997.

24

Infant Mortality in Japan and the United States

Michele Kiely, Munehiro Hirayama, Helen M. Wallace,
Woodie Kessel, Y. Nakamura, John L. Kiely,
and Audrey H. Nora

At the beginning of the 20th century, infection was the cause of most morbidity and mortality in infants and children. Health supervision of children consisted of examinations capable of identifying contagious diseases, but not sufficient for adequate treatment.[1] Until the development of immunizations, public health measures such as pasteurization, improved nutrition, and sanitation accounted for most reductions in childhood mortality.

Although we made significant advances in the medical care and treatment, in many areas such as infectious disease, we face new and difficult challenges. Over the past several decades, major economic, social, and demographic changes have significantly affected American families. These include a decline in the time parents spend with their children, less direct contact between children and their extended families, increased geographic mobility, a shortage of high-quality child care services, a reduction in neighborhood cohesiveness and social supports, and an extensive restructuring of family relationships.[2,3] These changes have resulted in injuries, violence, abuse and neglect, and human immunodeficiency virus (HIV) infection. As every past century has born witness to the ills associated with poverty, so too at the outset of this new century, poverty and its consequences remain our most significant challenge.[4] In 1995, 20% of related children were living in families where their income was below the federal poverty level, and 64% lived in homes headed by a single parent. This group is among the most vulnerable of our population. Children in families headed by single mothers, African American children, and children living below 150% of the federal poverty level were much more likely to be in poor or fair health than children in two-parent families, white children, and children living in more affluent families.[4]

The concerns regarding infant survival in the United States date back to 1912, when the federal government established the Children's Bureau to "investigate and report . . . upon all matters pertaining to the welfare of children and child life among all classes of our people." Initially, the bureau sought to improve vital registration and to study infant mortality and the link between the health of mothers and that of their infants. In 1913 and 1914, the Children's Bureau published *Prenatal Care* and *Infant Care*, respectively. These books were designed to promote adequate prenatal care, good nutrition during pregnancy, and appropriate child care techniques. In 1930, The Children's Charter was produced by President Hoover's White House Conference on Child Health and Protection. The agenda it proposed was comprehensive. Many of the objectives contained in the Charter continue to challenge the public health field today, particularly those related to infant health and social justice.

A traditional method for assessing performance and potential is to compare maternal and child health outcomes in the United States and in countries around the world, especially with those countries with favorable outcomes, such as the lowest infant mortality rates. This approach allows for an assessment of the resources necessary to do a better job of improving the health and well-being of mothers and children as well as preventing morbidity and mortality. After World War II, Japan lowered its infant mortality rate (IMR). It is now the lowest in the world, and comparisons with the United States are revealing. During the post-war period, the economic and social situation of Japan also changed dramatically. There are few articles in the medical literature[5,6] to explain the contributions to the dramatic decrease in Japan's IMR. The information presented here focuses on the shift in the IMR in Japan after World War II, as well as a comparison of the decrease in the IMR in the United States over the same period of time.

INTERNATIONAL TRENDS IN INFANT MORTALITY

Since 1984, Japan has had the lowest reported infant mortality among the countries of the world. Countries with reported infant mortality rates lower than the United States have been located in Scandinavia, Western Europe, the United Kingdom, and the Pacific Rim (Table 24.1). Differences in the infant mortality rates among industrialized nations reflect differences in the health status of women before and during pregnancy and the quality of primary health care accessible to pregnant women and their infants. Although the United States has greatly reduced its infant mortality rate since 1965, in 1993 it still ranked 25th among industrialized countries. The risk of a Japanese child dying in infancy was 48% lower than that of a child in the United States in 1993.

A major difference between the United States and the other countries listed in Table 24.1 is that all the other countries have some form of national health program offering preventive and therapeutic coverage to their total population.

COMPARISON OF INFANT MORTALITY IN JAPAN AND THE UNITED STATES

In 1993, the infant mortality rates (IMRs) in Japan and the United States were 4.3 and 8.4 per 1,000 live births, respectively. Thus, in 1993, the IMR in the United States was 1.95 times the IMR in Japan. From 1979 to 1993, the IMR in Japan dropped 50%. Over the same time period, the IMR in the United States dropped 39.7% (Fig. 24.1).

TABLE 24.1

Live Births and Infant Mortality Rates for Countries with Population
Greater Than 1,000,000 and Infant Mortality Rates
Equal to or Less Than 10 per 1,000 Live Births in 1993

Country	Live Births	Infant Mortality Rate
Japan	1,208,989	4.35
Finland	65,032	4.40
Singapore	50,226	4.68
Hong Kong	68,291	4.76
Sweden	117,846	4.84
Norway	59,041	5.11
Denmark	67,442	5.40
Switzerland	83,700	5.55
Germany	794,950	5.84
Ireland	500,000	5.99
Australia	264,151	6.11
England and Wales		6.24
Netherlands	193,338	6.27
Canada	397,110	6.30
Austria	94,389	6.49
Scotland		6.50
France*	712,000	6.82
Northern Ireland		7.07
Italy	537,500	7.16
Spain†	386,708	7.19
New Zealand	58,868	7.24
Israel		7.80
Belgium*		8.20
Greece		8.30
United States	4,000,240	8.37
Czech Republic		8.47
Cuba		9.40
Portugal		9.57

Based on the latest data available for countries or geographic areas with at least 1 million population and with complete counts of live births and infant deaths as indicated in the United Nations Demographic Yearbook, 1994, and unpublished 1995 edition.
*Data for Belgium and France are for 1992.
†Data for Spain are for 1991.
Source: National Center for Health Statistics, Centers for Disease Control and Prevention. *Health, United States (1996–97).* Hyattsville, MD: DHHS, 1997.

In 1993, the neonatal mortality rates (NMRs) in Japan and the United States were 2.3 and 5.3 per 1,000 live births, respectively. Thus, in 1993, the NMR in the United States was 2.3 times the NMR in Japan. From 1970 to 1993, the NMR in Japan dropped 73.6%. Over the same time period, the NMR in the United States dropped 64.9%. In 1993, 53.5% of the total infant mortality in Japan occurred in the neonatal period. In 1993, in the United States 63.1% of the total infant mortality occurred in the neonatal period (Table 24.2).

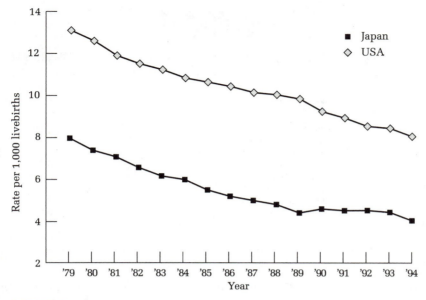

FIGURE 24.1
....

Infant mortality in Japan and the United States, 1979–1994.

In 1993, the postneonatal mortality rates (PNMRs) in Japan and the United States were 2.0 and 3.1 per 1,000 live births, respectively. Thus, in 1993 the PNMR in the United States was 1.6 times the PNMR in Japan. From 1970 to 1993 the PNMR in Japan dropped 54.5%. Over the same time period, the PNMR in the United States dropped 43.9%.

Major causes of infant death in Japan in 1992 were congenital anomalies, birth trauma, hypoxia, birth asphyxia and other respiratory

....

TABLE 24.2

....

Infant, Neonatal, and Postneonatal Mortality Rates (1950–1993)

Year	IMR		NMR		PNMR	
	Japan	U.S.	Japan	U.S.	Japan	U.S.
1950	60.1	29.2	8.7	20.5	NA	8.7
1960	60.7	26.0	4.9	18.7	NA	7.3
1970	13.1	20.0	8.7	15.1	4.4	4.9
1980	7.5	12.6	4.9	8.5	2.6	4.1
1991	4.4	9.8	2.4	5.6	2.0	3.4
1993	4.3	8.4	NA	5.3	NA	3.1

IMR, infant mortality rate; NMR, neonatal mortality rate; PNMR, postneonatal mortality rate.

TABLE 24.3

Infant Mortality Rates for the Nine Leading Causes of Infant Death: Japan, 1992

Rank	Cause of Death	Rate (1,000 Live Births)
1	Congenital anomalies	1.69
2	Birth trauma, hypoxia, birth asphyxia, and other respiratory conditions	0.81
3	Accidents and adverse effects	0.27
4	Septicemia (including newborn)	0.16
5	Pneumonia and bronchitis	0.12
6	Other external causes	0.06
7	Premature babies of unknown causes	0.05
8	Meningitis	0.22
9	Malignant neoplasms	0.22

conditions, and accidents (Table 24.3). Japan has made significant progress in the reduction of infant deaths due to gastrointestinal and respiratory infections.[7]

Infant Mortality in the United States

Infant mortality in the United States had dropped continually and reached a record low in 1994 of 8.0 deaths per 1,000 live births. The infant mortality rate for black infants was 15.8 per 1,000 live births, compared with a rate of 6.6 for white infants. Black infants died at a rate 2.4 times that of white infants. The infant mortality rate for Hispanic infants in 1994 was 6.5 per 1,000 live births. This rate is the same as for non-Hispanic white infants. However, the Hispanic population is not a homogeneous group. Cuban infants had an infant mortality rate of 4.5, Mexican infants had an infant mortality rate of 6.6, and Puerto Rican infants had an infant mortality rate of 4.5. The remaining group of Hispanic infants includes Central and South American as well as other and unknown Hispanics and had an infant mortality rate of 5.7. Factors contributing to the continued disparity between white infant mortality and that of the other populations need further research.

In 1994, there were 31,710 infant deaths. The 10 leading causes of death have not changed for several years. The decreases in sudden infant death syndrome and respiratory distress syndrome are considered responsible for the improved infant mortality rate. Sudden infant death syndrome dropped from the second most common cause of infant death to the third. Congenital anomalies, disorders related to short gestation and unspecified low birthweight, sudden infant death syndrome, and respiratory distress syndrome account for 52.7% of infant deaths. The next six leading causes of death (newborn affected by maternal complications of pregnancy; newborn affected by complications of placenta, cord, and membranes; accidents and adverse affects; infections specific to the perinatal period; pneumonia and influenza; and intrauterine hypoxia and birth asphyxia) account for 16% of infant deaths (Table 24.4). The remaining causes account for 31.3% of infant deaths. Congenital anomalies are the leading cause of death for white infants, whereas disorders related to short gestation and unspecified low birthweight are the leading cause of death for black infants, with congenital anomalies second.

The state of the economy has a significant impact on use of health care and on health status, especially in the populations of greatest concern. It is instructive to consider the following: one of four infants and toddlers and one older child in five lives in poverty. Between 1980 and 1995, the number of children living in poverty increased by almost 2.9 million. In 1995, 14 million children younger than 18 years lived in families with income below 100% of the federal poverty level. This group included 41.5% of African American children, 39.3% of Hispanic children, and 15.5% of white children. For families in economic distress, ensuring adequate food, clothing, and shelter will likely take precedence over seeking adequate health care. At the same time, the relative cost of seeking health care is greater for this population. Health care programs, in an attempt to maintain basic services in the face of shrinking resources, may be cutting out those services considered ancillary or expanded, such as outreach and home visiting.

TABLE 24.4

Infant Mortality Rates for the 10 *Leading Causes of Infant Death: United States,* 1994

Rank	Cause of Death*	Rate (1,000 Live Births)
1	Congenital anomalies	1.73
2	Disorders relating to short gestation and low birthweight	1.08
3	Sudden infant death syndrome	1.03
4	Respiratory distress syndrome	0.40
5	Newborn affected by maternal complications of pregnancy	0.33
6	Newborn affected by complications of placenta, cord, and membranes	0.24
7	Accidents and adverse affects	0.23
8	Infections specific to the perinatal period	0.21
9	Pneumonia and influenza	0.14
10	Intrauterine hypoxia and birth asphyxia	0.14

*Based on ninth revision of ICD, 1975.

In a 1995 report from the Centers for Disease Control, data were analyzed from the 1988 National Maternal and Infant Health Survey to examine the relationship between poverty and infant mortality in the United States. Among infants born to women living in poverty in 1988, the overall excess mortality risk was approximately 60% compared with infants born to women living above the poverty level. The infant mortality rate varied by poverty level and was 8.3 per 1,000 liveborn infants for women with incomes above the poverty level and 13.5 per 1,000 liveborn infants for women below the poverty level. The association between poverty and infant mortality was stronger for postneonatal deaths than for neonatal deaths.[8]

Japan's Infant Mortality Rate Compared with Selected Race of Mother in the United States

Because the racial composition of the United States is considerably more diverse than the racial composition of Japan, it may be instruc-

TABLE 24.5

Infant Mortality Rates in Japan and for Selected Races in the United States
(1950–1994)

Year	IMR			NMR			PNMR		
	Japan	U.S.		Japan	U.S.		Japan	U.S.	
		White	Japanese		White	Japanese		White	Japanese
1950	60.1	26.8		27.4	19.4		32.7	7.4	
1960	30.7	22.9		17.0	17.2		13.7	5.7	
1970	13.1	17.8		8.7	13.8		4.4	4.0	
1980	7.5	10.9		4.9	7.4		2.6	3.5	
1983	6.2	9.6	*	3.9	6.3		2.3	3.3	
1985	5.5	9.2	6.0*	3.4	6.0		2.1	3.2	
1988	4.8	8.4	7.0*	2.7	5.3		2.1	3.1	
1989	4.6	8.1	6.0*	2.6	5.1		2.0	2.9	
1990	4.6	7.6	5.5*	2.6	4.8		2.0	2.8	
1991	4.4	7.3	4.2*	2.4	4.5		2.0	2.8	
1993	4.3	6.8		2.3	4.3		2.0	2.5	

IMR, infant mortality rate; NMR, neonatal mortality rate; PNMR, postneonatal mortality rate.
*Infant and neonatal mortality rates for groups with fewer than 10,000 births are considered unreliable. Postneonatal mortality rates for groups with fewer than 20,000 births are considered unreliable. Infant and neonatal mortality rates for groups with fewer than 7,500 births are considered highly unreliable and are not shown. Postneonatal mortality rates for groups with fewer than 15,000 births are considered highly unreliable and are not shown.

tive to compare Japan's IMR with those U.S. racial groups with the best IMRs—whites and Japanese Americans. Data for U.S. infants of Japanese origin are available from the National Linked Files of Live Births and Infant Deaths. It can be seen that infants of Japanese origin in the United States have lower infant mortality rates than U.S. whites and higher infant mortality rates than Japanese. Because of the small number of deaths to infants of Japanese origin, multiple years of data are combined to help stabilize the mortality rates. This is particularly important when separating mortality into its component parts. It is noted that compared with U.S. white infants, infants of Japanese origin have consistently lower infant, neonatal, and postneonatal mortality rates (Table 24.5).

COMPARISON OF FACTORS CONTRIBUTING TO INFANT MORTALITY

Low Birthweight

The relationship between birthweight and mortality as well as between birthweight and morbidity is consistent between countries and for different ethnic groups within countries. In general, mortality rates are extremely high at very low birthweights. Mortality falls as birthweight increases, so that mortality is lowest at birthweights of around 3000 to 3999 grams. As birthweight increases beyond 4000 grams, mortality then rises.[9] Additionally, birthweight is related to maternal weight gain, with approximately a 20-gram gain in birthweight for every 1 kilogram of maternal weight gain.[10]

The incidence in Japan of very low birthweight, defined as less than 1500 grams, dropped from 0.4% in 1970 to 0.3% in 1975. It rose slightly since 1975 to 0.6% in 1994. Over the same time period, the U.S. percentage of very low birthweight rose from 1.2% to 1.3% (Table 24.6). The observed rise in very low birthweight for both countries may be a reflection of improvements since 1970 in technology's ability to keep very small infants alive.

Moderately low birthweight, defined as between 1500 and 2500 grams, has ranged in Japan from a low of 4.82% in the early 1980s to a high of 6.9% in 1994. In 1980, 7.9% of infants in the United States were moderately low birthweight. This decreased to a low of 6.8% in the early 1980s to a high of 6.0% in 1994. The percentages of moderately low birthweight infants in Japan and the United States are quite similar. However, Japanese women as a group are smaller than American women. Because maternal size is a strong predictor of birth-

TABLE 24.6

Incidence of Low and Very Low Birthweight

	Birthweight <2500 Grams		Birthweight <1500 Grams		Birthweight Between 1500 and 2500 Grams	
	Japan (%)	U.S. (%)	Japan (%)	U.S. (%)	Japan (%)	U.S. (%)
1970	5.7	7.9	0.4	1.2	5.3	6.7
1975	5.1	7.4	0.3	1.2	4.8	6.2
1980	5.2	6.8	0.4	1.2	4.8	5.6
1985	5.5	6.8	0.5	1.2	5.0	5.6
1990	6.3	7.0	0.5	1.3	5.8	5.7
1991	NA	7.1	NA	1.3	NA	5.8
1992	6.8	7.1	0.6	1.3	6.2	5.8
1993	7.0	7.2	0.6	1.3	6.4	5.9
1994	7.5	7.3	0.6	1.3	6.9	6.0

weight,[11] it is not surprising that Japanese women have relatively small babies.

Within the United States, the incidence of low and very low birthweight varies considerably by race or ethnicity. Black babies have the highest incidence of low and very low birthweight at 13.2% and 3.0%, respectively. This is three times the incidence of very low birthweight for white infants (1.0%) and 2.2 times the incidence of low birthweight for white infants (6.1%). American Indians, including Aleuts and Eskimos, have a very low birthweight incidence of 1.1% and a low birthweight incidence of 6.4%. Asian and Pacific Islanders have a very low birthweight incidence of 0.9% and a low birthweight incidence of 6.8%. Details of low and very low birthweight for specific ethnic groups are provided in Table 24.7.

Analyzing data from the 1988 National Maternal and Infant Health Survey, Parker and colleagues[12] compared associations between five indicators of socioeconomic status (maternal education, paternal education, maternal occupation, paternal occupation, and family income) and reproductive outcomes, including low birthweight. Nearly all socioeconomic indices were associated with low birthweight among both black women and white women.

Age of Mother

The Japanese have a very narrow maternal age distribution, which means that they do not have the number of young or older women delivering infants that the United States has. For example, in 1984, only

TABLE 24.7

Incidence of Low and Very Low Birthweight by Mother's Race

Race of Mother and Hispanic Origin of Mother	1970	1975	1980	1985	1990	1991	1992	1993	1994
Low Birthweight (<2500 grams)									
All mothers	7.9	7.4	6.8	6.8	7.0	7.1	7.1	7.2	7.3
White	6.9	6.3	5.7	5.7	5.7	5.8	5.8	6.0	6.1
Black	13.9	13.2	12.7	12.7	13.3	13.6	13.3	13.3	13.2
American Indian or Alaskan Native	8.0	6.4	6.4	5.9	6.1	6.2	6.2	6.4	6.4
Asian or Pacific Islander	—	—	6.7	6.2	6.5	6.5	6.6	6.6	6.8
Chinese	6.7	5.3	5.2	5.0	4.7	5.1	5.0	4.9	4.8
Japanese	9.0	7.5	6.6	6.2	6.2	5.9	7.0	6.5	6.9
Filipino	10.0	8.1	7.4	7.0	7.3	7.3	7.4	7.0	7.8
Hawaiian or part Hawaiian	—	—	—	—	7.2	6.7	6.9	6.8	7.2
Other	—	—	—	—	6.6	6.7	6.7	6.9	7.1
Hispanic origin	—	—	6.1	6.2	6.1	6.2	6.1	6.2	6.2
Mexican	—	—	5.6	5.8	5.6	5.6	5.6	5.8	5.8
Puerto Rican	—	—	9.0	8.7	9.0	9.4	9.2	9.2	9.1
Cuban	—	—	5.6	6.0	5.7	5.6	6.1	6.2	6.3
Central or South American	—	—	5.8	5.7	5.8	5.9	5.8	5.9	6.0
Other or unknown Hispanic	—	—	7.0	6.8	6.9	7.3	7.2	7.5	7.5
White, non-Hispanic	—	—	5.7	5.6	5.6	5.7	5.7	5.9	6.1
Black, non-Hispanic	—	—	12.7	12.6	13.3	13.6	13.4	13.4	13.4
Very Low Birthweight (<1500 grams)									
All mothers	1.2	1.2	1.2	1.2	1.3	1.3	1.3	1.3	1.3
White	1.0	0.9	0.9	0.9	1.0	1.0	1.0	1.0	1.0
Black	2.4	2.4	2.5	2.7	2.9	3.0	3.0	3.0	3.0
American Indian or Alaskan Native	1.0	1.0	0.9	1.0	1.0	1.1	1.0	1.1	1.1
Asian or Pacific Islander	—	—	0.9	0.9	0.9	0.9	0.9	0.9	0.9
Chinese	0.8	0.5	0.7	0.6	0.5	0.7	0.7	0.6	0.6
Japanese	1.5	0.9	0.9	0.8	0.7	0.6	0.9	0.7	0.9
Filipino	1.1	0.9	1.0	0.9	1.1	1.0	1.1	1.0	1.2
Hawaiian or part Hawaiian	—	—	—	—	1.0	1.0	1.0	1.1	1.2
Other	—	—	—	—	0.9	0.9	0.9	0.9	0.9
Hispanic origin	—	—	1.0	1.0	1.0	1.0	1.0	1.1	1.1
Mexican	—	—	0.9	1.0	0.9	0.9	0.9	1.0	1.0
Puerto Rican	—	—	1.3	1.3	1.6	1.7	1.7	1.7	1.6
Cuban	—	—	1.0	1.2	1.2	1.2	1.2	1.2	1.3
Central or South American	—	—	1.0	1.0	1.1	1.0	1.0	1.0	1.1
Other or unknown Hispanic	—	—	1.0	1.0	1.1	1.1	1.1	1.2	1.3
White, non-Hispanic	—	—	0.9	0.9	0.9	0.9	0.9	1.0	1.0
Black, non-Hispanic	—	—	2.5	2.7	2.9	3.0	3.0	3.0	3.0

1.3% of deliveries in Japan occurred to teenagers, whereas in the United States, 13.1% of deliveries occurred to teenagers (11.1% among whites and 23.6% among blacks). In 1992, only 1.6% of deliveries in Japan occurred to teenagers; in the United States, 12.7% of deliveries occurred to teenagers (10.9% among whites and 22.7% among blacks). In the United States, the percentage of births to teenagers is decreasing, so that in 1994 only 9.1% of births were to teenage mothers. Most children born in Japan today are conceived and delivered when their mothers are aged 20 to 34 years, with most mothers being between 25 and 29 years. Since 1950, the maternal age distribution has grown narrower.

Geographic Location

Until 1965, in Japan the rural areas had a higher infant mortality rate than the urban areas. Since then, the difference in infant mortality rates between rural and urban areas has become very small. The infant mortality rates of all prefectures are currently almost equal.

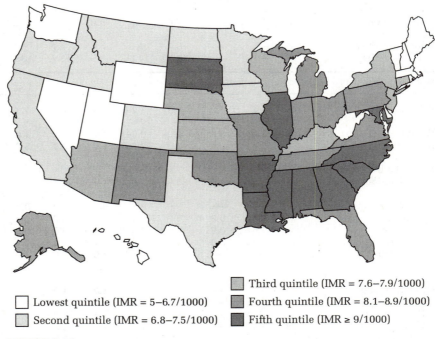

☐ Lowest quintile (IMR = 5–6.7/1000)
▨ Second quintile (IMR = 6.8–7.5/1000)
▨ Third quintile (IMR = 7.6–7.9/1000)
▨ Fourth quintile (IMR = 8.1–8.9/1000)
■ Fifth quintile (IMR ≥ 9/1000)

FIGURE 24.2

Infant mortality by state, 1994.

There are significant differences in the United States by geographic location. Certain states, especially those in the Southeast have a higher than average infant mortality rate (Figure 24.2). The states with the highest infant mortality rate were the District of Columbia, Mississippi, Louisiana, and Alabama; those with the lowest were Rhode Island, Massachusetts, Maine, New Hampshire, and Utah.

Prenatal Care

Quality prenatal care promotes the health and well-being of the pregnant woman, the fetus, the infant, and the family and provides an opportunity to look beyond pregnancy and delivery to identify the resources essential for further healthy development of parents and infant. It includes early and continuing risk assessment; health promotion and health behavior advice; medical and psychosocial interventions, referral, and follow-up; and delivery planning. Women who receive such high-quality prenatal care are less likely to have a low birthweight infant; this is particularly true for high-risk women. Because significant change in risk status can arise at any time during pregnancy, continuing risk assessment throughout pregnancy is necessary for all women, and the specific content and timing of prenatal visits, contacts, and education should vary depending on the risk status of the pregnant woman and her fetus.

Japan. In 1958, the challenge of providing health insurance for all was met by the enactment of the National Health Insurance Law. There are 177.9 physicians per 100,000 population. The number of physicians and hospitals in Japan is evenly distributed throughout Japan. Physicians in hospitals are considered employees and usually do not charge patients additional fees.

When women in Japan register their pregnancy with the municipality office, they receive a Maternal Child Health Handbook (MCH Handbook) and vouchers for two free prenatal examinations. Although almost 100% of pregnancies are registered, in 1993, only 58.4% were registered during the first trimester. This percentage has risen steadily from 21% in 1965. There are, on average, approximately 10 prenatal care visits. Aside from the two free prenatal examinations, medical insurance does not cover prenatal care. If women cannot afford to pay for prenatal care, systems are in place to cover their expenses.

United States. After rapid improvement in the 1970s, the 1980s, and the early 1990s, the percentage of women receiving first trimester prenatal care held steady at around 76%. In 1992, the percentage of women receiving first trimester prenatal care increased to 77.7%, in 1993 to 78.9%, and to 80.2% in 1994. The gains in the percentage of women receiving first trimester prenatal care between 1993 and 1994 were seen for mothers of all racial and ethnic groups, educational levels, and marital statuses. This was 3% to 4% for teenage mothers, unmarried mothers, mothers with less than a high school education, and black and Hispanic mothers. When reviewed by detailed race and ethnicity data, Japanese women in the United States have consistently had the highest rates of first trimester prenatal care.

Along with the increases in women receiving first trimester prenatal care, there was a concomitant decrease in the percentage of women delaying the initiation of prenatal care until the third trimester or who received no prenatal care. In 1989, 6.4% of women received late or no prenatal care. This percentage was as high as it had been in the early 1970s. Since then it has decreased steadily to a new low of 4.4% for 1994.

In 1992, the U.S. Maternal and Child Health Bureau within the Health Resources and Services Administration released a Health Diary, based on Japan's MCH Handbook. The book is approximately 80 pages long and provides health guidance as well as a place to record information from the beginning of the pregnancy until the child is 24 months old. The book is available to the public on request. State and local health departments can purchase the book for distribution or the camera-ready boards.[13]

Delivery

Place of Delivery. Since 1947, there has been a marked increase in in-hospital deliveries in Japan. In 1950, only 4.6% of deliveries occurred in hospitals. In 1958, the Ministry of Health, as part of its promotion of in-hospital deliveries, established the Maternal and Child Health Centers as facilities for deliveries in rural towns and villages. This strategy was successful as evidenced by the fact that, in 1965, 84% of births occurred in hospitals and, in 1990, 99.9% occurred in hospitals.

In 1989, 98.8% of births in the United States occurred in hospitals. In that same year, 95.4% of births were attended by physicians, 3.7% were attended by midwives, and 0.3% were attended by others and unspecified persons. By 1994, the percentage of births in hospitals had increased to 99.0%. Along with this was a decrease to 93.8% of births attended by physicians and an increase to 5.5% in births attended by midwives and 0.7% to births attended by others and unspecified persons.[14,15]

TABLE 24.8

Cesarean Section Rates: United States, 1989–1994

Year	Cesarean Rate		
	Total*	Primary[†]	VBAC Rate[‡]
1994	21.2	14.9	26.3
1993	21.8	15.3	24.3
1992	22.3	15.6	22.6
1991	22.6	15.9	21.3
1990	22.7	16.0	19.9
1989	22.8	16.1	18.9

*Percentage of all live births by cesarean delivery.
[†]Number of primary cesareans per 100 live births to women who have not had a previous cesarean.
[‡]Number of vaginal births after previous cesarean (VBAC) delivery per 100 live births to women with a previous cesarean delivery.

Type of Delivery. The cesarean section rate in Japan has been slowly increasing since 1984. In 1990, in hospitals, 10.2% of deliveries were cesarean sections and 89.8% were vaginal deliveries. In clinics, in 1993, 9.1% of deliveries were cesarean sections and 90.9% were vaginal deliveries.

In the United States, the cesarean section rate was at 22.8% of deliveries in 1989; this was the first year this item was coded on the birth certificate. This percentage has decreased steadily to 21.2% in 1994. Primary cesarean section rate has also declined each year from 16.1% in 1989 to 14.9% in 1994. The percentage of vaginal births after previous cesarean section (VBAC) increased from 18.9% in 1989 to 26.3% in 1994 (Table 24.8). Despite the 39.2% increase in VBAC rates, the percentage is still far below the goal of 35% that the United States Department of Health and Human Services set as part of the Year 2000 Health Objectives.

Length of Stay in Hospital after Delivery

Japan. In Japan, almost all mothers and babies remain in the hospital for 1 week following delivery. Health authorities believe that this week in the hospital makes it possible for physicians and nurses to identify symptoms and treat them early. Additionally, aside from the universal medical insurance, which covers 80% of medical expenses for everyone in Japan, a program exists that covers all medical expense for high-risk newborns.

United States. Over time there has been a shortening in the length of hospital stays for neonates and their mothers. Data indicate that between 1970 and 1992, the average length of hospital stay for all deliveries has consistently decreased. The average length of stay for vaginal deliveries decreased from 3.9 to 2.1 days; for those who delivered by cesarean section, the average length of stay decreased from 7.8 to 4.0 days. The trend toward shorter hospital stays was evident prior to the current insurance and managed care plans, which further limited the length of maternity stays. Although the overall length of stay following a vaginal delivery is approximately 48 hours, numerous cases of postpartum discharge of less than 24 hours (and even less than 12 hours) have been reported.

In 1980, approximately 30% of infants born in the United States were discharged at 2 days or less, 30% were discharged at 3 days, and the remaining 38.5 percent at 4 days or more. By 1993, 30% of newborns were discharged at 1 day, 38.5% at 2 days, 17% at 3 days, and only 14.3% at 4 days or more.

This reduction in duration of postpartum stay for women and their infants has aggravated and sharpened the focus on problems that have always been there: the inappropriate discharge of mothers and their newborns before they are prepared and ready, and inadequate follow-up care for this highly vulnerable population. Even with legislation mandating insurance coverage for 48-hour stays following a vaginal delivery and 96-hour stays following a cesarean delivery, such legislation will not resolve all problems related to inappropriate discharge and inadequate follow-up care.

There are no objective scientific data to determine appropriate length of stay now or in the past. The literature reviewing the early discharge practice has limited value because definitions of early discharge are variable and have changed over time. Regarding study methodology, it was observed that in many studies reported in the literature the sample sizes are too small to detect differences between the groups; there is rarely random assignment of groups; there is either no control group or the control group is not appropriate; the length of hospital stay is not necessarily as categorized (i.e., some persons in the short stay group have stays as long as those in the comparison group); and women and infants likely to have birth-related complications are excluded. Failing to prove that shorter hospital stays are unsafe (especially in the face of numerous methodologic flaws) is not the same as proving they are safe.[16]

In May 1995, Maryland became the first state to have legislation requiring insurance companies and health maintenance organizations in that state to pay for a minimum of 48 hours of care in the hospital after delivery. According to the National Conference of State

Legislators, many states have introduced or enacted legislation related to early discharge. Although many states have legislation, there are currently limitations of who is covered under these laws. Most state legislation exempts persons covered under Employee Retirement Income Security Act. Consequently, even in states with such laws, a significant number of women are not covered by legislation ensuring that they can remain in the hospital for 48 hours following delivery. In September 1996, federal legislation was enacted. Title VI (Newborns' and Mothers' Health Protection Act of 1996) of the Veterans Affairs–Housing and Urban Development and Independent Agencies Appropriations Act, 1996 (P.L. 104-204) became effective January 1, 1998. This law does not supersede state laws if the state law regulates such coverage. In order not to be preempted by the federal law, a state law must provide a minimum of 48 hours of inpatient care following a vaginal delivery and 96 hours following a cesarean delivery; meet guidelines established by the American College of Obstetricians and Gynecologists, the American Academy of Pediatrics, or other medical professional associations such as nurse midwives; and provide that the length of stay is determined by the woman's health care provider. In addition, insurers providing group health insurance may not restrict benefits to mothers or newborns to less than 48 hours following a normal vaginal delivery, nor may they restrict benefits to mothers or newborns to less than 96 hours following a cesarean section. However, the provider and mother may jointly decide that the mother and newborn may leave the hospital prior to the 48 or 96 hours. A health insurer is prohibited from denying eligibility to enroll or renew insured persons to avoid the requirements of this law; providing incentives to mothers to accept less than the minimum protections, penalizing providers for granting benefits allowed by this act, or giving incentives to providers to induce them to act inconsistent with this law. Conversely, a mother cannot be required to give birth in a hospital or to stay in the hospital for a fixed period of time. The federal law does not apply to insurers who do not provide childbirth benefits. Finally, the federal law allows insurers to impose deductibles, co-insurance, or other cost-sharing measures.

Table 24-9 lists the average length of stay in a number of countries, including the United States and Japan. There is a general trend to suggest that countries where women and infants have longer hospital stays also have lower infant mortality. It would be fallacious to assume without detailed study that there is a causal relationship between the length of hospital stay and the infant mortality rate. It is possible that there is some indirect relationship that reflects the value that society places on children.

TABLE 24.9

Current Average Length of Stay Post-Delivery

Country	Average Length of Stay	
	Vaginal Delivery	Cesarean Delivery
United States	2.1 days	4.0 days
Australia	3.0 days	N/A
Canada	2.4 days	4.7 days
France	3.0 days (private patients) 4.0 days (public patients)	7.0 days
Great Britain	3.0 days	N/A
Japan	6.5 days	N/A
Norway	4.5 days	10.0 days
Sweden	4.0 days	7.0 days

Sources: U.S. Department of Health and Human Services and Ministries of Health for their respective countries.

Family Planning

Japan. The main forms of contraception used by couples in Japan are the condom and induced abortion. The total contraceptive practice rate in Japan was 81.0% in 1992.

United States. In 1970, Title X of the Public Health Service Act was enacted, creating for the first time a comprehensive federal program providing family planning services on a national basis. By fiscal year 1983, $4,340,000 was spent to provide family planning services to 5 million women. The largest single source of funding is the federal-state Medicaid program (Title XIX of the Social Security Act). Clinic services are also partially supported in most states with federal funds from the Maternal and Child Health Block Grant (Title V of the Social Security Act) and the Social Services Block Grant (Title XX of the Social Security Act).

In 1990, 59.3% of women aged 15 to 44 were using some form of contraception. The percentage of women using contraception increases with age. Overall, women using contraception used the following methods as their primary means of contraception: 29.5% used female sterilization, 12.6% used male sterilization, 28.5% used birth control pills, 1.4% used an intrauterine device, 2.8% used a diaphragm, and 17.7% used condoms.

Although the benefits of publicly funded family planning services in the United States have long been recognized, only 84% of women in households with income below 200% of the poverty level were using contraceptives. Public health authorities have agreed on its demonstrated effectiveness not just in preventing pregnancy but in improving the health of women and their children.

Abortion

Japan. Abortion is one of the leading forms of birth control in Japan. Induced abortions are performed by obstetrician-gynecologists. The Japan Medical Association issues the special license required to perform abortions. They are performed in hospitals and occur mainly in the first trimester.

The reported number of induced abortions reached a peak in the years between 1955 and 1960, when more than 1 million abortions were performed annually. This number has declined steadily, with 413,000 abortions performed in 1992. Of these, almost 94% were performed in the first trimester.[17]

United States. In 1973, abortion was declared legal in the United States. This legalization brought with it a dramatic increase in the number of legal procedures and a concomitant decrease in maternal mortality. Each year more than 1.6 million women have an abortion in the United States. More than half of all abortions are performed at or before 8 weeks of pregnancy. In 1992 in the United States, the Centers for Disease Control (CDC) reported that there were 1,359,000 legal abortions, and the Allen Guttmacher Institute reported that there were 1,529,000 legal abortions.[18] The CDC acquires abortion service statistics from three sources: central health agencies, hospitals and other medical facilities, and the National Center for Health Statistics. The total number of abortions reported to CDC is about 11% less than the total estimated independently by the Allen Guttmacher Institute. (The Guttmacher Institute is a not-for-profit organization that does reproductive health research, policy analysis, and public education.) The abortion ratio (number of abortions per 100 live births) has been decreasing slightly from a high of 35.9 in 1980 to 32.1 in 1994. The abortion ratio decreases with age; ranging from a ratio, in 1994, of 70.4 per 100 live births for those younger than 15 years old to a low among 30-

to 34-year-olds of 17.2 per 100 live births. The ratio then increases, so that women older than 40 years of age have a ratio similar to that of 15- to 19-year-olds.

Eighty-four percent of counties in the United States have no abortion provider. The scarcity of abortion services is more marked in rural counties, with 94% of non-metropolitan areas having no abortion services. Despite the concentration of abortion services in urban areas, fully one third of metropolitan areas have no provider or have providers who perform fewer than 50 abortions per year. The number of providers performing abortions decreased 18% from 2,908 in 1982 to 2,308 in 1992. Almost half (49%) of all abortions in 1992 took place in the five most populous states: California (304,000), New York (195,000), Texas (93,000), Florida (85,000), and Illinois (68,000). In 1992, most abortions (69%) took place in the country's 441 abortion clinics. 20% took place in other clinics, 7% in hospitals, and 4% in physician offices.

Access to Care

Few of the interventions available in the United States can hope to be successful if a woman or infant cannot enter the health care system. Among the barriers that prevent access to the health care system is the continued inability to pay for comprehensive perinatal and infant care. At present, millions of women of childbearing age have neither private insurance nor Medicaid coverage. Additionally, many private policies either do not cover maternity costs or have large deductibles. Financial support for expanded services such as case management and outreach is tenuous. The number of practitioners available and willing to provide maternal and infant care does not meet the need. Of the more than 3,000 counties in the United Sates, more than 40% are identified as having no primary care provider and an additional 13% as having only partially met needs. Problems relating to lack of systems of comprehensive care, ease of entry into the system, convenient operating hours, child care services, and transportation continue to pose challenges. Cultural barriers, such as those resulting from inadequate provider language and cultural competency skills, inhibit access. Health information must be communicated in multi-language formats as well as in versions for illiterate individuals or those with low literacy.

Although more than half the counties have either no or not enough providers, most women in the United States are still managing to obtain prenatal care. Data from U.S. vital statistics between 1981 and 1995 indicate that receipt of prenatal care initiated in the first trimester has increased for pregnant women from approximately 76%

to 81% in the United States. There has been a concomitant decrease in the number of women who delay the initiation of prenatal care until the last trimester of their pregnancy or who received no care at all—a 40% decrease since 1981. In addition, the majority of pregnant women in the United States have been getting at least the amount of care recommended by the American College of Obstetricians and Gynecologists, with more pregnant women beginning care earlier.[19]

INFERENCES ASSOCIATED WITH JAPAN'S LOW INFANT MORTALITY RATE

Although Japan and the United States may be compared in many areas, the United States is 25.6 times as large as Japan, with a population twice as large as Japan's. The United States is ethnically diverse; Japan is not.[20] The Japanese have a very narrow socioeconomic status distribution, which means that they do not have the number of women in extreme poverty that the United States has. The monthly average income per worker's household was 554,000¥ (U.S. $5,600) in 1992. Poor people can get livelihood assistance by the social security system of 150,000¥ (U.S. $1,500) per month. In 1990, approximately 1 million people received this assistance. Additionally, there is a relative absence of financial barriers to receiving professional health services.

In 1958, Japan enacted the National Health Insurance Law. Good medical care is available almost any place in Japan. The building of paved roads allowed for the diffusion of medical care into rural areas. General hospitals providing secondary medical care, including neonatal intensive care units, are located in every area with a population of at least 300,000. Considerable emphasis has been placed on the importance of many aspects of health—prenatal care, continuous infant and child health care, personal hygiene, nutrition, and the use of community health services, including immunizations.

As noted earlier, when women in Japan register their pregnancy with the municipality office, they receive a MCH Handbook. This handbook was originated approximately 50 years ago. It has become important in both its instrumental and symbolic function. The MCH Handbook is pocket-sized and is approximately 75 pages long. It is designed to be a source of health education as well as a record of the mother's and child's health. Japan has a very high literacy rate, which makes utilization of the handbook easier.

Japan has population-based screening. Pregnant women are screened for hepatitis B antigen. If the mother tests positive, newborn babies are given immunoglobulin twice and hepatitis B vaccine three times at public expense. Newborn infants are screened for phenylke-tonuria, maple sugar urine disease, homocystinuria, galactosemia, adrenal hyperplasia, and congenital hypothyroidism. At 6 months, infants are screened for neuroblastoma.

The Maternal and Child Health Law prescribes that the health examination for children be done twice during the preschool period, at 18 months and at 3 years. In practice, almost all local governments implement health examinations for infants two to three times in the first year of life. After 3 years, more than 90% of children are in nursery school, and health supervision or guidance is provided in the school setting. Finally, there is a very high value placed on childbearing and children in Japanese society. This value is reflected in public and private policies.

IMPLICATIONS FOR OTHER COUNTRIES, INCLUDING THE UNITED STATES

The steps taken by Japan to reduce infant mortality may provide ideas that should be considered by other counties. General steps taken include improvement in the general standard of living for all people. This includes the standard of housing, water supply, general hygiene, and education. Additionally, all persons, including women and children, need to have health insurance.

There are specific steps Japan took related to the care of women, infants, children, and families. Japan developed and promoted the use of the MCH Handbook, including its use as a health education device. The handbook was used as a tool to collect data on the health of women, issues of pregnancy, and information on infants. Japan provided improved reproductive health care for all women of childbearing age and for their infants. This included high risk care, as needed, for women, continuous prenatal care, and education about infancy and early childhood for parents. Special programs were provided to communities with unusually high fetal loss and morbidity or with a high level of other unfavorable pregnancy outcomes. All fetal deaths are reviewed to ascertain the cause and to develop prevention strategies. Family planning education was instituted as well as the availability of ending unplanned or unwanted pregnancies. Finally, Japan increased the use of nurse midwives and public health nurses in hospitals, at health centers, and at home.

Japan has managed to focus increased attention on women and young children as a vulnerable group in the population. Additional resources have helped produce more favorable outcomes on indicators of maternal and infant health, in general, and on infant mortality in particular.

References

1. Cone, T.E., Jr. *History of pediatrics*. Boston: Little, Brown, 1979.
2. Green, M. (ed). *Bright futures: Guidelines for health supervision of infants, children, and adolescents*. Arlington, VA: National Center for Education in Maternal and Child Health, 1994.
3. U.S. Department of Health and Human Services, Public Health Service, Health Resources and Services Administration, Maternal and Child Health Bureau. *1997 Child health U.S.A. '96–'97*. (DHHS Pub. No. HRSA-M-DSEA-97-48). Washington, DC: U.S. Government Printing Office, 1997.
4. Montgomery, L.E., Kiely, J.L., and Pappas, G. The effects of poverty, race, and family structure on U.S. children's health: Data from the NHIS, 1978 through 1980 and 1989 through 1991. *American Journal of Public Health*. 1996;86:1401–1405.
5. Matsuyama, E. Saving the children: How Japan keeps down its infant mortality rate. JOICFP Documentary Series 18, Tokyo, 1986.
6. Ministry of Health. *Maternal and child health in Japan. Mothers' and children's health and welfare association*. Tokyo: 1992.
7. *Maternal and child health statistics of Japan*. Ministry of Health and Welfare, Tokyo, 1996, pp 52–53.
8. CDC. Poverty and infant mortality—United States, 1988. *Morbidity and Mortality Weekly Report*. 1995;44:922–927.
9. Golding, J. Epidemiology of perinatal death. In M. Kiely (ed). *Reproductive and perinatal epidemiology*. Boca Raton, FL: CRC Press, 1991.
10. Niswander, K., and Jackson, E.C. Physical characteristics of the gravida and their association with birth weight and perinatal death. *American Journal of Obstetrics and Gyncology*. 1974;119:306–313.
11. Kleinman, J.C., and Madans, J.H. The effects of maternal smoking, physical stature and educational attainment on the incidence of low birth weight. *American Journal of Epidemiology*. 1985;121:843–855.
12. Parker, J.D., Schoendorf, K.C., and Kiely, J.L. Associations between measures of socioeconomic status and low birth weight, small for gestational age, and premature delivery in the United States. *Annals of Epidemiology*. 1994;4:271–278.
13. U.S. Department of Health and Human Services, Public Health Service, Health Resources and Services Administration, Maternal and Child Health Bureau. *Health diary: My baby, myself*. (DHHS Pub. No. HRSA-MCHB-92-4). Washington, DC: U.S. Government Printing Office, 1992.
14. National Center for Health Statistics. Advance report of final natality statistics, 1989. *Monthly Vital Statistics Report*. 1991;40(suppl 8).
15. National Center for Health Statistics. Advance report of final natality statistics, 1989. *Monthly Vital Statistics Report*. 1991;40(suppl 8).
16. Kessel, W., Kiely, M., Nora, A.H., and Sumaya, C.V. Early discharge: In the end its judgment. *Pediatrics*. 1995;96:739–742.
17. Institute of Population Problems, Ministry of Health and Welfare. *Annual report*. Tokyo: Government of Japan, 1993.
18. U.S. Department of Health and Human Services, Public Health Service, Centers for Disease Control and Prevention, National Center for Health Statistics. *Health United States 1996–97*. (DHHS Pub. No. PHS-97-1232-7-0248). Washington, DC: U.S. Government Printing Office, 1997.
19. Kogan, M.D., Martin, J.A., Alexander, G.R., Kotelchuck, M., Ventura, S.J., and Frigoletto, F.D. The changing pattern of prenatal care utilization in the United States, 1981–1995, using different prenatal care indices. *JAMA*. 1998;279:1623–1628.
20. *Encarta concise encyclopedia*. Encarta Online, 1998 Edition.

25

Sexually Transmitted Diseases in the United States

ROBERT E. FULLILOVE

Sexually transmitted diseases (STDs) are a tremendous health and economic burden on the people of the United States. More than 12 million Americans are infected with STDs each year. In 1995, STDs accounted for 87 percent of all cases reported among the top ten most frequently reported diseases in the United States. Of the top ten diseases, five are STDs (i.e., chlamydial infection, gonorrhea, AIDS, primary and secondary syphilis, and hepatitis B virus infection).[1]

STDs: The Hidden Epidemic

Sexually transmitted diseases in the United States have a distinctly American character. Linked with sexual behavior, STDs are not discussed openly and frankly by policymakers or by the average American. As a result, *The Hidden Epidemic: Confronting Sexually Transmitted Diseases*[1] was produced by a 16-member committee of the Institute of Medicine (IOM) in order to bring to light a topic that remains in the shadows of public consciousness. Prominent among the committee's findings was that the rates of syphilis and gonorrhea in the United States were several times higher than those reported in other developed countries. (Table 25.1).

The report concludes that most American adults are poorly informed about STDs, apart from a general awareness of the causes of acquired immunodeficiency syndrome (AIDS). For example, most American women (89% according to a survey conducted in 1993) do not know that STDs are more harmful to women than they are to men. The consequences of this lack of awareness are considerable. It results in a

TABLE 25.1

Rates of Syphilis and Gonorrhea in the United States and Other Countries in the Developed World, 1995

	Syphilis Rates	**Gonorrhea Rates**
United States	6.3	149.5
Germany	1.4	4.9
England	1.0	34.1
Sweden	0.8	3.0
Canada	0.4	18.6
Denmark	0.4	5.5

Cases per 100,000 persons per year.
Source: Institute of Medicine. *The hidden epidemic: Confronting sexually transmitted diseases.* Washington, DC: National Academy Press, 1997.

failure to respond vigorously and effectively to a real and present threat. Lack of awareness on the part of clinical personnel also causes a failure to screen thoroughly and effectively for STDs, as evidenced by the high rates of STD infection in men and women who are both asymptomatic and unaware that they may have been exposed.[1]

The report also notes an alarming rise in viral STDs. Rates of herpes simplex, human papillomavirus (HPV), and viral hepatitis are particularly prevalent in the general population. An estimated 24 million Americans are infected with HPV; 200,000 to 500,000 cases of genital herpes are reported each year in the United States; and approximately one half of the 200,000 cases of hepatitis B reported each year result from sexual intercourse. The association between certain strains of HPV and a variety of genital and cervical cancers contributes to the already high mortality rates associated with the number one viral STD, human immunodeficiency virus (HIV).

Poverty and race are critical factors in the persistence of curable STDs such as syphilis and gonorrhea[2] among sexually active Americans. The residential patterns of rich and poor in the United States create geographically distinct pockets of poor people of color.[3] These areas are important predictors of where a variety of public health problems from violence to STDs are prevalent.[4] Aral concludes "Apparently, it is the combined effects of poverty, minority race-ethnicity, and geographic clustering that influence STD rates."[2]

Specifically, Aral's observations reflect the three most obvious trends in STD prevalence in the United States:

1. STD rates vary by age and race in the United States; gonorrhea, syphilis, and HIV, for example, are significantly more prevalent among young blacks and Hispanics than among whites.[2]

2. STDs cluster geographically in certain neighborhoods as well as within social networks that often do not have distinct spatial, neighborhood, or community boundaries.[5,6]

3. Poverty is an important risk factor in STD prevalence, particularly within communities with limited access to affordable screening and health care services.[1]

FACTORS DRIVING STD INFECTION IN THE UNITED STATES

Aral[7] cites seven behavioral trends that contribute to exposure to a sexually transmitted infection (Table 25.2).

TABLE 25.2

Seven Behavioral Risk Factors for STD Infection

1. Initiation of sexual behavior at an early age
2. Multiple sexual partners
3. One or more sexual partners at high risk for an STD
4. Frequency of intercourse (particularly anal intercourse)
5. Uncircumcised male partner
6. Use of vaginal douche
7. Failure to use condoms or barrier contraceptives consistently

Source: Aral as cited in Institute of Medicine. *The hidden epidemic: Confronting sexually transmitted diseases.* Washington, DC: National Academy Press, 1997.

Because STDs are preventable, the failure of many sexually active individuals to consistently use condoms and other means of barrier protection is frequently cited as a major contributing factor to STD epidemics in the United States as well as being an appropriate target for STD prevention programs. Catania and colleagues[8] observe that respondents to two waves of the National AIDS Behavioral Survey between 1990 and 1992 reported a significant increase in condom use among those with multiple sexual partners. The authors also cite data suggesting that total condom sales in the United States also increased during this period. Similar trends were reported by the IOM.[1]

However, despite the evidence of increased condom use, the majority of respondents to national surveys report that they use condoms rarely or never.[8] Moreover, the investigators raise concerns about patterns of movement into and out of the pool of persons at risk for HIV and other sexually transmitted diseases and the impact that this movement has on consistent condom use. Changes in risk behaviors, they note, may be the result of change in marital or sexual relationships in which an individual acquires a new partner (or loses one), concern about acquiring a sexually transmitted disease (and, as a result, changing one's sexual risk-taking behaviors), or exposure to an STD (and deciding to change one's risk-taking behavior to prevent a reoccurrence). Marriage, however, is not always associated with a positive change in risk behaviors.

We have found that heterosexuals with a history of risk factors for HIV seldom obtain testing prior to cohabitation or marriage and do not regularly use condoms after establishment of the relationship. Furthermore, the present study suggests that married people reporting extramarital sexual partners are typically the least likely to use condoms or obtain HIV testing.[8]

CONTROL STRATEGIES FOR THE MANAGEMENT OF STDS

Control of STDs in the United States has long been based on a dual strategy of case finding and treatment, a series of policies first recommended and instituted for the U.S. Public Health Service by Surgeon General Thomas Parran in 1936.[9] Case finding involves three basic steps:

1. Screening for infected individuals for the presence of disease
2. Testing and identification of those infected
3. The screening, testing, and treatment of the sexual contacts of those who have been infected

The tracing of sexual contacts is perhaps the most difficult of these steps. Two methods are typically used: notification of possibly exposed sexual partners by the infected individual and notification of partners by health workers. This strategy is based on a concept that likens sexual behavior to a branching tree with the infected person as the "trunk" and the individual's partners as the "branches."[6] If a public health worker, called a disease intervention specialist (DIS), could either convince the "case" to inform his or her partners or cases and contacts could be treated and the force of an epidemic outbreak might be significantly diminished.

The close connection between crack cocaine use, sexually transmitted disease,[6,10,11] and the social contacts between drug users and sex workers has helped STD researchers refine their notions about how STDs are propagated. The rapid expansion of crack use in the United States in the mid-1980s was associated with a new form of prostitution—the exchange of sex for drugs and/or money that typically occurred among members of neighborhood-based social networks. Men and women in these networks who were without the funds to support their cocaine addiction were often encouraged to provide "sexual favors" in exchange for the drug, thus creating a sexual barter system that coincidentally provided a new, efficient means for a variety of sexually transmitted infections to be disseminated. Outbreaks of syphilis in the rural South[12] and HIV infection within inner city communities[11] were reported among members of social networks linked by kinship and friendship ties and through networks of individuals who purchased and used drugs together. Ethnographic research that seeks to identify the "nodes" or "lots" within these networks (individuals who are considered links between cases and their contacts) became crucial for identifying the routes of transmission and dissemination of disease.[6]

One of the most effective examples of STD control was reported by Hibbs and Gunn in combating a crack cocaine–related outbreak of syphilis in Chester, Pennsylvania. The Health Department recognized that standard efforts to trace contacts and their partners would fail because of the anonymous nature of crack-related sex work. They targeted an aggressive screening program within the neighborhoods where crack was known to be widely sold and used. During a 6-day period in April 1989, 136 persons were screened, among whom 25 were found to have syphilis. Included within this group were a higher proportion of early latent cases than are typically reported using standard case finding techniques. The authors noted that there was an overall decline in cases after this aggressive campaign, suggesting that this targeted intervention may have played an important role in reducing the spread of infection.

A number of environmental settings have been created by the intersection of drug epidemics and sexually transmitted diseases that are natural targets for similar approaches. As Blank and colleagues noted, the nation's prisons are a particularly important locale for identifying men and women exposed to STDs.

New York City's only women's correctional facility admits about 12,500 women annually. Because prostitution and drug-related arrests are the most frequent charges, inmates are at high risk for having syphilis and, if not treated, for delivering congenitally infected babies.[13]

The authors described a very effective, aggressive screening campaign in which 685 remanded were given full medical examinations, screened for STDs during a 5-month period in 1993, further screened using the local syphilis case registry, and treated, if and when necessary. Results were dramatic: Syphilis treatment rates increased from 7% to 84% among women with indications for treatment and to 88% among pregnant women with indications for treatment.[13] More importantly, a prospective follow-up of pregnant inmates revealed no spontaneous abortions and eight live births. Of these eight births, only one infant required treatment for congenital syphilis, a finding that was directly attributed to the treatment received during incarceration.[13]

This study reflects a number of important lessons about how to remove barriers to providing syphilis and STD control in correctional facilities. First, aggressive screening, testing, and treatment must be instituted before inmates are released. Blank and colleagues[13] noted that the turnaround time for most serologies (5 to 7 days) was longer than the average time inmates were detained in the facility (median stay, 5 days); thus, inmates who would have been lost to follow-up were rapidly identified and treated because of the speed with which screening and testing were done. Second, having on-line computer access to the syphilis registry increased the efficiency of case finding and treatment efforts significantly. Third, and perhaps most importantly, these strategies are also likely to be particularly effective in other risk settings that are the unique product of the interaction between drugs, sexual behavior, and the economic decline of many United States inner city and rural communities.[4] Thus, in addition to correctional facilities, screening and treatment campaigns in homeless shelters, drug treatment facilities, and health clinics serving migrant populations should prove to be particularly effective in locating hard-to-reach populations that would not normally seek treatment at public STD clinics or in the offices of private medical providers.[13]

PREVENTION PROGRAMS

The IOM report[1] made recommendations for the formulation of a national strategy for STD control (Table 25.3).

The targets for behavioral change are largely individuals and health care facilities. Thus, programs to create healthy sexual relationships, to educate adolescents and members of underserved populations about STDs, and to conduct outreach and innovative service delivery programs arise from the view that the sexually active (or potentially active) individual must be the object of education, behavioral change, and improved clinical outreach and treatment programs.

Potterat,[5] however, takes a slightly different view. He cited the importance of the social network in the exposure to an STD and its role in the propagation of an infection to other network members. He described the concept of sociogeography to define the social and spatial location connections among individuals as they meet one another,

---

TABLE 25.3

Four Major Strategies Recommended by the Institute of Medicine (1997) to Establish a National System for STD Prevention

1. Overcome barriers to adoption of healthy sexual behaviors.
2. Develop strong leadership, strengthen investment, and improve information systems for STD prevention.
3. Design and implement essential STD-related services in innovative ways for adolescents and underserved populations.
4. Ensure access to and quality of essential clinical services for STDs.

share social experiences (including the use of alcohol and drugs, as well as dating and having sex), spend time at certain sites (bars, crack houses, community centers, churches, and schools, for example), and then repeat this cycle of activities with other individuals over a period of weeks, months, or even years. STD risk, he theorized, is best understood by examining how such behaviors are expressed and are embedded in the sociogeographic area that provides the critical niche for the survival of an STD epidemic. He concluded

The unit of STD transmission analysis and of intervention (including vaccination strategies) should be the social network rather than the individual. Core groups (of STD transmitters) are, after all, about groups, not individuals. Reaching the socially ("opinion leaders") and sexually (frequent partner change) important actors in core networks is crucial because individual behavior is best influenced by influencing network norms. As for resources to wage socio-geographic space wars against STDs, the need is for rifles, not shotguns.[5]

CONCLUSION

The "hidden epidemic" of STDs is one of the nation's most critical health problems. It is largely, but not entirely, driven by the set of social and economic changes that have dominated life in the United States during the latter part of the 20th century. Poverty, racism, drug use, crime, and incarceration are important factors in the propagation of syphilis, HIV, and other STDs, but the lack of awareness of the average American about these infections also contributes significantly to rising rates of viral STDs such as herpes and HPV.

The tragedy is that these infections can be prevented. Thus, the morbidity and mortality with which STDs are associated represent one of the principal ironies of modern life. Despite our technology, our advanced medical science, and improved detection capacity, many sexually active Americans fail to use condoms or other methods of barrier protection and needlessly expose themselves to infection. The fact that the majority of American adults know that condoms prevent HIV and other STDs makes the current rates of infection all the more unacceptable.

Our national inability to deal with the conditions that have made the nation's prisons a reservoir for HIV and other STDs must also be acknowledged. With the United States among the world leaders in the incarceration of its own citizens (only Russia imprisons a larger proportion), it is essential that we as a nation act aggressively to find alternatives to prisons, or, at the very least, to create programs that will effectively screen and treat the at-risk populations who find themselves in detention. The "hidden epidemic" is a threat that will not go away by itself; simply put, it cannot be ignored.

References

1. Institute of Medicine. *The hidden epidemic: Confronting sexually transmitted disease.* Washington, DC: National Academy Press, 1997.
2. Aral, S. The social context of syphilis persistence in the southern United States. *Sexually Transmitted Diseases.* 1996;23:9–16.
3. Massey, D.S., Gross, A.B., and Shibuya, K. Migration, segregation, and the geographic concentration of poverty. *The American Sociological Review.* 1994;59:425–445.
4. Wallace, R., Wallace, D., Andrews, H., Fullilove, R., and Fullilove, M.T. The spatiotemporal dynamics of AIDS and TB in the New York City metropolitan region from a socio-geographic perspective: Understanding the linkages of central city and suburbs. *Environment and Planning A.* 1995;27:1085–1108.
5. Potterat, J.J. Socio-geographic space and sexually transmissible diseases in the 1990s. *Today's Life Science.* 1992;12:16–31.
6. Rothenberg, R., and Narramore, J. Commentary: The relevance of social network concepts to sexually transmitted disease control. *Sexually Transmitted Diseases.* 1996;23:24–29.
7. Aral, S.O. Sexual behavior in sexually transmitted disease research: An overview. *Sexually Transmitted Diseases.* March–April, 1994;21(Suppl):S59–S64.
8. Catania, J.A., Binson, D., Dolcini, M., Stall, R., Choi, K.Y., Pollack, L.M., et al. Risk factors for HIV and other sexually transmitted diseases and prevention practices among U.S. heterosexual adults: Changes from 1990 to 1992. *American Journal of Public Health.* 1995;85:1492–1499.
9. Oxman, G.L., and Doyle, L. A comparison of case-finding effectiveness and average costs of screening. *Sexually Transmitted Diseases.* 1996;23:51–57.
10. Fullilove, R.E., Fullilove, M.T., Bowser, B.P., and Gross, S.A. Risk of sexually transmitted disease among Black adolescent crack users in Oakland and San Francisco, Calif. *Journal of the American Medical Association.* 1990;263:851–855.
11. Edlin, B.R., Irwin, K.L., Faruque, S., McCoy, C.B., Clyde, B., Word, C., et al. Intersecting epidemics—crack cocaine use and HIV infection among inner city young adults. *New England Journal of Medicine.* 1994;331:1422–1427.
12. Nakashima, A.K., Rolfs, R.T., Flock, M.L., Kilmarx, P., and Greenspan, J.R. Epidemiology of syphilis in the United States, 1941–1993. *Sexually Transmitted Diseases.* 1996;23:16–23.
13. Blank, S., McDonnell, D.D., Rubin, S.R., Neal, J.J., Brome, M.W., Masterson, M.B., and Greenspan, J.R. New approaches to syphilis control: Finding opportunities for syphilis treatment and congenital syphilis prevention in a women's correctional setting. *Sexually Transmitted Diseases.* 1997;24:218–228.

26

AIDS *in the United States: The Changing Epidemic*

Robert E. Fullilove

DEMOGRAPHICS

In 1996, a number of important changes were observed in the epidemic of human immunodeficiency virus (HIV) and acquired immunodeficiency syndrome (AIDS) in the United States. What had begun principally as an epidemic among gay white men in 1981 had become an epidemic of people of color by 1996. That year, of the 69,151 new cases reported, 38% of the patients were white, 19% were Hispanic, and 41% were black. The disproportionate impact of HIV disease in communities of color was also reflected in the variation in the rates of cases per 100,000 among the principal race/ethnic groups in the United States. Blacks were most significantly affected (89.7 per 100,000 as compared with 13.5 per 100,000 among whites); Asian/Pacific Islanders (5.9 per 100,000), by contrast, were least affected.[1]

Women constituted an increasing proportion of the cases reported in 1996 among adults and adolescents (20%), and the proportion of cases among men who have sex with men declined to 50% of this total. Black women accounted for slightly less than 60% of the 13,820 cases reported among women in 1996. Significantly, heterosexual contact with a person at risk for HIV was the exposure factor that accounted for the majority of cases among black women (37%), followed closely by history of intravenous drug use.[1] HIV disease among black women also was responsible for the high prevalence of black children (63%) among the 678 pediatric AIDS cases reported in 1996.

Despite the fact that every state in the United States reported at least one case in 1996, more than 50% of all cases reported that year were concentrated in five states: California, New York, Florida, Texas, and New Jersey. The epidemic has a distinctly urban character as well: Rates per 100,000 in metropolitan areas with 500,000 or more per population (36.9) were four times those in non-metropolitan areas (8.7). New York City, which has approximately 0.5% of the United States adult population, had 15% of the cases reported to the Centers for Disease Control and Prevention in 1996. Rates per 100,000 in two of the poorest neighborhoods of color in New York City—Central Harlem and the South Bronx—were 34 times those for New York City as a whole and 120 times the national average, according to the New York City Department of Health. Thus, although not formally identified as an exposure category for HIV infection in traditional AIDS surveillance reports, poverty must be considered one of the greatest risk factors for HIV/AIDS in the United States and throughout most of the developing world.[2]

CHANGING TRENDS

Despite the continued pattern of change in the profile of United States AIDS cases, the most important change in the character of the epidemic in the United States was the significant decline in the number of deaths among those infected with HIV.

Deaths among persons reported with AIDS declined 23 percent in 1996 compared with 1995, with the largest declines occurring during the last three quarters of 1996. From 1995 to 1996, deaths declined in all four geographic regions: (West [33%], Midwest [25%], Northeast [22%], and South [19%]), among men and women, among all racial/ethnic groups, and in all risk/exposure categories.[3]

These changes, although encouraging, do not necessarily signal the end of the epidemic or the moment to sound the "all clear." HIV disease was a leading cause of death in the United States among persons aged 25 to 44 in 1996, and the epidemic continues to expand within new populations of heterosexuals.[3]

Use of crack cocaine has been increasingly cited as a significant risk factor for HIV infection. Women with a history of engaging in sex work associated with crack cocaine use appear to be particularly at risk.[4,5] In an HIV seroprevalence study conducted in three inner-city neighborhoods (New York City, Miami, and San Francisco) in the early 1990s, the prevalence of HIV infection among crack-smoking women was reported to be 29.6% in New York City and 23% in Miami. Engaging in sex for drugs or money was the principal risk factor in both samples, but sexually transmitted diseases, including syphilis (reported by 80% of the crack smokers in this study) and herpes, were also independently associated with HIV infection. The study's authors concluded: "Thus, our data support the possibility that the spread of sexually transmitted diseases among crack smokers facilitates the spread of HIV."[5]

Prisons are also important factors in the dynamic that maintains the HIV/AIDS epidemic in poor communities of color, particularly in the New York metropolitan area.[6,7] The "War on Drugs," begun during the Reagan Administration in the 1980s, has been widely cited as a major factor in the dramatic increase in the adult prison population during that decade. In 1991, for example, 61% of the inmates in the federal prison system were serving time for a drug-related crime.[8] Given the intersection between drug use and HIV infection and national policies to create a criminal justice solution to the nation's drug problem, it was inevitable that prisons would become significant reservoirs for HIV infection.

Conclusive evidence of such a trend was provided by a 1994 survey conducted by the Centers for Disease Control and Prevention with the co-sponsorship of the National Institute of Justice among the 50 state prison systems for adults. The 5,270 AIDS cases reported in that survey among the national inmate population represented a rate of 5.2 per 1,000, six times that reported for the United States adult population. Four factors contributed to these rates:

1. A prison population with significant numbers of HIV infected persons and/or those with risk factors for such infection
2. The prevalence of risky drug use and risky sexual behavior in many prisons
3. The release of the vast majority of prisoners to their communities of origin
4. High rates of recidivism, re-incarceration, and reconfinement among this population[9]

The War on Drugs that created this population of inmates has public health consequences that are potentially devastating. The cycling of men and women in and out of the prison system and back to their communities seems certain to ensure that HIV will maintain its ecological niche in poor communities and perhaps provide the reservoir from which it can spread to more affluent communities as well.[10,11]

Ultimately, the War on Drugs has created a much bigger problem than the one it was designed to solve. It is entirely possible that out of a desire to provide a cost-effective, morally acceptable, criminal justice response to the nation's substance use and abuse, an effective engine for expanding and disseminating the devastation of the HIV epidemic has been created instead.[11]

Wallace has argued that the prevalence of large numbers of AIDS cases in poor communities in New York is a symptom of their social, economic, and political collapse. HIV/AIDS in areas such as the South Bronx is just one component of a series of calamities confronting this community, including high rates of homicide, tuberculosis, substance abuse, infant mortality, and violent crime. This "synergy of plagues" creates a highly unstable public health crisis that is likely to result, among other outcomes, in a failure of the epidemic to remain neatly confined within the inner city.[12,13]

The changing face of AIDS in the United States already provides such evidence. In addition to its geographic spread, HIV has demonstrated the capacity to leapfrog from one population to another (e.g., gay men to injection drug users) and to make use of a variety of risk behaviors (e.g., unprotected sexual intercourse, sharing infected drug injection equipment) in gaining access to new populations.[2]

TREATMENT ISSUES

For now, the principal hope for the containment of the epidemic rests in the recent development in antiviral drug therapies. As recent trends suggest,[3] these therapies have achieved remarkable results. The new drugs—protease inhibitors (PIs)—inhibit protease enzyme function, a necessary step in the creation of new HIV virus. Saquinavir (Invirase) was the first of these drugs to receive approval from the United States Food and Drug Administration (FDA), followed by ritonavir (Norvir) and indinavir (Crixivan).[14] In combination, these three protease inhibitors have demonstrated the capacity to reduce the amount of HIV RNA in the blood (referred to as the "viral load") to undetectable levels.

Stine[14] points out that it is probably much too premature to believe that the current effectiveness of these new medications will bring us one step closer to a cure. The long-term impact of the drugs on the body is not known, and the possibility remains that HIV simply takes refuge in the central nervous system or in the lymph nodes when under attack from antiretrovirals. Thus, the failure to detect it in the blood does not permit us to claim that its threat has been removed or that it will not re-emerge at some later point.

There are other, perhaps more significant, problems associated with these new drugs, however. They are only effective if a complex regimen is followed. It is not unusual, for example, to prescribe as many as 15 or more pills per day for some patients, and even the most assiduous pill takers report that they are, at times, confused as to what they have taken and which pill should be taken next. The consequences of failing to follow the regimen strictly can be severe. There is evidence that skipping the medication may result in the development of a strain of HIV that (1) is resistant to these drugs, (2) will be more virulent than the strains we are currently observing, and (3) may be passed on to others if safe sex and/or safe drug use practices are not used.[14]

The anger of a resistant new form of the virus and the possibility that it would be transmitted to a sufficiently large number of individuals is a frightening scenario. It invokes images of a more destructive epidemic than the one we are confronting at present and has led many clinicians to question the wisdom of giving these drugs to individuals who are, in their perception, very likely to be at high risk of failing to adhere to the strict regimen. Thus, many drug addicts, many individuals with a psychiatric disorder, and many homeless persons are believed to be treatment risks and are, in some places, denied these medications.

These beliefs appear to arise more from prejudice than from scientific evidence. Adherence to a complex drug regimen has been demonstrated to be uniformly difficult in studies of tuberculosis, hypertension, and diabetes, irrespective of race, class, ethnicity, or exposure status.[14] Thus, there are few data that suggest that drug users or homeless persons are greater treatment risks for antiretrovirals than any other group of individuals in treatment.

Refusal to treat poses enormous ethical dilemmas. There is the suspicion, for example, that the motivation to treat only certain patients arises from economic, rather than medical, considerations. Given the expense of the new therapies ($1,000 per month is not unusual for a patient on combination therapies), this suspicion is difficult to dispel. With the costs out of reach of all but the most well-to-do patients, many persons living with and/or affected by the disease can gain access to the newest treatments only if they are receiving government subsidies or if they are participants in a clinical trial.

The problem is dramatically exacerbated in the developing world, where there are many nations without the financial resources to pay for even very modest condom distribution programs, much less the expensive technologies necessary to test, monitor, adjust, and assess the progress of a patient receiving similarly costly combination drug therapies. The ethical questions surrounding who is entitled to such therapies and who should pay for them continue to be raised.[14]

Perinatal HIV/AIDS and the appropriate treatment of infants and mothers infected with HIV pose particularly challenging ethical issues. The first challenge is posed by the recognition that there is an effective prophylaxis for HIV disease in children, namely zidovudine (AZT). In clinical trial ACTG076 (AIDS Clinical Trial Group), researchers reported a dramatic reduction in the rates of babies born with an HIV infection.[15] Given the current recommendation that monotherapies (such as AZT) are "no longer a recommended option for treatment of HIV-infected persons," the first draft of the report of the NIH Panel to Define Principles of Therapy of HIV Infection noted

One exception is the use of zidovudine according to the ACTG076 (AIDS Clinical Trial Group) regimen specifically for the purpose of reducing the rate of perinatal HIV transmission in pregnant women who have not yet decided to initiate antiretroviral therapy based on their own health indications.[16]

A number of ethicists have criticized this draft report for its failure to explore more fully the problems created by asking mothers to make choices between their own health and that of their unborn child.

They note that the only contraindication for combination antiviral therapies arises when AZT should be used to reduce the risk of HIV infection in a neonate. With little clinical evidence about the impact of combination therapies on children or infants, critics have asserted that these recommendations speak more to our national biases against a woman's right to control her health and less to what can be based on sound, scientific recommendations.

What is known is that the risk of perinatal transmission is greatest during the first trimester of a pregnancy. Evidence suggests that perhaps as many as 90% of pediatric AIDS patients were infected during this period.[14] The NIH panel's recommendation, therefore, has been to suggest the initiation of viral therapies after the first 14 weeks, and to use AZT.

Treatment recommendations for HIV-infected pregnant women are based on the belief that therapies of known benefit to women should not be withheld during pregnancy unless there are known adverse effects on the mother, fetus, or infant that outweigh the potential benefit to the woman.[17] In general, pregnancy should not compromise optimal HIV therapy for the mother.[16]

The recommendations are directed to women who know their HIV status and who will be able to consult with treatment providers to make appropriate decisions about the best course of treatment to pursue during the first trimester. Many women do not know their status, however, and are not aware that they may be at risk. This lack of awareness combined with the advent of new drug therapies has dramatically increased the call for mandatory HIV testing of pregnant women, precisely because there now exist a variety of treatment options that were not previously available. The fear that mandatory testing would drive many women at risk to avoid both treatment and testing—out of the fear of being stigmatized and discriminated against—is no longer valid, critics assert, because early detection is essential to beginning an effective course of treatment.

The high rates of pediatric AIDS among blacks and Hispanics only complicate this debate. Although these two groups constitute less than 20% of the United States population, they account for 75% of the pediatric AIDS cases reported in the United States since the beginning of the epidemic. Mandatory testing policies will inevitably be directed to communities of color with high seroprevalence rates and high rates of pediatric AIDS cases. Thus, New York City, Newark, and Miami, the cities with the largest number of pediatric AIDS cases in the United States, are particularly important targets for such campaigns.

The political risks involved are considerable. Such a policy will have a disproportionately large impact on the small number of communities that are epicenters for HIV infection. These areas are likely to be confronted with a surge in the number of cases whose treatment will be the responsibility of an already overburdened public health system. But the call to increase surveillance efforts has already been made.

*Although AIDS surveillance continues to be essential for understanding reasons for the lack of timely access to HIV testing and care and the failure of treatment regimens to delay HIV disease progression, HIV surveillance is becoming increasingly important as more infected persons receive effective antiretroviral therapy. In June, 1997, the Council of State and Territorial Epidemiologists (CSTE) recommended that all states implement HIV case reporting **by name** from health-care providers and laboratories.*[18] [emphasis added]

CONCLUSION

The changing face of the AIDS epidemic brings with it a curious blend of optimism and ethical confusion. The continuing growth in the number of infected individuals in the United States in a variety of infected individuals in the United States in a variety of different geographic regions and among a variety of different population groups—particularly poor people of color—is mirrored by unprecedented improvements in the therapies used to combat the disease. HIV/AIDS remains an enormous drain on health care resources. The advent of effective but expensive new therapies is a cause for optimism among those who can afford them and despair among those who cannot. Meeting the needs of this population and containing the epidemic will force local, state, and federal governments to make a number of hard and potentially costly decisions. Mandatory testing of pregnant women (and eventually all persons at potential risk for HIV infection) will, with little doubt, become a public health necessity by the year 2000. Increasingly sophisticated methods for testing for HIV and for using diagnostic data to target effective medical interventions will make it ethically impossible not to diagnose and treat every potential case of HIV infection.

The costs of containment using aggressive diagnostic and treatment strategies will probably be less than the costs of treating individuals with AIDS who are diagnosed late in the progression of HIV disease. But the pressures on a democracy to respect individual rights, on the one hand, and respond effectively to a severe public health crisis, on the other, are considerable. The drama will ultimately play itself out in poor communities of color, already wary of a public health establishment that created and sanctioned programs such as the

Tuskegee Syphilis Study. There seems little doubt that the battle against HIV/AIDS during the close of the 20th century will, quite simply, define the practice of public health in the year 2000.

References

1. CDC (Centers for Disease Control and Prevention). *HIV/AIDS Surveillance Report.* 1996;8:1–39.
2. Mann, J., and Tarantola, D. *AIDS in the world II.* New York: Oxford University Press, 1996.
3. CDC. Update: Trends in AIDS incidence—United States, 1996. *MMWR.* 1997;46: 861–867, 884–885.
4. Institute of Medicine (IOM). *The hidden epidemic: Confronting sexually transmitted diseases.* Washington, DC: National Academy Press, 1997.
5. Edlin, B.R., Irwin, K.L., Faruque, S., McCoy, C.B., Word, C., Serrano, Y., et al. Intersecting epidemics—Crack cocaine use and HIV infection among inner-city young adults. *New England Journal of Medicine.* 1994;331:1422–1427.
6. Garrett, L. *The coming plague: Newly emerging disease in a world out of balance.* New York: Farrar, Strouss and Giroux, 1994.
7. Fullilove, R.E., and Fullilove, M.T. *Community disintegration and public health: A case study of New York.* (submitted for publication).
8. DiMascio, W.M., Mauer, M., ad DiJulia, K. *Seeking justice: Crime and punishment in America.* New York: Edna McConnell Clark Foundation, 1995.
9. CDC. HIV/AIDS education and prevention programs for adults in prisons and jails and juvenile confinement facilities: United States, 1994. *MMWR.* 1996;45:268–271.
10. Wallace, R., Wallace, D., Andrews, H., Fullilove, R., and Fullilove, M.T. The spatiotemporal dynamics of AIDS and TB in the New York metropolitan region from a sociogeographic perspective: Understanding the linkages of central city and suburbs. *Environment and Planning A.* 1995;27:1085–1108.
11. Fullilove, R.E. Substance abuse and public policy in the United States: A war on drugs or managed care for treatment. *Current Issues in Public Health.* 1996;2:68–73.
12. Wallace, R. A synergism of plagues: "Planned shrinkage," contagious housing destruction, and AIDS in the Bronx. *Environmental Research.* 1988;47:1–33.
13. Gould, P., and Wallace, R. Spatial structures and scientific paradoxes in the AIDS pandemic. *Geografiska Annaler.* 1994;76B:105–116.
14. Stine, G. *AIDS update 1997.* Upper Saddle River, NJ: Prentice Hall, 1997.
15. CDC. U.S. Public Health Service recommendations for HIV counseling and voluntary testing for pregnant women. *MMWR.* 1995;44:1–12.
16. National Institutes of Health. *Report of the NIH Panel to Define Principles of Therapy of HIV Infection.* [Draft Report]. Washington, DC: NIH, 1997, pp 10, 14.
17. Minkoff, H., and Augenbraun, M. Antiretroviral therapy for pregnant women. *American Journal of Obstetrics and Gynecology.* 1997;176:478–489.
18. Council of State and Territorial Epidemiologists (CSTE). 1997.

27

Nutrition Issues for Mothers, Children, Youth, and Families

MARY STORY AND LISA HARNACK

Nutrition is essential for sustenance, health, and well-being throughout the life cycle. For the past few decades, as the relationship between diet and health and disease has become more clear, increased attention has been placed on the importance of preventive nutrition. Nutritional status is associated with diet-related conditions such as overweight, high serum cholesterol levels, hypertension, and osteoporosis, which increases the risk of certain chronic diseases in adults such as coronary heart disease, stroke, type II diabetes, and bone fracture.[1,2] Among children, nutritional status can affect growth and development, resistance to disease, and risk for future chronic diseases.[3] Nutritional status both preconceptionally and during pregnancy has an impact on pregnancy and infant outcomes.

With the close of the 20th century, it is of interest to review the most pertinent nutrition-related concerns affecting Americans. This chapter reviews the public health nutrition concerns affecting populations in the United States, focusing primarily on pregnant women, children, adolescents, and families. The Healthy People 2000: Na-

---

TABLE 27.1

Healthy People 2000: Selected Key Nutrition-Related Objectives for Mothers and Children

---

- Reduce overweight to a prevalence of no more than 20% among people aged 20 and older and no more than 15% among adolescents aged 12–19.
- Reduce growth retardation among low-income children aged 5 and younger to less than 10%.
- Reduce dietary fat intake to an average of 30% of calories or less and average saturated fat intake to less than 10% of calories among people aged 2 and older.
- Increase complex carbohydrates and fiber-containing foods in the diets of people aged 2 and older to an average of 5 or more daily servings of vegetables and fruits and to an average of 6 or more daily servings of grain products.
- Increase calcium intake so at least 50% of people aged 11–24 and 50% of pregnant and lactating women consume an average of 3 or more daily servings of foods rich in calcium, and at least 75% of children aged 2–10 and 50% of people aged 35 and older consume an average of 2 or more servings daily.
- Reduce iron deficiency to less than 3% among children aged 1–4 and among women of childbearing age.
- Increase to at least 75% the proportion of mothers who breastfeed their babies in the early postpartum period and to at least 50% the proportion who continue breastfeeding until their babies are at least 5–6 months old.
- Increase to at least 85% the proportion of mothers who achieve the minimum recommended weight gain during their pregnancies.
- Reduce the incidence of spina bifida and other neural tube defects to 3 per 10,000 live births.

Source: U.S. Department of Health and Human Services. *Healthy People 2000: National health promotion and disease prevention objectives.* Washington, DC: Public Health Service, 1991.

tional Health Promotion and Disease Prevention Objectives[1,4] provide priority areas for public health efforts. The first part of this chapter focuses on the nutrition-related objectives (Table 27.1) that pertain to pregnant women, mothers, children, and adolescents. The second part of the chapter briefly describes the federal food assistance programs and the potential impact of the recent welfare legislation. The last part of the chapter presents strategic nutrition plans for the 21st century for improving diet and nutritional health.

PRIORITY NUTRITION CONCERNS

Overweight

Obesity is one of the most pervasive public health problems in the United States. Overweight adults are at increased risk for morbidity and mortality associated with many acute and chronic medical conditions, including hypertension, dyslipidemia, coronary heart disease, diabetes mellitus, gallbladder disease, respiratory disease, some types of cancer, gout, and arthritis.[5] Overweight during childhood and adolescence is associated with overweight during adulthood and has also been linked to subsequent morbidity and mortality in adulthood.[1] The United States is experiencing an epidemic of obesity among adults, children, and adolescents. Studies since the 1980s have shown a dramatic increase in the prevalence of overweight among all age groups.[5-7]

The prevalence of overweight varies considerably by age, gender, and race (Table 27.2). The most recent data on the prevalence of overweight in the United States are derived from the Third National Health and Nutrition Examination Survey, 1988–1994 (NHANES III) conducted by the National Center for Health Statistics. Among adults, 33% of men and 36% of women were overweight.[5] Overweight is particularly prevalent among women of color. Thirty-four percent of non-Hispanic white adult women were overweight, whereas 52% of non-Hispanic blacks and 50% of Mexican Americans were overweight.[5] Poverty is also related to overweight in women. For example, in NHANES II, 37% of women with incomes below the poverty level were overweight compared with 25% of those above the poverty level.[1]

In NHANES III, 8% of 4- to 5-year-olds, 14% of children aged 6 to 11 years, and 12% of adolescents aged 12 to 17 years were overweight[6,7] (see Table 27.2). The prevalence of overweight is particularly high among Mexican American youth and African American adolescent girls.

TABLE 27.2

Prevalence of Overweight Among Children, Adolescents, and Adults
(NHANES III, 1988–1994)

	Children (%)			Adolescents (%)	Adults (%)
	2–3 Yr	4–5 Yr	6–11 Yr	11–17 Yr	≥20 Yr
Both sexes	3.4	7.9	13.7	11.5	34.9
Males	2.1	5.0	14.7	12.3	33.3
White, non-Hispanic	1.1	2.7	13.2	11.6	33.7
Black, non-Hispanic	2.8	8.5	14.7	12.5	33.3
Mexican American	6.2	1.0	18.8	15.0	36.4
Females	4.8	10.8	12.5	10.7	36.4
White, non-Hispanic	2.8	9.0	11.9	9.6	33.5
Black, non-Hispanic	5.6	11.2	17.9	16.3	52.3
Mexican American	10.5	13.2	15.8	14.0	50.1

Overweight is defined as:

2–5-year-olds: Weight-for-stature above the 95th percentile of the NCHS reference growth curves.
6–17-year-olds: BMI at or above the sex-and age-specific 95th percentile from National Health Examination Survey cycles 2 and 3.
Adults (≥20 years): BMI ≥27.8 for men and ≥27.3 for women (85th percentiles from NHANES II for ages 20–29 years).
Source: National Center for Health Statistics. Update: Prevalence of overweight among children; adolescents and adults—United States, 1988–1994. *MMWR.* 1997;46(9):199–201; and Ogden, C.L., Troiano, R.P., Briefel, R.R., Kuczmarski, R.J., Flegal, K.M., and Johnson, C.L. Prevalence of overweight among preschool children in the U.S., 1971 through 1994. *Pediatrics.* 1997;99(4) (electronic version).

Overweight is a complex, heterogeneous condition in which genetic, metabolic, environmental, cultural, and socioeconomic factors are involved. Genetic influences largely determine whether a person can become obese, and environmental influences determine the manifestation and extent of the obesity. Overweight occurs as a result of a positive shift in energy balance, when energy intake from food exceeds energy expenditure.[5] It is not clear why the prevalence of obesity has increased substantially over the past several decades, but low physical activity and high-fat and high-calorie diets are likely to be predisposing factors. The food supply in the United States is plentiful, and high-fat, high-energy foods are palatable, inexpensive, and widely available. Results from NHANES III also documented a high prevalence of physical inactivity among adults, and rates of inactivity were greater for women than men and for non-Hispanic blacks and Mexican Americans than non-Hispanic whites.[5] A review of the literature suggests that overweight among children and adolescents may be less associated with increased energy intake than with low physical activity.[7]

To reverse the trend of increasing overweight, dual action is needed in the nutrition and physical activity areas to help Americans reduce their fat consumption, increase fruit and vegetable consumption, and pursue more physical activity.[4] Because overweight disproportionately affects low-income groups, and people of color, such as African American women, Hispanics, and Native Americans, culturally appropriate prevention and intervention programs should be targeted toward these groups. The increasing prevalence of overweight among children indicates that prevention activities aimed at encouraging healthy food choices and increased physical activity need to begin during childhood.

Inadequate or Excessive Dietary Intakes

Dietary Fat. The public health recommendation is that all healthy people older than age 2 reduce dietary fat intake to an average of 30% of calories from fat and average saturated fat intake to less than 10% of calories.[1] Considerable evidence associates diets high in fat with increased risk of obesity, some types of cancer, and gallbladder diseases. There is a strong relationship between saturated fat intake, high blood cholesterol, and increased risk for coronary heart disease.[1,2] The current dietary fat recommendations for children have been criticized because of the possible deleterious effects on growth and development. However, recent large-scale studies with children lowering dietary fat to 28% to 30% of calories, found that growth, sexual maturation, iron stores, or nutritional adequacy were not affected by the dietary intervention.[8,9] Still, given the importance of adequate calories and nutrients for growth and development, careful attention should be placed on ensuring dietary adequacy for children and adolescents.

Results from the most current national food consumption surveys indicate that intakes of total fat and saturated fats have decreased in recent years. In 1988 to 1991, median total fat intake as a percentage of calories was about 34%, down from 36% in 1976 to 1980.[2] Although improvements have been made for all age groups, intakes of total fat and saturated fatty acids remain above recommended levels for a large proportion of the population. Fewer than 20% of children 6 to 17 years of age and only 21% of adult males and 25% of adult females consumed diets containing recommended levels of total fat.[2] Median intakes of total fat and saturated fatty acids were similar for males and females of different racial and ethnic groups.[2]

Fruits and Vegetables. Public health recommendations are that people aged 2 and older consume a minimum of two servings of fruits and three servings of vegetables a day.[4] Higher intakes of fruits and vegetables are associated with reduced risk of a variety of cancers.[1] Increasing the consumption of fruits and vegetables is also likely to reduce overall fat intake. The most recent national estimates reveal that only 32% of adults and 20% of children and adolescents consume five or more servings of fruits and vegetables per day.[10,11] Moreover, nearly 25% of all vegetables consumed by young people were french fries. Fruits tend to be consumed less frequently than vegetables. Over a 3-day period, about 30% of adolescent and adult males and 24% of adult and adolescent females did not eat any fruits, and about 6% of individuals did not eat any vegetables.[2] Lower intakes of fruits and vegetables are even more pronounced in low socioeconomic groups, where cancer incidence among adults is higher.[2] A recent report from the National Cancer Institute compared food intake data collected in 1987 and 1992 surveys using the same food frequency questionnaires. Between 1987 and 1992, the proportions of Americans consuming high-fat foods decreased; however, there was no change in the consumption of fruits and vegetables.[12]

A recent national survey found that only about one quarter of the population is aware of the dietary recommendation for fruits and vegetables.[2] People who were aware that they should eat at least five servings a day consumed more fruits and vegetables than those who thought two or fewer servings were adequate. Future public health campaigns need to promote awareness and behavior change strategies. Special efforts and resources should be directed to low-income populations, addressing personal and environmental barriers to healthy eating, such as accessibility, cost, and quality issues.

Calcium. Calcium is essential for the formation and maintenance of bones and teeth. The level of bone mass achieved at skeletal maturity (peak bone mass) is a factor modifying the risk for developing osteoporosis.[1] Achieving peak bone mass appears to be related to adequate calcium intake in adolescence and early adulthood.[13]

Many people, particularly adolescents and adult females consume less than the recommended amount of calcium. Population-based survey data indicate that only about one half of children aged 2 to 10 met the average daily goal of two or more servings of milk and milk products. Only about one fifth of young people aged 11 to 24 and pregnant and lactating women met the average daily goal of three or more servings of milk and milk products.[4] The same proportion of people aged 25 and older met the average daily goal of two or more servings.[4] The low calcium intakes from food by many adolescents and adults, particularly females, suggest that many Americans are not getting the calcium they need to achieve and maintain optimal bone health and prevent age-related bone loss. Lower-income populations also have lower mean calcium intakes compared with higher-income groups.[2]

About 75% of calcium in the United States food supply is from milk products. Milk products contain about 300 mg calcium per serving (for example 8 oz of milk or yogurt or 1.5 oz of cheddar cheese). Other calcium-rich foods include calcium-set tofu, Chinese cabbage, kale, calcium-fortified orange juice, broccoli, and lime-processed tortillas.[13] Calcium supplements may be appropriate for children, adolescents, young adults, and pregnant and lactating women who are unable or unwilling to increase calcium intake through food sources.

In 1997, the Institute of Medicine[13] issued new dietary reference intakes (DRI) for calcium. These new recommendations were set at levels associated with maximum retention of body calcium. For several sex-age groups, the recommended calcium intakes are higher than the previous recommended dietary allowances. The new DRI for calcium for youth aged 9 to 18 years is 1300 mg/day and for adults 19 to 50 years is 1000 mg/day. The DRI for pregnant and lactating women is 1300 mg/day for women younger than age 19 and 1000 mg/day for women older than 19 years.

Given the importance of calcium to bone health, public health efforts are needed to increase awareness about the importance of calcium to health, recommended intakes (in terms of servings), and food sources of calcium, such as lower-fat dairy products. Culturally appropriate food sources of calcium should be recommended for ethnic and facial minority groups. High-risk groups, such as adolescent girls, should be the focus of targeted education efforts.

Folic Acid. Spina bifida and anencephaly are serious birth defects known as neural tube defects (NTDs). Strong evidence based on a number of clinical trials and case control studies has documented that folic acid can reduce the risk of NTDs.[4,14] As a result of these studies, in 1992, the U.S. Public Health Service recommended that "all women of childbearing age who are capable of becoming pregnant should consume 0.4 mg of folic acid per day for the purpose of reducing their risk of having a pregnancy affected with spina bifida or other neural tube defects."[15] Based on a synthesis of information from several studies, it was inferred that folic acid at levels of 0.4 mg/day will reduce the risk of NTDs in the United States by 50%.[15] In general, NTDs occur between postconceptional days 15 and 28.[14] This critical period for NTDs occurs at a time when most women are unaware of their pregnancy. Because about 50% of pregnancies are unplanned in the

United States, to maximize NTD prevention it is necessary to recommend that all women who are capable of becoming pregnant consume 0.4 mg of folic acid daily. However, current intakes of folate among women of childbearing age are considerably less than the recommendations; usual daily intake of folate for U.S. women is about 0.2 mg.[4]

At present there are three complementary strategies to increase intakes of folic acid: (1) eating more folate-rich foods; (2) multivitamin/folic acid supplementation; and (3) food fortification.[14,16] A diet rich in folate can be achieved by increased consumption of folate-rich vegetables (e.g., green leafy vegetables), fruits (e.g., orange juice), and fortified breakfast cereals (e.g., Total, Product 19). Such a diet is rich in several other nutrients and would have multiple health benefits. However, this strategy would require a major dietary change on a population level. Increased folate intakes can also be achieved with supplementation (most multivitamin preparations contain 0.4 mg folate). Although many women planning a pregnancy may take a folic acid supplement periconceptionally, it is unlikely that all women of childbearing age would take a folic acid supplement on a regular basis during all their childbearing years. The most effective public health strategy appears to be fortification of some staple foods with folic acid.[16] This is comparable to the prevention of goiter by the addition of iodine to salt. Fortification of food (such as flour, bakery products, juice) with folic acid would reach a large proportion of women, including those with unplanned pregnancies and low-income women who have difficulty buying supplements or nutritious foods.[14] In 1996, the U.S. government approved food fortification of all "enriched" grain products with folic acid starting in 1998. Increased intakes of folic acid may be of benefit to many segments of the population, not just women of childbearing potential. Recent research has linked low folic acid levels with increased blood levels of homocysteine, which in turn are associated with higher risk of heart disease and other chronic diseases.[4]

Educational efforts are needed to increase the awareness of folic acid NTD prevention among the general population. Results from 1995 and 1997 national surveys conducted by the Gallup Organization on behalf of March of Dimes indicate there has been a modest increase in awareness and use of folic acid by women of childbearing age.[17] In 1997, 66% of women sampled had read or heard about folic acid, compared with 52% in 1995. Awareness that folic acid helps prevent birth defects increased from 5% in 1995 to 11% in 1997, and the proportion of women who knew that folic acid should be taken before pregnancy increased from 2% in 1995 to 11% in 1997. Thirty percent of 1997 survey respondents who were not pregnant at the time of the survey reported that they were taking a multivitamin containing folic acid on a daily basis, compared with 25% in 1995. These results, although encouraging, suggest that more educational campaigns are needed emphasizing the benefits of folic acid and presenting the various ways for achieving adequate intakes of folate.

Iron Deficiency

Iron deficiency is the most prevalent nutritional deficiency disorder in the United States. Iron deficiency refers to a lack of iron that is severe enough to impair the production of red blood cells but not necessarily to the extent that the hemoglobin concentration falls below the normal reference range.[3] Iron deficiency can progress to iron deficiency anemia, which refers to an anemia that is associated with additional laboratory evidence of iron depletion. The most vulnerable populations for iron deficiency include infants and young children, women of childbearing years, and pregnant women.[1] Among infants and young children, iron needs are primarily for growth. Women of childbearing age are at increased risk for iron deficiency because of iron loss in menstruation. Pregnancy imposes increased iron needs for the growth of the fetus and for expansion of maternal blood volume.[3]

Current population-based prevalence data on iron deficiency anemia are not yet available from NHANES III. In NHANES II (1976–1980), the prevalence of iron deficiency anemia (defined as having abnormal results for two or more of the following tests: mean corpuscular volume, erythrocyte protoporphyrin, and transferrin saturation) was about 9% in children 12 to 24 months of age and 5% for non-pregnant women of childbearing age.[18] No national population survey data on iron deficiency anemia are available for pregnant women. However, data on low-income women are available from the Pregnancy Nutrition Surveillance System (PNSS) of which the Special Supplemental Food Program for Women, Infants and Children (WIC) is the primary source of data. In 1990, the prevalence of iron deficiency anemia was 10%, 14%, and 33% in the first, second, and third trimesters of pregnancy, respectively, for low-income pregnant women.[3]

The prevalence of iron deficiency is substantially higher in low-income children. For women between 20 and 44 years of age, a higher prevalence of iron deficiency anemia is associated with poverty, low educational attainment, and high parity.[3] The prevalence of iron deficiency among infants and young children has been declining since the 1980s. The improvements are attributed to changes in infant feeding practices, specifically, the later introduction of cow's milk and greater use of iron-fortified formula and cereal.[1,3,18] The incorporation of iron-fortified formula in the WIC food package for infants is believed to have played a major role in the decline of anemia among infants from low-income families. Substantial progress has been made in preventing iron deficiency anemia among infants and children; however, the prevalence among pregnant women and non-pregnant women of childbearing age has not changed appreciably over the years.[18]

Iron deficiency anemia in children and adults can impair energy metabolism, temperature regulation, and immune function. However, the consequence of greatest concern for infants and young children is impairment of mental and psychomotor development, which is associated with even mild iron deficiency anemia.[1] Infants and toddlers who have iron deficiency anemia consistently perform less well on tests of mental and motor development than their peers whose body iron stores are replete.[19] Compared with controls, preschoolers and older school-age children with iron deficiency scored lower on cognitive tests and performed less well on school tests. Iron supplementation led to significantly improved performance on measures of overall intelligence and on tests of specific cognitive processes among iron-deficient children. Also, iron deficient children who are exposed to lead have an increased risk of lead poisoning due to increased absorption of lead.[19] Prevention of iron deficiency anemia is a cost-effective method for decreasing the risk of lead poisoning.

Adults with iron deficiency have increased lactic acid levels and tachycardia with exercise and impaired work performance. Among pregnant women, studies have shown that anemia early in pregnancy is associated with prematurity and low birthweight, which are the most common causes of infant morbidity and mortality.[3] Iron deficiency anemia may also be associated with poor maternal weight gain during pregnancy.[18]

The prevention of iron deficiency merits a high priority because of its high prevalence and serious consequences. Prevention programs should be targeted to those subpopulations at greatest risk, such as those in poverty and recent immigrants. Two approaches can be used to reduce the prevalence of iron deficiency anemia: a population-based approach and an individual-based approach.[18] The population-based approach seeks to lower the population's risk by enriching and fortifying the food supply and by modifying individual food choices through education and dietary change programs. The individual-based approach seeks to identify those at highest risk and provide preventive interventions and treatment. Both approaches are complementary means of achieving lower rates of iron deficiency anemia. A reduction in the prevalence of iron deficiency among infants and young children can be achieved by increasing the proportion of women who breast-feed post partum, increasing the use of iron-fortified formulas when formulas are used, and delaying the introduction of whole cow's milk feedings until 9 to 12 months.[1] For children and women, dietary iron intakes can be improved by increasing the consumption of iron-rich foods (meat, fish, poultry, iron-fortified cereals). Consuming foods that contain vitamin C (e.g., citrus fruits/juice, strawberries, green pepper, broccoli) with meals increases the absorption of non-meat sources of iron by maintaining the iron in its reduced, more soluble form. Items that inhibit absorption of iron (tea, coffee, whole grain cereal [particularly bran], unleavened whole wheat bread, and dried beans) should be consumed separately from iron-rich foods. For prevention of iron deficiency anemia and depletion of maternal iron stores in pregnant women, supplementation with 30 mg elemental iron per day is recommended for all women during the second and third trimesters of pregnancy.[20]

Adequate Weight Gain and Nutrition During Pregnancy

Nutrition plays a critical role in maternal health, and attention to diet and nutritional status both before and during pregnancy may reduce the risk of adverse pregnancy outcomes. An infant's birthweight is a major determinant of survival potential. Nutrition-related risk factors for low infant birthweight include prepregnancy weight, gestational weight gain, and iron deficiency anemia.[3] Women who begin pregnancy underweight are at greater risk for the delivery of a low birthweight infant than those who are normal weight or overweight. Inadequate weight gain during pregnancy also increases the risk of low birthweight. A low prepregnancy weight in combination with inadequate gestational weight gain is associated with the highest incidence of low birthweight.[20] About one third of all mothers gain inadequate weight during their pregnancies.[1] About 14% of low birthweight births in the United States can be attributed to inadequate gestational weight gain.[3] The Institute of Medicine[20] has established prenatal weight gain recommendations based on prepregnancy body weight (Table 27.3). Weight gains at the higher end of the range are recommended for young adolescents and African-American women, as both groups are at increased risk for having a low birthweight infant.

During pregnancy, increased energy and nutrients are needed for the growth and maintenance of the fetus, maternal tissues, and the placenta. Therefore, healthy eating practices during pregnancy are important to ensure a healthy outcome for the pregnant woman and her developing fetus. Data on the dietary intakes of pregnant women in the United States indicate that mean intakes from food were lower than recommended levels for several key nutrients (folate, calcium, vitamin

TABLE 27.3

Gestational Weight Gain Recommendations Based on Prepregnancy BMI

BMI	Weight Gain (lb)
Low (<19.8) (underweight)	28–40
Normal (19.8–26.0)	25–35
High (26.1–29.0) (overweight)	15–25
Very High (>29) (obese)	≥15

BMI, body mass index (wt/ht²).
Source: Institute of Medicine. Nutrition During Pregnancy: Part I. Weight Gain, Part II. Nutrient Supplements Committee on Nutrition Status During Pregnancy and Lactation, Food and Nutrition Board. Washington, DC: National Academy Press, 1990.

B_6, iron, zinc, and magnesium).[2] The Dietary Guidelines for Americans[21] are appropriate guidelines to meet the nutrient needs of pregnant women. A recommended daily food guide for pregnancy may include 6 to 11 servings of grain products, two to four servings of fruit, three to five servings of vegetables, two to three servings of meat or meat alternatives, and two to three servings of dairy products. With the exception of iron, the increased nutrient needs of pregnancy can be met by most women with a nutritionally balanced diet.[20]

Breastfeeding Promotion

The recent policy statement on Breastfeeding and Use of Human Milk from the American Academy of Pediatrics (AAP)[22] summarizes the considerable advances that have occurred in breastfeeding research and sets forth principles to guide health care providers in the initiation and maintenance and support of breastfeeding. The AAP statement concludes that "human milk is the preferred feeding for all infants including premature and sick newborns, with rare exceptions." It is further stated, "exclusive breastfeeding is ideal nutrition and sufficient to support optimal growth and development for approximately the first 6 months after birth. . . . It is recommended that breastfeeding continue for at least 12 months, and thereafter for as long as mutually desired." The advantages of breastfeeding range from biochemical, immunologic, enzymatic, and endocrinologic to psychosocial, developmental, hygienic, and economic.[1] Human milk is uniquely superior for infant feeding and contains the ideal balance of nutrients, enzymes, immunoglobulin, anti-infective and anti-inflammatory substances, hormones, and growth factors to provide physiologic benefits for the newborn infant. Research shows that human milk and breastfeeding of infants provide advantages with regard to general health, growth, and development, while decreasing the risk for a large number of acute and chronic diseases.[22] For example, a recent longitudinal analysis of infant morbidity and the extent of breastfeeding in the United States found that breastfeeding protects infants against the development of diarrhea and ear infection in a dose-response manner.[23] The more breast milk an infant received in the first 6 months of life, the less likely that diarrhea or an ear infection developed. Breastfeeding also provides a time of intense maternal-infant interaction.

Breastfeeding rates suffered an abysmal decline in the 1940s, 1950s, and 1960s, following the introduction of infant formulas. Beginning in the early 1970s, breastfeeding rates steadily increased, reaching a peak in 1982 (62%) and then declining to 52% in 1989.[19] However, during the 1990s there has been a resurgence of breastfeeding in the United States. In 1995, 60% of mothers initiated breastfeeding and 22% continued breastfeeding at 6 months of age. Compared with rates in 1989, the initiation of breastfeeding increased more than 14%, and the rate of breastfeeding at 6 months of age increased by 19%.[24] Breastfeeding rates continue to be highest among women who are older, college educated, relatively affluent, and live in the western states. Among those least likely to breastfeed are women who are low-income, black, younger than age 20, and live in the southeastern region of the United States. Between 1989 and 1995, the largest increases in the initiation of breastfeeding and continued breastfeeding to at least 6 months of age occurred among groups of women who traditionally have been the least likely to breastfeed. For example, there was a 36% to 42% increase in breastfeeding initiation among mothers who were younger than 20 years, grade school educated, and in the WIC program. There has also been an increase in breastfeeding among women of color. Between 1989 and 1995, breastfeeding during the early postpartum period increased from 23% to 37% among black women and 48% to 61% for Hispanic women.[24]

The increase in breastfeeding seen among less educated and younger women is due in large part to the WIC program.[24] In the last decade, the WIC program has put forth much effort to develop community-based breastfeeding promotion programs for WIC participants. Continued efforts must be made to encourage more mothers to initiate breastfeeding and to breastfeed longer. A major barrier to meeting the Healthy People 2000 objective for breastfeeding is the lack of work policies and facilities that support breastfeeding.[1] Given the large percentage of mothers of young children who work outside the home, and the recent changes in the welfare program, which will require parents to find jobs, efforts to support breastfeeding will need to focus on work and school policies to provide assistance, such as extended maternity leave, part-time employment, provision of facilities for pumping and storing breast milk or breastfeeding, and on-site child care.[1] Another barrier is the portrayal of bottle feeding rather than breastfeeding as the social norm. The media can play an important role in promoting positive attitudes about breastfeeding and helping to establish breast-feeding as a socially acceptable and preferred pattern of infant feeding. Finally, there is a need to provide resources (home visits, breast pumps) and social support (such as peer counseling) for low-income women.

Growth Retardation

Retardation in linear growth in preschool children serves as an indicator of overall health and development but may especially reflect the adequacy of a child's diet.[1] Although inadequate nutrition is generally the first cause considered in growth retardation, other factors include infectious diseases, chronic diseases, or extreme psychosocial stress. Inadequate weight gain during pregnancy and low birthweight may also affect the prevalence of growth retardation among infants. Growth retardation or stunting is defined as height-for-age below the fifth percentile of children in the National Center for Health Statistics' reference population.[3] Given this definition, 5% of healthy children are expected to be below the fifth percentile of height for age as a result of normal biologic variation. A prevalence of more than 5% indicates that, on a population level, full growth potential is not being reached by children of that subgroup.[1] This prevalence is exceeded by low-income children in the United States, suggesting that inadequate nutrition or poor health may be a problem.[1] NHANES III data on growth retardation by poverty status are not yet available; however, NHANES II (1976 to 1980) data showed that 13% of 2- to 5-year-olds below the poverty level were under the fifth percentile in height for age, compared with only 5% of same-age children above the poverty level.[1]

The Pediatric Nutrition Surveillance System (PedNSS) of the Centers for Disease Control and Prevention (CDC) is designed to monitor the nutritional status of low-income children served by various publicly funded health and nutrition programs, with WIC being the largest program represented. In 1991, the overall prevalence of stunting for PedNSS children younger than 24 months of age was 10%, twice the expected level of 5%.[3] For children 2 to 5 years of age, the prevalence was 7%, slightly higher than the expected 5%. Among blacks and Native American children in this age group, the prevalence of stunting was 5% to 6%; for both whites and Hispanics the prevalence was 7% to 8%; and for Asians the prevalence was 12%.[3] During the 1990s, the prevalence of stunting has been stable among most of the populations monitored by PedNSS. However, among Asian children, primarily Southeast Asian refugees, there has been a drastic decrease in the prevalence of low height-for-age. Among Asian children younger than 2 years of age, the prevalence of stunting decreased from 22% in 1982 to 10% in 1991, a relative reduction of 54%.[3] This improvement in height suggests a positive change in the nutritional, health, and socioeconomic status of Southeast Asian refugee families since their arrival in the United States in the late 1970s and early 1980s.

Although growth retardation is not a problem for the vast majority of young children in the United States, the consequences of growth stunting and malnutrition are serious. Chronic undernutrition during infancy and early childhood has significant adverse effects on subsequent cognitive development and school performance.[19] Studies have shown that supplementary feeding during pregnancy and during the first 2 years of life enhances the development of nutritionally at-risk children and improves cognitive competence as measured 10 years later.[25]

Interventions to reduce growth retardation in children include better nutrition; improvements in the prevention, diagnosis, and treatment of infectious and chronic diseases; and the provision and use of fully adequate health services.[1] Special attention should be given to poor and homeless children as well as children with disabilities and other special needs. Good nutrition is a first step in ensuring that children reach their full growth potential, both in terms of physical health and cognitive development. Given the importance of adequate nutrition and the higher prevalence of growth retardation among low-income children, health professionals need to advocate for continued funding of the federal nutrition programs.

Hunger and Food Insecurity

There was not a year 2000 objective for hunger because national baseline data were unavailable.[1] During the 1990s considerable research has been conducted on the measurement of hunger, and it is expected that there will be a new year 2010 nutrition objective related to hunger and food insecurity. The first comprehensive measurement of food insecurity and hunger from a nationally representative sample was completed by the U.S. Bureau of the Census.[26] The study represents the first national prevalence estimate for food insecurity and hunger for the 12-month period ending April 1995. The study sought to measure resource-constrained or poverty-linked food insecurity and hunger. Food security is defined as "access by all people at all times to enough food for an active, healthy life." Food insecurity is defined as "limited or uncertain availability of nutritionally adequate and safe foods or limited or uncertain ability to acquire acceptable foods in socially acceptable ways." Hunger is defined briefly as "the uneasy or painful sensation caused by a lack of food." The report defines four categories of food security status: food secure, food insecure without hunger, food insecure with moderate hunger, and food insecure with severe hunger. The study found that the large majority of American households (88% of the approximately 100 million households in the United States) were food secure in 1995. About 11.9 million households experienced food insecurity at some level during that year. Of these 11.9% of households, 7.8% are classified as food insecure without hunger, 3.3% as food insecure with hunger, and 0.8% as food insecure with severe hunger.[26] Food insecurity is clearly related to income and poverty, and rates are higher in female-headed households, in households with children (especially young children), in black and Hispanic households, and in central city areas.

FOOD ASSISTANCE PROGRAMS

The United States Department of Agriculture (USDA) administers the nation's major domestic food-assistance programs. These programs, which served an estimated one in six Americans in 1996, provide a nutritional safety net to people in need and play an important role in reducing food insecurity in U.S. households.[27] Federal outlays for USDA's food-assistance programs totaled $38 billion in 1996. The food-assistance programs can be categorized into four general areas: (1) the Food Stamp Program; (2) child nutrition programs; (3) WIC program; and (4) food donation programs.

Food Stamp Program

The Food Stamp Program was created in 1964 to help low-income households obtain a more nutritious diet by using government-issued stamps to purchase foods in the marketplace. The Food Stamp Program is the single largest federal food-assistance program with 64% of all USDA expenditures and is the primary source of nutrition assistance for low-income Americans.[27] An average of 25.5 million people per month, or about 1 in every 10 Americans, received food stamps in 1996 at a cost of $24.4 billion. The Food Stamp Program is an entitlement program, which means that all who meet criteria have the right to receive benefits. The most common participating household is a family with children.

Child Nutrition Programs

The child nutrition programs were designed to subsidize meals served to children in schools and a variety of other institutions and consists of five programs: the National School Lunch, School Breakfast, Child and Adult Care, Summer Food Service, and Special Milk Programs. Combined outlays for these programs were $8.4 billion in 1996. The largest of these programs is the National School Lunch Program (NSLP), which had outlays of $5.3 billion in 1996.[27]

The NSLP was created in 1946 as a response to the discovery during World War II that many young recruits to the armed forces were in poor physical condition because of poor nutrition. The NSLP operates through federal reimbursements as cash and commodity foods to schools for lunches that meet federally defined meal pattern requirements. Each school day, about 26 million children, representing about 58% of all children in nearly 94,000 schools, participate in the program. About 50% of children receive a free school lunch; another 8% receive a reduced-price lunch.[27] Although school meals have been successful in meeting meal-specific RDA goals for protein, energy, vitamins, and minerals, levels of fat and saturated fats have exceeded national recommendations. In 1993, only 1% of schools offered lunches providing an average of 30% or less of calories from fat.[4] Recent legislation mandated that schools participating in the NSLP meet the goals in the Dietary Guidelines for Americans for lower fat content.

Congress established the School Breakfast Program in 1966, to provide funding for breakfast in "poor areas and areas where children had to travel a great distance to school." In 1996, government spending for the program was $1.1 billion. About 80% of all school breakfasts were served free and another 6% were served at reduced prices in 1996.[27] Studies have shown improvements in academic functioning among low-income elementary school breakfast participants.

More than 125 million meals or snacks were served to low-income children during summer vacation under the Summer Food Service Program. During the peak month of July, an average of 2.2 million children in 28,000 sites participated each day at a cost of $246 million.[27]

WIC *Program*

The Special Supplemental Food Program for Women, Infants and Children (WIC) is targeted to low-income pregnant or lactating women and infants and children up to age 5 who are certified as having health or nutritional risks. The program was created in 1974 to supplement diets in specific nutrients by providing milk or cheese, iron-fortified cereal, vitamin C juice, eggs, and peanut butter or dry beans. Iron-fortified formula is provided to infants who are not breastfed. Participants receive an average of $31 per month in food benefits. In addition to the specified packet of supplemental foods, the program provides nutrition education.

WIC program costs totaled $3.7 billion in 1997. Because WIC is not an entitlement program, participation is limited by federal funding levels, which have never been adequate to serve all eligible applicants. Increases in appropriated funds and cost-containment measures such as infant formula rebates have allowed WIC to serve more eligible people. In 1996, WIC served 7.2 million participants per month, of whom three fourths were infants or children.[27] Numerous studies have documented the effects of prenatal WIC participation on increasing newborn birthweight and preventing low birthweight, preventing preterm delivery, and reducing Medicaid costs.

Food Donation Programs

Food donation programs consist of six separate government programs: Food Distribution on Indian Reservations, Emergency Food Assistance, Food Distribution for Charitable Institutions and Summer Camps, Food Donations to Soup Kitchens and Food Banks, Disaster Feeding, and Nutrition for the Elderly. Since the late 1980s, these programs have been reduced substantially. Modifications in the price stabilization and surplus removal programs have resulted in less surplus food being available for distribution through these programs.[27]

Nutrition and Food Assistance Programs Under Welfare Reform

Federal food assistance programs are an important means of ensuring that all Americans have access to an adequate, safe, and nutritious food supply at adequate cost. These programs are being cut back, however, under the new welfare reform law, P.L. 104-193, the Personal Responsibility and Work Opportunity Reconciliation Act

(PRWORA) of 1996. Although states, under the new law, are assuming authority over many programs, the federal government remains custodian of the food assistance programs. A variety of program changes are slated to save $30 billion through 2002, according to the Congressional Budget Office—$27 billion is to come from the Food Stamp Program, and $3 billion from child nutrition programs. PRWORA changed the basic set of safety net programs for families with children in fundamental ways that jeopardize the entire safety net concept.[28] Changes in the food assistance programs may have widespread impact in increasing food insecurity, especially among families with young children.

IMPROVING NUTRITION FOR THE 21ST CENTURY

Although Americans are slowly changing their eating patterns toward more healthful diets, considerable gaps remain between public health recommendations (Healthy People 2000 objectives and the Dietary Guidelines for Americans) and actual practices. Progress has been made in decreasing total fat intakes and saturated fatty acids; however, they still remain above recommended levels. Fruit and vegetable consumption has not increased substantially in recent years and is below recommended levels. Mean calcium intakes from food also have not changed appreciably over the 1990s and are below recommended values, particularly for adolescents and adult females.[2] In addition to dietary intakes, nutritional status continues to be of public health concern. The prevalence of overweight has increased dramatically over the past few decades among all age groups but is especially high among low-income women and black and Mexican American adolescent and adult females. Although improvements have been made in decreasing the rates of iron deficiency among infants and young children, prevalence rates have not changed among pregnant women and non-pregnant women of childbearing age. Progress has also been made in the proportion of women who breastfeed. There has also been a positive change in the prevalence of low-income children who are low height-for-age, especially among Asian children. Overall progress toward healthier eating practices and nutritional status will depend on improvements for people of color and low-income populations—two subgroups who are at greatest risk for nutrition-related problems and conditions.

The challenge for health professionals is to implement public health programs and policies to protect and promote healthy eating and nutritional health of Americans. Kumanyika[29] stresses that health professionals need to advocate more aggressively for adherence to dietary recommendations within federal agencies, for example by ensuring the healthfulness of school meals and foods distributed to low-income women and children and also the inclusion of nutrition education in core services provided in publicly funded health clinics. Advocacy efforts are also needed to strengthen in-kind safety net programs to better meet children's and families' needs for adequate food.[30] The effects of PRWORA cuts in the Food Stamp Program and Child Nutrition Programs on food security of families and nutritional status of pregnant women and children should be monitored carefully. Health and social service professionals need to advocate that all Americans be guaranteed food security. Programs such as WIC, which has been found to be effective in improving the health and nutritional status of pregnant women and infants, should be fully funded.

Health professionals also need to help individuals become aware of and implement the dietary guidelines. Providers such as obstetricians, pediatricians, and nurse practitioners can educate women of childbearing age on choosing healthy diets, new mothers about breastfeeding their infants, and children and their parents on healthful food choices to support growth and development. Because many people in low-income and minority communities have limited reading skills, targeted educational programs using more audiovisual material and fewer printed materials are needed in health care and community settings.[29] More evaluative research and demonstrative projects are needed on behavior change interventions and prevention programs. A better understanding of barriers to behavior change among high-risk populations is also needed.

Continued work is needed toward the development and implementation of nutrition surveillance and monitoring systems at the local, state, and national levels. Data are currently lacking on the nutritional status of youth with chronic and disabling conditions, youth and women in correctional facilities, families in homeless shelters, children in child care facilities, and Native American families on reservations. To improve surveillance and research efforts, more sensitive dietary assessment methods are needed.

If Americans are to meet dietary recommendations, sufficient food choices must be available. Considerable progress has already been achieved by the food industry in increasing the availability of food products with lowered sodium and fat, and these efforts need to be continued. These products, along with quality fruits and vegetables, need to be made available to schools and other institutions and low-income families. With food safety issues receiving national attention, ensuring a safe and wholesome food supply will be of high priority.

References

1. U.S. Department of Health and Human Services. *Healthy People 2000: National health promotion and disease prevention objectives.* Washington, DC: Public Health Service, 1991.
2. Federation of American Societies for Experimental Biology, Life Sciences Research Office. *Third report on nutrition monitoring in the United States: Executive summary.* Washington, DC: U.S. Government Printing Office, 1995.
3. Wilcox, L.S., and Marks, J.S. *From data to action: CDC's public health surveillance for women, infants, and children.* Atlanta, GA: Centers for Disease Control and Prevention, 1995.
4. U.S. Department of Health and Human Services. *Healthy People 2000: Midcourse review and 1995 revisions.* Washington, DC: Public Health Service, 1995.
5. National Center for Health Statistics. Update: Prevalence of overweight among children, adolescents and adults—United States, 1988–1994. *MMWR.* 1997;46(9):199–201.
6. Troiano, R.P., Flegal, K.M., Kuczmarski, R.J., Campbell, S.M., and Johnson, C.L. Overweight prevalence and trends for children and adolescents: The National Health and Nutrition Examination Surveys, 1963–1991. *Archives of Pediatric and Adolescent Medicine.* 1995;149:1085–1091.
7. Ogden, C.L., Troiano, R.P., Briefel, R.R., Kuczmarski, R.J., Flegal, K.M., and Johnson, C.L. Prevalence of overweight among preschool children in the U.S., 1971 through 1994. *Pediatrics.* April, 1997;99(4) (electronic version).
8. Luepker, R.V., Perry, C.L., McKinley, S.M., Nader, P.R., Parcel, G.S., Stone, E.J., Webber, L.S., Elder, J.P., Feldman, H.A., Johnson, C.C., Kelder, S.H., and Wu, M. Outcomes of a field trial to improve children's dietary patterns and physical activity. *JAMA.* 1996;275:768–776.
9. Lauer, R.M., Obarzanek, E., Kwiterovitch, P.O., et al. Efficacy and safety of lowering dietary intake of fat and cholesterol in children with elevated low-density lipoprotein cholesterol. *JAMA.* 1995;273:1429–1435.
10. Krebs-Smith, S.M., Cook, A., Subar, A., Cleveland, L., and Friday, J. U.S. adults' fruits and vegetable intakes, 1989–1991: A revised baseline for the Healthy People 2000 objective. *American Journal of Public Health.* 1995;85(12):1623–1629.
11. Krebs-Smith, S.M., Cook, A., Subar, A., Cleveland, L., Friday, J., and Kahle, L.L. Fruit and vegetable intakes of children and adolescents in the United States. *Archives of Pediatric and Adolescent Medicine.* 1996;150:81–86.
12. Breslow, R.A., Subar, A.F., Patterson, B.H., and Block, G. Trends in food intake: The 1987 and 1992 National Health Interview surveys. *Nutrition and Cancer.* 1997;1: 86–92.
13. Food and Nutrition Board, Institute of Medicine. *Dietary reference intakes. Calcium, phosphorus, magnesium, vitamin D, and fluoride.* Washington, DC: National Academy Press, 1997.
14. Czeizel, A.E. Folic acid-containing multivitamins and primary prevention of birth defects. In A. Bendich and R.J. Deckelbaum. *Preventive nutrition: The comprehensive guide for health professionals.* Totowa, NJ: Humana Press, Inc., 1997.
15. CDC. Recommendations for the use of folic acid to reduce the number of cases of spina bifida and other neural tube defects. *MMWR.* 1992;41:1233–1238.
16. Bower, C. Folate and neural tube defects. *Nutrition Reviews.* 1995;53(9):S-33–35.
17. Johnston, R.B., and Staples, D.A. Knowledge and use of folic acid by women of childbearing age—United States. *MMWR.* 1997;46(3):721–723.
18. Food and Nutrition Board, Institute of Medicine. *Iron deficiency anemia. Recommended guidelines for the prevention, detection, and management among U.S. children and women of childbearing age.* Washington, DC: National Academy Press, 1993.
19. U.S. Department of Health and Human Services. *Surgeon General's report on nutrition and health.* Washington, DC: Government Printing Office, 1988.
20. Institute of Medicine. *Nutrition during pregnancy.* Committee on Nutrition Status During Pregnancy and Lactation. Food and Nutrition Board. Washington, DC: National Academy Press, 1990.

21. U.S. Department of Agriculture. *Dietary guidelines for Americans.* Washington, DC: U.S. Department of Health and Human Services, 1995.

22. American Academy of Pediatrics Work Group on Breastfeeding. Breastfeeding and the use of human milk. *Pediatrics.* 1997;100(6):1035–1039.

23. Scariati, P.D., Grummer-Strawn, L.M., and Fein, S.B. A longitudinal analysis of infant morbidity and the extent of breastfeeding in the United States. *Pediatrics.* June, 1997;99(6):e5.

24. Ryan, A.S. The resurgence of breastfeeding in the U.S. *Pediatrics.* April, 1997;99(4) (electronic version).

25. Politt, E. (ed). Task Force on Nutrition and Behavioral Development of the International Dietary Energy Consultative Group. A reconceptualization of the effects of undernutrition on children's biological, psychosocial and behavioral development. Social Policy Report. *Society of Research in Child Development.* 1996;X(5):1–25.

26. USDA. Food and Consumer Service, Office of Analysis and Evaluation. *Household food security in the United States in 1995. Executive summary.* Washington, DC: U.S. Department of Agriculture, September, 1997.

27. Oliveira, V. Food assistance spending held steady in 1996. *Food Review.* 1997; 20(10):1–10.

28. Lewit, E.M., Terman, D.L., and Behrman, R.E. Children and poverty: Analysis and recommendations. *The Future of Children.* 1997;7(2):4–24.

29. Kumanyika, S. Improving our diet—Still a long way to go. *New England Journal of Medicine* 1997;335(10): 738–740.

30. Politt, E. Does breakfast make a difference in school? *Journal of the American Dietetic Association.* 95:1134–1137.

28

Oral Health in Maternal and Child Health

PAUL S. CASAMASSIMO

Major gains have been made in the oral health of Americans in the last half of this century. Women and children have been beneficiaries of many improvements in oral health, including a dramatic decrease in dental caries and increased availability of fluoridated water supplies. Despite better oral health for many, others within the maternal and child health (MCH) community continue to experience significant disease and limited access to care. Minority groups, the poor, recent immigrants, the uneducated, and those living in non-fluoridated communities constitute segments of society who have not benefited equally from advances in oral health science and practice and whose access to care remains limited. This chapter reviews the advances in oral health status of the MCH population and briefly discusses issues that have affected and will likely continue to affect it into the next century.

The major oral health issues facing the MCH population can be summarized, using a variety of sources,[1–6] as the following:

1. The need to reduce preventable infectious diseases of dental caries and periodontal disease, with particular emphasis on the distribution of disease in certain MCH populations

2. Problems with access to oral health care, particularly for poor and minority MCH populations

3. Limited availability of public health measures such as early dental screenings, dental sealants, water fluoridation, and referral of special needs populations to established care pathways

4. Inadequate systemic infrastructure that is necessary to deliver consistent services nationally, establish standards and policies, and advocate for MCH oral health issues

5. Weak integration of oral health services into general health at all levels

REDUCTION OF ORAL DISEASES

Dental caries and periodontal disease are the major conditions affecting MCH populations. Both are preventable infectious diseases that affect all age groups.

Dental Caries

Dental caries is an infectious disease of teeth causing acid breakdown of enamel and dentin, abscess formation, and eventual loss of teeth.

Treatment and prevention of dental caries account for most dental expenditures in this country. Since the 1970s, dental caries in permanent teeth has declined dramatically in children so, on average, about 50% of children do not have dental caries in their permanent teeth.[7] This statistic belies the fact that dental caries remains the most common infectious disease and is now clustered in selected populations in high acuity.

Caries is primarily a disease of childhood, but its effects reach into adulthood. By age 17, more than 80% of children have dental caries of their permanent teeth. Employed women, 18 to 19 years of age, have almost 13 decayed or filled tooth surfaces (DFS, a measure of mean caries experience). This climbs to a DFS of 25 by age 35 to 39 years.[1] Black women in this age group have a lower caries rate, but they also have a lower rate of filled surfaces, suggesting less access to care.

Overall, minorities tend to have more untreated disease, and the historical trend of having less dental caries than whites appears to be reversing.

Several other trends in dental caries appear to be developing in MCH populations that have implications for the future. First, studies have noted a clustering of dental caries into a smaller group of children, so that roughly 25% of children experience 75% of dental caries.[3] Many of these children are from at-risk populations, including the poor and minorities. Clustering represents an opportunity to identify risk factors and apply risk profiling to those with varying susceptibility, so resources can be used more efficiently. Unfortunately, the care system's approaches to management of dental caries lag well behind the clustering phenomenon. For example, many public health measures remain global rather than targeted at high-risk groups. Insurance and entitlement programs are not designed to offer risk-based benefits to those most severely affected.

Early childhood caries (ECC) is a new term to address dental caries in primary teeth. Data from this country and from other industrialized nations suggest that primary dentition caries is no longer declining.[8] The explanation for this remains elusive but may relate to increasing use of inappropriate bottle feeding, inability of this segment of the population to gain access to preventive measures like fluoride or professional visits, and increasing numbers of immigrants. A major factor may also be the prevailing standard of care that delays the first dental visit until 3 years of age.[9] Those most severely affected are poor and minority children. Native American children, for example, routinely experience dramatically high rates of primary caries, often double that of white children of similar age. Poor black children also often have higher rates of primary caries as well.[10]

The third trend notable for children is the continued presence of baby bottle tooth decay (BBTD) as a subcomponent of ECC. BBTD occurs when very young children are pacified with a bottle containing a liquid with fermentable carbohydrate, most often sugar. This is usually done at night but also occurs during waking hours when parents or caretakers use the bottle for behavior modification. Studies place the prevalence of BBTD at well over 50% among Native American children and at 20% of other at-risk groups such as Head Start children. BBTD creates immediate and long-term consequences for oral health. The caries pattern created is rapid and severe in many cases, requiring expensive restorative treatment. The age of the affected child often mandates that treatment be done using sedation or general anesthesia to manage behavior, adding expense and risk. A 1996 study of Iowa Medicaid reported that the average additional (non-dental) cost of treatment was $1,812 in 1994 for 317 children 5 years of age and younger, adding more than $500,000 to overall treatment charges.[11]

Just as troubling for future caries management in this youngest segment of the MCH population afflicted with BBTD is the well documented phenomenon of increased susceptibility of these children to future caries throughout childhood[12] even when intensive caries preventive strategies are used. Current preventive strategies stress education, but it should be noted that recent research suggests that BBTD has deep cultural link and a strong relationship to societal stresses on parents and thus may be resistant to preventive education.[13]

Periodontal Disease

Periodontal disease is the other major infectious disease of concern in the MCH population. Periodontal disease is an umbrella term to describe infections and deteriorating conditions of the gingival tissues and bone supporting teeth. Gingivitis is a minor form affecting the gums and is reversible in most cases with good oral hygiene. Periodontitis involves irreversible destruction of bony support of teeth as the result of infection by oral microorganisms. In adults, periodontal disease accounts for more tooth loss in later decades than dental caries.

For the majority of young children, gingival problems are minor. However, periodontal conditions affect one of two adolescents,[1] and the first signs of bone loss (as measured in millimeters of loss of gingival attachment to the tooth) appear during this period. Early onset periodontitis (EOP), defined as attachment loss of more than 3 mm, is not common, but most recent national data suggest that 10% of African Americans, 5% of Hispanics, and 1.3% of whites are affected in the 15- to 17-year age group. EOP is also associated with increased caries.[14]

Women of childbearing age experience periodontal problems that increase with age. National data available from the 1985–1986 Oral Health Survey of Adults and Seniors show gingival bleeding in 37% to 46% of employed women 18 to 39 years of age. In this same group, up to 15.7% had periodontal pockets suggestive of attachment loss.[1] Periodontitis is a finding in diabetes, a systemic condition that occurs in higher rates in minorities. Very recent research suggests that there may be an association between periodontal disease in mothers and prematurity in their offspring.[15] In addition, there may be an association between periodontal disease and heart disease.[16]

The implications of these most recent associations could be significant and make prevention of periodontal disease a major oral health priority in the next decade and beyond. At present, periodontitis prevalence in adults seems stable as compared with 1986 levels.[5] The concern that periodontal disease, like dental caries, is higher in the poor and minority populations may also direct future policy and programmatic decisions. Recent emphasis placed on research into this disease and its prevention may be more a factor of the baby boom generation's aging than the disease's impact on oral health.

In summary, oral health has improved, but many within the MCH population have seen only minor gains and others have experienced none. Clearly some children and many women have benefited from the decline in permanent tooth dental caries. Racial and income differentials continue to exist for dental caries and periodontal disease, particularly for untreated disease.

ACCESS TO CARE

In 1996 to 1997, 63% of women had a dental visit within a year, with a slightly lower percentage for those 25 to 34 years of age. Higher percentages were noted for those with higher education and income levels. Whites tend to seek dental care more often than non-whites[17] and tend to seek it more frequently with shorter intervals between visits.[4]

The cost of care is a major factor in access. In 1992, dental care accounted for a little over 5% of health care expenses.[4] Data from the 1995 Behavior Risk Factor Surveillance System indicate that about 44% of adults do not have dental insurance,[18] yet all but 3% of total expenditures for oral health services are private dollars. Only 38% to 48% of women 18 to 44 years of age have dental insurance. About 50% of 5- to 17-year-olds have some form of dental insurance, primarily through an employed parent. Reaching the age of majority causes a dip in insurance coverage that takes about 6 years to reverse.

TABLE 28.1

Oral Health Status and Utilization of Dental Services for U.S. Children and Adults

Condition or Variable	Poor*		African American		Hispanic		U.S. Mean	
	Ch	*Ad*	*Ch*	*Ad*	*Ch*	*Ad*	*Ch*	*Ad*
Percentage with untreated coronal dental caries	—	—	27.2	22.1	—	23.0	15.3	8.12
Percentage with private dental insurance	7.8	13.3	31.9	35.6	28.7	31.2	44.3	43.9
Percentage with dental sealants	4.3		4.2		5.1		10.9	
Percentage with at least one visit in preceding year	48.8	42.7	49.9	43.9	47.9	45.2	61.7	57.7
Average number dental visits per year	1.1	1.4	1.0	1.3	1.6	1.5	2.1	2.1

Ch, children; Ad, adults.
*Income less than $10,000.

Table 28.1 provides an overview of age, race, insurance, and oral health care seeking for U.S. children and adults.

Medicaid

Any discussion of access to oral health care for MCH populations must include consideration of Medicaid. The establishment of Medicaid in 1965 was intended to ensure access to health care for the poor. The Early and Periodic Screening Diagnosis and Treatment (EPSDT) Program of Medicaid requires states to pay for oral health services for children and to ensure that they are delivered. States may or may not offer dental services for adults and have the discretion to limit services. Dental per capita expenditures under Medicaid actually decreased between 1975 and 1998 in contrast to all other medical benefits of the program.[4] Edelstein[19] reported summary statistics for the program period 1993 to 1995 that are reflective of the limited success of the Medicaid dental program:

- Only 18 percent of all Medicaid-eligible recipients (children, adults, handicapped, and elderly) received any dental treatment.
- Combined state and federal spending for dental services was $1 billion annually.

- Dental expenditures accounted for 1% of total Medicaid expenditures.
- Annual expenditures per enrolled beneficiary were $43, and for each beneficiary who had at least one dental visit were $241.

Some states have converted dental programs to managed care/health maintenance organization (HMO) style programs. None of these has operated long enough to make conclusions about their effect on oral health of recipients. Success of HMO-driven systems, capitation, carve-outs, gate-keeping, and other aspects of managed care remains to be seen. The additional layer of administration provided by such arrangements can hinder participation by both recipient and provider.

Numerous state and government reviews of Medicaid dental services have noted consistent problems with the program.[20,21]. Providers cite low fees, extensive paperwork, rigorous regulation, poor patient compliance, and limitation of allowable services creating a dual standard of care and ethical dilemmas for dentists. More recently, participating dentists have left the system because of concerns about audits that question treatment decisions and use extrapolation techniques that project billing errors across an entire practice Medicaid population. Recipients complain of limited access because of lack of providers and transportation costs to reach providers who will accept Medicaid.

If Medicaid is to work, these problems need to be addressed. Creative approaches to attract providers, such as stipending training programs to develop sensitive providers, are needed. Fees need to approach usual and customary private fee structures to be competitive. Quality standards that eliminate the dual standard of care need to be developed and disseminated. Formative rather than punitive auditing practices need to be developed and applied. Acuity needs to be factored into populations, and appropriate steps should be taken to account for the higher disease rates in the covered population. On a national and state level, regular evaluation of program success needs to be instituted. A consistent and comparable database must be developed for this purpose.

State Child Health Insurance Program

In 1997, Congress enacted the State Child Health Insurance Program (Title XXI), also called S-CHIP or CHIP, entitling states to federal monies for child health assistance. States can expand Medicaid or create new programs to cover children with family incomes of up to 200% of the poverty level. Children from "working poor" families unable to purchase health insurance will benefit from CHIP. When Medicaid is the vehicle chosen by a state for CHIP, dental benefits, including EPSDT, must be provided. However, states choosing alternatives to Medicaid need not offer dental benefits. At the writing of this chapter, 12 of 14 proposed state plans included dental benefits of some type, which on face value suggests better access to care.[19]

Oral health advocates have expressed concerns with each of three coverage options—Medicaid, no dental coverage, or new programs that include dentistry. If Medicaid is expanded, the program brings with it the problems noted earlier in this chapter. It is possible that access will not be improved, even though more children are eligible, because the forces keeping away providers remain. In addition, the sudden addition of eligible recipients, many of whom have significant treatment needs, may overwhelm and drive away existing providers. A state opting for no dental coverage ignores the significant treatment needs of the very populations the legislation intends to serve. States choosing new programs, such as "benchmarks" equivalent to those dental plans offered their state employees, may inadvertently impose restrictions or limit services because of co-payment provisions, gate-keeping, and other subtle benefit limitations.

In summary, improvement of access to oral health for MCH populations is a complex problem well beyond the scope of this chapter. When considering that about 35% to 40% of the MCH population lives below or within 175% of poverty, improved access will revolve around improvement in public programs. Significant issues stand in the way of meeting access goals, including but not limited to

1. Decreased funding for public health clinical programs
2. Competing programs within states for limited dollars, such as within state MCH Block Grants
3. Inadequate provider pool, particularly pediatric dentists and dentists willing to be Medicaid providers
4. Complex and conflicting eligibility requirements affecting women and dependent children
5. Dependency of a disproportionate percentage of the MCH population on publicly funded clinical care programs

PUBLIC HEALTH MEASURES

Fluoride

Fluoride is the public health measure that can be credited with reducing the dental caries rate in this century. About 144 million Americans (56%) have access to fluoridated water, with most of these served by public water systems. This includes more than 60 million children. In addition, estimates are that 93% of children 2 to 16 years of age use a fluoridated dentifrice. Almost all toothpaste sold in the United States contains fluoride.[22]

Fluoride consumed during tooth development strengthens enamel against carious attack by food acids after eruption. Fluoride consumed daily acts on teeth already erupted to remineralize, thus arresting or reversing early caries. Some antibacterial effect has been attributed to fluoride as well. Its negative effects in this country are limited to fluorosis or tooth mottling and toxicity when consumed in concentrated form. The MCH population thus benefits from fluoride passively in drinking water and foodstuffs produced within fluoridated communities. Dentifrice swallowed also contributes to the fluoride load of young children. Topical effects of fluoride are also gained from foodstuffs and water consumed as well as from home application in dentifrice and professionally applied fluoride treatments.

The major fluoride issues for the MCH population relate to increasing the percentage of the population receiving optimal fluoride in communal water systems and addressing increasing fluorosis in the population due to a halo effect caused by ubiquitous sources in the food chain and dentifrices. Although clearly a public health issue, fluoride has been pushed into the political spotlight by various groups across the political spectrum, including environmentalists and those concerned with government's intrusion into privacy. It is unlikely that major changes will occur in the availability of fluoride in water supplies. A more likely scenario is a relatively stable percentage of Americans exposed to fluoridated water and more exposed to topical and systemic fluoride via existing and new personal and professionally applied vehicles, such as fluoride varnishes.

Dental Sealants

The other major anti-caries preventive measure is dental sealants. These are plastic coatings applied to teeth by dentists or other trained professionals before dental caries begins. Since most dental caries of posterior teeth occurs in their pits and grooves, sealants offer a potential major anti-caries effect.

Sealants can be applied in private offices as well as in public health settings such as mobile clinics or school-based programs. A Year 2000 goal is to have 50% of children with sealants on at least one tooth.[23] Currently, only about one in five 5- to 17-year-old children have dental sealants on the permanent teeth. The number of children with sealants has risen since 1986 to 1987, when about 7% to 8% of children had sealants. Access to care plays an important role in obtaining sealants; racial differences in who has sealants tend to disappear when access to care is equaled.[24]

Public funding provides sealants to those in low-income groups who are also the ones who experience most dental caries. Thus, policies and programs providing sealants are important. Similarly, sealants represent a sound, low-cost preventive measure that needs to be a part of all private and public dental coverage programs. When combined with fluorides, which protect enamel surfaces between teeth, a major caries reduction can be anticipated.

INFRASTRUCTURE FOR ORAL HEALTH

Dental disease can be debilitating. In 1989, more than 164 million hours of work were missed because of dental problems. In addition, 117 hours of school were lost per 100 students.[4] Despite the morbidity associated with oral problems, the lack of life-threatening consequences makes it a low priority when compared with other social and health issues. This second-class status may contribute to the lack of emphasis given dental health in many arenas and, to some degree, the infrastructural problems[1,5] at local, state and national levels.

Dental health is administered by dozens of federal agencies. At the state level, resource allocation varies greatly, as does the oversight of oral health issues. Although diversification and decentralization have some benefit, they also put oral health at risk not to have critical mass for effective programming, advocacy for funding, and other important administrative functions. An additional theme in dealing with infrastructural weakness in MCH oral health is the lack of a cohesive family focus for oral health. This has resulted in fragmentation of effort and failure to formulate standards or to generate minimal and consistent guidance for clinical care programs.

An important consideration for the future is consolidation of efforts to develop a strong infrastructure for policy, clinical programming, research, development of standards, advocacy, and health care promotion. The creation of the National Oral Health Resource Center[25] is a beginning in consolidating information within a single database.

INTEGRATION OF ORAL HEALTH INTO GENERAL HEALTH

In recent years, some effort has been made to integrate oral health into general health considerations. Although such an effort establishes competition for interest and resources, it also consolidates oral health as an important health component. One notable example is the Bright Futures project to establish preventive health supervision guidelines for children.[26] This joint project of the Health Care Financing Administration and the Maternal and Child Health Bureau of the Department of Health and Human Services incorporated oral health into overall health considerations. Another example is the inclusion of oral health in state block grants. Seventy-five percent of federal funding for state dental programs comes from MCHB Block Grants to states, or about $12 to 15 million in the most recent budget cycle.[25]

Additional integration is occurring slowly through networking with groups sharing MCH focus. Oral health is integrated in the Special Supplemental Food Program for Women, Infants and Children (WIC) and Head Start. Professional and child advocacy groups advocating for children have established coalitions, and oral health–related organizations have become a part of these efforts. In the private sector, professional groups like the American Academy of Pediatric Dentistry and the American Academy of Pediatrics have co-developed guidelines on sedation, child abuse, and other aspects of MCH that are shared.[27]

Management of children with craniofacial deformities, most commonly cleft lip and palate, represents one of the most successful models of integration of oral health into a health pathway. In most states, multidisciplinary teams manage the care of children with these deformities. Physicians, psychologists, speech and language therapists, and other health providers join with orthodontists, pediatric dentists, oral surgeons, and prosthodontists to render care to these children, beginning as early as in the first year of life. In response to a 1987 Surgeon General's report on children with special health care needs,[28] national standards were developed to guide the care of these children.[29] Although strict protocols vary from team to team, these standards describe the appropriate interventions in the disciplines of surgery, audiology, dentistry, genetics, nursing, otolaryngology, pediatrics, psychology/social work, and speech and language, as well as credentialing and quality assurance. Some states utilize a handicapped children's service or bureau to ensure access and payment for services as well as to coordinate services in areas where team access is limited or non-existent.

Future improvement of oral health will require that integration continue and expand, and that the role of oral health in such MCH areas as systemic health, school readiness, behavior, and early development be clarified and better understood.

References

1. Steffensen, J.E.M., and Brown, J.P. Public Health Service Workshop on Oral Health of Mothers and Children: Background issues papers, September 10–12, 1989. *Journal of Public Health Dentistry*. 1990;50:355–472 (special issue).

2. USDHHS. *Equity and access for mothers and children: Strategies from the Public Health Workshop on Oral Health of Mothers and Children. September 9–12, 1989.* DHHS Publication No. HRS-MCH-90-4. Washington, DC: NCEMCH; 1990.

3. Association of Maternal and Child Health Programs. *Position statement on oral health in children and youth.* Washington, DC, 1993.

4. USPHS Oral Health Coordinating Committee. *Toward improving the oral health of Americans: An overview of oral health status, resources, and care delivery.* (final draft). March, 1993.

5. Gift, H.C., Drury, T.F., Nowjack-Raymer, R.E., et al. The state of the nation's oral health: Mid-decade assessment of healthy people 2000. *Journal of Public Health Dentistry.* 1996;56:84–91.

6. Nowak, A.J., Johnsen, D., Waldman, H.B., et al. *Pediatric oral health.* Washington, DC: Center for Health Policy Research, George Washington University, 1992.

7. Brunelle, J.A. *Oral health of U.S. schoolchildren. National and regional findings.* DHHS Publication No. (NIH) 89-2247. Washington, DC: U.S. Government Printing Office, 1989.

8. Brown, L.J., Kingman, A., and Brunelle, J.A. Most U.S. schoolchildren are caries free: This is no myth. *Public Health Reports.* 1995;110:531–533.

9. American Academy of Pediatrics, Committee on Psychosocial Aspects of Child and Family Health. *Guidelines for health supervision.* Elk Grove, IL: AAP, 1988.

10. Edelstein, B.L., and Douglass, C.W. Dispelling the myth that 50 percent of U.S. schoolchildren have never had a cavity. *Public Health Reports.* 1995;110:522–530.

11. Damiano, P.C., Kanellis, M.J., Willard, J.C., et al. *A report on the Iowa Title XIX Dental Program.* Iowa City, IA: Public Policy Center and College of Dentistry, University of Iowa, April, 1996, pp 21–22.

12. Nowak, A.J. Rationale for the timing of the first oral evaluation. *Pediatric Dentistry.* 1998;19:8–11.

13. Benitez, C., O'Sullivan, D., and Tinanoff, N. Effect of a preventive approach for the treatment of nursing bottle caries. *ASDC Journal of Dentistry for Children.* 1994;61:46–49.

14. Albandar, J.M., Brown, L.J., and Loe, H. Clinical features of early-onset periodontitis. *Journal of the American Dental Association.* 1997;128:1393–99.

15. Offenbacher, S., Katz, V., Fertig, G., et al. Periodontal infection as a possible risk factor for preterm low birthweight. *Journal of Periodontology.* 1996;67:1103–13.

16. Loesche, W.J., Schork, A., and Terpenning, M.S. Assessing the relationship between dental disease and coronary heart disease in elderly U.S. veterans. *Journal of the American Dental Association.* 1998;129:301–311.

17. Bloom, B., Gift, H.C., and Jack, S.S. Dental services and oral health; United States, 1989. National Center for Health Statistics. *Vital Health Statistics.* 1992;10(183).

18. Centers for Disease Control and Prevention. Preview. *MMWR.* December 19, 1997;46(50):1199–1203.

19. Edelstein, B.L. *Public funding of dental coverage for children: Medicaid, Medicaid managed care and state programs.* Washington, DC: Children's Dental Health Project, 1998, p 11.

20. U.S. Congress, Office of Technology Assessment. *Children's health services under the Medicaid program—background paper.* OTA-BP-H-78. Washington, DC: U.S. Government Printing Office, October, 1990.

21. Department of Health and Human Services, Office of Inspector General. *Children's dental services under Medicaid, access and utilization.* OEI-09-93-00240. Washington, DC: U.S. Government Printing Office, April, 1996.

22. Pendrys, D.G. Risk of fluorosis in a fluoridated population. *Journal of the American Dental Association.* 1995;126:1617–24.

23. PHS, Office of the Assistant Secretary for Health, Office of Disease Prevention and Health Promotion. *Healthy People 2000: National health promotion and disease prevention objectives.* DHHS Publication No. (PHS) 91-50212. Washington, DC: U.S. Government Printing Office, 1990.

24. Brown, L.J., Kaste, L.M., Selwitz, R.H., et al. Dental caries and sealant usage in U.S. children 1988–91: Selected findings from the third national health and

nutrition examination survey. *Journal of the American Dental Association.* 1996;127:335–343.

25. Rosetti, J., and Maternal and Child Health Bureau. *Oral health activities and projects.* Unpublished report, 1998.

26. Green, M. *Bright futures: Guidelines for health supervision of infants, children and adolescents.* Arlington, VA: National Center for Education in Maternal and Child Health, 1994.

27. American Academy of Pediatric Dentistry. Reference manual 1994–95. *Pediatric Dentistry.* 1994;16:1–96.

28. Office of Maternal and Child Health. *Surgeon General's report: Children with special health care needs.* Washington, DC: USDHHS, PHS. June, 1987.

29. American Cleft Palate-Craniofacial Association. *Parameters for evaluation and treatment of patients with cleft lip/palate or other craniofacial anomalies.* March 1993.

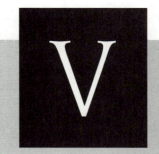

Programs
and Initiatives

29

The Future of Prevention

James S. Marks and Lynne S. Wilcox

The right way to begin is to pay attention to the young and make them as good as possible. Socrates as quoted in Plato's Euthyphro

What affects the well-being of a child, of a family? A discussion of prevention must begin first with a determination of what it is the society, public health systems, and clinical medicine want to improve on. Focusing the question on well-being fits with the World Health Organization (WHO) definition of health as the state of complete physical, mental, and social well-being and not merely the absence of disease. Yet in practice we often define prevention very narrowly, focusing primarily on one-on-one clinical interventions such as immunizations and the early detection of specific illnesses. We have been too narrow in what we have thought and too narrow in what we have studied, and, accordingly, we are too limited in what we know works and what we do. To address fully the concept of prevention and family health, one cannot deal merely with the prevention of disease but rather with the promotion of well-being.

What do children and their families require to live a full and satisfying life, to participate in family and community, and to contribute to society? Any list of conditions, life stages, or other context necessarily limits and draws boundaries around our thinking. In looking to the future, past limitations should not constrain us. In fact, it is more appropriate that we think expansively regarding prevention as befits the broad definition of health adopted by the WHO, which means that we must recognize and foster the contributions to personal health made by societal policies and community structures and supports as well as clinical services. In this chapter, we address some of the broader issues of prevention and the contexts for policies, programs, and supports. Specific examples, when provided, are meant to serve as examples only and not as a complete list. Much more information related to specific preventive interventions can be found in other chapters in this text.

THE NATURE OF PREVENTION

One of the paradoxes of our times is that by all the usual measures we have achieved unprecedented levels of health yet many in our society feel ill at ease about their health and well-being and that of their children. This is due in part to the broadening definition of health. However, it also reflects the ephemeral nature of prevention. Prevention is successful when nothing happens—it is hard to make a well person feel better. It is very difficult to point to an individual and say that person would have contracted measles except he had received the vaccine, would have failed in school except that he was in Head Start, would have become a smoker except that he had health education in school. In addition, prevention requires a mindset that is optimistic about the future, with the belief that actions taken now will lead to personal advantage. The advantage must be of significant magnitude to warrant taking the action and accepting the delay in the outcome, which is in fact only a possibility and rarely assured.

Prevention is classified as primary, secondary, or tertiary according to when the preventive intervention is applied in the course of the disease or condition. *Primary prevention* is a maneuver or activity that prevents the onset of disease. More specifically, primary prevention is directed at people who are susceptible before they develop the condition. Generally, but not always, the causes or risk factors for a disease must be well known for primary prevention efforts to be feasible. Examples include immunization, automobile seat belts, and school health education to prevent tobacco use. Epidemiologically, primary prevention lowers disease incidence and is what is usually thought of by the public as prevention. *Secondary prevention* involves the early detection and treatment of the disease, presumably permitting greater likelihood of cure, or at least longer survival with the disease than would have been possible with later diagnosis. Secondary prevention is directed at persons who are asymptomatic or whose symptoms are non-specific for the disease or condition but have developed early biologic evidence of the disease. It generally does not reduce the incidence of disease, but if treatment is curative, can reduce prevalence. Because the disease is not yet manifested, secondary prevention is usually thought of in the context of screening asymptomatic persons. Common examples of this would include testing for iron deficiency, lead screening, and screening for metabolic diseases such as phenylketonuria. *Tertiary prevention* occurs in the person with the disease and is aimed at reducing the complications of that disease, thus improving the quality of life for the person with the condition. It does not change incidence and, rarely, prevalence except to the extent that, if reduction of complications lengthens survival with the disease, prevalence may increase. An example of tertiary prevention would be aggressive treatment of early rheumatoid arthritis to prevent joint destruction or the close management of blood glucose levels in persons with type 1 diabetes to delay onset of renal disease.

A newer concept advanced by some is *primordial prevention*, which refers to genetic modifications, prenatally or early in life, to prevent the susceptibility to important clinical conditions. The explosion in genetic research of the last few years and the promise of the Human Genome Project make this concept both plausible and also attractive.

SPECIFIC PREVENTION OPPORTUNITIES

Because all future aspects of prevention cannot be addressed in this chapter, we focus on those critical issues that operate at the levels of society and the health care system.

Genetic Counseling and Gene Therapy

First, we want to expand on the opportunities related to new genetic knowledge. It is clear that in the future we will have unprecedented opportunities for prevention of many severe conditions of infants and children. This will operate through not only single gene defects but also polygenic predisposition that could fundamentally change much of preventive efforts in the future.

Identification of genetic variance that places individuals at high risk for adverse health outcomes is likely to lead to substantially more targeted and individualized counseling regarding primary preventive interventions and guidelines regarding screening recommendations in those whose risk is much greater than the general population. This kind of targeted preventive intervention that does not itself relate to direct alteration of genetic risk will likely occur sooner than specific genetic therapies or alterations and will be applicable to many more conditions. The expectation, essentially unproven but likely, is that persons and families who are made aware of their substantial risk for an adverse health event because of their genetic makeup would be more likely to engage in health promoting behaviors and practices than they would if provided more general counseling or even counseling that recognized past family history but did not tie it explicitly to genetic risk.

It is also likely that for some conditions, especially very severe single gene defects, there will be direct genetic manipulation developed early and provided widely. It is likely that manipulation of multiple genes to minimize predispositions will be developed much more slowly and with greater caution to ensure that the principle of primum non nocere is respected and that these manipulations do not cause unforeseen, untoward problems for the individuals or families so treated.

Nevertheless, the tremendous promise here is likely to be one of the dominant prevention forces of the 21st century, with the ramifications for clinical care and broader societal policies only crudely perceived at this time. If the Human Genome Project's promise is to be realized in prevention, it will require a systematic effort to widely apply the findings of the research through counseling and instruction for those at high risk, interventions that are not widely supported in our health care system currently. The future of genetic prevention issues will also be driven by a host of ethical issues that have yet to be grappled with in any fundamental way: confidentiality, genetic testing when no intervention exists, implications when testing several family members is, in essence, testing them all, and genetic discrimination in health care and employment, to name but a few.

Familial Dynamics and Rearing

There is also great preventive potential developing around the body of behavioral research on intrafamily dynamics, rearing styles, and disciplinary practices. There is a growing understanding of the influence of these issues on behaviors during childhood and adolescence and carrying on into adulthood. Studies have shown the protective effect of certain family styles and a sense of connectedness to family on a wide variety of risk behaviors in adolescents. In those families that have a greater sense of connectedness, children are less likely to engage in behaviors that put their health at risk than children who do not have that sense. Conversely, there is also increasing evidence that children raised in families where they were abused or children who saw their mother being abused, had an alcoholic parent, or the like, are more apt to report higher rates of a wide variety of personal risk behaviors and outcomes such as smoking, alcohol abuse, drug use, teenage pregnancy, obesity, and violent behavior. This risk increases in a dose-response fashion as the severity and variety of adverse childhood experiences increase. There is also some evidence that intervention programs, such as home visiting programs for new mothers, can lead to improvements in parenting skills and disciplinary practices, and for those mothers identified as potentially at high risk for child abuse, can lower rates of child abuse.

This broad array of behavioral research into family dynamics, if pursued and expanded, offers the potential for intervention and fundamental changes in many of the most disturbing areas of current societal concern for children and adolescent health and well-being. With increasing specificity, we are now learning what puts children at risk and what can be done to diminish those adverse outcomes. It is striking that, in contrast with the explosion in genetic knowledge, this is far less biomedical and technology driven but is as fundamentally important for health and social outcomes. However, it is also an area where there are few models of widespread application of the interventions. Unlike in clinical care (where we can readily envision new genetic therapies being offered), the current health care system makes it unlikely that such family services will be provided without fundamental changes in how prevention is promoted, supported, and practiced.

Community-Based Prevention

Through the 1980s and 1990s, there has been a growing sense that community approaches are an essential means for achieving major public health goals. Any important health problem of our time is not going to be solved by medical care alone, public health alone, or any other single segment of society. Rather, problems like teen pregnancy, drug abuse, and physical inactivity will require the engagement of all our major community institutions and the public at large. This interdependence means that a fundamental strategy for prevention of such serious health problems requires the formation of a wide network of partnerships and collaborations among the leadership institutions in communities, including schools, major employers, churches, health departments, health care organizations, and volunteer groups.

Promising research is being done in the area of social capital or collective efficacy. This is basically a measure of social cohesion and trust among community members and their willingness to intervene on behalf of the common good. Work in this area is still in its earliest stages as far as determining how best to measure social capital and linking these measures with important health outcomes. We know that some poor communities have much better health indices than others of similar socioeconomic status and access to medical care. Recent studies suggest that at-risk children who are in families that have links to their communities do better developmentally and behaviorally than similar children in similar situations but whose parents do not have these links. Other research has found lower rates of violence in neighborhoods where residents feel there are informal mechanisms of social control and higher assessments of social cohesion than in similar neighborhoods whose residents rate these measures lower.

An underlying principle in a science-based approach to public health and medical care is that differences between individuals, families, and communities are not random occurrences but rather are outcomes based on causes that are ultimately measurable and potentially responsive to intervention. We need to understand those features of communities that support and promote health and understand the ways to foster their development.

Specific examples of engagement of community institutions can be observed in school health systems, where there is now a substantial body of controlled trials that show that school health education performed by trained teachers and engaging parents and the community can substantially reduce the rate of tobacco use initiation, increase physical activity in school settings, improve nutrition choices made by children in school settings and at home, and substantially lower the rate of teen pregnancy. This kind of infrastructure development and engagement of schools may offer in the 21st century a whole new way of supporting community institutions to foster the development of trust and the empowerment of community members to resolve important health and social problems.

CHALLENGES TO PREVENTION

Just as the opportunities for prevention are growing, so also are some of the challenges. We are in time of rapid evolution of our health care system from a cottage industry where individuals or small groups of practitioners provided health care and were reimbursed on a fee-for-service basis to a corporate model where individual practitioners become employees or contractors providing the health care of individuals for a fixed fee. In theory, this structure should be an incentive for prevention by diminishing future need for therapeutic intervention. However, in practice—at least thus far—the incentives are set up to operate only in the short-term. That is, providers of care compete principally on cost over only a 1- or 2-year period. Individuals and families, as well as employers and other purchasers, change providers frequently, based on minor cost differences, so that the advantages of prevention cannot accrue. There will have to be a longer term horizon for cost and outcome benefits for the health care system to deliver the prevention it is capable of. If this happens the pressures for it will likely come from employers and employees who recognize that they will eventually have to pay for ill health that could have been prevented.

Prevention issues in the future will also require the close linkage of clinical, public health, and community approaches. Increasingly, more is known about interventions that can reduce the risk of injury, illness, and hospitalization but often require behavioral change on the part of the parent, other caretaker, health care provider, and/or child. For many of these areas, specific clinical studies show effectiveness of counseling efforts in changing those behaviors; examples include use of infant car seat, bicycle helmets, and asthma education. What is less clear is the effectiveness of counseling as *routinely offered* in usual care settings and the role and value of education in other settings and by other means (e.g., via the Internet).

Unlike with programs aimed at specific "dreaded" clinical conditions (e.g., cancer, HIV, etc.), it is hard to "put a face on prevention."

The public at large, policymakers, and providers of care can easily think of friends and relatives who have these diseases and died from them. It is much harder to identify the person who would have died or become seriously ill but instead is now healthy because he or she never took up cigarettes, stayed physically active, or received their immunizations. This difficulty in putting a face on prevention means that people find it easier to become passionate about and committed to treatment or research for a cure regardless of cost effectiveness but find it harder to become passionate about and committed to prevention of the disease or condition, even when those efforts are highly cost effective.

At the most macro-level, the future of prevention will be heavily influenced by more comprehensive measurements of health rather than just mortality and disease rates. Recently there has been a major effort, the Global Burden of Disease project sponsored by WHO and the World Bank, that has attempted to measure in a single construct the mortality and disability burden of many diseases and conditions worldwide. Using disability adjusted life years (DALY), the investigators took into account: mortality by age and both disability severity and duration, and then projected forward the changes in burden until the year 2020. The net effect makes a case for a better balance between the preventive, public health, and primary care approaches to health versus technology-intensive, care-driven approaches that now characterize health care around the world. A U.S.-specific analysis is currently under way that will provide a DALY-based measure by which to assess preventive potential for many diseases and principal risk factors.

CONCLUSION

The 21st century could become the Prevention Century, but only if we move our efforts firmly and clearly beyond the walls of the clinic and even beyond the constraints of traditional public health. A tremendous amount of the needed scientific research has been completed, but it awaits widespread application. It is unclear, however, whether the societal will is present, especially because there are clearly cost implications at the front end. But the only true investment in health is in our children—to make them the best we can.

General References

1. Khoury, M.J., and the Genetics Working Group. From genes to public health. The applications of genetic technology in disease prevention. *American Journal of Public Health*. 1996;86:1717–1722.

2. Wertz, D.C., Fanos, J.H., and Reilly, P.R. Genetic testing for children and adolescents: Who decides. *JAMA*. 1994;272:875–881.
3. Felitti, V.J., Anda, R.F., Nordenberg, D., Williamson, D.F., Spitz, A.M., Edwards, V., Koss, M.P., and Marks, J.S. The relationship of childhood abuse and household dysfunction to many of the leading causes of death in adults: The adverse childhood experiences (ACE) study. *American Journal of Preventive Medicine*. 1998; 14:245–258.
4. Resnick, M.D., Bearman, P.S., Blum, R.W., Bauman, K.E., Harris, K.M., Jones, J., Tabor, V., Beuhring, T., Sieving, R.E., Shew, M., Ireland, M., Bearinger, L.H., and Udry, J.R. Protecting adolescents from harm: Findings from the National Longitudinal Study on Adolescent Health. *JAMA*. 1997;278:823–832.
5. Straus, M.A., Sugarman, D.B., and Giles-Sims, J. Spanking by parents and subsequent antisocial behavior of children. *Archives of Pediatric and Adolescent Medicine*. 1997;151:761–767.
6. Runyan, D.K., Hunter, W.M., Socolar, R.R.S., Amaya-Jackson, L., English, D., Landsverk, J., Dubowitz, H., Browne, D.H., Bangdiwala, S.I., and Mathew, R.M. Children who prosper in unfavorable environments: The relationship to social capital. *Pediatrics*. 1998;101:12–18.
7. Sampson, R.J., Raudenbush, S.W., and Earls, F. Neighborhoods and violent crime: A multi-level study of collective efficacy. *Science*. 1997;277:918–924.
8. Vincent, M.L., Clearie, A.F., and Schluchter, M.D. Reducing adolescent pregnancy through school and community-based education. *JAMA*. 1987;257:3382–3386.
9. Luepker, R.V., Perry, C.L., McKinlay, S.M., Nader, P.R., Parcel, G.S., Stone, E.J., Webber, L.S., Elder, J.P., Feldman, H.A., Johnson, C.C., Kelder, S.H., Wu, M., for the CATCH Collaborative Group. Outcomes of a field trial to improve children's dietary patterns and physical activity: The Child and Adolescent Trial for Cardiovascular Health (CATCH). *JAMA*. 1996;275:768–776.
10. Murray, C.J.L., and Lopez, A.D. (eds). *The global burden of disease*. Cambridge, MA: Harvard University Press, 1996.

30

The Healthy Start
Initiative

THURMA McCANN GOLDMAN AND DAVID S. DE LA CRUZ

Giving people a voice in the systems that affect their lives can be very powerful. When a community is able to redesign its health and social service systems, both the community and its members are transformed. But community participation in reshaping systems does not just happen. If members of a community are truly to have an impact, they must have an organized voice. Collaborative efforts, including coalitions, are becoming that voice.

OVERVIEW OF COALITIONS

A coalition is a union of people and organizations working to influence outcomes on a specific problem.[1] Coalitions are useful for accomplishing a broad range of goals that reach beyond the capacity of any individual member organization. These goals range from information sharing to coordination of services, from community education to advocacy for major environmental or policy changes.[2,3]

Coalitions offer numerous potential advantages over individuals or organizations working independently.[1] The broader purpose and breadth of coalitions give them more credibility than individual organizations and can reduce the suspicion of self-interest. Among the many benefits of coalitions are the following:

1. Conserve resources, which are becoming more limited
2. Reach more people within a community than a single organization can
3. Accomplish objectives beyond the scope of any single organization
4. Have greater credibility than an individual organization
5. Provide a forum for sharing information
6. Provide a range of advice and perspectives to the lead agency
7. Foster personal satisfaction and help members understand their jobs in a broader perspective
8. Foster cooperation among grassroots organizations, community members, and diverse sectors of a large organization

Coalitions build trust and consensus among people and organizations that have similar responsibilities and concerns within a community.

However, a coalition is not appropriate in every situation and is only one of a variety of tools for accomplishing organizational goals.[1,4] A lead agency should consider carefully the responsibilities of developing and coordinating a coalition. The success of a coalition is usually uncertain. In addition, lead agencies tend to underestimate the requirements needed to keep coalitions functioning well, especially the commitment of substantial staffing resources. Coalitions also require significant commitment from the members, who frequently must weigh coalition membership against other important work. Potential results need to be measured against their costs, keeping in mind that results of coalition efforts often diverge from the initial expectations of the organizations that created them. Furthermore, some tasks are inappropriate for coalitions because they may require quick responses that are unwieldy for coalitions or they may require an intensity of focus that is difficult to attain with a large group.[3,5]

Also, before initiating a coalition, it is important to determine whether related groups already exist within the community.[6,7] At times, it will be far more effective to participate in an already existing group with compatible goals than to form a new coalition. Finally, people and organizations often define terms differently. It is important to define clearly the type of group that will be set up, including its mission, membership, and structure, and to make sure that all participants understand and agree with this definition.

There are eight steps to building an effective coalition[1,8]: 1) analyze the program's objectives and determine whether to form a coalition; 2) recruit the right people; 3) devise a set of preliminary objectives and activities; 4) convene the coalition; 5) anticipate the necessary resources; 6) define elements of a successful coalition structure; 7) maintain coalition vitality; and, 8) make improvements through evaluation.

A federally funded initiative that has used coalitions and community collaboration to successfully implement its activities is Healthy Start. The following description of the Healthy Start Initiative includes the ways in which coalitions have been used.

THE HEALTHY START INITIATIVE

For many years, infant mortality has been used as a key indicator of a society's health status. The fact that in 1989 the United States ranked 21st among industrialized nations in infant mortality rates challenged maternal and child health experts. This led the White House Task Force to Reduce Infant Mortality to convene and make recommendations that were adapted by the Interagency Committee on Infant Mortality in 1990. This targeted approach to infant mortality reduction was one of the most recent efforts, among many through the years, of tackling a problem that, although showing signs of some improvement, seemed far from the Healthy People 2000 goal (Objective 14.1a) of no more than 7.0 infant deaths per 1,000 live births.

Despite recent gains in reducing infant deaths, infant mortality remains a serious and tragic problem that can be solved only if all stakeholders—community members (including its leaders), businesses, health care professionals, and policymakers—work together to find answers. To help find these solutions, and put them into practice across the country, the Healthy Start Initiative was first developed as a national demonstration program in 1991. The Initiative was founded on the premise that community-driven strategies were needed to attack the causes of infant mortality and low birthweight, especially among high-risk populations.

Healthy Start, a community-based initiative, uses a systems development approach to reduce infant mortality and improve the health and well-being of women, infants, children, and families. Healthy Start strengthens and enhances community systems of maternal and infant care while challenging communities to fully address the medical, behavioral, and psychosocial needs of women, infants, and families. Healthy Start concentrates on the provision of community-based, culturally sensitive, family-centered, comprehensive perinatal services to women, infants, and their families in communities with high rates of infant mortality. Healthy Start also focuses on the integration of these services into existing systems of perinatal care.

The principles guiding the planning and operation of the Healthy Start Initiative are innovation, community commitment and involvement, increased access to services, service integration, and personal responsibility. A unique hallmark of Healthy Start is the development and mobilization of strong coalitions—composed of consumers, local and state governments, the private sector, schools, health care providers, and neighborhood organizations—to address infant mortality reduction and make their community more healthy.

At its inception, the Healthy Start Initiative was designed to determine the unmet needs within the communities' geographic catchment area and to devise a comprehensive plan that would decrease infant mortality over a 5-year period. The motivation behind this effort was the promise of unprecedented resources ($140 million), which would be awarded directly to local communities in exchange for the development and implementation of programs that would lower the infant mortality rate by 50% during the funding period.

Applicants for the Healthy Start demonstration grants were sought among urban and rural communities with infant mortality rates at least 1.5 times the national average. In late 1991, 15 applicants (13 urban and 2 rural) were awarded planning grants. The initial grants supported year-long comprehensive planning activities through fiscal year 1992; the projects began serving clients in fiscal year 1993. In late 1994, seven additional communities (five urban and two rural) received Healthy Start demonstration Special Project Grants. These communities also had infant mortality rates higher than 1.5 times the national average.

As a demonstration initiative, Healthy Start had the responsibility to develop, demonstrate, disseminate, and replicate strategies for reducing infant mortality. Although the 22 Healthy Start communities vary widely, over the course of the 5-year demonstration nine models have taken shape and have been implemented in ways that address each community's special needs. That is, in designing its unique approach to reducing infant mortality, each Healthy Start community has examined the factors that have contributed to infant mortality within its own neighborhoods and identified the community's needs and resources. As a result of this process, Healthy Start communities have developed nine models of effective intervention, along with community-specific strategies to implement the models successfully:

- Community-based consortia
- Outreach and client recruitment
- Care coordination/case management
- Family resource centers
- Enhanced clinical services
- Risk prevention and reduction
- Facilitating services
- Training and education
- Adolescent programs

These nine models are a means of empowering communities to reduce the incidence of low birthweight, preterm births, and infant mortality and to increase access to prenatal care. These models are Healthy Start's legacy and all focus on the same goal: community-based infant mortality reduction. The models accomplish this through community-based services integration, including consortium development, especially for those at highest risk.

Soon after receiving funding, members in each of the Healthy Start communities began analyzing how to identify needs, involve the community, work with consortia, establish and maintain an array of program initiatives, and evaluate their efforts. At the end of the demonstration phase, these teams—including consumers, consortia members, and Healthy Start project staff—had learned many lessons and were able to share their experiences and lessons learned.

Healthy Start has now entered the replication phase, during which the lessons learned and experiences gained during the first 6 years of the initiative are being disseminated to other communities.

The purpose of the Healthy Start replication phase is to implement successful infant mortality reduction strategies developed during the demonstration phase and to launch Healthy Start projects in other rural, urban, and inner-city communities currently without a Healthy Start–funded project.

During the replication phase, the Healthy Start Initiative is supporting cooperative agreements to 41 new communities for the replication and/or adaptation of successful Healthy Start strategies, along with those individual programs already under way from 20 of the demonstration phase communities. Furthermore, an additional 14 communities have been designated Planning Grantees and are being supported in their year-long comprehensive planning activities.

The Healthy Start communities funded during the demonstration phase are mentoring the new replication sites on the models and strategies that the demonstration sites were successful in implementing. Successful strategies are those that have achieved the agreed on program performance for an activity. More scientific measures of outcomes from the demonstration phase will be forthcoming via special comprehensive reports of the national evaluation and individual local studies.

The replication of a demonstration project provides a unique opportunity to use and refine the lessons learned by the now mentoring project sites. The sharing of information among the replication and mentoring sites is occurring in a variety of ways, including formal meetings and conferences. Regional mentoring conferences and open houses have enabled new Healthy Start projects to experience and address implementation issues associated with each of the nine intervention strategies.

Although the demonstration phase was valuable to the 22 Healthy Start communities, the lessons learned during the demonstration phase are not applicable only to those communities funded by the Healthy Start Initiative. There are more than 300 communities across the United States that have an infant mortality rate greater than one and a half times the national rate. These lessons can prove valuable to the 300 communities, as well as to other maternal and child health professionals.

As more communities try to change their health and social systems to make them more responsive to the needs of the community members, collaborative efforts are becoming recognized as potent vehicles for transformation.[9,10] The federal Healthy Start Initiative has recognized that power and has placed collaboration, in the form of community-based coalitions, at the center of its efforts. A key component of the Healthy Start Initiative is to reduce infant mortality by helping communities assess their needs and decide which interventions work best to meet their individual and unique needs.

Although Healthy Start focuses on reducing infant mortality, its efforts to involve the community in collaboration can be replicated to tackle other public health problems. As health care reform continues to alter the health and medical system in the United States, the benefit of collaboration becomes even more relevant: as a community transforms its systems to meet its needs, the community is empowered.

By emphasizing the consortia model, the Healthy Start Initiative focuses the power of collaboration on the problem of infant mortality. A well-organized community can lead to benefits that ultimately reduce maternal and infant mortality and morbidity rates. These benefits include increasing the public's understanding of the problem, strengthening the public's commitment to deal realistically with the problem, using existing resources more efficiently and effectively, and mobilizing additional resources.

HEALTHY START COMMUNITY CASE EXAMPLES

At the heart of the Healthy Start Initiative is the belief that the community, guided by a consortium of individuals and organizations from many sectors, can best design and implement the services needed by the women, children, and families in that community. The key reason that collaboration is essential to fighting infant mortality is found in the complexity of the problem itself. Because infant mortality is affected by socioeconomic conditions such as poverty, inadequate housing, unemployment, racism, and violence, no single organization can solve the problem. A collaborative, multidisciplinary approach within the community can create the long-term vision needed to attack the problem from a variety of angles.

The following are case examples from 5 of the Healthy Start communities funded during the demonstration phase of the Initiative. These examples are meant to show how the different communities used their consortium to collaborate and build coalitions that have helped them in their fight against infant mortality.

Savannah Healthy Start Initiative

The Savannah Youth Futures Authority functions as the consortium to monitor progress on all aspects of their project. The collaborative structure precedes the Healthy Start Initiative and was created by legislation adopted by the State of Georgia to achieve the following mandate for children in Chatham County:

Adopt and amend a comprehensive plan to improve the conditions for children in Chatham County; coordinate, evaluate and administratively support the implementation of the plan; and, contract with public and private agencies to implement and monitor the plan.

The Authority functions under the structure of its enabling legislation and by-laws for a nonprofit corporation. During the 1990s, they have evolved a process of consensus decision-making among the members of the Authority. Interagency agreements provide the framework for the mutual commitments of partners to specific initiatives. This comprehensive approach has created a culture of collaboration among the Authority's members and partners that facilitates interagency operations and planning for results-based interventions. The Annual Profile of Children shows significant improvement on many indicators of child and family well-being, including significant reductions in infant mortality and percentage of women delivering with inadequate prenatal care and increases in adequate infant immunization.

Consumer participation is a valued component of the Savannah project, and consumer input is obtained in several ways. An advisory council, the Community Change for Youth Development Neighborhood Council, has been established that serves as the liaison between the community, their Family Resource Center, and the grantee. This group was pulled together to identify and implement priority activities such as a gymnasium renovation project; at the completion of this project, the gymnasium became available for meetings and other community events. Also, several participant focus groups have been held to obtain community input on planning and evaluation. For example, before childbirth classes were initiated, focus groups were held with both teens and adults to determine what they thought about the health education they had previously received. This input was used to determine preferred days of the week and times, childbirth curriculum content, and the approach to be used with pregnant teens. Additionally, a Moms Recommendation/Implementation Advisory Group has been developed by the Fetal and Infant Mortality Review program to receive perceptions from mothers and pregnant women on what activities should be pursued and suggestions on the types of follow-up that should occur. Occasional retreats for planning and leadership development have been used to strengthen group cohesion and commitment.

Chicago Healthy Start

The purposes of the Chicago Healthy Start (CHS) consortium are to advise the Illinois Department of Public Health (IDPH) on the implementation of CHS activities in the target area; to encourage full integration of all core services; to monitor the quality of service delivery; to encourage accurate and comprehensive data collection and evaluation; to assist in the identification of funding to sustain the initiative; and to refine the committee structure to accomplish these purposes. The consortium structure was designed to ensure representation from the communities being served. Seven Healthy Start standing committees were established over the first 5 years of the project: Systematic Change, Case Management, Family/Community Mobilization, Community Economic Development, Public Education/Media, Data and Evaluation, and Substance Abuse. The committees are composed of providers and non-provider residents and are a collaboration of key agencies that impact the maternal and child health of the community residents. The committees elected the members of the Healthy Start consortium.

In addition to the committees, the consortium also receives input from the Executive Committee, which is composed of two IDPH representatives, two Chicago Department of Public Health representatives, two Cook County Bureau of Health Services members, two members from each of the five Family Centers, task force chairs, six community representatives, and the consortium chair, vice chair, and secretary. This coordination with city, county, and state health departments has been invaluable in fostering the relationships needed to coordinate the multi-funded maternal child health services offered to residents of the project area. The current consortium roster includes 43 service providers, five representatives from state government, a consumer, and three others.

Since the initial planning of Chicago Healthy Start, consumers have been encouraged to participate in the consortium. One of the major problems, however, has been getting consumers to participate on the Standing Committees, thus becoming eligible to be elected to the consortium and to function as voting members. Although attendance by consumers has been good, their willingness or comfort with participating on subcommittees has not been at the level desired or anticipated by CHS. The community-based agencies have tried many approaches to encourage consumer participation. Barriers to attendance include child care and transportation.

Another successful tool has been offering practical incentives. These mechanisms have increased initial participation, and once consumers attend the consortium meeting and see that their opinion is not only respected but solicited, they return and bring their pregnant friends. Although they are not formally members of the consortium, consumer participation has increased to the point that the consumers have outnumbered the providers at several meetings. Provider and non-provider resident input has been respected and accepted. There is extensive documentation of consortium recommendations that have been implemented. The Chicago Healthy Start Initiative is programmatically sound because it took the time to build trust between its participants by listening to its committees and consortium.

Currently the consortium's mission focuses on the use of "one-stop shopping" as the principle for the delivery of health and social services to families living in the project area. The consortium is convinced that collaboration between managed care providers, hospitals, and community-based case management agencies will make the best use of existing resources and improve access to services. Regarding sustainability, the consortium and IDPH leaders have received technical assistance on marketing the Family Centers to health maintenance organizations (HMOs), hospitals, and other providers who deliver services to large numbers of Medicaid recipients. Proposals to include the five Family Centers collectively in managed care panels or other forms of affiliation with hospitals or other health care providers have been developed. The consortium and the IDPH are engaged in ongoing discussions about sustaining the Family Centers.

Boston Healthy Start Initiative

The Boston Healthy Start Initiative (BHSI) has one consortium, which regularly meets at different locations throughout the project area. This structure has been formalized through by-laws that include a conflict of interest statement. Another accomplishment has been the development of a culturally diverse consortium that coordinates on-going focus groups to develop educational materials for Latino, Haitian, and East Asian communities; they developed a domestic violence brochure in Spanish and English that has received national recognition. The project has encouraged meaningful involvement of, and input from, consumers, and through pairing new consumers with an experienced Board member, they have been able to provide a less threatening orientation to the consortium.

Consumers are involved in BHSI policy development, implementation, and evaluation of all activities through their participation in the consortium, focus groups, public information forums, and a number of other community-based activities. The consortium has six committees with which consumers are encouraged to become involved to further enhance their input; much project business occurs through the work of these committees. Consumers represent 60% of the consortium membership; on the 25-member Executive Committee of the consortium, 70% are non-provider residents, with a 37% consumer representation. Resident and consumer training has been provided in stages: initial sessions focused on structure of the organization—the goal and objectives and mission statement; information on general health issues affecting the project area were provided next; then community residents completed a survey identifying other health issues on which they wanted more. The BHSI has received a foundation grant for further consortium development, which has been used to train 15 consumers to become community organizers and trainers. Through this grant, the consortium is hoping to replicate this organizational model in other initiatives throughout the city.

The consortium has been successful in creating an interface between a number of city agencies, including city government, hospitals, and the community. Mistrust between these agencies and the community had to be addressed by having cultural sensitivity training and an opportunity to learn what residents and consumers with a public health focus are capable of doing. Similarly, a number of community health centers and small community-based organizations have focused on the larger issue of infant mortality by working with each other. BHSI has learned that it is easier to approach the private sector with ideas for specific activities (preferably those occurring annually) that they can sponsor and for which they receive public exposure, such as health fairs and annual meetings. They have been able to negotiate with companies to match purchases; for example, the public transit company donated five bus posters when Public Information Committee members and project staff agreed to purchase five. There have been similar successes with buying air time for the radio and having stations match additional commercials without charge.

Regarding sustainability, the consortium is actively involved with project staff in hosting a series of 10 roundtables with seven other initiatives within the project area on joint sustainability; this includes programs with a focus on reduction of juvenile crime, mental health delivery reform, job readiness, and small business development. The consortium and project are also looking to universities and community health centers for resources; seven community health centers have received community benefits funding as a result of their work with the project.

Healthy Start/New York City

The Healthy Start/NYC project has a project-wide consortium and one consortium in each of its three service areas. This structure has been formalized through the development of by-laws that define the roles and responsibilities of each of the principals, including the grantee, subcontractor agencies, and project committees. Creation of these by-laws through a group process at the inception of the project has helped fortify a team approach in New York City and mitigated turf and control issues among key stakeholders. In addition to this accomplishment, the four consortia have provided an important vehicle for collaboration among disparate organizations, including grassroots and well-established public and private sector organizations, as well as providers and local residents within a large city with a complex service infrastructure. These four consortia have also helped increase community awareness of the Healthy Start/NYC project, services that are available, and the multiple causes of infant mortality. The project area–wide consortium's public information committee, which was chaired by the executive director of the Greater New York March of Dimes, was instrumental in developing successful public information campaigns to raise awareness and involvement in the project. The Healthy Start/NYC project, through its consortium's governance structure, also recognized the need for infrastructure development within its participating subcontractor organizations. Training has been provided that included strategic planning, board development, program planning and sustainability, and financial management.

Consumer involvement within the Healthy Start/NYC project is most evident at the service area consortium level. Consumers participate in management and governance and program development and planning. Each of the three Healthy Start/NYC targeted communities has developed strategies to involve consumers. Participation of consumers can range up to 30 or more who are involved on a regular basis. Consumer participation has been elicited through focus groups, client satisfaction surveys, outreach, volunteer services, community conferences, and involvement in consumer advisory groups. Consumers are also involved in developing programs such as a farmer's market, community awareness breakfasts, youth conferences, advocacy and public speakouts, and domestic violence trainer workshops.

Consumers receive critical training, including workshops on the importance of male involvement in parenting and strengthening relationships; job development, such as the Harlem Works program, which helps move welfare clients to work; self-esteem building; and entrepreneurial skills.

Healthy Start/NYC has approached businesses and the private sector and has received funding from major corporations in the project, including Consolidated Edison of NY, Pfizer Inc., Chase Manhattan Bank, and Banco Popular. Foundation support includes the New York Community Trust and the New York Yankees Foundation.

Healthy Start/NYC plans to continue its consortia through the support of private funders. The project area–wide consortium will focus on increasing consumer involvement, joint resource development, and advocacy during the replication phase. The project's consortia are unique in that they are the only New York City–based venues in which experts from the community and city administration come together on a regular basis.

Richmond Healthy Start Initiative

The purpose of the Richmond Healthy Start Initiative (RHSI) consortium is to establish a comprehensive and coordinated approach to reduce infant mortality throughout Richmond with a special focus on three high-risk target zones (South Zone, North-West Zone, and East Zone). The goal is to enable and empower these communities to create permanent institutional responses to the problem of infant mortality and to improve access to health care and social services for women and their families. Meetings are held quarterly at various locations throughout the targeted areas; the standing committees also meet regularly each quarter. This organization has been formalized with by-laws that emphasize that the role of the consortium is to enhance, not compete with, maternal and child health–focused activities in Richmond. Meaningful involvement from Healthy Start consumers has been encouraged, and RHSI contractors are asked to invite and assist their consumers to participate. Twelve representatives from contractors, human service agencies, consumers, universities, and the public health department constitute the Steering Committee membership. Other consortium committees include Consumer Involvement, Data and Evaluation, Sustainability, Program Year-End Review, Public Education, and Conference Planning. These committees actively participate in decision-making, planning objectives, and charting the course of the consortium.

Membership composition of the consortium includes consumers, social service agencies, volunteer agencies serving women and their families, hospitals, members of the business community, churches, and community health centers. Representatives from State Title V agencies, the Department of Social Services, and Richmond Public Health are also included in the membership. The RHSI continues to focus on increasing and strengthening the consumer representation. Consumers take the lead in setting the agenda and determining the objectives of the Consumer Involvement Committee. Members of this committee are currently receiving training on leadership and group development. Home visitor training for mothers who are moving from welfare to work has been provided to project participants, including committee members.

Sustainability efforts of RHSI have included a series of events. RHSI held a community-wide conference, "Richmond's Challenge:

Give Every Baby a Healthy Start." Three major components for the day-long event were a corporate breakfast roundtable, community summit, and conference. The purpose of the corporate roundtable was not only to make the corporate sector aware of the RHSI and its mission, but more importantly to reach out to them for support in sustaining and increasing the work of the project. At the community summit, there was strong representation from the consumers, who identified issues and needs in their communities that are related to families, especially to children. More foundation and corporate roundtables are planned for this next year. One outcome of the corporate roundtable has been having a large law firm volunteer to establish an independent nonprofit status for RHSI. Marketing teams have been created from consortium membership and are receiving training from a marketing specialist to assist them in promoting funding support from the business community. The RHSI project director has created a grant writing team within the Richmond City Department of Public Health, the project grantee, to aggressively seek additional grant funding related to maternal and child health.

CONCLUSIONS AND RECOMMENDATIONS

The local Healthy Start consortia identified several actions to foster collaborative efforts. Although the following actions are a result of lessons learned during the demonstration phase of the Healthy Start Initiative, they are also applicable to any agency or organizations involved with consortium development:

1. *Bring together all those involved in Healthy Start programs who are working on developing the consortia and the local councils as part of a community summit meeting.* At the very least, those already working on these issues in the various communities should be brought together to discuss their concerns and strategies. Consumers and activists need to be part of that discussion; they are the individuals involved in the front-line of community organizing.

2. *Provide information on other efforts in collaboration and community organizing.* There are many other collaborative efforts occurring around the country that might have lessons for the Healthy Start Initiative. Disseminating this information on a regular basis would be helpful. It would be even more valuable if opportunities were created for Healthy Start staff to meet with some of the leaders of these other efforts, either

through visits to their communities or through attendance at national conferences that deal with these issues.

3. *Provide help for training staff and community members in coalition/consortium building and community organizing.* Healthy Start staff and consumers need training in building coalitions and organizing their communities. Staff and consortium members at all levels should be involved. Leaders of the local councils as well as leaders of the project consortia could benefit from training. Consumers also need to be part of the training.

4. *Federal office provide support and guidance, while being receptive and understanding to the unique needs of each community.* The Division of Healthy Start should continue to strive to be receptive to comments and suggestions from the Healthy Start project sites. Open communication and dialogue is necessary to support the consortium development effort.

Many diverse factors contribute to our national infant mortality rate. Considerable progress has been made in identifying these factors and meeting the challenges they present, but much more work still needs to be done. Through the years of the Healthy Start Initiative, disparities—racial, economic, and geographic—in access to early prenatal care have been reduced, resulting in a trend toward healthier birth outcomes. But the work must continue. The Healthy Start communities have identified community-based strategies that can significantly and effectively reduce infant mortality, thereby increasing our knowledge of successful approaches to guarding the health of both mother and infant. During the replication phase, Healthy Start will continue its fight against infant mortality.

Kevin L. Thurm, Deputy Secretary U.S. Department of Health and Human Services, spoke at a Healthy Start conference in 1996. An excerpt of his remarks follow, summarizing the importance that Healthy Start invests in collaboration:

From community leaders to clergy, from parents to teachers, from health care providers to corporations, it will take all of us working together to do right by our children and our families, to reach parents where they read, work, and live, to reach them in their homes and at their jobs, on buses and in the streets, to reach across boundaries of culture and geography, race and income, providing hope and healing for all parents, all families, all Americans.

If we continue to stand together and work together, we can win the fight against infant mortality—the fight for the future of our children and our country.[11]

References

1. Cohen, L., Baer, N., and Satterwhite, P. Developing effective coalitions: An eight step guide. *Injury Awareness and Prevention Centre News*. 1994;4(10).
2. Butterfoss, F.D. Coalitions for alcohol and other drug abuse: Factors predicting effectiveness (unpublished doctoral dissertation). School of Public Health, University of South Carolina, 1993.
3. Goodman, R.M., Wandersman, A., Chinman, M., Imm, P., and Morrissey, E. An ecological assessment of community-based interventions for prevention and health promotion: Approaches to measuring community coalitions. *American Journal of Community Psychology*. 1996;24(1).
4. Chinman, M.J. Benefits, costs and empowerment in community coalitions (unpublished doctoral dissertation). Clinical/Community Psychology Program, University of South Carolina, 1995.
5. Wandersman, A., and Florin, P. Careful community research and action. *The Community Psychologist*. Summer, 1990;4–5.
6. Amherst H. Wilder Foundation. Factors influencing the success of collaboration. In *Collaboration: What makes it work*. 1992.
7. Butterfoss, F.D., Goodman, R.M., and Wandersman, A. Community coalitions for prevention and health promotion. *Health Education Research*. 1993;8(3):315–330.
8. Wandersman, A., Valois, R., Ochs, L., de la Cruz, D.S., Adkins, E., and Goodman, R.M. Toward a social ecology of community coalitions. *American Journal of Health Promotion*. 1996;10(4):299–307.
9. Bracht, N., and Gleason, J. Strategies and structures for citizen partnerships. In N. Bracht (ed). *Health promotion at the community level*. Vol. 15. Newbury Park: SAGE Publications, 1990, pp. 109–124.
10. Kumpfer, K.L., Turner, C., Hopkins, R., and Librett, J. Leadership and team effectiveness in community coalitions for the prevention of alcohol and other drug abuse. *Health Education Research*. 1993;8(3):359–374.
11. Thurm, K.L. Presentation at Winning the Fight Against Infant Mortality: A National Summit on Community and Corporate Initiatives. Washington, DC, September, 1996.

31

Head Start

ANNE COHN DONNELLY AND FREDERICK C. GREEN

The History and Intent of Head Start

As recounted by Ed Zigler, one of the founders and later steward of Head Start, the federal Head Start Program began in 1965 with very high expectations and high hopes that it would significantly improve the chances that poor children would succeed in life. The idea was hatched during the "War on Poverty" in response to one simple statistic—in 1964 nearly half of the nation's poor people were children and most were younger than age 12. Program designers understood that a War on Poverty must address the needs and conditions of these poor children; they also knew that a War on Poverty that would benefit children was a war most of the public would support. Head Start was the only weapon in the war targeting the problems of children; the other programs were for adults and older teens.

In its conception, and from its inception, Head Start was seen as a comprehensive program: a child care and education facility for preschoolers that would address the need for systematic evaluation of the health status of children through episodic screening for hearing and eye care, proper nutrition, the provision of immunization and other facets of young children's physical and mental health. It would also focus on motivating children and creating a climate that would help in the development of children's mental processes and skills. In other words, it would address all facets of child development. At the same time, it would involve parents as integral parts of the children's lives and education for their children's as well as their own benefit. An emphasis would be placed on employing the parents and other poor people in the program.

In its inception, Head Start was to be a summer-only program, with the plan that poor preschool children from low income families would be ready to begin kindergarten or first grade and communities would use otherwise closed school facilities and provide summer jobs for teachers. It did not take long to see the benefits of year-round support for these children, and the program expanded toward a full year (i.e., 10 months) in its second year, sprouting up in churches and storefronts and other available community facilities.

The program was to be for all poor children of preschool age. Although not a part of the initial design, in response to the special needs of handicapped and disabled children, a set proportion of enrollment (i.e., 10%) was assigned for handicapped children.

Unlike special initiatives today, when Head Start began, the idea was that it would serve a significant portion of the target population—at least 100,000. It would be launched as an instant nationwide program. The movers and shakers behind Head Start and the rest of the

War on Poverty were ready for action, not pilots and demonstrations and evaluations. Once the President's wife Lady Bird Johnson signed on as the Honorary Chairperson and a kick-off reception was held at the White House, enthusiasm grew, and in its first year Head Start in fact served more than one half a million children. This nationwide implementation gave instant visibility to the program and gathered grassroots support virtually across the country (or, as some like to point out, in every congressional district). It was this widespread community support that has stood this federal effort in good stead through repeated federal reauthorizations.

Of course, not everyone embraced Head Start. Some segments of the community saw federally supported child development programs as "contrary to the American ethos." Some felt that child care programs should target parents directly by helping them off the welfare rolls rather than targeting children to enhance their developmental potential. Despite these competing views, Head Start flourished.

Community enthusiasm for the program was matched by the enthusiasm of volunteers in Washington, DC, and across the country—volunteers to help representatives from poor neighborhoods write proposals, volunteers to help government officials review proposals, volunteers to help set up and operate funded efforts. This enthusiasm was widespread—from spouses of high-ranking government officials to pastors in local churches to all manner of health and education professionals (e.g., doctors and dentists who would do free checkups). High-visibility national groups such as the American Academy of Pediatrics joined the cause. To help maintain and promote this volunteerism, part of the 20% local match required of grantees could consist of volunteered time. Health and hospital facilities and others were urged to have community advisory committees, a form of community control. This was in contrast to most such community facilities, which were typically governed by non-neighborhood residents.

The original push for parental involvement in Head Start was in many ways revolutionary: the concept was that children would benefit from their parents' direct involvement in the program. The parents could learn about child development and facets of child learning and also fill many of the staff positions. The concept initially was that parents would not totally control Head Start but that with 51% membership on the programs' policy councils, parents would have shared control in planning and administration. The roles of parents in program direction and community activism emerged later. (In 1973, for example, the national Head Start Association was formed by the Head Start directors; a year later, in recognition of the importance of parents, parents were admitted to the Association.)

In order to ensure that there was a cadre of trained caregivers to meet children's development needs and who were more affordable than teachers with bachelor's degrees, Head Start established opportunities for parents and other community people to be trained as Child Development Associates (CDA) so they could provide quality child care in Head Start and other child care programs. This would be the beginning of a career ladder for many of these people. Over the years, there have been many ups and downs in the implementation of this training initiative. (Today it is proposed that Head Start Centers be required to have at least one teacher in every classroom of 17–18 children with a recognized credential in child development or at least an associate's degree in early childhood education.)

INNOVATIONS IN HEAD START

From the outset, there have been a number of program innovations in Head Start, in addition to efforts to move the program from a part-day summer program to a full-year full-day one. The idea was to provide continuity of support—from the earliest year through Head Start and thereafter. The three most significant innovations are (1) efforts to follow children into elementary school after Head Start, (2) efforts to reach children before they enter Head Start (i.e., from pregnancy or birth), and (3) efforts to reach out to families in their homes as well as through Center-based programs.

In 1967, a Follow Through program was designed and initiated to extend comprehensive services to Head Start children when they entered kindergarten and through third grade. Efforts like this, which were never fully funded, have continued throughout Head Start's history. As such, in the early years, Follow Through became an experiment to develop and compare the effectiveness of various curriculum models. (Today, this effort is embodied in the Head Start Transition Project.) Also in 1967, still the early years of Head Start, Parent and Child Centers were set up in 33 of the Head Start communities to serve families with young children from birth to 3 years. Centers like these, which have continued ever since, are the precursors to Early Head Start. One of Head Start's most successful innovations, which also began in the early years, was Home Start, an effort designed to offer all the benefits of Head Start but in the home. This home-based intervention, which was especially well suited to rural areas, has continued as an option to any Head Start program. (Today, the home-based component is as integral a part of Early Head Start as it is of Head Start in general.)

EARLY HEAD START: PROMISE FOR THE FUTURE

By the early 1990s, recognition that children need positive child development experiences starting at birth was widespread. The reauthorization of the Head Start Act in 1994 made it possible for Head Start to include an "early" Head Start component for babies and toddlers. The Early Head Start program, which officially began in 1995, pooled Head Start's existing programs for families with infants and toddlers with the Parent and Child Centers, the Head Start home-based component, and the government's Comprehensive Child Development Program. The hope was that Early Head Start would finally establish the beginnings of a full continuum of support for low income children and their families.

The idea behind Early Head Start was to direct resources into supports and services that would build communities while providing healthy child and family development. The concept was to offer a constellation of services (health, social services, early childhood education) to families with newborns through age 3, while maintaining a commitment to training, quality, service coordination, and evaluation. In many ways, the specific goals for Early Head Start were no different than those of Head Start, although there was recognition that support to and education of parents of these very young children were essential features. Further, Early Head Start recognized that for infants and toddlers to develop optimally, they must have healthy beginnings and the continuity of responsive and caring relationships with the primary adults in their lives. The program reflects research from the previous three decades, which has shown that when programs focus on both the child *and* the parent and family, through early high-quality, comprehensive, intensive services, even the most vulnerable children and families can develop in positive ways.

The Early Head Start program thus was designed with the benefit of 30 years of experiences with the Head Start program. Early Head Start was at its inception founded on a set of principles that matured slowly for its parent program:

- A commitment to excellence
- A focus on prevention and promotion
- A commitment to developing strong, caring continuous relationships
- Strong involvement of parents
- The inclusion of children with disabilities, and their families
- Comprehensive, flexible, responsive, and intensive services

- A smooth transition from Early Head Start to Head Start or other high-quality preschool programs
- Collaboration with other community providers and institutions that affect children and their families

In order to accomplish these goals, Early Head Start efforts are concerned with the development of the child, the family, the staff, and the community. In its first year, 143 Early Head Start projects were supported, serving 22,000 children younger than age 3. One year later, the number of projects doubled.

VARIATION ACROSS HEAD START PROGRAMS: A QUESTION OF QUALITY

In recognition that the poor were not a homogeneous group and that poor communities each had their own "culture," at the outset Head Start was not a precisely defined program. There was no prescribed curriculum. Rather, each grantee was given latitude in shaping the form of the program. As a result, Head Start programs early on varied significantly; the lack of a consistent set of standards and also the lack of a specific set of beliefs about early childhood contributed to this variability. Although a variety of models were suggested in the early years, the variability in who was hired as a teacher—and the general lack of trained teachers in some communities—contributed to the variability.

Variability across Head Start sites was seen over time, and questions about quality were raised. Certainly the uneven training of teachers and the low pay contributed to these concerns. But other issues surfaced as well. The class size in Head Start rooms was uneven. The delivery of health services to children was not consistent. The services offered to families identified with multiple problems was not always comprehensive. Even the facilities within which Head Start programs found themselves were varied; many were temporary and not all met codes for safety. As a result, over time, standards were set and imposed on Head Start grantees, and programs began to look more comparable and began to address issues of quality.

WHAT HEAD START HAS ACCOMPLISHED

The story of Head Start's accomplishments can be told in two ways— through numbers and through measured outcomes. The numbers alone are impressive.

The Numbers

Since its inception in 1965 (when it was launched as a summer-only program) through 1996, more than 16 million children and their families have been served (Table 31.1). It is important to note that enrollment dropped dramatically after the first 5 years; Head Start achieved the 1965 enrollment size again in 1991. By 1996, federal appropriations grew from $96 million to $3.5 billion. In contrast to this growth

TABLE 31.1

Head Start Enrollment and Appropriation History

Fiscal Year	Enrollment	Congressional Appropriation
1965 (Summer Only)	561,000	$ 96,400,000
1966	733,000	$198,900,000
1967	681,400	$349,200,000
1968	693,900	$316,200,000
1969	663,600	$333,900,000
1970	477,400	$325,700,000
1971	397,500	$360,000,000
1972	379,000	$376,300,000
1973	379,000	$400,700,000
1974	352,800	$403,900,000
1975	349,000	$403,900,000
1976	349,000	$441,000,000
1977	333,000	$475,000,000
1978	391,400	$625,000,000
1979	387,500	$680,000,000
1980	376,300	$735,000,000
1981	387,300	$818,700,000
1982	395,800	$911,700,000
1983	414,950	$912,000,000
1984	442,140	$995,750,000
1985	452,080	$1,075,059,000
1986	451,732	$1,040,315,000
1987	446,523	$1,130,542,000
1988	448,464	$1,206,324,000
1989	450,970	$1,235,000,000
1990	540,930	$1,552,000,000
1991	583,471	$1,951,800,000
1992	621,078	$2,201,800,000
1993	713,903	$2,776,286,000
1994	740,493	$3,325,728,000
1995	750,696	$3,534,128,000
1996	752,077	$3,569,329,000

A total of 16,098,000 children have been served by the program since it began in 1965.

Source: Head Start Bureau, DHHS, Washington, DC, 1997.

TABLE 31.2

The Head Start Child in 1996

Ages	
5-year-olds and older	6%
4-year-olds	62%
3-year-olds	29%
Younger than 3 years of age	4%
Income	
Less than $9,000 1 per yr.	62%
Less than $12,000 per yr.	78%
Racial/Ethnic Composition	
American Indian	3.5%
Hispanic	25.2%
Black	36.0%
White	32.3%
Asian	3.0%

Total Enrollment in 1996 was 752,077.

Source: Head Start Bureau, DHHS, Washington, DC, 1997.

in dollars, the increase in numbers of children served has been more gradual. In 1965, 561,000 were served during the summer; in 1996, the number was just over 752,000 year round, with 20% now receiving full-day services year round. (This percentage is slowly increasing through collaborations with local child care providers.)

A profile of the children served in 1996 tells an important story (Table 31.2). The program serves a diverse population with a significant representation of pre-kindergarten children (4-year-olds). These children were served in 16,636 centers, which in turn were supported through 1,440 grantees. There were more than 146,000 paid staff supported by more than 1,239,000 volunteers. Of the paid staff, 30% were parents of current or former Head Start children. And, according to the Head Start Bureau, 75% of the volunteers were parents.

In terms of raw numbers, the program has touched literally millions and millions of lives. Yet today, with these large numbers, only about one third of the eligible poor children are served by the program.

The Outcomes

From the very outset of Head Start, evaluation or outcome data were recognized as important. However, most would agree that the hasty evaluation of the first summer's program was of little value. In fact, the evaluations in the earliest years were problematic if for no other reason than because of their narrow scope. Early political supporters had believed (and promised) that Head Start would improve children's IQ, and early evaluations studied this specific outcome rather than the broader issues of child development Head Start was really intended to address. More recent evaluations have addressed these broader issues.

The early evaluation studies did demonstrate gains in IQ, but the gains were only temporary. Initial IQ gains declined over time, and Head Start in those early years was found to have no measurable impact on later school achievement or performance. (These early studies, coupled with the political climate, help explain years of shrinkage or at least no or minimal growth in the program size as shown in Table 31.1.)

Later studies, which looked at child development more globally and at Head Start *and* comparable programs, resulted in findings that supported the ability of intensive, carefully implemented interventions to produce important changes. Findings showed children who were less likely to be held back in school and less likely to require remedial education. Overall, Head Start children had better health, immunization rates, and nutrition as well as enhanced socioemotional traits and family relationships. Parents reported improved relationships with their children. Further, studies of comparable programs documented cost savings—for every dollar spent on preschool programs like Head Start, taxpayers save up to $7.

Thus, overall the findings about Head Start are positive. They show a variety of salutary effects for families, children, and communities. Head Start advocates have used these findings to support the continuation of the program, to promote Early Head Start and the Follow Through program, and to leverage support to strengthen and tighten the standards for all Head Start programs.

HEAD START'S FUTURE: WELFARE REFORM AND BEYOND

The environment in which Head Start operates helps define the future needs of Head Start. Of the many social, economic, and political changes over Head Start's more than 30-year history, many look to recent reforms in the welfare system as pivotal for Head Start's future. Certainly, on the face of it, as more and more parents of preschool children rotate off the welfare rolls to work, the need for child care—and for the unique assistance of Head Start—will grow. The demand on the Head Start program will increase in a number of ways:

1. *There will undoubtedly be a need to expand the size of the program.* There was major growth in Head Start in 1990 when the nation's governors established as the top national educational goal for the year 2000 that all children will be ready to learn when they enter school. The growth in Head Start since 1990 in no way meets the need. Today, about one third of the eligible population is served.

2. *There is a need to make available full-year (12 months) and full-day services at all Head Start Centers.* Most Head Start is half-day, 10 months a year. It takes little thought or discussion to understand that such availability is inadequate for a parent working full time. The proposal has been made to use Head Start funds to combine with other public funds from other child care programs to achieve this. The barriers to such collaboration are substantial. There are more than five separate federal funding streams for child care (not to mention state and local funding streams), and each has its own set of eligibility and funding requirements. Indeed, one could argue that there are not enough child care dollars in the first place to meet the need.

3. *There is a need to find a way to care for the youngest children.* The advent of Early Head Start opens the door for serving this population; now there is a need to give local communities the flexibility to spend as much of their Head Start expansion funds on infants and toddlers as needed. The more discretion local programs have in allocating their dollars by age group, the more able they will be to respond to local need.

4. *There is a need to work to sustain Head Start benefits in elementary schools.* The Transition Project opens the door for making sure that Head Start students continue to receive support as they grow older. With more and more of their parents working, the need increases.

5. *There is a need to maintain vigilance over the quality of all Head Start services and most especially its teachers.* Uneven quality has plagued the program from the beginning. As with most any preschool (or school) program, the individual site may only be as good as the teacher. Qualified teachers need to be well trained; they also need to be individuals with compassion and understanding in order to work with young children and their families. With low wages, it has been hard to attract and retain such qualified workers. The future success of the program depends on innovations to change this, which may focus on the parents themselves.

In addition to these five issues, as more and more parents in general are working, it may well be time to consider the benefits to society of raising the eligibility requirements for Head Start so that more than just the very poor can benefit from the program.

CONCLUSION

Since its inception, Head Start has had the constant support of people involved in the program within the community. Despite the fact that Head Start has fallen in and out of favor with policymakers—in some large measure because of evaluation studies with designs too narrow to capture the comprehensive nature of the program—the program today thrives, maintains bi-partisan support and appears to have important impacts on the vast majority of the population served. It can be argued that with welfare reform and increased understanding about the needs of children in their earliest years of life, it is now time to take Head Start and programs like it to a larger scale, so the benefits of this comprehensive child development program can universally reach all of America's youngest citizens.

References

1. Zigler, E., and Muenchow, S. *Head Start: The inside story of America's most successful educational experiment.* New York: Basic Books, 1992.
2. Zigler, E., and Styfco, S.J. *Head Start and beyond: A national plan for extended childhood intervention.* New Haven, CT: Yale University Press, 1993.
3. Zigler, E., and Valentine, J. (eds). *Project Head Start: A legacy of the War on Poverty.* 2nd ed. Alexandria, VA: The National Head Start Association, 1997.
4. *The statement of the Advisory Committee on Services for Families with Infants and Toddlers.* Washington, DC: U.S. Department of Health and Human Services, 1994.

32

Childhood Immunizations

LANCE RODEWALD AND JOEL KURITSKY

IMPORTANCE OF CHILDHOOD IMMUNIZATION

Routine immunization is a health intervention that saves both lives and dollars. The decline in vaccine-preventable disease incidence in the past several decades has been dramatic, saving the lives and improving the health status of millions of children. In the United States, compared with no vaccination program, vaccination saves about $2 (for hepatitis B vaccination) to $30 (for diphtheria and tetanus toxoids and pertussis [DTP] vaccination) for every dollar spent, and compared with prevaccination-era disease levels, the current U.S. disease levels are from 97% to 100% lower. Failure to vaccinate not only places children at risk of vaccine-preventable disease but also is associated with failure to receive other important aspects of primary care. For example, compared with completely immunized children, underimmunized children make fewer health supervision visits, are up to six times more likely to not be screened for anemia, and are twice as likely not to be screened for lead exposure.

TABLE 32.1

Number of Cases of Vaccine-Preventable Diseases Targeted for Elimination by the Childhood Immunization Initiative, United States, 1988–1992 and 1996

Vaccine-Preventable Diseases	Total Reported Cases, 1988–1992						1996 Cases	
	1988	1989	1990	1991	1992	Total	Children Indigenously Acquired Cases	Aged <5 Years
Diphtheria	2	3	4	5	4	4*	4*	0
Hib invasive disease[†]	NN	NN	NN	1,540	592	165	165	165
Measles	3,396	18,193	27,786	9,643	2,237	508	443	109
Poliomyelitis[‡]	0	0	0	0	0	0	0	0
Rubella	225	396	1,125	1,401	160	213[§]	196	9
Tetanus[‖]	2	2	3	3	3	0	0	0
Mumps	4,866	5,712	5,292	4,264	2,572	751	725	154

Hib, *Haemophilus influenzae* type B; NN, not nationally notifiable.
*Including 2 cases reported to National Immunization Program but not reported as 1996 cases to the National Notifiable Diseases Surveillance System.
[†]Among children <5 years of age; includes type b and unknown serotype. Data are provisional as of July 22, 1997.
[‡]Indigenously acquired cases due to wild poliovirus.
[§]Confirmed and unknown case status only.
[‖]Among children <15 years of age.
Source: CDC. Status report on the Childhood Immunization Initiative: Reported cases of selected vaccine-preventable diseases—United States. *MMWR.* 1997;46(29):665–671.

From 1989 to 1991, there was a resurgence in measles in the United States, which was caused by low immunization coverage levels in preschool children. The resurgence demonstrated that high immunization coverage levels in school-age children were insufficient to prevent epidemics and that coverage in preschool children must also be high in order to prevent disease transmission. Major efforts were undertaken to understand barriers to preschool immunization, to de-

---

TABLE 32.2

Vaccination Coverage Levels Among Children Aged 19–35 months, by Selected Vaccines, United States, 1992[1] and 1996[2]

Vaccine/Dose	Childhood Immunization Initiative 1996 Goals	NHIS* (January–December 1992) % (95% CI)	NIS[†] (January–December 1996) % (95% CI)
DTP/DT			
≥3 Doses	90%	83 ± 2.2	95 ± 0.4
≥4 Doses	—	59 ± 2.9	81 ± 0.7
Poliovirus			
≥3 Doses	90%	72.4 ± 2.3	91 ± 0.5
Haemophilus influenzae type b (Hib)			
≥3 Doses	90%	28.2 ± 2.6	92 ± 0.5
Measles-containing vaccine (MCV)[‡]			
≥1 Dose	90%	82.5 ± 2.3	91 ± 0.5
Hepatitis B			
≥3 Doses	70%	—	82 ± 0.7
Combined Series			
4DTP/3Polio/1MMR[§]	—	55.3 ± 2.8	78 ± 0.8
4DTP/3Polio/1MMR/3Hib [‖]	—	—	77 ± 0.8

CI, confidence interval; DTP, diphtheria and tetanus toxoids and pertussis vaccine; DT, diphtheria and tetanus toxoids.
*National Health Interview Survey (NHIS), household data only; children in this survey year were born between February 1989 and May 1991.
[†]National Immunization Survey (NIS), household and provider data; children in this survey year were born between February 1993 and May 1995.
[‡]Goals are for MMR (measles-mumps-rubella vaccine); estimates are for MCV.
[§]Four or more doses of DTP/DT, three or more doses of poliovirus vaccine, and one or more doses of MCV.
[‖]Four or more doses of DTP/DT, three or more doses of poliovirus vaccine, one or more doses of MCV, and three or more doses of Hib.
Source: CDC. Status report on the Childhood Immunization Initiative: National, state, and urban area vaccination coverage levels among children aged 19–35 months—United States, 1996. *MMWR.* 1997;46(29):657–664.

velop interventions that raise coverage levels, and to add capacity to the immunization delivery system.

In 1994, the Childhood Immunization Initiative (CII) was launched. The three goals of the CII to be achieved by 1996 were to (1) reduce most vaccine-preventable disease to zero, (2) increase vaccination levels for 2-year-old children to at least 90% for the initial and most critical doses in the vaccine series and to 70% for a more recent vaccine, hepatitis B, and (3) build a vaccine delivery system to maintain these achievements in the United States. A fourth goal is that by the year 2000 a comprehensive infrastructure will be in place to provide the full series of vaccines for at least 90% of all children.

As a result of programmatic interventions, vaccination coverage levels rose. Currently, for preschool children, coverage levels are at record highs, and incidences of vaccine-preventable disease are at record lows. The disease reduction goals of the CII were met or nearly met, as shown in Table 32.1. The immunization coverage goals were met or exceeded, as shown in Table 32.2. In fact, the coverage goals were met or nearly met among the five major race/ethnicity groups in the United States.[1]

Despite these successes, much work remains. Even though the gap in coverage by race/ethnicity has been substantially narrowed, there remains a persistent 10% to 11% gap in coverage between children residing in families above the poverty threshold and those residing in impoverished families.

The third CII goal—to build a system to sustain high coverage—is still in process and is the primary topic of this chapter. We will describe the current status of the U.S. immunization delivery system and the changes that it is undergoing as a result of health care reform measures and state and federal policy initiatives.

What Prevents Timely Vaccination of Preschool Children

Since the recent measles resurgence, a great deal of research has been conducted to understand barriers that prevent timely immunization of preschool children.[2] Barriers to vaccination are predominantly confined to preschool children because all states have school vaccination requirements that effectively ensure that more than 95% of all children entering school have completed their recommended series. Thus, the problem is failure to receive timely vaccination, not failure to eventually be vaccinated.

There are several potential barriers that turn out *not* to be significant barriers when examined closely. First, many have speculated that parental attitudes toward vaccination can explain underimmunization. However, the evidence shows otherwise[3]—parents are very supportive of protecting their children through vaccination. Second, attitudes of providers have remained very positive toward routine vaccination. And third, the vast majority of preschool children have access to an immunization provider. For example, according to the 1993 National Health Interview Survey, 93% of undervaccinated children 19 to 35 months of age had a usual source of primary care. Having access to a primary care provider does not guarantee using the services, however.

Findings in the recent literature about significant barriers to vaccination are several. First, poverty with its associated factors, such as residence in a single-parent family, transportation difficulties, and large family size, has consistently been identified as a barrier to timely immunization.

Second, cost of vaccination is a barrier that is mediated through referral to health department clinics. Parents prefer to have their children receive their immunizations by the same provider that delivers other components of primary care. For example, Lieu and colleagues[4] showed that 62% of parents of families at health department clinics had a source of preventive care other than the immunization clinic and that most would have preferred to receive their vaccines at these sources. Cost was named by these parents as the main barrier to immunizations at primary care sources. The RAND Health Insurance Experiment showed that less health insurance coverage for vaccination resulted in lower vaccination rates.[5] More recent data have shown that immunization delay is greatest for children lacking insurance coverage,[6] and that once previously uninsured children receive full insurance coverage for vaccination services, their use of health department clinics drops dramatically, their use of primary care providers increases significantly, and their immunization coverage levels improve.[7]

A third barrier is the role that provider practices play in underimmunization. Few providers assess their performance on immunizations; few operate recall/reminder systems; and many opportunities to immunize children are missed in primary care offices.

A fourth barrier is an information gap in the knowledge of children's vaccination status. Providers generally overestimate the immunization coverage levels of their patients, and parents tend to believe that their children are up-to-date on their immunizations. For example, in the 1994 National Health Interview Survey, 78% of parents of underimmunized children thought that their child was completely immunized. A prerequisite for vaccination is to know who is in need of vaccination. Thus, the role of individual-specific information is critical.

PROGRAMMATIC STRATEGIES TO ADDRESS VACCINATION BARRIERS

A number of strategies were developed to address the barriers to timely immunization and were implemented by state immunization programs as part of the Childhood Immunization Initiative. A key point in these initiatives was the recognition that system- and provider-based interventions held more potential to improve coverage levels than strategies to enhance parents' belief in the value of immunization. These beliefs were already high—the system was where the repairs were needed.

System-Based Interventions

The CII contained action steps to (1) improve the quality and quantity of vaccination delivery services; (2) reduce vaccine costs for parents; (3) increase community participation, education, and partnerships; (4) improve monitoring of disease and vaccination coverage; and (5) improve vaccines and vaccine use.

To address vaccine cost and referral to health department clinics, the Vaccines for Children Program (VFC) was created in 1994. The VFC Program is an entitlement program that provides free vaccine for children without health insurance, children receiving Medicaid, and children who are Alaskan Indians or Native Americans. Children with commercial health insurance that does not cover vaccination can receive VFC vaccine in federally qualified health centers. Providers enrolled in the VFC Program benefit by not having to pay for vaccine and by being able to charge a state-determined fee for the administration of the vaccines. The VFC Program has been shown to reduce the rate of referral from private providers to health department clinics for immunizations.[8]

Accountability is an important part of VFC. It is challenging because state programs must balance administrative requirements against the need to ensure that VFC vaccine reaches only VFC-eligible children. Details on the VFC Program can be obtained from the National Immunization Program at its Internet home page (http://www.cdc.gov/nip). Currently, there are more than 50,000 provider practices enrolled in the program.

To improve monitoring of vaccination coverage levels, measurement systems were established at three levels: clinic-based, state and urban area–based, and national. In 1991, an immunization supplement to the National Health Interview Survey was initiated that asked parents about the immunization status of their children younger than 7 years of age. This survey measured coverage at the national level. In 1994, the National Immunization Survey was started. This survey measures state and urban area coverage, and the aggregated results have been used to monitor progress toward the Healthy People 2000 goals. An important aspect of these surveys is that the vaccination histories are verified against the provider records.

For clinic-level management, the Centers for Disease Control and Prevention (CDC) developed the Clinic Assessment Software Application (CASA) to measure clinic-based immunization coverage levels and to help clinics diagnose problems with their immunization practices. Goals with a system to measure progress was a powerful combination to improve preschool immunization coverage levels.

Provider-Based Interventions That Raise Coverage

In 1993, the Standards of Pediatric Immunization Practices were developed and endorsed by the major provider organizations in the United States. The Standards, listed in Table 32.3, address 18 important aspects of childhood vaccinations, including methods to improve practice-based coverage levels. These standards have been shown to be effective at raising coverage[9] and have proved to be a practical set of guidelines for immunization programs to use to enhance their service delivery and that of local area providers.

Additional research has expanded the evidence base of interventions to raise immunization coverage. Three strategies have been shown to substantially raise vaccination coverage levels: (1) recall and reminder systems to bring underimmunized children back to the provider for vaccination, (2) assessment of provider practice coverage levels with ranked feedback to the providers, and (3) linkage with the U.S. Department of Agriculture's Special Supplemental Food Program for Women, Infants and Children (WIC). Recall and reminder systems have been known to be effective prevention interventions for decades (there are more than 50 randomized controlled trials just for immunizations), so the following discussion concentrates on office assessments and WIC linkages.

Conducting practice-based assessments of immunization coverage levels and feeding this information back to the providers in a format that allows them to see how they rank against their peers has been

TABLE 32.3

Standards of Pediatric Immunization Practices

Standard 1	Immunization services are **readily available**.
Standard 2	There are **no barriers** or **unnecessary prerequisites** to the receipt of vaccines.
Standard 3	Immunization services are available **free** or for a minimal fee.
Standard 4	Providers utilize all clinical encounters to **screen** and, when indicated, **immunize** children.
Standard 5	Providers **educate** parents or guardians about immunization in general terms.
Standard 6	Providers **question** parents or guardians about **contraindications** and, before immunizing a child, **inform** them in specific terms about the risks and benefits of the immunizations their child is to receive.
Standard 7	Providers follow only true **contraindications**.
Standard 8	Providers administer **simultaneously** all vaccine doses for which a child is eligible at the time of each visit.
Standard 9	Providers use accurate and complete **recording procedures.**
Standard 10	Providers **co-schedule** immunization appointments in conjunction with appointments for other child health services.
Standard 11	Providers **report adverse events** following immunization promptly, accurately, and completely.
Standard 12	Providers operate a **tracking system**.
Standard 13	Providers adhere to appropriate procedures for **vaccine management**.
Standard 14	Providers conduct semi-annual **audits** to assess immunization coverage levels and to review immunization records in the patient populations they serve.
Standard 15	Providers maintain up-to-date, easily retrievable **medical protocols** at all locations where vaccines are administered.
Standard 16	Providers operate with **patient-oriented** and **community-based** approaches.
Standard 17	Vaccines are administered by **properly trained** individuals.
Standard 18	Providers receive **ongoing education** and **training** on current immunization recommendations.

Source: CDC. Standards for pediatric immunization practices. *MMWR*. 1993;42(No. RR-5).

shown to raise coverage levels in health department clinics. For example, in the Georgia Health Department clinics, median clinic coverage increased from 53% to 89% over a period of 6 years,[10] and the coverage gains have been sustained since that time. The CDC has produced the previously mentioned assessment tool CASA (Clinic Assessment Software Application), which is available on the Internet at http://www.cdc.gov/nip/casa/index.htm. This assessment tool standardizes the definitions of immunization status and practice membership, allowing for meaningful comparisons among sites.

Clinic assessments are now required of all health department clinics in the United States. There is less experience with private practice assessment to date; however, some localities do assess private provider practices, and they have found these programs to be effective. Examples include Boston, where median coverage among two groups of private providers has increased from 60% to 80% and from 52% to 77% over a 4-year period.[11] One of the difficulties in conducting assessments of private provider offices is the expense associated with the assessment. Research is currently under way to develop more cost effective sampling methods.

Linkage between the WIC Program and immunizations has been shown to be a highly effective method to raise immunization coverage levels rapidly. WIC currently enrolls approximately 44% of the nation's infant birth cohort, and because it is a "means-tested" program, it captures a large proportion of the nation's poor children. The specific interventions that have been shown to be effective in randomized controlled trials include (1) assessment of each child using a documented immunization history, (2) referring underimmunized children to their immunization provider, and (3) requiring more frequent visits to the WIC clinic for underimmunized children until they become completely immunized. Other WIC-based interventions are currently being tested, including the use of outreach, recall, and reminder programs to identify WIC clients in need of vaccination.

CHALLENGES FOR THE IMMUNIZATION DELIVERY SYSTEM

There are a number of challenges that will require substantial effort to address. Many of these challenges stem from changes in health care system organization.

Changes in Public/Private Split in Service Delivery

Delivery of vaccinations to preschool children is being privatized through a set of convergent policy and financial reforms—the VFC Program, state-based health insurance reform, and the rise of Medicaid managed care. All three of these initiatives have incentives for children to receive their immunizations in their medical home for primary care. The VFC Program has an explicit goal of enabling children to receive free vaccine at a private provider office, thus "recoupling" immunizations and primary care for children previously referred to health department clinics for vaccination. State-based insurance reform includes a requirement that health insurance benefits cover the entire cost of vaccination. Managed Medicaid programs are privatizing immunization delivery by requiring vaccination at the child's assigned primary care provider.

The new federal Child Health Insurance Plan, designed for uninsured children in families with incomes less than 200% of the poverty index, will further privatize the immunization delivery system by providing coverage for vaccination at the primary care provider office. States have the choice between expanding Medicaid eligibility or using private insurance plans to cover non–Medicaid-eligible children. Experience in New York showed that when immunizations were covered for children of the working poor, immunization visits at health department clinics decreased by 67%, immunization visits at primary care provider offices increased by 27%, and immunization coverage levels increased by 5%.[7]

Recent evidence from the National Health Interview Survey shows that approximately 22% of children were immunized by health department clinic providers, and 68% were immunized by private providers. Thus, one can expect that as the impetus for privatization continues, the proportion of vaccinations delivered by health department clinics will decline.

Given that this privatization is consonant with programmatic goals, the challenge for the public health community will be to assess and ensure the adequacy of vaccination services delivered by others. This is a major challenge because there are more than 125,000 private providers. Typical tools for assessing the adequacy of service delivery for health department clinics (e.g., CASA) may need to be modified to assess private providers.

Vaccinating Adolescents

As a result of recently adopted recommendations for hepatitis B vaccination, adolescents are the largest group of children in need of one or more vaccinations. The Advisory Committee on Immunization Practices (ACIP) recommended that all children should be protected with hepatitis B vaccine before their 13th birthday. Because universal infant immunization has been highly successful (with recent immunization coverage levels of 82%), there is a cohort of children who were born prior to the universal hepatitis B recommendation and who are younger than 18 years of age. Time is critical, because as this cohort ages, it becomes more difficult to access them with the health care system, and some members of this cohort will begin behavior patterns that place them at high risk of disease. In other words, every day approximately 11,000 children pass the recommended vaccination age. There are millions of children in this cohort, and the time that it takes the health care system to gear up for this service delivery translates to children unprotected from hepatitis B.

Some of the decisions regarding optimal strategies for reaching all adolescents will revolve around who should provide and pay for the vaccinations. School-based clinics have the potential to vaccinate large groups of children. Managed care organizations and private providers, however, have responsibility for vaccinating their patients. A few states have adopted school entry regulations that require initiation of hepatitis B vaccination prior to middle school entry, regardless of who provides the vaccinations; some states plan to conduct school-based vaccination clinics.

Improving Disease Surveillance

As disease incidence falls, collecting and reporting complete and accurate information on the remaining cases become increasingly important in order to better understand the factors that allow disease transmission to continue in spite of high vaccination coverage. The occurrence of vaccine-preventable diseases in a community may be a sentinel event that signals the presence of an underimmunized population within the community. Such populations may be small, access health care infrequently, or be otherwise difficult to identify.

As vaccination and other disease control efforts reduce disease incidence in the United States, the quality of surveillance data begins to limit the precision with which progress toward disease elimination can be monitored; data quality has become a major limitation. Surveillance indicators that allow monitoring of diagnostic effort are needed to ensure that the absence of reported cases reflects the true absence of disease, rather than the absence of effort to detect disease. In addition, adequate laboratory evaluation of suspected cases is essential. For example, complete serotyping of *Haemophilus influenzae* isolates from cases of invasive disease in children is essential to define the factors that allow these cases to continue to occur.

New Vaccines

Until the late 1980s, routine childhood vaccination had been a field marked by slow but steady progress. Since that time (and into the foreseeable future), routine vaccination has been anything but routine (see http://www.aap.org/family/parents/immunize.htm for an always up-to-date vaccination schedule). Advances in biotechnology are bringing new combination vaccines, vaccines against additional diseases, improvements in existing vaccines, and changes in the vaccination schedule. There are currently more than 20 combination vaccines at various stages of development and testing. Although vaccine purchase may be more complicated, eventually these combinations will not only allow protection from disease with fewer injection, but they will greatly facilitate vaccination against additional diseases by piggybacking new vaccines onto accepted and fully-implemented vaccines—for example, by including hepatitis A vaccine in a combination vaccine. Thus, technology will come to the aid of the immunization delivery system.

Licensing new vaccines against diseases that were previously not vaccine-preventable is one of the more exciting aspects of these advances. Vaccines against rotavirus, Lyme disease, and herpes simplex may be licensed in the near future. An important vaccine for infants will be one against respiratory syncytial virus, as it is a leading cause of hospitalization of infants. Research and development is being conducted to produce a pneumococcal conjugate vaccine to protect children younger than 2 years of age, who have the greatest burden of pneumococcal meningitis and otitis media.

Disease Eradication

A goal to eradicate polio was set in 1988 by the World Health Assembly, and the program is on track to eradicate the disease near the year 2000. Recent successes in measles elimination in the United States and South America, along with supporting molecular epidemiologic studies, have made the eradication of measles worldwide appear to be feasible. Studies are under way to determine whether measles can be eradicated using the health care infrastructure that is in place for the polio eradication program.

VISION OF THE FUTURE IMMUNIZATION DELIVERY SYSTEM

What should the immunization delivery system look like in order to address the challenges and opportunities of childhood immunization? First, vaccinations should be delivered in the context of a medical home for comprehensive primary care, referral for routine vaccination from the medical home because of vaccine cost or availability should not be necessary, a link between every child and a primary care provider implies accountability for vaccination, and changing primary care providers should imply a hand-off of responsibility, accountability, and information (vaccination histories). Second, providers should practice in accordance with the Standards for Pediatric Immunization Practices and make available to their patients all of the universally recommended vaccines. And, finally, an information system should exist that (1) monitors vaccination coverage levels among defined groups, such as provider patient panels and communities, (2) supports recall and reminder systems, (3) identifies children in need of vaccination at all provider and assessment sites, (4) supports disease surveillance and monitoring of vaccine adverse events, and (5) facilitates dissemination of new vaccine recommendations to immunization providers.

State and local health departments have responsibilities that go beyond the provision of care to individuals. Consistent with the Institute of Medicine's 1988 report on the future of public health, health departments have core functions of assessment, policy development, and assurance. For the immunization delivery system, these health department functions translate into the following core functions:

1. Monitor the incidence of vaccine-preventable diseases.
2. Monitor immunization coverage levels. Included in this function are the programmatic activities of conducting assessments of provider practices and coverage levels and monitoring coverage of children entering school.
3. Diagnose, investigate, and control outbreaks of vaccine-preventable diseases.
4. Inform and educate providers and patients about vaccines and vaccine-preventable diseases.
5. Mobilize community partnerships to help immunize the population.
6. Develop policies and plans that support individual and community-based immunization strategies.
7. Develop, implement, promote, and utilize laws, rules, and regulations that pertain to vaccine-preventable disease control.
8. Link people to health care providers who immunize, and ensure the provision of immunization services when otherwise available.
9. Ensure a competent public health and personal health care workforce through training.
10. Evaluate the effectiveness, accessibility, and quality of personal and population-based immunization services.
11. Procure and manage vaccines.

A key aspect to having a sustainable immunization program is having strong partnerships. The National Immunization Program has partnerships that promote and support international and national programs. These include voluntary organizations, such as Rotary International, which has played a key role in raising funds and promoting the efforts at worldwide polio eradication. In addition to voluntary organizations, partnerships with provider groups are essential. All the major provider groups, including the American Academy of Pediatrics, the American Association of Family Physicians, the National Medical Association, and the Interamerican College of Physicians and Surgeons, have supported immunization goals.

Other partnerships are those among federal programs. Currently, the immunization program is partnering with the Health Care Financing Administration to promote the VFC Program, with United States Department of Agriculture to promote WIC linkages, and with the Department of Housing and Urban Development and the Corporation for National Service to promote immunizations of residents of housing authorities.

Through a competitive process, the National Immunization Program has developed partnerships with the following organizations: (1) Association of State and Territorial Health Officials; (2) Healthy Mothers, Healthy Babies Coalition; (3) Congress of National Black Churches; (4) National Coalitions of Hispanic Health and Human Services Organizations; (5) Ambulatory Pediatric Association; (6) American Nurses Association; (7) Interamerican College of Physicians and Surgeons; (8) National Association of Community Health Centers; (9) National Medical Association; (10) National Council of La Raza; and (11) American Pharmaceutical Association. Each of these organizations works with its local affiliates and at the national level to provide appropriate educational and communications activities with its members. The National Immunization Program, working with its state partners, also helps promote immunization coalitions. There are currently 64 active state and local coalitions. These entities have members from all constituency groups who promote and facilitate immunization activities.

References

1. CDC. Vaccination coverage by race/ethnicity and poverty level among children aged 19–35 months—United States, 1996. *MMWR*. 1997;46(41):963–969.
2. The National Vaccine Advisory Committee. The measles epidemic: The problems, barriers, and recommendations. *JAMA*. 1991;266:1547–1549.
3. Strobino, D., Keane, V., Holt, E., Hughart, N., and Guyer, B. Parental attitudes do not explain underimmunization. *Pediatrics*. 1996;98:1076–1083.
4. Lieu, T.A., Smith, M., Newacheck, P., Langthorn, D., Venkatesh, P., Herradora, R. Health insurance and preventive care sources of children at public immunization clinics. *Pediatrics*. 1994:373–378.

5. Lurie, N., Manning, W.G., Peterson, C., Goldberg, G.A., Phelps, C.A., and Lillard, L. Preventive care: Do we practice what we preach? *American Journal of Public Health.* 1987;77:801–804.

6. Zimmerman, R., and Janosky, J. Immunization barriers in Minnesota private practices: The influence of economics and training on vaccine timing. *Family Practice Research Journal.* 1993;13:213–224.

7. Rodewald, L., Szilagyi, P., Holl, J., Shone, L., Zwanziger, J., and Raubertas, E. Health insurance for low-income working families. *Archives of Pediatric and Adolescent Medicine.* 1997;151:798–803.

8. Zimmerman, R., Medsgar, A., and Ricci, E. Impact of free vaccine and insurance status on physician referral of children to public vaccine clinics. *JAMA.* 1997;278: 996–1000.

9. Pierce, C., Goldstein, M., Suozzi, K., Gallaher, M., Dietz, V., and Stevenson, J. The impact of the Standards for Pediatric Immunization Practices on vaccination coverage levels. *JAMA.* 1996;276:626–630.

10. LeBaron, C., Chaney, M., Baughman, A., et al: Impact of measurement and feedback on vaccination coverage in public clinics, 1988–1994. *JAMA.* 1997;277:631–635.

11. Link, D. Chart audits to promote community-wide childhood immunization. Presented before the 31st National Immunization Conference, Detroit, MI, May, 1997.

33

Adolescent Health and Welfare Reform

JENNIFER C. MAEHR AND MARIANNE E. FELICE

By the year 2000, there will be approximately 40 million young people between the ages of 10 and 19 years in the United States, constituting about 14% of the general population. This proportion of adolescents to the rest of the nation's population has remained relatively steady for the last two decades. Approximately one third of the adolescent population are members of minorities, and that proportion is expected to grow to about 45% over the next few decades. Nearly one fifth of all adolescents live below the poverty line, and in most cases, in one-parent families headed by women.[1,2]

Adolescent health problems have been the focus of much media attention over the past several years. Issues related to adolescent sexuality and violence have been the most problematic for the general population because these are areas that touch everyone in a given community. Although birth rates have gradually decreased in the past few years, the United States still has the highest birth rates to 15- to 19-year-olds than any developed country.[3,4] In 1996, there were 54.7 live births per 1,000 women aged 15 to 19 years.[5] Most of these young mothers are unmarried and on welfare. Compared with their peers who delay childbearing, they are less likely to finish high school or hold a steady job. Their infants are more likely to die in the first year of life, have a low birthweight, and develop psychosocial problems such as poor school performance when compared with children born to older women.[2]

About half of this country's 15- to 19-year-old female adolescents have had sexual intercourse.[6] Up to 40% of teens do not use any form of birth control at their first sexual encounter.[2] Despite an increasing trend in condom use, only half of high school seniors report using condoms.[2,7] Given these behaviors, teens account for 25% of all new cases of sexually transmitted diseases (STDs), with black females accounting for a disproportionately high percentage of these cases.[2] Unlike the population of adults with acquired immunodeficiency syndrome (AIDS), 46% of the new adolescent AIDS cases are female, the majority of whom acquired the human immunodeficiency virus (HIV) from heterosexual sex, often with a partner who is an intravenous drug user. AIDS is now the sixth leading cause of death for Americans between the ages of 15 and 24 years.[7]

Adolescent drug use, sex, and violence are often intertwined. Although illicit drug use among teens decreased in the 1970s and 1980s, there is the suggestion that rates may be increasing again in the 1990s. Alcohol and cigarettes were the drugs most widely used in 1993, followed by marijuana, smokeless tobacco, and inhalants.[2,8] Homicide and suicide are the second and third leading causes of death among young people and often are related to substance abuse. Homicide rates for black male adolescents and suicide rates for white male adolescents are dramatically higher than the rates for the general adolescent population.[2,9-11]

With respect to the health of the nation's adolescents, approximately 6% of teens have a chronic medical condition that limits their daily activities, and 12% are overweight.[2,12] In 1988, almost 25% of all teens aged 10 to 17 had not received routine health care within the previous 2 years.[13] Accidents and unintentional injuries are now the leading cause of death among adolescents, the majority from motor vehicle accidents and often indirectly from risk-taking behavior such as drinking alcohol and not wearing a seat belt. Despite these health issues and the apparent need for preventive health counseling, about 5 million teens in this country between 10 and 18 years of age (15%) have no health insurance.[2]

These figures are worrisome, and it is clear that programs are needed to both prevent and intervene in these problems. In addition to balancing the budget and reducing welfare costs, federal and state legislatures are also concerned about these problems and their effects on public coffers. Across the country, many laws have been passed with the intent to curb problems related to adolescent behavior and health, specifically their lack of health insurance, the high rates of teen pregnancy and STDs, and escalation of youth violence and drug trafficking. Unfortunately, many of these legislative efforts may cause more problems than solutions. In this chapter, we address the effect of recent legislative actions on adolescent health in four areas: teen parenting, statutory rape, sexual education, and health insurance coverage. After reviewing these areas, we offer some suggestions for legislatures to consider for future action.

WELFARE REFORM AND TEEN PARENTING

The Personal Responsibility and Work Opportunity Reconciliation Act of 1996 (P.L. 104-193), enacted in 1997, affects adolescents in several different ways. Overall, the intent of the Act is to reduce the nation's welfare population by making public assistance a temporary rather than lifelong or extended benefit with more rigorous eligibility requirements that vary by state. The Act is anticipated to save the federal government $54.5 billion through the year 2003. The scope of the Act is broad and affects assistance for poor families, families with teen parents, and recipients of Supplemental Security Insurance (SSI) and food stamps, and it indirectly affects Medicaid.[14]

The Act repeals the Aid to Families with Dependent Children (AFDC) program and replaces it with block grants to states called Temporary Assistance for Needy Families (TANF). Section 408(a)(4-5) of the Act prohibits states from using TANF grant funds for assisting unmarried custodial parents younger than 18 who have not graduated from high school and who have a child at least 12 weeks old in their care unless they attend school or an alternative training program and also live with either a parent or parent equivalent. Exceptions can be made in specific circumstances, such as abusive settings.[14]

It is unclear how commonly exceptions will be made. Potentially, a teen mother may be forced to leave her child in the care of another person less competent than herself while she is attending school, or she may be forced to live in a setting not conducive to the stability of both herself and her children because of exposure to drugs, abuse, or neglect. Current research has shown that continued shared residence with the baby's grandmother among teen mothers is associated with increased stress. The grandmother's child care assistance in a non–shared living arrangement, however, appears to be advantageous to the teen mother's parenting and the outcomes for the child.[15]

Teen mothers are at risk for short interval repeat pregnancies: almost 30% of all first-time adolescent mothers have a second child within 2 years of the first delivery.[15] TANF has restrictions that may affect teens with repeat pregnancies. There now is a 5-year lifetime limit on receipt of any TANF benefits regardless of interruptions in services, and adults in families receiving TANF will be required to work in some capacity after receiving 24 months of assistance.[14] Given these restrictions, the teen who has her first baby at 17 years and her second baby by 19 years may be required to work part-time and may lose all assistance by the time the second baby is 3 years old.

Research does not support the idea that welfare payments exert an important influence on non-marital childbearing.[16] Although it is unclear whether these restrictions will have any impact on the birth rate for teens, welfare reform will limit the services available to some of these teens and their babies.

WELFARE REFORM AND STATUTORY RAPE

In the attempt to further reduce teen birth rates and related welfare costs, Section 906 of P.L. 104-193 encourages states and local jurisdictions to strongly enforce existing statutory rape laws with emphasis on predatory older men. These laws vary markedly by state and recently have been expanded in some states to be more inclusive with tougher penalties. These legislative changes are in response to increased public attention on studies showing that in a majority of teenage births the babies are fathered by adult men (i.e., men older than 19 or 20 years). More recent analyses, however, suggest that the extent of the problem is not as prevalent as once thought.[17,18]

In the study by Lindberg and co-workers, data were analyzed from the National Maternal and Infant Health Survey conducted by the National Center for Health Statistics between 1988 and 1991. Of all births to 15- to 19-year-old girls in 1988 in the United States, 8% were to unmarried girls between 15 and 17 years of age and their partners who were at least 5 years older.[18] Data from the 1995 National Survey of Family Growth show that 13% of all women who had their first voluntary intercourse before they were 16 had first partners who were 20 years of age or older.[6] These percentages reflect those cases that approximate the legal criteria in most states for statutory rape.

The teen mothers who had older partners were more likely to engage in "problem behavior" than teen mothers with more closely aged-matched partners. These problems include repeat pregnancies and alcohol use. Nonetheless, 35% of these teen mothers had been living with their older partner during the pregnancy, and 49% were living with their partner at the time of the interview (up to 30 months after the birth), which seems to suggest involvement in a stable relationship.[18] If these older partners living with the teen mothers are prosecuted, the teen mother and her family may potentially lose housing and financial support.

States currently do not require health care providers to report the age or identity of the sexual partners of adolescent patients unless abuse is suspected. Nonetheless, fear of being reported may jeopardize the health care for the teenager who is involved with an older man. In an attempt to avoid prosecution, adult men may discourage their teen partners from seeking health care, including prenatal care, postnatal care, and pediatric care for their children. Because of uncertainty regarding confidentiality, the teen may not want to disclose pertinent information to her physician, which represents an obvious barrier in the patient-physician relationship. The older partner who wants to be involved may be deterred from attending prenatal and pediatric visits and may become less involved in the care of his teen partner and baby.

Although statutory rape laws may increase the prosecution of older men who coerce the younger more vulnerable teens into sexual relationships, they will unlikely change teen birth rates. These laws may actually jeopardize the socioeconomic and health status of some of these teen mothers and their children.

WELFARE REFORM AND ABSTINENCE PROMOTION

In an effort to reduce teen pregnancy rates, Section 912 of P.L. 104-193 provides grant money to every state that applies for abstinence-only education aimed at groups most likely to have children out-of-wedlock. This federal legislation was enacted without proof that such programs are effective. A similar adolescent pregnancy prevention initiative in California, Education Now and Babies Later (ENABL), was implemented in 1992 and canceled soon after in 1996 for failure to meet its objectives.[19]

This California program included education aimed at seventh and eighth graders, community and school-based activities, a statewide media campaign, $15 million in funding for the first 3 years, and a rigorous evaluation component. Overall, the program curriculum was taught to 187,000 youths in California. At that time, ENABL was the largest statewide pregnancy prevention program ever initiated.[19,20]

The educational base of the program was the Postponing Sexual Involvement (PSI) curriculum, which previous research had shown was effective in delaying the onset of sexual intercourse for youths in areas of high teenage pregnancy rates. The PSI curriculum in previous programs, however, had included information on contraception, which the ENABL program decided not to include.[19,20]

For evaluation, 9,000 surveys and 75 individual and 50 focus group interviews were reviewed. Youths, parents, and community representatives, in general, supported the program, although most wanted changes to the curriculum. Almost 90% of the girls wanted more information on contraception. Eighty-two percent of all the youths wanted additional topics on prevention of STDs, including HIV. The majority of parents who completed the survey also endorsed the expansion of the curriculum to include more information on STD and pregnancy prevention.[19]

At 17 months into the program, the evaluation showed that youths in the treatment groups (PSI curriculum) were equally likely to have become sexually active and were not less likely to report a pregnancy or STD than youths in the control groups. As a result, California's Governor Pete Wilson, who had formerly launched ENABL, canceled the program and was quoted as saying, "I have concluded that we need a much more comprehensive strategy to deal with out-of-wedlock pregnancy."[19,20]

Although there is a definite need to teach abstinence as an option, middle school youths, especially girls, want information on contraceptive methods. Teens also want to know about STDs. Parents, in general, seem to support contraceptive as well as STD education. Programs that have been shown to be effective in reducing pregnancy rates include information on contraception.[16] With the alarming increase in AIDS cases among male and especially female adolescents,[7] it is harmful to keep children uneducated about safe sex.

A great deal of money, time, and effort was placed in the ENABL program. The grant money provided by P.L. 104-193 for abstinence-only programs totals $50 million per year for 5 years. In order to obtain this funding, states have to match funds by supplying $3 in cash or "in kind" for every $4 supplied by the federal government. The grand total for states and federal funding combined for 5 years would come to $437.5 million.[21] It is hoped that states will avoid errors made previously and, before investing their money or reallocating their resources from other programs into abstinence-only education, carefully research the possible results of such an undertaking. The intent of this policy (i.e., reduced teen pregnancy) may not be reached if funds and resources are taken from currently successful health education programs.

ADOLESCENT HEALTH CARE AND INSURANCE COVERAGE

Adolescents have the lowest rate for utilization of health care services and are the least likely to receive care in outpatient, office-based settings. The reasons for this are numerous. Cost of care and lack of health insurance impede many teens from obtaining medical attention. Other barriers to health care include the teens' concerns about confidentiality, embarrassment over their health issues, potential need for parental consent for treatment, clinician availability, and transportation problems.[2,22]

In 1994, the percentage of uninsured children younger than 18 years of age reached its highest level, 14.2%, since 1987, accounting for 10 million uninsured children. This drop in health coverage was felt greatest by children living in low-income, working families. Of the 4.1 million poor teens between 13 and 19 years of age, 1.3 million, or 32%, were uninsured in 1994.[23] Teens who are underinsured are more likely to be in fair to poor health, from poor or near-poor households, and in a minority group.[2] Without health insurance, children and teens are less likely to seek and receive routine preventive health care, immunizations, and dental care as well as treatment for chronic illnesses and injuries.[23] In fact, uninsured teens are twice as likely as insured teens to not have seen a doctor in the previous 2 years.[2]

Medicaid coverage of children younger than 18 years of age has increased to cover 18.4% of all children in this age range. This increase, however, was not enough to offset the steady drop since 1987 in private health insurance for this group, which reached its lowest level, 65.6%, in 1994. The number of teens covered by Medicaid will increase yearly until 2002, when all poor children up to 19 years of age will have to be covered. Current law states that Medicaid cover all pregnant women, infants, and children up to 6 years of age with a family income at or below 133% of the federal poverty level as well as children 6 years or older born after September 30, 1983 with a family income at or below 100% of the federal poverty level. Many states, however, expanded Medicaid to cover teens born before 1983.[23]

In 1993, 13.8 million children met the federal age and poverty income requirements for Medicaid. Of these children, 8.4 million were on Medicaid, approximately 3 million had other health insurance, and 2.3 million remained uninsured even though eligible for Medicaid.[24] Of all uninsured children in 1994, 30% were Medicaid-eligible.

For those who are eligible for Medicaid, many potential barriers may keep them uninsured. Parents may think erroneously that they are not eligible because one or both parents are working or because both parents live at home. Completing the Medicaid enrollment process can be difficult. Half of all Medicaid denials are for failure to supply required documentation.[23]

It is often the case that eligible teens have no Medicaid coverage because of failure of a parent or guardian to complete the Medicaid process. Most older teens are capable of enrolling themselves, but a guardian is required for this process. As a result, doctor visits and immunizations are missed and medications, including birth control, are not obtained. This lack of insurance is most critical for chronically ill teens (e.g., asthmatics) and sexually active teens who put themselves at risk for pregnancy and STDs. In fact, a teen can become eligible for and enroll herself in Medicaid once pregnant, but that same teen 1 month previously and not pregnant may not have been able to obtain contraception because of ineligibility for or non-enrollment in Medicaid. Some young men may never be eligible.

Health care for children and adolescents is critical and less expensive compared with adults. In 1994, non-disabled children younger than 21 years of age accounted for 49% of Medicaid recipients but only 16% of all Medicaid expenditure for medical care.[23] Preventive care, in particular, is cost effective for this age group, including the prevention of tobacco use, drug and alcohol abuse, and adolescent pregnancy. The cost of clinical preventive services for adolescents on average is $73 to $120 per adolescent per year. The cost of select adolescent morbidities, however, is approximately $859 per year for each adolescent between 11 and 21 years of age.[25,26]

For example, $185 million was spent in 1987 on adolescent alcohol and drug treatment. In 1992 dollars, $882 million was spent on the approximately 3.8 million reported cases of STDs among adolescents aged 15 to 19 years. With respect to adolescent pregnancy, the hospital and physician costs for live births to mothers 15 to 19 years of age totaled close to $2.5 billion in 1989. Of those infants born to women younger than the age of 20 years, 9% were low birthweight; the hospital costs for these infants are estimated to have been approximately $1.172 million.[26]

An estimated 1.2 to 2.1 million unintended pregnancies are prevented yearly by publicly funded reproductive programs. For every government dollar spent on family planning services, an average of $4.40 is saved on medical services, welfare, and nutritional services. On a broader scope, for every dollar spent on school-based clinics, $1.38 to $2.00 is saved as a result of reductions in the use of emergency room care, lower pregnancy rates, early prenatal care, and increased diagnosis and treatment of STDs.[26] If adolescents are provided routine health maintenance, it can actually save the government money.

The future does look brighter for this nation's children. The balanced budget agreement allocates $24 billion in additional money over the next 5 years to extend medical coverage to uninsured children through the age of 18, primarily those from working poor families. States will receive funding through the State Children's Health Insurance Program (S-CHIP) depending on the number of uninsured children in that state. States will have more freedom to determine eligibility, reimbursement rates, contractors, and inclusive benefits such as medical, dental, transportation, and counseling services covered. The new law prohibits states from decreased spending on Medicaid below current levels.[27,28]

Estimates from the Congressional Budget Office (CBO) and Children's Defense Fund show that the money allocated will allow health insurance for as many as 2.2 to 5 million currently uninsured children. A percentage of the federal money has been provided specifically for media campaign and recruitment. The states were given little time to make the changes necessary to enact the new law, which had its first installment in October 1997.[27] Due to state-to-state flexibility, however, it is impossible to predict which uninsured teens will benefit from this new legislation and what specific services will be provided.

Despite these recent gains in legislation for child and adolescent health, P.L. 104-193 revises the eligibility criteria for children and teens on SSI, making it more difficult to qualify, especially for those with emotional or behavioral problems. Currently, more than 1 million children receive SSI benefits. To be considered disabled according to the new legislation, a child must have "a medically determinable physical or mental impairment, which results in marked and severe functional limitations, and which can be expected to result in death or which has lasted or can be expected to last for a continuous period of not less than 12 months." No child younger than 18 who "engages in substantial gainful activity" will be considered disabled.[14,29]

The leading single cause of disability for adolescents is mental disorders (32% of all disabilities). Approximately 5 million teens between 12 and 17 years of age are significantly impaired due to emotional or behavioral problems. Recent estimates show that 7.5 million children younger than age 18 need mental health services, but less than one third actually receive them.[2] The CBO predicts that by 2002, 315,000 children who would have previously qualified for SSI will no longer be eligible.[30] One can therefore assume that the number of children needing services but not receiving them will only increase.

Historically, SSI has been linked to Medicaid in such a way that when SSI is terminated, Medicaid is also terminated. Legislators, however, used the recent budget agreement to ensure that those children losing SSI will still be guaranteed Medicaid coverage.[28] Older teens, born before September 30, 1983, may remain at risk for losing Medicaid when they lose SSI if the state in which they reside has no alternative eligibility pathway for Medicaid and has not enacted optional coverage of all low-income children younger than the age of 19 in Medicaid.[29] Those losing SSI will have to know that they are still eligible for Medicaid and may have to reapply in order to receive benefits.

Unless previously enrolled in SSI prior to August 22, 1996, teens who are legal aliens are no longer eligible under the new Act for SSI. Teens who suffer from disabilities related to alcohol or drug abuse are also not eligible for SSI.[28,29]

RECOMMENDATIONS

Based on the previous discussion, we would make the following suggestions to state and federal legislatures.

Teen Parenting

This nation needs to support the teen who is already a parent, while preventing future, unintended teen pregnancies. Legislation that makes it more difficult for a teen parent to obtain federal assistance will have repercussions that impact not only on her health but the health of her child(ren).

2. TANF benefits should be extended beyond 5 years for young mothers.
2. If teen mothers are to finish high school and/or obtain jobs, child care should be available at schools and places of employment, and more innovative job training programs need to be federally funded.

3. Government cannot legislate family communication. By requiring teen mothers to live at home with a "parent," laws may unintentionally cause more harm than good.

4. Comprehensive health care should be available to both the teen mother and her child(ren) in order to reduce repeat pregnancies and infant morbidity by allowing unlimited access for an extended period of time to medical, nursing, psychosocial, and nutritional services.

5. All teen parents, male and female, should be encouraged to attend federally funded parenting classes designed specifically for them.

Statutory Rape

There is a need to prosecute adult men who coerce young teenage women into having sex, especially those men who are repeat offenders and who have no intention of fathering their children. This scenario, however, certainly is not true of all men who have teen partners.

1. This country needs better mechanisms besides age discrepancy to discern those situations in which teens are being coerced into a sexual relationship that is unwanted.

2. We need to provide safe havens for teens living in dangerous, abusive, or neglectful settings that often force them to turn to unhealthy solutions.

3. Rather than punishing older partners, legislatures should concentrate on promoting programs for high-risk teenage girls and their children.

4. Locally and federally funded community and school programs that promote self-respect, teach useful skills, and provide healthy alternatives to early sexual activity and pregnancy should increase in number, especially in areas of high teen pregnancy rates.

Sex Education

A more thorough approach besides teaching abstinence only is required for school-based sexual education.

1. Before legislatures launch a major educational program, such as abstinence-only promotion, there needs to be strong evi-

dence that such a program will work. More research is needed in this area, including smaller pilot programs. Mechanisms for evaluation and the flexibility for change must be built into the legislation for these programs.

2. We need to understand teenagers' feelings and attitudes regarding sex, pregnancy, and parenting in order to better tailor programs to their needs and to uncover the underlying issues behind early sexuality and unprotected intercourse.

3. School-based sexual education is imperative and should include information on reproductive anatomy, childbirth, parenting, STDs, and contraceptive options including abstinence, barrier methods, hormonal contraception, and emergency contraception.

4. We cannot rely on school-based sexual education alone to convey safe-sex practices to teenagers. We need to educate the public so that friends and family can feel comfortable advising teens on these topics. The media need to take responsibility and better promote safe-sex and STD prevention rather than giving children mixed messages about sex. Health care providers should take every opportunity to initiate discussion on sexuality issues and contraception with their adolescent patients.

Adolescent Health Care and Insurance Coverage

Prevention is cost effective and can reduce adolescent morbidity and mortality. The recent expansion in health insurance for children will help some teens 18 years old and younger obtain care, but gaps in coverage will still remain.

1. An aggressive media campaign and public outreach will be required to educate those who are now eligible for federally and state-supported health insurance. To ensure enrollment, the application process must be simplified, and competent teens should be able to enroll themselves.

2. All teens in this country should have health insurance and easy access to care. School-based clinics, community health centers in the rural and urban settings, academic-based adolescent clinics, and mobile vans providing health care to the inner cities will continue to be valuable resources for teens who fall through the cracks.

3. Employers should be encouraged by tax benefits and other legislative measures to provide affordable health care for depen-

dents of employees and for teen employees. State and federal incentives need to exist for families to purchase private health insurance for their children.

4. We must acknowledge that adolescents have disabilities. It is difficult at best for families to cope emotionally and financially with the problems related to chronic illnesses, mental and behavioral disorders, and substance abuse. We must continue to support programs that enable disabled youth to receive appropriate health care without exhausting all financial resources of their families.

It is said that a society is judged by how it cares for those unable to care for themselves, such as children and youth. Although many adults are generous when it comes to children, they may feel that adolescents do not need the same types of care and concern. In reality, the adolescents we are caring for today are the adults of tomorrow. Many of their problems are a reflection of the problems facing all American society. It is in all our best interests to ensure that the youth of today are supported, educated, and protected with access to the best health care that we can offer. Legislators are in a unique position to make that happen.

References

1. National Adolescent Health Information Center. Fact sheet on adolescent demographics. In *Adolescent fact file*. San Francisco: University of California, June, 1995.
2. Ozer, E.M., Brindis, C.D., Millstein, S.G., Knopf, D.K., and Irwin, C.E. *America's adolescents: Are they healthy?* San Francisco: National Adolescent Health Information Center, University of California, 1997.
3. Henshaw, S.K., Kenney, A.M., Somberg, D., and Van Vort, J. *Teenage pregnancy in the United States: The scope of the problem and state responses.* New York: Alan Guttmacher Institute, 1989.
4. Jones, E.F., Forrest, J.D., Goldman, N., et al. *Teenage pregnancy in industrialized countries.* New Haven, CT: Yale University Press, 1986.
5. Moore, K.A., Romano, A.D., Gitelson, L.B., et al. *Facts at a glance.* Washington, DC: Child Trends, Inc., October, 1997.
6. Centers for Disease Control and Prevention. Fertility, family planning, and women's health: New data from the 1995 National Survey of Family Growth. DHHS Publication No. (PHS)97-1995. *Vital and Health Statistics.* Series 23: No. 19, May, 1997.
7. Collins, C. *Dangerous inhibitions: How America is letting AIDS become an epidemic of the young.* Monograph Series #3. San Francisco: University of California, Center for AIDS Prevention Studies, February, 1997.
8. National Adolescent Health Information Center. Fact sheet on adolescent substance abuse. In *Adolescent fact file*. San Francisco: University of Califoria, November, 1995.
9. National Adolescent Health Information Center. Fact sheet on adolescent homicide. In *Adolescent fact file*. San Francisco: University of California, February, 1995.
10. National Adolescent Health Information Center. Fact sheet on adolescent suicide. In *Adolescent fact file*. San Francisco: University of California, June, 1995.

11. Woods, E.R., Lin, Y.G., Middleman, A., et al. The associations of suicide attempts in adolescents. *Pediatrics.* 1997;99(6):791–796.

12. Berg, F.M. Three major U.S. studies describe trends. *Healthy Weight Journal.* 1997;11(4):67–74.

13. National Adolescent Health Information Center. Fact sheet on adolescent health care utilization. In *Adolescent fact file.* San Francisco: University of California, April, 1996.

14. CityMatCH. Federal welfare reform highlights. *City Lights.* Spring, 1997;6(2):4.

15. East, P.L., and Felice, M.E. *Adolescent pregnancy and parenting: Findings from a racially diverse sample.* Mahwah, NJ: Lawrence Erlbaum Associates, 1996.

16. Brown, S.S., and Eisenberg, L. (eds), for Institute of Medicine. *The best intentions: Unintended pregnancy and the well-being of children and families.* Washington, DC: National Academy Press, 1995.

17. Donovan, P. Can statutory rape laws be effective in preventing adolescent pregnancy? *Family Planning Perspectives.* 1997;29(1):30–34,40.

18. Lindberg, L.D., Sonenstein, F.L., Ku, L., and Martinez, G. Age differences between minors who give birth and their adult partners. *Family Planning Perspectives.* 1997;29(2):61–66.

19. Cagampang, H.H., Barth, R.P., Korpi, M., and Kirby, D. Education Now and Babies Later (ENABL): Life history of a campaign to postpone sexual involvement. *Family Planning Perspectives.* 1997;29(3):109–114.

20. Kirby, D., Korpi, M., Barth, R.P., and Cagampang, H.H. The impact of the postponing sexual involvement curriculum among youths in California. *Family Planning Perspectives.* 1997;29(3):100–108.

21. Anglin, T.M. Adolescent policy considerations. Presented at Adolescent Health 2000 Conference. Washington, DC, June 13, 1997.

22. Klein, J.D., Slap, G.B., Elster, A.B., et al. Access to health care for adolescents. A position paper of the Society for Adolescent Medicine. *Journal of Adolescent Health.* 1992;13(2):162–170.

23. U.S. General Accounting Office. *Children's health insurance in 1994* (GAO/HEHS-96-129).

24. U.S. General Accounting Office. *Medicaid and uninsured children* (GAO/HEHS-95-175).

25. Gans, J.E., Alexander, B., Chu, R.C., and Elster, A.B. The cost of comprehensive medical services for adolescents. *Archives of Pediatric and Adolescent Medicine.* 1995;149:1226–1234.

26. National Adolescent Health Information Center. Fact sheet on investing in preventive health services for adolescents. In *Adolescent fact file.* San Francisco: University of California, San Francisco, July, 1994.

27. Jeter, J. Budget deal creates health care quandary: States must scramble to insure more children. *The Washington Post.* August 4, 1997, Section A, pp. 1,6.

28. Tharp, M., and Benoza, G. Pediatricians urged to "grab a seat at the table," advise states on $24 billion for child health care. *AAP News.* September, 1997;13(9):1,6.

29. Rosenbaum, S., and Darnell, J. Special issue: An analysis of the Medicaid and health-related provisions of the Personal Responsibility and Work Opportunity Reconciliation Act of 1996. *Health Policy and Child Health.* Summer, 1996;3(3):1–12.

30. Koppelman, J. Impact of the new welfare law on Medicaid. *National Health Policy Forum.* 1997;Issue Brief/No. 697:1–9.

34

The Progress and Potential of Injury Prevention

G. ALLEN BOLTON, MARTHA STOWE, AND PAUL J. BOUMBULIAN

The authors of this chapter gratefully acknowledge the research efforts of Rob Elston, former Communications Specialist for the Greater Dallas Injury Prevention Center, toward the preparation of this material.

An injury is physical damage to the body caused by acute exposure to mechanical, chemical, thermal, or electrical energy or by the absence of essentials such as heat or oxygen. Without a transfer of energy, trauma does not occur.[1,2] In this chapter, we use the words *injury* and *trauma* interchangeably.

Injuries are not accidents. *Accident* implies randomness or unpredictability, traits that are uncharacteristic of injuries.[2–5] Robertson writes that "accident is also intertwined with the notion that some human error or behavior is responsible for most injuries." That focus precludes examinations and interventions that would include the multitude of other factors that contribute to injuries and their severity.[6] These other factors are often more amenable to change than is human behavior, thereby breaking the causal chain of events that would otherwise lead to injury. The causal chain, or epidemiologic triangle, is explained later in this chapter.

Injuries are a public health problem. In a landmark publication, public health leader Dr. William Foege stated, "Injury is the principal

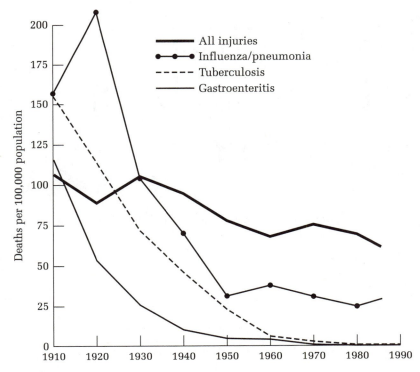

FIGURE 34.1

Death rates from injuries and infectious diseases by year, 1910–1986.

public health problem in America today [1985]." His statement was based on the impact of trauma on the health of the population. He and the National Committee for Injury Prevention and Control explained that, historically, trauma and infectious diseases have been the major causes of premature death throughout the world.[2] Since the beginning of the 20th century, public health measures have significantly reduced infectious disease mortality. However, public health has devoted relatively little attention and few resources to the prevention of injury. Figure 34.1 illustrates significant downturns in death rates from four infectious diseases between 1910 and 1986, while virtually no progress was made in the reduction of injury deaths.[3] Public health interventions were key to each dramatic decrease in these infectious disease categories. For example, enactment of the nation's first Water Quality Standards Act and the widespread adoption of pasteurization of milk in the early 20th century contributed to large reductions in the death rate from gastroenteritis.[7] Public health, as is pointed out later, did not become significantly involved in injury prevention until the 1980s.[5,8,9]

RATES AND TYPES OF INJURIES IN THE UNITED STATES

In 1994, there were 150,956 injury deaths in the United States.[10] In 1995, that number was 147,891, resulting in an age-adjusted death rate of 51.5 per 100,000 population. This represents 6% of all deaths in the United States. Additionally, 8% of all hospital discharges and 37% of all emergency room visits in 1995 were due to injury.[11] There were 14.2 emergency department visits for trauma per 100 U.S. residents.[12] Office-based physicians treated another 81.6 million trauma patients during the same year. This is equal to 31.2 visits per 100 persons and represents 11.7% of all physician office visits.[13] Overall, injuries are responsible for 12% of medical spending in the United States, or about $44 billion in direct health care costs per year.[8,14] Medical care for trauma represents the second largest category of medical expenditures in the United States.[15] Figure 34.2 depicts the volume of injuries reported in our health care system in 1995.

Trauma is the fourth leading cause of death for the entire human life span, but it has a disproportionate impact on the young. Between the ages 1 and 34, it is the leading cause of death in our country.[10] In fact, injuries are the leading cause of life-years lost.[3,16] For children aged 1 to 4, injuries account for 40% of all deaths. For older children and youth, aged 5 to 19, they are responsible for 70% of all deaths. Twenty percent of childhood hospitalizations are related to trauma.[17]

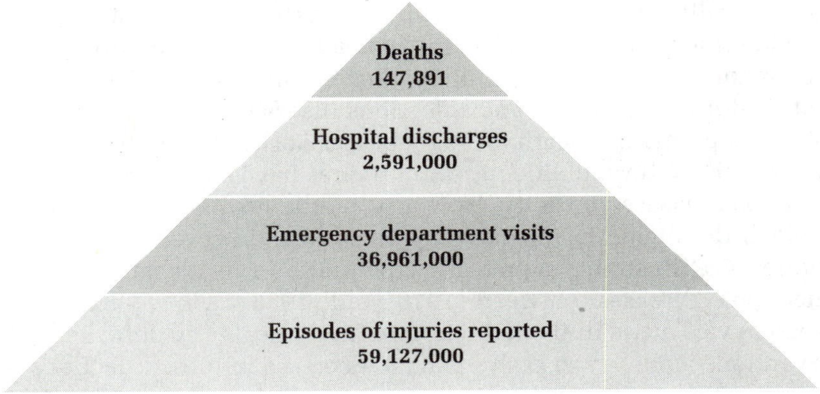

Deaths
147,891

Hospital discharges
2,591,000

Emergency department visits
36,961,000

Episodes of injuries reported
59,127,000

FIGURE 34.2

Burden of injury: United States, 1995.

Injuries are also the leading cause of death for young adults aged 20 to 24. From ages 25 to 34, injuries are the second leading cause of death, after death from human immunodeficiency syndrome (HIV)/acquired immunodeficiency syndrome (AIDS), and from ages 35 to 44, fatalities from trauma rank fourth behind HIV/AIDS, malignant neoplasms, and heart disease. By ages 45 to 54 and 55 to 64, deaths from heart disease and malignant neoplasms are two and eight times the total number of injury deaths in those respective age groups.[11] For the population older than age 65, the incidence of injury is lower than in any other age groups, but elderly patients are more likely to die from their injuries. Trauma is the fifth leading cause of death among this age group.[18]

Unintentional injuries were responsible for 61% of trauma deaths in 1994. The leading cause of fatal unintentional injuries was motor vehicles followed by falls, poisonings, burns, and drownings. In each of these categories there were also fatalities classified as intentional. Among intentional injury deaths, 56% are classified as suicides. Firearms are the leading mechanism of fatal injury for homicides and suicides, representing nearly three quarters and two thirds of the deaths in these categories, respectively.[10]

In 1994, motor vehicle injuries represented 28% of all trauma deaths (79% of which were to motor vehicle occupants, 15% to pedestrians, and 4% to motorcyclists). Firearms were responsible for 26% of the fatalities. Poisonings were third, with 11% of the total; and falls accounted for 10%. Drownings and burns were virtually tied for fourth place with approximately 3% of the deaths in each category.[10]

Leading causes or mechanisms of injury vary by age categories. Table 34.1 details the leading causes of fatal and non-fatal injury for different age groups.

TABLE 34.1

Leading Fatal and Nonfatal Injuries by Age

	Ranking of Mechanism of Injury	
Age	*Fatal*	*Nonfatal*
0–1	Suffocation Motor vehicle	
1–4	Motor vehicle Drowning	Falls Struck by person/object
5–14	Motor vehicle Firearms	Falls Struck by person/object
15–24	Firearms Motor vehicle	Motor vehicle Struck by person/object
25–64	Motor vehicle Firearms	Falls Motor vehicle
65+	Falls Motor vehicle	Falls Motor vehicle

Data from Baker, S.P., O'Neill, B., Ginsburg, M.J., and Li, G. *The injury fact book.* 2nd ed. New York: Oxford University Press, 1992; and *Health, United States, 1996–1997, and injury chartbook.* Hyattsville, MD: National Center for Health Statistics, 1997.

Risk of injury and death also varies greatly by sex and race. Unintentional and intentional injury death rates are higher for males than for females in each age group except infancy, where rates are similar.[3,11] The rate of nonfatal injury is also higher for males in all age categories up to age 65. At that point, the rate for females begins to exceed that for males.[11]

In 1995, the age-adjusted injury death rate in the United States was 21% lower than in 1980.[11] The majority of this decrease occurred in the early-1980s and can be largely attributed to improvements in transportation safety. In Table 34.2, the age-adjusted death rates for unintentional injuries show impressive reductions for all ethnic categories during the past half century. Data on Hispanic residents were not reported for 1950. Homicides have increased dramatically among all ethnic groups and continue to be over-represented in the black and Hispanic populations. Suicide rates have remained relatively stable during this period.

A significant risk factor for unintentional and intentional injuries is alcohol. For motor vehicle–related incidents, approximately 20% of serious injuries and 50% of fatalities are related to alcohol use. Like-

TABLE 34.2

Age-Adjusted Death Rates for Injury by Ethnicity

	All Races	White	Black	Hispanic
Unintentional Injuries				
1950	57.5	55.7	70.9	NA
1995	30.5	29.9	37.4	29.8
Homicide				
1950	5.4	2.6	30.5	NA
1995	9.4	5.5	33.4	15.0
Suicide				
1950	11.0	11.6	4.2	NA
1995	11.2	11.9	6.9	7.2

Data from *Health, United States, 1996–1997, and injury chartbook.* Hyattsville, MD: National Center for Health Statistics, 1997.

wise, studies indicate that alcohol may be involved in as many as half of all residential injury deaths. For intentional injuries, alcohol is also a major contributor. Various studies of violence have found alcohol to be involved in 33% to 60% of homicides and in a high proportion of non-fatal injuries. The contributory effect of the use of other drugs on the incidence of trauma has also been documented; however, the role of alcohol is better understood and more prevalent.[2]

HISTORY OF INJURY PREVENTION

Tracing Its Roots

In the early part of the 20th century, injury prevention efforts focused largely on the "fault" or behavior of the victims, with little consideration or understanding of other variables that helped produce trauma. Hugh De Haven in 1942 first looked at methods of preventing injury other than changing human behavior. As a World War I pilot who survived a crash, he studied how vehicle and restraint system designs could minimize the damage done by crash forces. He demonstrated that humans can be "crash packaged" in automobiles so that, in the event of a crash, the human body can be protected.[2]

A few years later in 1949, John E. Gordon was the first to characterize injuries like classic infectious diseases. He identified epidemic episodes, seasonal variation, geographic, socioeconomic, and rural-urban distributions for trauma. Gordon recognized that injuries are not caused by a single cause but by the interaction of forces between an agent and host in a permissive environment. Although this line of thinking was correct and significantly advanced the understanding of injury epidemiology, Gordon's description of agents was not accepted.

In 1961, James Gibson, an experimental psychologist at Cornell University, was the first to actually delineate the agents of injuries as physical energy, "either mechanical, thermal, radiant, chemical or electrical.[1] Shortly after Gibson's paper was published, William Haddon, Jr. modified the description of energy transfer to include negative agents, e.g., the absence of heat or oxygen.[2] Haddon, a physician-epidemiologist, developed his analysis into preventive approaches. He is widely regarded as the founding father of injury prevention. In 1966, Haddon became the first administrator of what is known today as the National Highway Traffic Safety Administration. For many years after that government appointment, he was the president of the Insurance Institute for Highway Safety. In both roles, he made significant contributions to the safety of transportation in the United States.

By 1983, a handful of professionals across the country were conducting research on the causes and prevention of trauma. In that year, Congress commissioned a study on the state of injury, injury research and the role of government in injury prevention and treatment. In response, the National Academy Press convened a Committee on Trauma that published its findings and recommendations in the landmark publication *Injury in America*.[9] Congress responded to the Committee's recommendations by appropriating funds for the establishment of a federal lead agency for injury prevention at the Centers for Disease Control and Prevention (CDC). The Division of Injury Epidemiology and Control (DIEC) was established at the CDC in 1985.

In 1989, a Committee was reconvened to review the progress of DIEC. The result was a recommendation to Congress that the issue warranted Center rather than Division status at CDC. In 1992, the National Center for Injury Prevention and Control (NCIPC) was created from the DIEC. It is the primary federal agency responsible for injury prevention research outside of transportation safety. In 1997, another Committee on Trauma was convened by the IOM for the purpose of reviewing progress within the field since 1985 and making recommendations about the future of injury prevention. Their report is due at the end of 1998.

Basic Concepts and Underlying Principles

Haddon, Baker, Robertson, and others have explained that the epidemiologic triangle that has been applied to the study of diseases is also applicable to injuries.[1,3,6,19,20] The epidemiologic triangle has as its three points (1) agent, (2) host, and (3) environment. All three factors must interact to cause disease or injury. Every injury is produced when an *agent* transfers energy to a *host* or human body in an *environment* that permits and even facilitates trauma. For example, a speeding, unhelmeted, teenage motorcyclist (host) driving a bike that is capable of speeds over 150 mph (agent) on a dark, rain-slick rural road (environment) is a scenario in which injury is probable. Thus, interventions to prevent diseases or injuries alter or eliminate one or more of these factors.

Haddon further refined our understanding of injury causation when he conceptualized the Haddon matrix. The matrix examines agent, host, and environmental factors over three time periods relevant to injury production and severity: pre-event, event, post-event. The matrix clearly shows the preventive value of the epidemiologic view in traumatic events.

Haddon Matrix
(Example using a motor vehicle collision)

	Factors		
Phases	Agent/Energy	Host/Human	Environment
Pre-event	Exceeding speed limit	Drinking alcohol	Poor visibility
Event	No airbag	Unrestrained occupant	
Post-event		Frail elderly occupant	Rapid Emergency Medical Service (EMS) time

The pre-event phase covers factors that determine whether a potentially injury-producing event will occur. The event phase includes factors that determine whether injuries are produced by the event. And, the post-event phase includes factors that determine whether injury severity can be reduced.[2]

Applying epidemiology to trauma underscores the preventable nature of injuries. Injuries are not random events. They are caused by the alignment of factors that can be both anticipated and altered. In other words, injuries are predictable and controllable.

There are three possible prevention stages, sometimes called injury control. The first stage, primary prevention, is the prevention of the incident that might have caused trauma. Avoiding a car wreck by using a designated (sober) driver exemplifies primary prevention. The second stage, secondary prevention, involves preventing or reducing the severity of injury once a traumatic incident (e.g., a car wreck, a fight) occurs. The deployment of airbags in a collision and the proper extrication of vehicle occupants by trained EMS personnel are two examples of secondary prevention techniques. The third stage, tertiary prevention, consists of efforts to reduce morbidity after injury and restore trauma victims to maximum functional potential. Proper nursing care using special cushions, special beds, and weight relief techniques are tertiary prevention methods aimed at preventing pressure sores in patients with spinal cord and traumatic brain injuries.[21-23]

Prevention Strategies

Injury prevention or control strategies can be categorized as active or passive. Generally, passive strategies, or those that work automatically and do not require any action on the part of the individual(s) being protected, have been most successful. Engineering changes that have made roadways less hazardous are passive strategies that have saved thousands of lives since the 1960s. Active strategies require that people alter their behavior and repeat the new, safer behavior every time they are exposed to a certain risk. Wearing a helmet when riding a motorcycle is an active injury prevention strategy that requires considerable effort and expense on the part of the motorcyclist. Those at risk must believe the justification for this safe behavior, select and buy the safety device, and wear the helmet each time they ride. Most injury prevention strategies combine both active and passive elements, but those that emphasize a passive approach have resulted in greater sustained reductions in injury.[1,20,21,24]

In addition to the active/passive categorization, injury prevention countermeasures fall into one of three strategies: (1) engineering or technology, (2) enforcement of policies/regulations, and (3) education.[2,5,16]

Engineering is a passive injury prevention strategy that has led to significant reduction in injuries throughout the 20th century. Safer roads, safer automobiles, safer toys, safer residential and commercial construction, safer drug packaging all are examples of engineering or technological interventions that have reduced injury.

Safety policies or regulations and their enforcement are important for the reduction of certain types of trauma. In 1978, Tennessee became the first state to pass a law requiring small children to be transported in child safety seats. Passage of the law resulted in a modest increase in child safety seat usage. However, the greatest impact came after law enforcement agencies in the state began enforcing the law. Regulatory interventions are effective, but somewhat less so than technological interventions. One reason is that with regulations there is some action required by the individual being protected, which means that individuals cannot assume an entirely passive role. Additionally, the effectiveness of policies may be highly dependent on the manner and consistency of enforcement efforts, or on the public's perception of their enforcement.[8]

Educational interventions can be effective, especially in combination with other strategies, but alone are the least effective of the three single strategies. Education is an active strategy. After safety information is communicated to at-risk individuals, it is necessary for those receiving the message to change personal behavior each time they are at risk. Some well-designed, well-executed educational interventions have been shown to be effective at reducing trauma. The Willy Whistle pedestrian safety curriculum and The Injury Prevention Project (TIPP) of the American Academy of Pediatrics are two such examples.[2,25] However, education is most effectively used as a complementary effort to other types of injury countermeasures.

Between 1962 and 1970, Haddon developed and refined a list of ten strategies to interfere with the transfer of energy that produces injury. These strategies are inclusive of the active/passive categorization and address primary, secondary, and tertiary prevention:

1. Prevent the creation of the hazard.
2. Reduce the amount/quantity of the hazard.
3. Prevent the release of a hazard that already exists.
4. Modify the rate or spatial distribution of the hazard.
5. Separate, in time or space, the hazard from that which is to be protected.
6. Separate the hazard from that which is to be protected by a material barrier.
7. Modify relevant basic qualities of the hazard.
8. Make what is to be protected more resistant to damage from the hazard.
9. Begin to counter the damage already done by the hazard.
10. Stabilize, repair, and rehabilitate the object of the damage.[1,2]

FUTURE OF INJURY PREVENTION

How will the relatively young field of injury prevention evolve into the 21st century? Given authoritative estimates on several factors that are likely to influence trauma, a picture of how the future should look begins to emerge.

To further define our vision of the field, in Spring 1997 the Institute of Medicine reconvened the Committee on Trauma to examine recent accomplishments in injury prevention and to make recommendations for the future. The Committee will complete its work nearly 15 years after the initial Committee on Trauma penned *Injury in America*. Students of this textbook are encouraged to examine the new Committee's summary after it is available in late-1998 or 1999. Their recommendations will help position the filed of injury prevention for the challenges of the 21st century.

Factors That Will Shape the Future of Injury Prevention

Population Demographics. Between 1995 and 2050, the population of the United States is expected to increase 150% from 263 million to 394 million. With this increase, the population will become more racially diverse and the number of those older than age 65 is expected to grow 240% (Fig. 34.3). Among ethnic groups, the projected growth among the Hispanic population, from 10.2% of the population in 1995

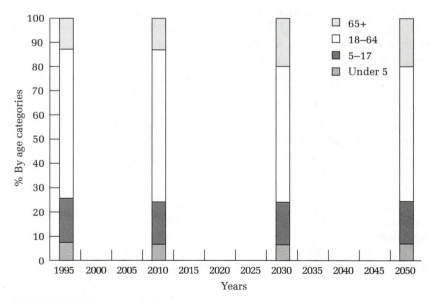

FIGURE 34.3

U.S. population projections by age.

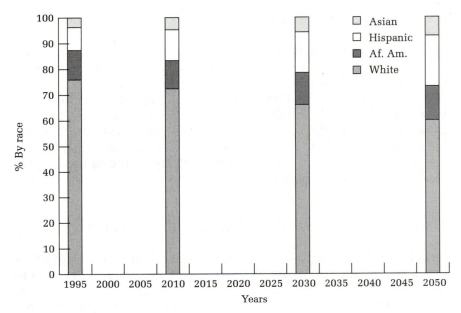

FIGURE 34.4

....

U.S. population projections by race.

to 24.5% of the population in 2050, is particularly impressive (Fig. 34.4). During the second decade of the 21st century, the proportion of elderly residents will rise dramatically.[26] By 2030, one in five Americans will be older than age 64.[27]

These population projections will affect the future of trauma care and trauma prevention, because injury patterns vary across age categories and ethnic populations. Although each age group will grow during the next 50 years, particularly challenging from an injury prevention standpoint will be the increase in the number of residents older than age 64. The elderly have the highest rates of hospitalization for injury and the highest fatality rates for injury than any other age groups.[3]

The growth in the proportion and number of Hispanic residents will also be challenging from an injury perspective. Hispanics are at disproportionate risk for transportation-related injuries, injuries resulting from violence, and injuries involving alcohol.[11] In fact, the increasing diversity of the U.S. population is expected to amplify existing cultural and attitudinal differences among racial and ethnic groups in regard to injury prevention. A new "breed" of injury prevention professionals who are competent to deal with these differences will be needed.

Managed Care. As was established in Chapter 18, managed care will be a significant force in the delivery of health care in the 21st century. Managed care plans, particularly health maintenance organizations (HMOs), are becoming the primary sources of employer-funded health care and of Medicare and Medicaid coverage. In 1994, 51 million U.S. residents were enrolled in HMOs, up from 6 million in 1976. For private employers and the government, managed care plans are less costly than traditional fee-for-service indemnity plans.[28]

Most managed care plans assume some, if not all, of the responsibility (or risk) for the health of the insured population. That is, the plan negotiates a premium or price per enrollee. Whatever health problems affect the population of enrollees, the plan is responsible for providing health care. It is in the best interest of the managed care plan to protect the health of its enrollees. A few plans, typically in areas where managed care has a large share of the health care market, have begun to realize savings from the implementation of injury prevention programs. In an effort to decrease bicycle-related head injuries among its pediatric enrollees, the Group Health Cooperative of Puget Sound, a 490,000-member HMO, implemented an injury prevention program in 1987. Its efforts to increase bicycle helmet use among children reduced bicycle-related head injuries by 67% over 5 years.[28] Because trauma care is particularly costly, injury prevention can be viewed as a means of lowering the financial risks of managed care plans.

Programming Strategies

The Medical Model—Intervening at the Clinical Level

The Ongoing Provision of Trauma Care. Trauma care systems are regional or statewide networks of acute care facilities that treat trauma patients. Fully developed trauma care systems provide injury prevention strategies through policy and education, prompt recognition of injurious events with rapid response by EMS, advanced communication and medical control for EMS, on-scene triage and transportation to appropriate medical facilities, designated trauma care facilities, interfacility transfer agreements, rehabilitation facilities, and standardized trauma care data systems.[29] Studies have shown that preventable trauma deaths decrease after implementation of trauma care systems. Nevertheless, less than one quarter of the United States population is served by these systems.[30,31]

Trauma centers, particularly Level I trauma centers, are the hub of trauma systems. One of the main reasons for fledgling efforts to develop trauma care systems is the economic instability of designated trauma centers. A study of trauma center closures identified the level of uncompensated care, high operating costs, and inadequate reimbursement from government medical assistance programs as the three primary reasons hospitals discontinue trauma services.[15] Particularly vulnerable from an economic standpoint are trauma centers located in large urban areas. Their vulnerability is due to the large volume of poor and uninsured injured patients they treat.[32,33]

The survival of trauma centers and the expansion of trauma systems in the United States are desirable and will depend on the ability to manage the demand for trauma care services. Demand management limits the number of people who need the service and provides only the appropriate level of care for those who are in need of it. The key strategy for managing the demand for trauma care services is to prevent injuries.[15,33-35]

Incorporation of Prevention into Clinical Practice. By providing routine medical care to injured patients, medical personnel are involved in tertiary prevention (as described in the section Basic Concepts and Underlying Principles). However, studies and expert opinion indicate an increasing need for and efficacy of physician involvement in primary prevention of injuries.[16,22,25,36-39] There are at least three roles for physicians in injury prevention.

Screening and counseling patients to modify high-risk behaviors is a proven strategy to reduce injuries and is a role that should be expanded for physicians. Particularly impressive is the involvement of pediatricians in this role over the past decade. Evaluation of The Injury Prevention Program (TIPP), an office-based counseling schedule developed by the American Academy of Pediatrics, has shown a 13:1 benefit-cost ratio.[25]

A second role is advocacy. Physicians can influence public policy regarding trauma prevention. Abraham Bergman, a Seattle pediatrician, was instrumental in the adoption of national standards for fire-retardant material in children's sleepwear, and Robert Sanders lobbied the Tennessee legislature (and subsequently many other state legislatures) to achieve passage of the nation's first mandatory child safety seat law.[2]

A third role for physicians is collaborative research. While scientists in other areas (e.g., epidemiology, economics, sociology) can contribute to injury prevention research, the physicians who treat injured patients have perspectives and insights that are valuable to scientific inquiry. Each of these three roles, however, will require significant modification in the manner in which physicians are trained currently.[16,29] They will also require institutions to examine and perhaps alter how physicians' performance and compensation are determined.

The Public Health Model—Intervening at the Community Level.
David Satcher, director of the CDC, stated, "If public health doesn't
work at the level of the community, it doesn't work."[40] He was referring to a new initiative at CDC, Safe America, which is aimed at transferring knowledge about injury prevention into action within communities. It is no coincidence that 2 years before Satcher's statement,
Ricardo Martinez, Administrator of the National Highway Traffic
Safety Administration, unveiled Safe Communities, an initiative with
the same ideals and goals for transportation safety.

Public health leaders are acknowledging that many "easy gains"
have come through passive strategies such as technology and the semi-
passive strategy of legislation and enforcement. Although there is still
work that can be done to advance these types of strategies, the very active strategy of community participation is a primary direction for the
field into the next century.

Community participation is "the involvement of people in designing and implementing research and interventions intended to benefit them."[41] There are varying degrees of participation from shared decision making at one end of the spectrum through passive compliance
to tokenism. Green emphasizes that the more engaged community
members are, the more successful the project is likely to be.[42] Although the concept has been around health care since at least the
1960s, the power of community participation was first recognized in
the 1980s North Karelia Project. This program sought to reduce cardiovascular disease risk factors such as smoking, cholesterol, and obesity
in a community in Finland. Residents became alarmed to learn of their
community's excessive mortality rates and initiated the project's
media efforts, counseling and education programs, food labeling efforts, and other activities with the aid of health professionals. After 15
years of experience, the North Karelia Project not only reduced risk
factors, it actually produced a decrease in heart disease mortality.[43]
Examples of injury prevention programs that have incorporated community participation to change risky behavior and reduce the incidence of trauma are emerging.[43–48] The World Health Organization
began testing and promoting such community level strategies in Sweden in 1978.[45] And now that the U.S. government's two lead agencies
on injury prevention, the National Center for Injury Prevention and
Control and the National Highway Traffic Safety Administration, have
embraced this type of intervention method, we can expect to experience a rapid growth in the number of, and knowledge from, community-based injury prevention projects.

The three primary challenges facing injury prevention professionals as we begin an era of working with communities to reduce
trauma are (1) evaluation, (2) health systems bias, and (3) a breakdown
in society's traditional sense of community.

Research needs for the future are outlined later in this chapter. Especially appropriate for evaluation of community participation programs are the recommendations made for more prevention research and analytic epidemiologic studies. Schwab and Syme claim the information we gather from participatory interventions is not "normal science" because it is not driven by scientists but by the community. It does not seek universal truths but local or situational truths. Nevertheless, practitioners must embrace the "experience and partnership of those we are normally content simply to measure."[41]

The second major obstacle is health systems bias. Injury prevention professionals typically receive little or no training in community development, and few seem to appreciate the skills necessary to be successful in such an uncontrolled environment. The majority of injury prevention professionals are affiliated with health systems, i.e., hospitals, academic medical centers, health departments, etc. This is likely to set up working barriers because there is a stark contrast between the values of such a system and the values of communities. Systems value hierarchical order (i.e., top-down), whereas communities value active consent of the people. Systems depend on clients or consumers, and communities depend on citizens. In Greek, the root word for client means "one who is controlled"; citizen means "one who holds the power." Another difference is that health systems define people and communities by disease or injury problems. This perspective is that communities are a collection of deficiencies; communities define themselves according to their capacities or assets. Finally, systems produce standardized outcomes, whereas communities require creativity to produce unique outcomes.[49]

The third obstacle is a growing loss of society's traditional "sense of community." Communities have traditionally been a group of individuals with a high degree of interconnectedness provided by geographic proximity and shared economic, religious, cultural, ethnic, or political values.[39] This interconnectedness is what we define as a "sense of community." The continuing breakdown of extended family networks and the increasing mobility of individuals are factors that negatively impact this interconnectedness among citizens.

Injury prevention professionals must understand these fundamental differences and seek to work through them. McKnight suggests this is possible and will even enhance the strength of communities. Successful health system–community interactions appear to depend on at least four practices of professionals with the systems: (1) professionals should not take a lead role in community programs, and they must demonstrate that they respect the wisdom of the community; (2) professionals have useful health information for citizens that should be shared in understandable form; (3) professionals should use their resources to expand the power of citizens and the community instead of bringing attention or resources to the health system; and (4) the professional should not look at the injury (or deficit) as what is important but should look at the community's capacities (or assets) to deal with such issues.[49]

Needs Within the Field of Injury Prevention

Research. Ultimately, injury prevention efforts have one or more of the following goals: to reduce the incidence of trauma, the severity of trauma, or the costs associated with trauma. To accomplish any of these ideals, research to determine the effectiveness of injury prevention efforts must be increased.[5,9,36,50] This type of prevention research should be conducted with community-level practitioners in mind. The feasibility of replicating, within communities, prevention initiatives that have fared well under "study conditions" is itself a research question that should be factored into prevention studies. Injury prevention programs must be subjected to rigorous process and outcome evaluation methods and the results reported in the professional literature and disseminated widely to practitioners at the community level.

Although descriptive epidemiologic studies have dominated injury prevention research to date and continue to have some value, Rivara and Wolf advocate a larger commitment to analytic epidemiology. Analytic epidemiology uses case-control or cohort designs to discern causal factors that influence the risk of injury. By identifying causal factors, these types of studies are more likely to yield information that will result in the development of effective intervention strategies.[50] These types of studies require more resources, planning, and analytic capabilities than descriptive studies but yield superior information for prevention.

Descriptive epidemiologic studies continue to be warranted if they address significant injury issues within the population. Much of the previous research of this type has focused on injury issues that are of academic interest yet of little interest or value to communities. Research that examines injuries that are "frequent but of low severity, infrequent and severe, or both infrequent and not severe" is common, costly, and has relatively little value in the actual prevention of trauma.[50] However, injuries that are frequent, severe, and for which there are not definitive descriptive studies are important to investigate.[25,40,50] The involvement of trauma care personnel, including EMS, emergency physicians, trauma surgeons, emergency nurses, or medical examiners/coroners, in the selection of injury prevention research issues may help investigators avoid conducting irrelevant descriptive studies.

The primary question to be asked of any injury prevention researcher, whether conducting a prevention, analytic epidemiologic, or descriptive epidemiologic study, is "Does the study provide *new* information that will lead to the better understanding of and prevention of trauma within the population?" With extremely limited research resources in this area, if the answer to this question is "no," the study should be abandoned in favor of more practical research applications.[3,50]

Data. Implicit in the discussion so far is the need for data on which to base injury prevention priorities and judge the effectiveness of injury prevention efforts. There are currently significant gaps in our understanding of the incidence, causes, and costs of injuries. To improve the quality of the information available to injury prevention practitioners, the following actions are necessary.

The International Classification of Disease Codes (ICD-9 and ICD-10 codes), a worldwide classification system for diagnoses used by health care facilities, includes a Supplemental Classification of External Causes of Injury and Poisoning (E-codes). ICD-9 is the ninth revision of the classification system, which has been in use since 1980. ICD-10 is the tenth revision, released in 1993, and is not yet being extensively used.[38] ICD codes are widely used by health care facilities largely because they are directly tied to reimbursement. The supplemental E-codes provide information on the mechanism of injury (e.g., automobile crash, bicycle crash, fall) and are not widely used. Increasing the reporting of E-codes on emergency department and hospital admission/discharge databases is a priority for the next century.[2,5,29,38,51]

Linking various injury databases would also provide information that would enhance the prevention of injuries. The first category in which this linking capacity is being developed is motor vehicle crashes.[52,53] Traffic crash records from law enforcement are being successfully linked to medical records from EMS, hospitals, and, in some cases, coroners. Other categories of injury such as fires and violence are also appropriate targets for linkage efforts.[38,39,51,53] Although efforts to link such information raise concerns about issues of confidentiality and propriety, advances in computer technology and in society's ability to manage information over the next several years are expected to make the linkage of such injury databases commonplace.

Another pressing data need is the development and implementation of uniform data sets for trauma care and rehabilitation. Currently, we do not know the extent to which acute care and rehabilitation systems are used. Nor do we know the overall efficacy, including the cost-effectiveness, of such systems. To realistically look at the continuum of injury prevention from primary through tertiary phases, such a uniform system is necessary.[29,51]

In each of the enhanced injury surveillance systems described in this section, there is needed a uniform method for assessing and coding injury severity and data from which injury costs can be calculated.[36,38]

Human and Financial Resources. Finally, no discussion on the future of injury prevention would be complete without the admonition that more resources are needed in order for the field to meet its life- and cost-savings potential. Resources are needed in two areas: personnel and funding. The need for additional training of medical personnel has already been cited. There is also a need for increasing the number of other scientists whose primary research focus is injury prevention and for increasing the number of community-level injury prevention practitioners. Without a properly trained "work force" in this area, the field cannot advance. Training will come from a combination of the increasing number of colleges and universities that offer courses in injury prevention, health departments and other agencies that offer workshops and seminars, and an explosion of injury prevention information available through professional publications and electronic media such as the Internet.

Financial resources are also necessary. It was estimated in the early 1990s that approximately 3% of health care funding was spent on prevention of any kind. The proportion spent on injury prevention was a fraction of 1%.[5,16] In perspective, in the 1980s injuries were the leading cause of premature life-years lost, followed by cardiovascular diseases and cancers. Yet, federal funding for injury prevention was one tenth that for cancer and one sixth that for cardiovascular diseases.[5,9,36] Since the 1980s, HIV/AIDS has become a leading cause of premature death, and funding for AIDS research has grown commensurate with its increasing threat to society. Injury prevention should receive funding in proportion to its impact on the health of the nation. It is recommended that governments not be the only sources to increase their spending on injury prevention. The corporate and non-profit sectors also have a lot to gain from investing in injury prevention research and programs.

References

1. Haddon, W. Advances in the epidemiology of injuries as a basis for public policy. *Public Health Reports.* 1980;95:411–421.
2. National Committee for Injury Prevention and Control. *Injury prevention, meeting the challenge.* New York: Oxford University Press, 1989.
3. Baker, S.P., O'Neill, B., Ginsburg, M.J., and Li, G. *The injury fact book.* 2nd ed. New York: Oxford University Press, 1992.

4. Christoffel, T., and Teret, S.P. *Protecting the public, legal issues in injury prevention.* New York: Oxford University Press, 1993.

5. National Research Council and the Institute of Medicine. *Injury in America, a continuing public health problem.* Washington, DC: National Academy Press, 1985.

6. Robertson, L. *Injury epidemiology.* New York: Oxford University Press, 1992.

7. Hanlon, J.J., and Pickett, G.E. *Public health administration and practice.* 8th ed. St. Louis, MO: Times Mirror/Mosby College Publishing, 1984.

8. Bolton, A., Boumbulian, P., and Anderson, A. Public health enemy number one: Injury in America. *Metropolitan Universities.* 1995;6:23–34.

9. Committee to Review the Status and Progress of the Injury Control Program at the Centers for Disease Control. *Injury control.* Washington, DC: National Academy Press, 1988.

10. Rivara, F.P., Grossman, D.C., and Cummings, P. Injury prevention (first of two parts). *New England Journal of Medicine.* 1997;337:543–548.

11. National Center for Health Statistics. *Health, United States, 1996–1997, and injury chartbook.* Hyattsville, MD: National Center for Health Statistics, 1997.

12. Stussman, B.J. *National hospital ambulatory medical care survey: 1995 emergency department summary.* Advance data from vital and health statistics, no. 285. Hyattsville, MD: National Center for Health Statistics, 1997.

13. Woodwell, D.A. *National hospital ambulatory medical care survey: 1995 summary.* Advance data from vital and health statistics, no. 286. Hyattsville, MD: National Center for Health Statistics, 1997.

14. Miller, T.R., Lestina, D.C., Galbraith, M.S., and Viano, D.C. Medical care spending—United States. *MMWR.* 1994;43:581–586.

15. Elliott, D.C., and Rodriguez, A. Cost effectiveness in trauma care. *Surgical Clinics of North America.* 1996;76:47–62.

16. Martinez, R. Injury prevention, a new perspective (editorial). *JAMA.* 1994;272:1541–1542.

17. Rodriguez, J.G., and Brown, S.T. Childhood injuries in the United States. *American Journal of Diseases of Children.* 1990;144:627–646.

18. Smith, D.P., Enderson, B.L., and Maull, K.I. Trauma in the elderly: Determinants of outcome. *Southern Medical Journal.* 1990;83:171–177.

19. Robertson, L.S. *Injuries: causes, control strategies, and public policy.* Lexington, MA: Lexington Books, 1983.

20. Waller, J.A. *Injury control: A guide to the causes and prevention of trauma.* Lexington, MA: Lexington Books, 1985.

21. Stanford, G.G., and Bolton, A. Injury prevention—the ultimate solution for reducing death and disability for traumatic injury in Dallas. *Dallas Medical Journal.* 1994;80:454–457.

22. Institute of Medicine. *Disability in America, toward a national agenda for prevention.* Washington, DC: National Academy Press, 1991.

23. Teutsch, S.M. A framework for assessing the effectiveness of disease and injury prevention. *MMWR.* 1992;41:1–12.

24. Rivara, F.P., Grossman, D.C., and Cummings, P. Injury prevention (second of two parts). *New England Journal of Medicine.* 1997;337:613–618.

25. Miller, T.R., and Galbraith, M. Injury prevention counseling by pediatricians: A benefit-cost comparison. *Pediatrics.* 1995;96:1–4.

26. Day, J.C. *Population projections of the United States by age, sex, race, and Hispanic origin: 1995 to 2050.* Washington, DC: U.S. Government Printing Office, 1996.

27. Hackler, C. (ed.) *Health care for an aging population.* Albany, NY: State University of New York Press, 1994.

28. Centers for Disease Control and Prevention. Prevention and managed care: Opportunities for managed care organizations, purchasers of health care, and public health agencies. *MMWR Supplement.* 1995;44:1–12.

29. Waxweiler, R.J., Rosenberg, M.L., and Fenley, M.A. (eds). *Injury control in the 1990s, a national plan for action: A report to the second world conference on injury control.* Association for the Advancement of Automotive Medicine, 1993.

30. Eastman, A.B. Blood in our streets: The status and evoluation of trauma care systems. *Archives of Surgery.* 1992;127:677–681.

31. Goldfarb, M.G., Bazzoli, G.J., and Coffey, R.M. Trauma systems and the costs of trauma care. *Health Services Research.* 1996;31:71–95.
32. Bazzoli, G.J., Meersman, P.J., and Chan, C. Factors that enhance continued trauma center participation in trauma systems. *Journal of Trauma.* 1996;41:876–885.
33. Cornwell, E.E., Berne, T.V., Belzberg, H., Asensio, J., Velmahos, G., Murray, J., and Demetriades, D. Health care crisis from a trauma center perspective, the LA story. *JAMA.* 1996;276:940–944.
34. Skolnick, A.A. Injury prevention must be part of nation's plan to reduce health care costs, say control experts (commentary). *JAMA.* 1993;270:19–24.
35. Fries, J.F., Koop, E., Beadle, C.E., Cooper, P.P., England, M.J., Greaves, R.F., Sokolov, J.J., and Wright, D. Reducing health care costs by reducing the need and demand for medical services. *New England Journal of Medicine.* 1993;329:321–325.
36. Rice, D.P., and Mackenzie, E.J. *Cost of injury in the United States, a report to Congress, 1989.* San Francisco: Institute for Health and Aging, University of California and Injury Prevention Center, The Johns Hopkins University, 1989.
37. Tengs, T.O., Adams, M.E., Pliskin, J.S., Safran, D.G., Siegel, J.E., Weinstein, M.C., and Graham, J.D. Five hundred life-saving interventions and their cost-effectiveness. *Risk Analysis.* 1995;15:369–390.
38. Berger, L.R., and Mohan, D. *Injury control, a global view.* New Delhi, India: Oxford University Press, 1996.
39. Bolton, A., Stanford, G., and Elston, R. *Summary of an international congress: safe communities, the application to large urban environments.* KI Red Report 358. Sundbyberg, Sweden: Karolinska Institute, 1997.
40. National Center for Injury Prevention and Control. CDC's director shares his vision of Safe America. *Injury Control Update.* 1997;2:2–4.
41. Schwab, M., and Syme, S.L. On paradigms, community participation, and the future of public health (commentary). *American Journal of Public Health.* 1997;87:2049–2051.
42. Green, L.W., and Kreuter, M.W., eds. *Health promotion planning: An educational and environmental approach.* 2nd ed. Mountain View, CA: Mayfield, 1991.
43. Gielen, A.C., and Collins, B. Community-based interventions for injury prevention. *Family and Community Health.* 1993;15:1–11.
44. Baker, E.L., Melton, R.J., Stange, P.V., Fields, M.L., Koplan, J.P., Guerra, F.A., and Satcher, D. Health reform and the health of the public, forging community health partnerships. *JAMA.* 1994;272:1276–1282.
45. Svanstrom, L., Schlep, L., Ekman, R., and Lindstrom, A. Falkoping, Sweden, ten years after: Still a safe community? *International Journal of Consumer Safety.* 1996;3:1–7.
46. DiGuiseppi, C.G., Rivara, F.P., Koepsell, T.D., and Polissar, L. Bicycle helmet use by children: Evaluation of a community-wide helmet campaign. *JAMA.* 1989;262:2256–2261.
47. Plautz, B., Beck, D.E., Selmar, C., and Radetsky, M. Modifying the environment: A community-based injury reduction program for elderly residents. *American Journal of Preventive Medicine.* 1996;12:33–38.
48. Bablouzian, L., Freedman, E.S., Wolski, K.E., and Fried, L.E. Evaluation of a community based childhood injury prevention program. *Injury Prevention.* 1997;3:14–16.
49. McKnight, J.L. Two tools for well-being: Health systems and communities. *American Journal of Preventive Medicine.* 1994;10:23–25.
50. Rivara, F.P., and Wolf, M.E. Injury research: where should we go from here? (commentary). *Pediatrics.* 1989;84:180–181.
51. U.S. Department of Health and Human Services. *Healthy People 2000: National health promotion and disease prevention objectives.* Washington, DC: U.S. Government Printing Office, 1991.
52. Johnson, S.W., and Walker, J. *The crash outcome data evaluation system (CODES).* DOT Pub. HS 808 338. Washington, DC: National Highway Traffic Safety Administration, 1996.
53. National Highway Traffic Safety Administration. *Getting started: a guide to developing safe communities.* DOT Pub. HS 808 404. Washington, DC: National Highway Traffic Safety Administration, 1996.

35

Emergency Medical Services for Children

JEAN L. ATHEY

HISTORY OF EMERGENCY MEDICAL SERVICES SYSTEMS

Advanced, highly organized emergency medical services (EMS) systems are relatively new. The existing network of lifesaving resources and technology entered its early stages of development barely 30 years ago. EMS systems evolved as a result of military experiences, which demonstrated that survival rates could be greatly increased through appropriate triage, timely transport, and prehospital care.[1] During the 1960s, civilian medical and surgical communities began to recognize the possibilities of developing an organized EMS system. The modern era of EMS and the start of a systems approach to improved trauma care were stimulated by the 1966 benchmark report *Accidental Death and Disability: The Neglected Disease of Modern Society.*[2]

The first EMS systems were designed to provide rapid intervention for sudden cardiac arrest in adults and rapid transport for motor vehicle crash victims. Because children suffer from a different spectrum of disease and injury than adults, and because children's physiologic responses to illness and injury are different, their treatment demands specific training, equipment, and techniques. The systems that were developed initially made no allowance for children's unique medical needs—a critical omission that decreased the quality of pediatric emergency care. Children's minority status within EMS (children account for only 10% to 15% of prehospital runs and 20% to 30% of emergency department visits) contributed to the lower quality of care they received.[3] Although outcomes for adults in emergency situations improved dramatically as a result of new EMS systems, children's outcomes did not keep pace.[4]

Beginning in the late 1970s, pediatricians and pediatric surgeons began to advocate on behalf of their patients and worked to obtain for children the same positive results that EMS had achieved for adults. For example, Martin Eichelberger pioneered a model pediatric trauma system for the Washington metropolitan area in the early 1980s. Research by James Seidel from Harbor-UCLA Medical Center showed that outcomes for critically ill and injured children improved when they were cared for in specialized pediatric centers. He also determined that many EMS providers did not have the training or equipment to care for pediatric patients.[5] At the same time, Max Ramenofsky's study of pediatric trauma deaths showed that errors in care resulted in an increased mortality rate for pediatric patients.[6] These studies spurred the development of the Emergency Department Approved for Pediatrics-Pediatric Critical Care Center (EDAP-PCCC) System in Los Angeles County—a model subsequently used by many states to improve pediatric emergency care in EMS systems.[7]

With documentation of the problems in hand and with models to address them available, the American Academy of Pediatrics began to urge multifaceted EMS programs that would decrease morbidity and mortality in children. The federal Emergency Medical Services for Children (EMSC) program was established in 1984 with the passage of legislation co-sponsored by Senators Daniel K. Inouye of Hawaii and Orrin G. Hatch of Utah.

Modestly funded since that time, the EMSC program has provided grants to states to address all the issues special to children in EMS systems, from injury prevention to prehospital care to emergency department care to rehabilitation. In addition, the program has increased our knowledge of how to treat children in emergency situations and has provided materials for educational programs and systems development that can be used by EMS systems in the absence of special grant funds. However, a 1993 study by the Institute of Medicine identified the many remaining gaps and deficiencies in pediatric emergency medical services,[3] and research undertaken in 1997 to obtain baseline data for the EMSC program's 5-year plan further documented and quantified many of these gaps. In short, much has been accomplished, but much more remains to be done.

WHY CHILDREN NEED SPECIAL ATTENTION

There are many reasons why children should be singled out for special attention within the EMS system if we are to provide them the same level of care we can provide to adults.

Assessment and Treatment

The EMS provider trained primarily in the care of adults must reassess normal and abnormal when dealing with a child's anatomy and physiology. For example, the child's larger surface area–to–mass ratio creates higher normal breathing and heart rates and lower blood pressure measurements than those of adults, and these vary with age. Children are also at higher risk of hypothermia.

Assessment of the child is further complicated by the fact that the underlying causes of symptoms and the array of problems that children present to EMS systems are different from those of adults. Assessment-based treatment protocols derived from adult experience may not be appropriate for children, as the underlying causes may be different. Chest pain or syncope, for example, are rarely due to primary cardiac causes in children. Thus, adult-oriented advanced life support training does not provide adequate guidance for treating children. Furthermore, the younger the child, the more subtle or nonspecific are the signs of illness; irritability, vomiting, fever, and lethargy are symptoms that may accompany a wide range of pediatric conditions, some life-threatening, some trivial.

Equipment

Treatment of the child is also complicated by the fact that "one size fits all" equipment designed for adults, such as blood pressure cuffs, intravenous needles, and bag-valve mask devices, do not fit infants and small children. Children require different equipment to accomplish the same ends. Hospital emergency departments and ambulances often do not have the full complement of equipment in sizes to fit all children. Beyond the need for different equipment is the need for training in use of that equipment, because many of the techniques for treating children differ from those of adults.

Communication with Children

Information about the child must frequently be obtained secondhand from the caregiver, especially when the child is very young. A child may not be able to cooperate with EMS providers because of anxiety, anger, or age. Parents also may be distressed, often without direct correlation to the severity of their child's condition, and so may not always be reliable sources of information.

Emotional and Cognitive Development

In assessing and treating the pediatric patient, EMS providers must recognize that a child's understanding of an illness or injury and the emotional response to that condition will vary with age. For example, the younger the child, the more distress is displayed during a painful medical procedure. This heightened distress may be related to the meaning a child attributes to experiences, for example, as punishment for misdeeds. Young children may take their cues primarily from the adult caregivers they know best, but at any given developmental stage, their response and understanding may be affected by curiosity, need for autonomy, desires for modesty and privacy, fears of death or mutilation, guilt, or misinterpretation of overheard discussions. Furthermore, parents share uniquely in their child's illness or injury and may react differently than when faced with a similar crisis in an adult family member. Parents feel helpless, afraid, and often guilty, sometimes devastatingly so. The concept of "injured child/injured family" reflects our understanding that when a child becomes acutely injured or ill, every member of the family is affected. Health care workers need to respond appropriately to the child's, as well as to the family's, emotional needs.

THE EMSC CONTINUUM OF CARE

EMS is sometimes thought of as prehospital care only—an ambulance and a paramedic. However, that paradigm has shifted in recent years, most notably with the development of a consensus document published in 1996 entitled *Emergency Medical Services: Agenda for the Future,*[8] which more broadly defines the EMS role to include prevention, especially of injury, and community health monitoring. EMSC advocates have always viewed emergency services as a continuum: prevention is its first goal, and when prevention fails, there should be a seamless, high-quality system of emergency treatment that includes prehospital care, emergency department care, access to specialty care, rehabilitation, and reintegration into the community.

Prevention

Prevention of illness and injury is obviously preferable to treatment. Several childhood illnesses are preventable through immunizations, although the United States still has far to go in adequately immunizing its children. Other illnesses develop rapidly, sometimes from inadequate or delayed treatment of a less serious condition.[3] Better understanding of how children's illnesses progress, among both parents and general practitioners, could help prevent illness from progressing to an emergency.

Injury is the leading cause of death among children and adolescents, claiming some 20,000 lives each year. Non-fatal injuries occur far more frequently: more than 13 million emergency department visits for children and adolescents per year are attributable to injury.[9] Injuries are preventable, although effective prevention requires a multifaceted approach targeting specific injury categories, such as motor vehicle and pedestrian injuries, residential fire, firearm violence, and child abuse. Such activities as heightening public awareness, enacting legislation, altering the environment to make it safer, and advocating the use of safety devices (e.g., smoke detectors, child safety seats, bike helmets, and gun safety locks) can over time lead to a reduction in child death and disability caused by injury.

Prehospital Care

When prevention fails, immediate quality care is needed for child health emergencies. The first component of prehospital care is a trained and informed layperson who can deliver "bystander care"—CPR, rescue breathing, and procedures to stop bleeding. Knowledge of when and how to call for help is also critical—911 (or the local emergency number) or a poison control center.

When an ambulance (or other transport vehicle) arrives, it should have proper equipment and the emergency medical technicians (EMTs) or paramedics should be skilled in treating children. A 1997 study found that only five states require all EMSC-recommended pediatric equipment on ambulances.[10] Training is a more complex issue; before recent modifications to the basic curriculum taught to EMTs, pediatric content was woefully inadequate. Improvements have now been made to that curriculum. However, because children represent a relatively low proportion of cases, EMTs have little opportunity to maintain their skills. One study found that skills degraded within 6 months.[11] Yet no state requires refresher courses in pediatrics as a condition of recertification for EMTs. It is therefore not surprising that a 1996 survey of EMTs found that treating children generated the highest concerns among these health care providers.

Once an ambulance arrives on scene, it should ideally transport a child to the nearest hospital ready to receive children, that is, sufficiently staffed with adequately trained personnel. Transport protocols should provide such guidance; yet only 11 states have disseminated guidelines for acute care facility identification.[10]

Emergency Department and Inpatient Care

Not all emergency departments have nurses and doctors trained in pediatric emergency care, nor do all have the basic equipment needed to treat children. In fact, one study found that only 46% of hospital emergency departments have all the equipment necessary to stabilize ill or injured children.[10] Other important features of an emergency department responsive to children's needs include the following:

1. Transfer guidelines, if the hospital does not have a pediatric intensive care unit: Not all hospitals can be expected to be

fully staffed and equipped to handle serious child emergencies. However, if a hospital is not prepared to treat such emergencies, procedures and protocols need to be in place so that children can be quickly and efficiently transferred to a "higher" level of care—otherwise, delays in definitive treatment result that can seriously compromise a child's recovery. Currently, only six states have guidelines for interfacility transport of children.[8]

2. Access to pediatric specialists: A hospital that treats children should have quick access to an array of physicians trained in pediatrics, from surgeons to physiatrists to anesthesiologists.

3. Family-centered policies: Emergency departments that are "family-centered" work proactively to ensure that families are respected, are given choices (e.g., to remain with a child during resuscitation), are provided support, and are viewed as partners in caring for a child.

4. Coordination of care and early referral: Unfortunately, many children are not referred for rehabilitation services following an acute illness or injury, regardless of their ability to do such things as walk, eat, dress, bathe, or communicate. Protocols for early involvement of a rehabilitation professional can ensure coordination of care and enhanced recovery.

Rehabilitation

Prior to release of a child from the hospital, a rehabilitation plan needs to be in effect to ensure that the child makes as full a recovery as possible and to avert future emergencies. This plan needs to include information about the child's medical condition, needed medications, and proper emergency intervention strategies. Parents and health care professionals need to work together to ensure that children receive ongoing rehabilitation services.

FACTORS AFFECTING CHILDREN'S EMERGENCY MEDICAL SERVICES

Probably the most important factor currently affecting children's emergency medical care is the movement to reduce the costs of health care and the revolutionary changes in the delivery system that have resulted. In particular, the move to managed care is fostering dramatic changes. There is growing concern that market-based health care reform may negate many of the improvements that have been made to the EMS system and/or delay continued improvements. Access to care and special services and EMS system development are particularly critical issues.

Access to 911 and Emergency Departments

The country has worked hard to provide an easily recognizable and widely known telephone number for quick and ready access to immediate emergency care. Although 911 is still not universal, it is available in most urban communities. In some cases, managed care companies have instructed their patients specifically not to call 911 but to use a different number in an emergency. Others have required a call to the managed care organization (MCO) for preauthorization of an ambulance. Such attempts to cut costs have the effect of undercutting the community's emergency response system while making the plan's participants unsure about what to do when a serious emergency occurs. In fact, parents are sometimes confused as to what process to follow in an actual emergency. Access to care may be delayed in some emergency situations, with devastating results.

MCOs also strive to reduce unnecessary emergency department visits. Currently, methods to control visits to emergency departments vary among MCOs. Many have established procedures to redirect patients with acute problems to sites other than emergency departments, but the triage protocols used for determining the appropriate treatment setting may not be pediatric-specific. Moreover, it is not easy to distinguish between an emergency, an urgent condition, and a nonurgent one, especially in children. Even health care professionals generally do not agree about the need for urgent care among emergency department patients;[12] a telephone triage system, as many MCOs have established, is likely to be even less accurate. It is important that a quality emergency system be available and that reducing inappropriate use of emergency care not lead to restrictions in appropriate and necessary use.

Hospital Designation Protocols

MCOs typically have a limited number of hospitals that their patients are authorized to use. These "participant providers" may not have adequate equipment or training to manage children's emergencies. Some hospitals are clearly superior in terms of treatment of children and others inferior. Using insurance coverage as opposed to quality considerations in choosing hospital destination in emergency situations may lead to poorer quality care for children.

Quality Improvement Activities

The challenge of delivering health care efficiently and effectively has accelerated the quality improvement activities of MCOs, purchasers, and federal, state, and local governments. Activities generally involve developing performance measures and clinical guidelines to produce improved outcomes; improving accreditation processes designed to evaluate the system of care delivery; and assessing consumer satisfaction. Many of the efforts are not routinely inclusive of pediatric emergency care. Quality improvement activities must be designed to encourage and monitor access to emergency care, pediatric subspecialty care, and injury prevention activities.

Primary Care Physicians as Front-Line Emergency Providers

A goal of EMSC and other child advocates is for every child to have an accessible primary care provider—a "medical home"—and, in fact, this is the foundation of most managed care plans. However, some MCOs are now performing triage of patients to doctors' offices for problems that used to be seen mainly in emergency departments. Many primary care providers are not adequately prepared to manage the increased acuity of the child who has been diverted from the EMS system. For example, it is estimated that only 10% of family health care providers maintain a minimum complement of pediatric emergency equipment and supplies in their offices.[10]

Increased Emergencies Among Children with Special Health Care Needs

Shorter hospital stays for seriously ill or injured children mean that these children are at risk for complications that once would have been dealt with prior to hospital release. Newborns are also sent home early, and they too may have emergencies previously controlled in the hospital setting. Increased numbers of children are living at home with special equipment, such as ventilators; these children are subject to severe emergency situations. In fact, children have died because of the lack of knowledge on the part of prehospital health care providers of how to deal with a child's specialized equipment in an emergency;

these providers are rarely trained in how to handle complex emergencies in children with special needs.

Access to Specialists

Managed care protocols may not be specific as to when a child needs a specialist, and a physician may find it difficult to refer a child, even when he or she considers it to be medically necessary and an emergency situation. Disincentives for specialty care are typically part of a managed care contract with a provider. Authorization for specialty care from the plan may not be forthcoming or may be approved only after prolonged dispute. Such delays can have devastating results in an emergency. Children can lose timely access to needed services from specialists and receive inferior care.

Access to Mental Health Services

Serious emergencies create tremendous stress for both parents and children. In a study in Tennessee, Glisson[13] found serious resource limitations within the hospital that prevented needed mental health services: individuals responsible for dealing with mental health problems are overworked and often unable to deal with family problems and emotional issues related to pediatric emergencies. Similarly, emergency department personnel have become increasingly busy as a result of personnel cuts implemented by hospitals to effect cost-saving, leaving health care providers little time to deal with families and the emotional concerns of pediatric patients. Even for children or adolescents treated for self-destructive behavior, it is estimated that only 24% of hospitals provide or arrange mental health services.[10]

Thus, the revolution in health care financing is affecting all aspects of EMSC. In addition to health care changes, however, other important policies and trends may well affect children's emergency care.

Welfare Reform

Under welfare reform, more children will need day care. However, adequate, quality, and affordable day care does not currently exist in the amount that is required. Some children in day care are already in unsafe situations, and day care providers are typically not well trained in how to prevent or handle an emergency. For example, only 25 states require licensed child care providers to be trained in CPR.[10] If strict safety standards in day care settings are not adopted and adhered to, children will be at increased risk for injury and for poor outcome from emergency situations, such as allergic reaction or asthma attack.

Another possible impact of welfare reform on children's emergencies is the effect on parents of leaving or taking time off from work to care for a sick child: the parent may risk losing his or her job and thus the family's only source of income. Without job protection, low-income parents with few economic options face a terrible choice, that of either securing health care for a sick child or maintaining the means to feed that child. With new managed care restrictions being placed on the use of emergency departments for after-hours non-emergency care, it may be that children will have diminished access to health care, leading to more emergencies.

Expansions in Child Health Insurance

The 1997 law granting more children access to health insurance *may* help improve child health and reduce emergencies through prevention and early treatment, but many access barriers will remain unless states are extremely diligent in addressing them. For example, in Pennsylvania one third of uninsured children were eligible for Medicaid prior to the new law but were still not enrolled. Barriers to enrollment include lack of information about eligibility, fear of stigma, and complicated enrollment procedures.[14]

It is expected that many, perhaps most, states will provide coverage for uninsured children under this law through managed care plans, as is happening with Medicaid. Both Medicaid beneficiaries and poor persons without health care coverage have traditionally been heavy users of emergency departments, for primary, urgent, and emergency care. Factors that impel these patients to use emergency department care include work schedules, transportation, and safety.[15] Even with the new law, if emergency department care becomes more limited because of MCO restrictions, but the other barriers to care are not addressed, children may still not have access to care, and the incidence of preventable child health emergencies may remain the same or even increase.

A VISION FOR THE FUTURE

Imagine this: A young child has her first asthma attack. The father panics as the child struggles to breathe. He calls 911 for emergency assistance. The emergency medical dispatcher guides the father in calming his child and positioning her to ease her breathing. A pediatric-trained emergency medical technician and paramedic arrive within minutes and, following a rapid assessment, recognize the immediate need to move this child to the emergency department. The emergency team gives the child oxygen and transports her, with her father, to a well-equipped emergency department. The staff, informed of the patient's condition, is ready for her arrival. Nurses and physicians who are trained to treat children with the most up-to-date procedures provide prompt, appropriate care that relieves the attack. Soon, the child is able to return home with no serious consequences. The emergency department forwards a report to the child's pediatrician, who will work with the family and teach them preventive measures to minimize future occurrences.

This is the vision for EMSC. To achieve that vision, many groups have been working together over the past few years to identify and correct the most glaring deficiencies in services and quality of care, at both the local and national levels. Successes include development of pediatric equipment guidelines for ambulances and emergency departments; development and adoption of pediatric treatment protocols; designation of certain hospitals as pediatric specialty facilities; increased training in pediatric emergency care by EMTs, nurses, and doctors; and enhanced attention to injury prevention, resulting in documented decreases in injury rates. However, no community has successfully addressed all the problems.

If children are to receive emergency health care that is of the highest quality, the sustained efforts of many groups are needed—community groups and professionals, health care organizations and parents. Each has a role to play in ensuring that the EMSC vision for the future can become a reality nationwide.

References

1. Gonsalves, D. Historical background of emergency medical services in the U.S. *Emergency Care Quarterly.* 1989;4(3):73–82.
2. National Academy of Science, Division of Medical Science. *Accidental death and disability: The neglected disease of modern society.* Washington, DC: National Academy of Science/National Research Council, 1996.
3. Durch, J.S., and Lohr, K.N. (eds). *Emergency medical services for children.* Washington, DC: National Academy Press, 1993.
4. Mullner, R., and Goldberg, J. The Illinois trauma system: Changes in patient survival patterns following vehicular injuries. *Journal of the American College of Emergency Physicians.* 1977;6:393–396.
5. Seidel, J.S., Hornbein, M., Yoshiyama, K., Kuznets, D., Finklestein, J.Z., and St. Geme, J.W. Emergency medical services and the pediatric patient: Are the needs being met? *Pediatrics.* 1984;73(6):769–777.

6. Ramenofsky, M.L., Luterman, A., Quindlen, E., Riddick, L., and Curreri, W. Maximum survival in pediatric trauma: The ideal system. *Journal of Trauma.* 1984;24(9): 818–823.
7. Henderson, D.P. The Los Angeles pediatric emergency care system. *Journal of Emergency Nursing.* 1988;14(2):96–100.
8. National Highway Traffic Safety Administration. *Emergency medical services: Agenda for the future.* DOT Pub. HS 808 441. Washington, DC: National Highway Traffic Safety Administration, 1996.
9. Weiss, H.B., Mathers, L.J., Forjuoh, S.N., and Kinnane, J.M., *Child and adolescent emergency department visit databook.* Pittsburgh, PA: Center for Violence and Injury Prevention, Allegheny University of the Health Sciences; 1998.
10. U.S. Department of Health and Human Services, Health Resources and Services Administration, Maternal and Child Health Bureau. *5-Year plan, midcourse review: Emergency medical services for children, 1995–2000.* Washington, DC: EMSC National Resource Center, 1998.
11. Su, E. *Final report: Pediatric prehospital critical care skills retention.* Unpublished report. U.S. Department of Health and Human Services, Health Resources and Services Administration, Maternal and Child Health Bureau, Grant no. MCJ-410649, 1997.
12. Gill, J.M., Reese, C.L., and Diamond, J.J. Disagreement among health care professionals about the urgent care needs of emergency department patients. *Annuals of Emergency Medicine* 1996;28(5): 474–479.
13. U.S. Department of Health and Human Services, Health Resources and Services Administration, Maternal and Child Health Bureau. *Emergency medical services for children: Abstracts of active projects FY 1997.* Torrance, CA: National Emergency Medical Services for Children Resource Alliance, 1997.
14. Jewish Health Care Foundation of Pittsburgh. *Annual report.* Pittsburgh, PA: Jewish Health Care Foundation, 1997.
15. Rask, K.J., Williams, M.V., Parker, R.M., and McNagny, S.E. Obstacles predicting lack of a regular provider and delays in seeking care for patients at an urban public hospital. *JAMA.* 1994;271:1930–1933.

36

Immigration
and Health

Mary Lou Valdez

IMMIGRATION IN THE UNITED STATES

The United States always has been a country of immigrants. Estimated at 9% of the current total population, Hispanics are the second largest minority group, after African Americans.[1] As the fastest growing minority group, they are made up of Mexican Americans, Puerto Ricans, Cuban Americans, Central and South American immigrants, and other Spanish-surnamed/Spanish-speaking persons. About 11 million Asian American and Pacific Islanders constitute the third largest U.S. minority group.[1] Immigrants have created a mosaic of cultures, languages, and mores that have become integral parts of U.S. society. As the world grows smaller through globalization, the ease with which immigrants may travel to the United States becomes more commonplace, and the opportunities increase for immigrants to visit and stay, either through legal or illegal means. What has remained constant for many immigrants over the years is the desire for opportunity and a hope for a better life, if not for them, then for their children. It is these very beliefs that have helped to build our nation.

More than 1 million immigrants enter the United States each year, with almost 30% of these arriving through illegal means.[2] The majority of legal immigrants enter the United States as immediate relatives of U.S. citizens. Almost 916,000 immigrants were granted legal permanent status during fiscal year 1996; 65% of these were family-sponsored immigrants.[3] Twenty-five percent fall within the age range of 25 to 34 years, and 41,780 (4.6%) were older than 60 years of age. Women represented 53.8% of the total.[3] In fiscal year 1996, approximately 8.2% of the total legal immigrant population was considered to hold professional specialties or technical occupations, although the majority of immigrants (60.3%) either had no occupation or did not report one.[3]

The current wave of immigrants is not expected to decrease. Some federal sources estimate that by the year 2010, 20% of school-age children in the United States will be recent immigrants.[2] The majority of immigrants live in California, Florida, Illinois, New Jersey, New York, and Texas.[2] Two of these states, California and Texas, as part of the U.S.-Mexico border, serve as gateways for many Latin American immigrants. A common characteristic of immigrant families residing in these two states is that, although parents or heads of households may be residing in the United States illegally, their children are U.S. citizens and thus entitled to the rights and benefits of all U.S. citizens.

An influx of immigrants adds to the complexity of sociocultural and economic challenges facing the United States today. In many ways, immigrants are viewed as adding positively to the American social fabric: sturdy familial networks, commitments to education for children, strong work ethics, healthy birth outcomes, and lower drug use rates when compared with various U.S. population groups. Conversely, immigrants complicate existing U.S. problems, including an increase in demands upon shrinking federal and state budgets, restricted public services, and increased poverty rates, which already disproportionately affect U.S. minority populations. While immigrants, with their larger family numbers, tend to add to the current child/adolescent population, the United States is grappling with the complexities of an aging population as the numbers of persons 65 years and older increase. The North American Free Trade Agreement (NAFTA) has added another aspect to this issue; many Americans consider NAFTA a disappointment and a drain on jobs and opportunities for U.S. communities. Other recent phenomena in the United States exacerbate the immigration dilemma, including the human immunodeficiency virus (HIV)/acquired immunodeficiency syndrome (AIDS) crisis and the continuing illegal drug problem.

In the midst of such burgeoning stresses, all immigrants (legal and illegal) have increased the need for public education, public health services, and diverse linguistic capacity at federal, state, and local levels. At the same time, the belief that immigrants, or "foreigners," have created a drain on U.S. communities has become more prevalent. It is common for U.S. citizens and policymakers to believe that immigrants take away from U.S. society much more than they contribute, and many consider the stresses that immigration places on communities too burdensome for any state or local community to tackle effectively.

The decisions made in dealing with immigrant populations will have long-term effects on U.S. populations, sociocultural trends, and economic health. The challenge for the 21st century is for the United States to protect and improve the well-being of its citizenry without destroying the diverse cultural fabric its society represents. The challenge is a tremendous one.

IMPACT OF WELFARE AND IMMIGRATION REFORM

The recently enacted U.S. Public Law 104-193, Personal Responsibility and Work Opportunity Reconciliation Act of 1996 (PRWORA), places stringent restrictions on legal immigrants. Most non-citizens are no longer eligible for Supplemental Security Income (SSI) and food stamp benefits. New immigrants arriving after August 22, 1996, are barred from federal means-tested benefits for 5 years; and after the 5-

year bar, those new immigrants with sponsors must include their sponsors' income when applying for federal means-tested benefits. Some programs are exempt from the 5-year bar, including emergency medical assistance, national school lunch benefits, child nutrition act benefits (including the Supplemental Food Program for Women, Infants and Children [WIC]), the Head Start program, public health assistance for immunizations, and testing and treatment of communicable diseases. At a state level, states will have the option to determine current immigrants' eligibility for Medicaid, Temporary Assistance for Needy Families (TANF), and Social Services Block Grants (SSBG). States also have the option to bar state-funded programs for current and new immigrants. Undocumented immigrants are, in large part, ineligible for federal, state, and local public benefits.[4] From a state level, an earlier predecessor to P.L. 104-193 is California's Proposition 187, which required publicly funded health care facilities to deny care to illegal immigrants and to report them to government officials.[5,6]

The consequences of these recent measures is not yet fully known. What is known, however, is that fear among immigrants— legal and illegal—will likely increase, and the gap between the haves and the have-nots will expand. To many immigrants, the United States represents hope and a future. Many immigrants come from war-torn countries or countries which offer little more than basic subsistence. When many immigrants arrive in the United States, they come not for public benefits, but for an opportunity to work and to create a new life for themselves and their families. P.L. 104-193 can easily create several scenarios, including increases in communicable disease, illiteracy, violence, and poverty and the development of an expanding subgroup of uneducated youth. Equally important, the creation of destructive attitudes and punitive policies that emphasize not only citizenship differences but differences in color, culture, and language may emerge. Current immigrants can expect U.S. racial and cultural divisions to widen. Despite the various scenarios that may result, the influx of immigrants will not likely diminish.

PUBLIC HEALTH ISSUES

The recent welfare reform legislation impacts no area more strongly than public health. By limiting access to health care and social services, these reform measures will increase the vulnerability of immigrants and their families, while increasing the susceptibility of the health status of the U.S. at-large population. Regardless of citizenship status, immigrants need their basic health needs covered, including basic food and shelter and immunization, testing, and treatment for diseases. If immigrants are afraid to seek care, medical conditions and diseases will exacerbate until the infected person has no choice but to seek emergency medical treatment. Such actions can potentially infect a larger segment of a population and increase the very medical costs such communities are trying to avoid. Prevention services are more cost effective than the billions of dollars spent in medical treatment costs. Although federally funded community and migrant health centers have historically been havens and sources of health care for the undocumented immigrant, the recent reform measures may destroy even the trust among this long-standing client population.

Existing U.S. stresses, such as homeless populations, HIV/AIDS-infected groups, and increasing numbers of runaway children, provide fertile environments for the spread of infectious diseases. If the recent welfare reform legislation results in larger numbers of persons living in poverty, infectious disease risks will likely increase. Negative lifestyle factors can only intensify the situation for populations that are disadvantaged economically and educationally. Disparities in death, diseases, and disability rates for these special populations will increase, especially among racial and ethnic populations, lower-income groups, and persons with disabilities. Immigrants, legal and illegal, fall within these special populations, and unless public health policies can target such groups, their situation can only worsen.

The public health issues for immigrants must be addressed jointly at local, state, and federal levels. Public health disease prevention through vaccinations not only benefits the direct recipients of the immunizations but also helps protect the at-large communities in which such persons may reside or pass through. Immunizations are cost-effective, positively influence health outcomes, and help avoid disease outbreaks and costly treatments. It is only in recent times that the region of the Americas has been free from the wild polio virus. The challenges of other preventable diseases such as measles, influenza, and hepatitis remain.

Another cost-effective prevention strategy against disease is good nutrition. Balanced and adequate diets and safe drinking water positively influence a person's mental and physical capacity and help empower persons to overcome personal burdens. If the United States wants to progress toward improving the life quality for Americans, then basic living standards should be within the grasp of all persons within our borders, regardless of citizenship. Similarly, a public health area of critical importance is sanitation. Inadequate basic sanitation and unhealthy living environments are major factors in the incidence of certain diseases, and in a general sense, thwart the opportunity for a basic standard for life quality.[7] The current welfare reform legislation, for affected citizens and non-citizens alike, could have a negative impact on their tenuous living conditions, create more communal living situations, and erect barriers to block even the most basic sanitary practices to be followed, including hand washing and other hygiene practices. Such conditions tend to strip away what little dignity people may be able to maintain and pull them further into the downward spiral of poverty.

Increases in the incidence of communicable and vector-borne diseases are a primary public health concern. Again, the public health risks expand past the infected person and have the capacity to affect much larger populations and communities. Among immigrant populations, such diseases as tuberculosis, sexually transmitted diseases, and HIV/AIDS may go undetected, especially if a person fears exposure, denial of care, and possible deportation. By the time a person would finally seek treatment, many unsuspecting persons may have been exposed to infection, and treatment costs have increased many-fold. For minority populations, including immigrant populations, effective outreach strategies can help increase awareness and detect potential cases early. If outreach workers identify possible at-risk persons, only to have to ascertain citizenship status and perhaps to deny services, then any public health strategy may be rendered ineffective.

It is also important to note that with increased globalization, emerging and reemerging diseases continue to multiply and are expanding risks for immigrants and non-immigrants alike. Communicable diseases like dengue, cholera, *Hantavirus*, and tuberculosis are again becoming threats throughout the world and in the Americas. Without public health strategies that universally impact the populations within our borders, the disease risk to the U.S. public looms larger.

MATERNAL AND CHILD HEALTH ISSUES

To achieve the public health and safety of U.S. populations, the United States works to improve the health of all Americans through a comprehensive approach that focuses on an increase in the span of healthy life, a reduction of health disparities, and access to preventive services. Among the subgroups that are particularly at risk for health problems are the uninsured, persons living in poverty, minority populations, and alien groups. The risk factors are even more acute with women and children, and the long-term effects of health problems can be especially devastating because many conditions are preventable.

There are various public health areas that will be directly affected by current welfare reform legislation. Maternal and child health issues, however, may have far-reaching implications over generations and may result in even higher health care costs to the U.S. taxpayer. For women and children, policymakers must evaluate the cost effectiveness of good prevention practices versus the soaring costs of emergency health care, regardless of legal status.[8]

For pregnant women, lack of prenatal care, infectious diseases, sexually transmitted diseases, and poor nutrition are among the many risks that can contribute to adverse birth outcomes. Regardless of a pregnant mother's citizenship status, complications from delivery may result in publicly funded, long-term medical costs for the newborn U.S. citizen. As policymakers tackle the effects of welfare reform, the cost effectiveness of good prevention practices versus the spiraling costs of health care, for the mother and/or the child, needs to be carefully evaluated.

Community and migrant health centers, the WIC program, and special federally funded programs under the Maternal and Child Health Services Block Grant have historically provided undocumented mothers and their children with a strong public health safety net to provide preventive services and primary health care.[8] For many of these prevention-type programs, citizenship was never an issue, and recipients could take advantage of such programs without fear of detection and deportation. With welfare reform, however, such programs, which have positively impacted the undocumented population, are in jeopardy. By denying care to indigent illegal alien females, especially pregnant women, U.S. communities may be inheriting even larger complications, such as congenital malformations, learning disabilities, and other poor birth outcomes for newborn U.S. citizens.

Additional factors emerge for foreign-born women and children that impact communities. In addition to the historical caretaker role, women, including foreign-born women, have become heads of households, with extended family networks dependent on them for income and livelihood. Public health issues such as mental health and psychological stresses, domestic violence, and sexually transmitted diseases are part of the dynamics confronted by documented and undocumented women. Again, with a fear of deportation or detection, undocumented women may avoid seeking care until their problems reach emergency proportions. The long-term effects on such women and their children could also be considerable in terms of life quality and health care costs.

Children in the United States, legal and illegal alike, face a myriad of difficulties in our current socioeconomic environments. Immunizations, illiteracy, child abuse, poor nutrition, substance abuse, and sexually transmitted diseases are just some of the public health challenges children face, not to mention educational or socialization obstacles. It would seem judicious to attempt to provide all U.S. children, regardless of citizenship, with hope for a new day and to enable them to create a viable productive future. Federal and state policy should advance, not inhibit, the opportunity to look ahead and plan for a better tomorrow.

As the 21st century approaches, U.S. federal, state, and local governments must work together to develop public policies and public health strategies that are cost-effective, sustainable, and supportive of the at-large citizenry. All persons within our borders—legal and illegal alike, permanent and transitory—can either be viewed as a risk or a benefit. Policymakers must work toward reducing the risks and expanding the gains that can result from those who come in search of the American dream.

References

1. U.S. Department of Health and Human Services. *Healthy People 2000 report*. DHHS Publication No. (PHS) 91-50212. September, 1990. Washington, DC: U.S. Government Printing Office, 1990.
2. Lamberg, L. Nationwide study of health and coping among immigrant children and families. *JAMA*. 1996;276:1455.
3. U.S. Immigration and Naturalization Service. *Statistical yearbook of the immigration and naturalization service, 1996*. Washington, DC: U.S. Government Printing Office, 1997.
4. W&A: Welfare reform and immigrants (P.L. 104-193, signed 8/22/96). Available at: http://www.ncsl.org/statefed/q&a.htm. Accessed September 2, 1997.
5. Ayres, B.D., Jr. Californians pass measure on aliens; courts bar it. *New York Times*. November 10, 1994, p B7.
6. Ziv, T.A., and Lo, B. Sounding board. Denial of care to illegal immigrants. Proposition 187 in California. *New England Journal of Medicine*. 1995;332.
7. Pan American Health Organization. *Health people, healthy spaces: Annual Report of the Director, 1996*. Official Document No. 283. Washington, DC, 1997.
8. Flowers-Bowie, L. *Funding prenatal care for unauthorized immigrants. Challenges for the states*. Washington, DC: National Conference of State Legislatures, 1997.

37

Ensuring Substance Abuse Services for Families

ELLEN HUTCHINS

Substance abuse is a significant problem affecting many families in the United States. During the 1990s, there was an increase in the need for both prevention and treatment services, especially for women and adolescents. As new programs are being developed for these populations, there is a need to ensure that services provided are gender-specific and address issues relevant to the population. Both managed care and welfare reform have given states new options as to how they will address substance abuse. This chapter examines the problem of substance abuse as it affects the maternal and child health population, provides some historical context for current trends, and discusses what the impact of managed care and welfare reform may be.

The problem of substance abuse within families, whether it involves a pregnant woman, an adolescent, or a male whose substance abuse affects other family members, should concern all maternal and child health professionals. Often it is unclear whose responsibility it is to address substance abuse and what role health providers and policymakers have to play. Frequently, health providers do not ask their patients about substance use and miss an opportunity to provide basic information and/or referrals to their patients who may be at risk for or using harmful substances.

Substance abuse is commonly viewed as an important social problem with health consequences for the individual; however, it also should be seen as a policy issue. Economic implications come into play when government resources are used to pay for drug prevention and treatment or building more prisons. Clearly, maternal and child health professionals should have a role in ensuring that substance abuse prevention and treatment services are available in their communities and that clients are not deterred from using these services because of punitive sanctions. This is even more important now as some managed care plans will not pay for substance abuse assessments and/or treatment and as states decide how to address substance abuse treatment under their welfare reform programs.

ADOLESCENT SUBSTANCE USE

Among adolescents, alcohol is frequently the drug of choice. However, many adolescent alcohol abusers are also polydrug users.[1] Amphetamine use is prevalent among adolescents to promote weight loss, a common goal for teenage girls. Inhalants, which are found in adhesives, lighter fluid, spray paint, cleaning fluids, and cooking spray, may have been tried by as many as 22% of teenagers.[2,3] Some adolescents develop destructive behavior because of substance abuse. The risk of pregnancy and sexually transmitted diseases increases when using substances. Studies have shown that the previous use of substances, including cigarettes, greatly increases the risk of early sexual involvement by adolescents. The higher the stage of drug use, the greater the likelihood of early sexual activity.[4]

PREVALENCE OF SUBSTANCE USE AMONG WOMEN, INCLUDING PREGNANT WOMEN

The problem of substance use during pregnancy significantly increased during the mid to late 1980s with the popularity of the inexpensive, smokeable form of cocaine called "crack" among women of childbearing age. Prior to this time, substance abuse was seen as affecting primarily men. Both the highly addictive properties of cocaine and its popularity among women of childbearing age have contributed to large numbers of pregnant women giving birth to drug-exposed infants. Current nationally cited estimates report that 5.5% of all pregnant women use an illicit drug during pregnancy.[5] The development of drug-exposed infants may be compromised by either the biologic effects of prenatal exposure to cocaine or by social factors related to having a substance-using mother.[6]

RESEARCH FINDINGS

African American women have the highest rates of use for cocaine and other illicit substances, with the exception that white women younger than 25 have higher rates for marijuana use. Total rates of alcohol use are highest among whites. Substance users frequently use several drugs rather than only one substance such as cocaine. Although media attention has focused primarily on cocaine use among women, alcohol use during pregnancy also deserves the attention of health professionals, because fetal alcohol syndrome is completely preventable. In addition, the abuse of prescription drugs such as stimulants, sedatives, and analgesics has been frequently reported, although data are not reliable.

There is a need for more research to better understand the contribution of various factors to a pregnant woman's substance use during pregnancy. In one study examining psychosocial risk factors in the backgrounds of pregnant cocaine users, it was found that substance-using women were more likely to have a family history of alcohol or other drug problems, to have been introduced to drugs by a male partner, to be depressed, to have a less social support, to have a current male partner who uses drugs or alcohol, and to have a less stable living situation.[7]

Additionally, there is a need for further evaluations to examine the most effective prevention and treatment strategies. Drug prevention strategies are usually school-based, thereby targeting only those adolescents who attend school. The most commonly cited prevention strategies include the Drug Abuse Resistence Education (DARE) program, conducted by police officers who talk to students about the dangers of drug use, and prevention approaches that teach adolescents about dealing with peer pressure and decision-making. Experimentation with alcohol, tobacco, and/or marijuana at early ages may lead to more serious illicit drug use. It is widely believed that pre-adolescents as well as adolescents need to be targeted in school-based prevention programs.

By the end of 1994, 95% of all cases of pediatric acquired immunodeficiency syndrome (AIDS) in New York State were being attributed to perinatal human immunodeficiency virus (HIV) from an infected mother.[8] The major contributing factors were the mother's intravenous drug use with contaminated needles or unprotected sex with an intravenous drug user.

TREATMENT SERVICES

Frequently the debate has focused on whether addicted persons are worthy of services, because many view addiction as a moral weakness rather than a disease and believe that the government should not be spending funds on people who deliberately choose to ingest illicit substances. The public health point of view is that addiction is a chronic, relapsing condition that may require multiple admissions to a drug treatment program but is worth the investment.

A 6-month follow-up of women who completed substance abuse treatment found that more were employed.[9] At the Families in Transition (FIT) program in Miami, Florida, all of the women were receiving welfare at the time of admission. Six to 12 months after discharge from treatment, 33% of the women moved off the welfare rolls, and an additional 19% reduced their welfare benefits through employment.[10]

Many women substance abusers are the primary caretaker for their children, and research suggests that pregnant and postpartum women may not enter treatment if child care is not available.[11] Szuster and colleagues[12] report better retention rates for women who participated in treatment with their children compared with those in treatment without their children.

STATES' RESPONSES TO THE PROBLEM

There have been more than 160 cases in 23 states (including the District of Columbia) of prosecution of pregnant drug-using women, primarily involving cocaine use. However, many of these convicted cases have now been overturned. Many states have interpreted child protective laws to apply to this situation and have removed newborns from maternal custody on the basis of neonatal urine toxicology results.[13] Over the past decade, the trend has been to either incarcerate the drug-using woman or remove the child from her care, rather than expand drug treatment capacity. Most states do not have sufficient drug treatment capacity for addicted women seeking help. Only recently has there been more of an emphasis on expanding women's treatment programs to include their children.

Although incarcerating an addicted woman during her pregnancy may seem like the simplest and cheapest solution to the problem, treatment for one woman costs less than half the annual cost of incarceration.[14] Incarcerated women rarely receive drug treatment and may leave prison without having gotten any assistance with their drug problem. There is a need to increase the number of comprehensive, gender-specific treatment programs for substance abusing pregnant women and mothers and their children. Services that need to be addressed include psychosocial support, health care, child care, and aftercare support. Efforts to prosecute pregnant women who use alcohol and other drugs need to be eliminated, and more efforts need to be made to refer them into treatment. The experience of leading experts throughout the United States is that removal of infants in these cases is usually unnecessary and can be harmful to the child.[15]

By the early 1990s, women constituted the fastest growing segment of the American population involved with the criminal justice system. More than 80% of the cases brought to prosecution involved women of color, specifically African American women. This may be due to the fact that these women rely on public hospitals and clinics more for their care, and more drug testing is done there.

Currently, seven states have reporting requirements for drug-exposed infants.[16] It is believed that punitive approaches by some states may have deterred some pregnant women from receiving prenatal care.

In a study by Chavkin,[17] it was found that the most common reasons for not seeking care were "having felt bad about using drugs" and having "felt guilty or embarrassed about being a drug-using woman." Chavkin found that women were in need of aftercare, services for children, education and training, addiction services, on-site health care, and housing and food.

Successful programs based on the family unification model should be expanded. One example is Operation PAR (Parental Awareness and Responsibility) in St. Petersburg, Florida. Through its long-term residential program, children from infancy to 10 years can live with their mother while she is receiving treatment.

SCREENING ISSUES

Staff training is important to address staff attitudes toward serving substance-using adolescents and women. Staff should include representation from the culture served, as well as provide bilingual services when needed. Consumer input is also desirable to ensure that services and approaches are reaching the population targeted.

Prenatal and family planning clinics need to screen all women for alcohol and illicit substances using simple self-report questionnaires. Staff need to be trained in how to administer these questionnaires in a non-judgmental way. The purpose of screening should be to identify women in need of counseling or referral, not to use this information to report them to authorities.

Innovative outreach services are important to identify those who may not access services on their own and should include homeless and battered women's shelters.[18] Alcohol and drug treatment are successful strategies that need to be addressed to end welfare dependency and increase employment-related outcomes. Outreach programs are especially important now with states developing Medicaid managed care contracts, which frequently do not cover outreach to those clients who do not seek medical services on their own.

WELFARE REFORM

A key goal of the new welfare program is to move recipients from welfare to work. Temporary Assistance for Needy Families (TANF) imposes strict work requirements and sets a 5-year lifetime limit on benefits. Studies have reported that between 15% and 20% of welfare recipients have alcohol and drug problems. Addiction is a significant barrier to self-sufficiency and the ability to maintain a job. If untreated, alcohol and drug problems may keep many welfare recipients from leaving welfare within their allotted time limits, so that states may then have to support them through state-only welfare programs or criminal justice and foster care. Treatment could result in cost savings at both federal and state levels. The new law provides states with opportunities for identifying substance-using women within the welfare system and coordinating treatment services.[19] Providing drug treatment is a necessary step toward job readiness.

One issue that states are confronted with is whether to test welfare recipients for drugs. Data indicate that it is costly and does not yield reliable information. A more reliable method would be to train caseworkers to administer self-report screening instruments. Treatment needs to be promoted as a first step toward being able to work. The welfare system generally consists of two groups of welfare recipients, those that use it intermittently and those who stay on for long periods. Those deemed "harder to serve" include those with alcohol and other drug problems. They will need assistance with social problems in order to succeed.

One provision of the new law is a lifetime ban on cash payments and food stamps to anyone with a drug felony conviction after August 22, 1996, unless the state enacts legislation "opting out" of the ban. A few states have already opted out of imposing this restriction.

If untreated, alcohol and drug problems keep many welfare recipients from working, and states could face penalties for not meeting the new law's work participation requirements, which rise from 25% to 50% between 1997 and 2002.

SUMMARY

Many of the policies enacted to deter substance abuse by imposing punitive sanctions have in fact deterred women from coming into the health system. More policies need to be developed that encourage women to seek preventive and treatment services. As states refine their strategies for preparing welfare recipients for self-sufficiency through work readiness, it will be essential that the problem of substance abuse be addressed. Similarly, it is important that managed care plans include assessment and treatment of addiction problems. Substance abuse affects an entire family, and if untreated, has extensive consequences. Maternal and child health professionals have a role in ensuring that policies and services encourage the identification and early treatment of this problem.

References

1. Martin, C.S., Arria, A.M., Mezzich, A.C., and Bukstein, O.G. Patterns of polydrug use in adolescent alcohol abusers. *American Journal of Drug and Alcohol Abuse.* 1993;19(4):511–521.
2. Dinwiddie, S.H. Abuse of inhalants: A review. *Addiction.* 1994;89(8):925–939.

3. National Institute on Drug Abuse. *Drug use among 8th, 10th, and 12th graders.* NIDA Notes 11(1). (NIH Publication No. 96-3478). Washington, DC: U.S. Government Printing Office, 1996.

4. Gilmore, M.R., Butler, S., Lohr, M.J., and Gilchrist, L. Substance use and other factors associated with risky sexual behavior among pregnant adolescents. *Family Planning Perspectives.* 1992;24:255–261.

5. U.S. Department of Health and Human Services. *Drug use among women delivering live births: 1992.* (NIH Publication No. 96-3819). National Institute on Drug Abuse, National Pregnancy and Health Survey, Rockville, MD: 1996.

6. Hutchins, E. Drug use during pregnancy. *Journal of Drug Issues.* 1997;27(3): 463–485.

7. Hutchins, E., and DiPietro, J. Psychosocial risk factors associated with cocaine use during pregnancy: A case-control study. *Obstetrics and Gynecology.* 1997;90(1): 142–147.

8. *Program advisory: Use of zidovudine to reduce perinatal HIV transmission in HRSA-funded programs.* U.S. Department of Health and Human Services, Rockville, MD: 1995.

9. Stevens, S., and Arbiter, N. A therapeutic community for substance-abusing pregnant women and women with children: Process and outcome. *Journal of Psychoactive Drugs.* 1995;27(1):49–56.

10. Young, N.K. *Alcohol and other drug treatment: Policy choices in welfare reform.* Washington, DC: National Association of State Alcohol and Drug Abuse Directors, 1996.

11. Smith, I.E., Dent, D.Z., Coles C.D., and Falek, A. A comparison study of treated and untreated pregnant and postpartum cocaine-abusing women. *Journal of Substance Abuse Treatment.* 1992;9(4):343–348.

12. Szuster, R.R., Rich, L.L., Chung, A., and Bisconer, S.W. Treatment retention in women's residential chemical dependency treatment: The effect of admission with children. *Substance Use and Misuse.* 1996;31:1001–1113.

13. Layton, C., Breitbart, V., Rawding, N., Chavkin, W., Fisher, W., and Wise, P. *Integrating the needs of women and children: Addressing perinatal drug exposure and perinatal HIV infection.* Washington, DC: National Association of County Health Officials, 1994.

14. Young, N.K., and Gardner, S.L. *Implementing welfare reform: Solutions to the substance abuse problem.* Washington, DC: Children and Family Futures and Drug Strategies, 1996.

15. National Council of Juvenile and Family Court Judges. *Protocol for making reasonable efforts to preserve families in drug-related dependency cases.* Reno, NV: National Council of Juvenile and Family Court Judges, 1992.

16. National Center on Child Abuse and Neglect. *Special reporting procedures: Drug-exposed infants.* Washington, DC: National Clearinghouse on Child Abuse and Neglect, 1996.

17. Chavkin, W., Paone, D., Friedman, P., and Wilets, I. Reframing the debate: Toward effective treatment for inner city drug-abusing mothers. *Bulletin of the New York Academy of Medicine.* 1993;70:50–68.

18. Jones, V., Hutchins, E., and Grason, H. Meeting the needs of addicted mothers and their children. *The Counselor.* November/December, 1990;13–16.

19. Legal Action Center. *Making welfare reform work: Tools for confronting alcohol and drug problems among welfare recipients.* New York: 1997.

38

Social Policy Reform and America's Cities: Risk and Opportunity for Maternal and Child Health

MAGDA G. PECK

Acknowledgments are due to William Sappenfield, Edward Ehlinger, Rob Fulton, Patrick Simpson, Paul Nannis, and Peter Morris, who provided guidance, insights, and thoughtful comments in the preparation of this chapter. Thanks also to Diana Fisaga for secretarial support and Maureen Duncan for assistance in literature review.

Major changes underway are modifying long-standing approaches to health and human services in place for more than a half century. Although current reforms affect every community, America's cities provide the principal stage upon which the current drama of changing social policy is playing out. Sharing the spotlight in this drama are managed care, welfare reform, and the newly enacted State Children's Health Insurance Program (Title XXI of the Social Security Act).

In less than a decade, managed care has become a permanent part of nearly every major urban community and a cornerstone to state Medicaid policy. City and county health departments, long-standing safety net providers to the most vulnerable, are shifting their service role from direct delivery to low-income families and children to population-based assurance and assessment. Welfare reform mandates able-bodied citizens to work first, eliminating entitlement to public sector support for those most in need. The State Children's Health Insurance Program gives states the opportunity to extend insurance coverage to large numbers of children who remain uninsured. Forthcoming social reforms not yet known also will need to balance further restraining costs and ensuring a safety net for those most vulnerable.

This chapter describes the social, economic, and demographic factors that converge in urban communities to form the vulnerable human stage on which recent changes in national health and social policy are being played out. It next identifies underlying issues that intensify the vulnerability of urban women, children, and families under current reforms—devolution of decision-making authority to states and localities for major social programs, public demand for greater public sector accountability, and public perception of the role of government to protect the vulnerable. It examines the impact of three current reforms—managed care, welfare reform, and child health insurance legislation—on health and human services for families and children in America's cities. Last, it outlines broad recommendations to ensure the health of women, children, and families in America's cities into the next century, in anticipation of continued social policy reform.

THE URBAN CONVERGENCE OF MATERNAL AND CHILD HEALTH RISKS

Urban communities (those found within the city limits) host populations with a disproportionate burden of adverse maternal and child health risks and outcomes. America's central cities are home to 25% of all children younger than 21 years and 15 million families, or 23.5% of all families in the U.S.[1] Recent demographic and economic trends in American cities amplify the already considerable risks associated with U.S. urban residence. The child poverty rate in the 50 largest cities increased from 18% to 27% between 1969 and 1989. The largest 25 cities have the highest numbers of female-headed households and the highest employment rates.[2] One half of all children in the United States who live in distressed neighborhoods (defined as communities with high concentrations of poverty, female-headed families, unemployment, and welfare dependency) reside in the 50 largest cities. Minority Americans are more likely to live in cities (60% of African Americans and 70% of Hispanics vs. 46% of whites).[3] According to 1990 Census data, 45% of all blacks and 40% of all Hispanics lived in the 100 largest cities, compared with 17% of whites. Thirty percent of blacks and 28% of Hispanics lived in the 25 largest cities, compared with 9% of whites. Residential segregation and concentrations of poverty are the hallmarks of urban minority poverty. In 1990, about 28% of the urban poor in the largest 100 cities in the nation lived in census tracts in which 40% or more of the population was poor, and 69% lived in census tracts in which 20% or more of the population was poor. This poverty concentration was found to be most intense for African Americans, of which 42% of those living in the 100 largest cities lived in census tracts in which 40% or more of the residents were poor. Urban minority populations are concentrated within poor communities that cannot support an economic base to nurture a neighborhood fabric of commerce and services.[3]

The greatest proportion of beneficiaries of the programs transformed by welfare reform are concentrated in its largest cities. Residents of the 23 central cities with more than 500,000 residents account for only 12% of the nation's population, yet 17% of the nation's poor live in these cities. The counties that contain the 10 largest cities in the United States accounted for 22% of the entire national Aid to Families with Dependent Children (AFDC) caseload in 1993, but only 14% of the population. The pattern of urban concentration is most pronounced in states with a single large city (e.g., New York and Chicago).[4]

There is no national system for compiling important indicators of wellness or morbidity at the city level.[5] However, compiled secondary data suggest that the largest cities have the highest rates of infant mortality, low birthweight, asthma, acquired immunodeficiency syndrome (AIDS), and firearm homicides.[2,5,6–9] According to the 1997 report City Kids Count: Data on the Well-being of Children in Large Cities,[10] all 10 leading measures of child well-being in the 50 largest U.S. cities were worse than measures for the nation as a whole.

FACTORS INTENSIFYING THE URBAN IMPACT OF SOCIAL REFORMS

The social, demographic, and economic conditions previously described are intensified by three factors underlying health and welfare reform in America's cities: public perception of government's role and capacity to meet the needs of vulnerable populations; demand for increased public sector accountability for measurable outcomes; and devolution of decision-making authority for social programs to the states. These issues will heighten the challenges facing urban communities into the next century.

Public Perceptions of Government's Role

Americans differ from citizens in other industrialized countries in their attitudes about the role of government in caring for the poor. A 1991 poll of Western nations showed that in the other countries studied, at least 50% of adults completely agreed with the statement: "It is the responsibility of the government to take care of very poor people who can't take care of themselves"; only 23% of American adults surveyed completely agreed.[11] This uniquely American view underscores the public's ambivalence about the role of their government in caring for those who may not be able to care for themselves. Blendon and colleagues[12] have described underlying beliefs that have shaped the public's policy preferences in social reform. One key belief identified is that both government and people share responsibility for self-sufficiency. According to recent polls, a majority (57%) of Americans said that the responsibility for making sure that non-working low-income people have a minimum standard of living should be shared between the government and the people themselves, friends, and volunteer agencies.

How well the sharing of responsibilities works depends in part on the size of governmental share and the capacity of others to make up the difference. This balance is most fragile in America's cities. Medicaid and the new Title XXI child health insurance require significant state cost sharing, principally to come from state appropriations. In an era of increased pressure to reduce the size of government and cap state and local taxes, public perception will influence in part the magnitude of state revenue allocated to health insurance for low-income women and children. Similarly, welfare reform policy in each state is being shaped in part by public opinion about those dependent on the public sector. Beliefs about whether welfare encourages teenage

childbearing, undermines families, or inhibits the work ethic and social values about key social issues such as mothers of small children
working outside the home, quality child care, and benefits to resident
immigrants will fuel the public debate. States' legislative responses
may leave significant gaps in coverage and funding, which localities
are left to fill. Urban county governments are the traditional provider
of last resort; their coffers may not be adequate to ensure a safety net
for urban families and children. The capacity of the religious, nonprofit, and philanthropic sectors already is being stretched by health
and welfare reform, and the goodness of friends, neighbors, and volunteers will be tested into the 21st century.

Accountability: Increased Public Demand for Measurable Results

Increasingly, the public is asking its government at all levels to account for the resources being given to it, to ensure that their dollars are
being well spent. Similarly, the United Way and other community-
based human service organizations are being asked by donors to
demonstrate clear results for the contributions made. This demand for
accountability—to know what public and private dollars are buying
and what effect these expenditures are having—is partially responsible for health and welfare reform. It suggests public doubt about government's capacity to efficiently provide effective services to the poor
and needy that will make a measurable difference.

The twin challenges in measuring maternal and child health outcomes in an era of reform are (1) ensuring capacity to measure community-wide results and (2) agreeing on appropriate outcomes to measure. Unless there is community-wide capacity to measure outcomes
of eligible and enrolled Medicaid beneficiaries, accountability to the
public for its public sector investments is incomplete. For example,
managed care organizations under contract with Medicaid have the capacity to measure prenatal care adequacy, percentage of women with
age-appropriate mammograms, and immunization in 2-year-olds for
those women and young children continuously enrolled in their plan.
From an urban public health perspective, these measures are necessary but insufficient to describe the health and well-being of the larger
population of Medicaid women, children, and families. The core function of state and local health departments to monitor the health of the
broader maternal and child health population is key to ensuring accountability.[13] Another key is community-wide acceptance of appropriate measures to determine "success." Although the sharply reduced
number of able-bodied adults on the welfare roles is hailed by the

highest level of elected leadership as "success" for welfare reform,[14] welfare reform's full story will remain untold in terms of its intended and unintended consequences without additional measures.

The New Federalism: Devolution of Authority to States

The term *new federalism* describes the changing relationship between national and state governments based on the theory that state and local governments can do a better job of providing services for their residents. Devolution entails passing policy responsibilities from the federal to state and local governments, thus enhancing the responsiveness and efficiency of government.[15] This wave of devolution is shifting the most difficult decisions about how to meet the health and social needs of vulnerable populations from the federal to state level. Most recently, welfare and child health insurance responsibilities have been devolved to the states, accompanied by legislated block grants (see section on Recent Health and Welfare Reforms).

Political forces will affect whether and how well each state addresses its urban health and social needs. Decades of increasing suburbanization and urban flight, and subsequent redistricting of state legislatures after the 1990 Census, have fueled new regional politics, with greater Republican strength and a decline in urban power in many state houses. The cities' push for programs for the urban poor and their efforts to shift their disproportionate burden for general assistance to the states have become less successful amid divisive regional politics. In those states where state policymakers may respond inadequately to the urban agenda and where governors push tax cuts and reduced social spending to attract new business, cities and urban counties will be left to bear the many costs of social transformation. Given the convergence of urban beneficiaries and uninsured, urban counties and cities are unlikely to muster proportional political will to safeguard their populations.[4]

Under welfare reform, the fulcrum of decision-making about eligibility, services, and administration of the capped federal block grant shifts to the states. Meeting local social needs rests in the hands of state policymakers, who have the authority to decide which individuals and groups in the state's welfare caseload will be exempted from time limits, whether the state will fund its own programs for those excluded by federal law, and whether the state will exercise its option of exempting unmarried teen mothers younger than 18 from having to live at home to receive welfare support when it is not deemed in their interest. States also are the center of decision-making for the new State Children's Health Insurance Program. Under Title XXI of the Social

Security Act, each state will decide whether to expand its existing Medicaid program to further extend coverage to uninsured children or to design its own insurance product for children. Choosing the Medicaid route requires continued compliance with all federal Medicaid conditions about eligibility and benefits, requires beneficiary protections and consumer safeguards for enrollees of managed care plans, and prohibits the exclusion of qualified alien children who are not citizens. States that create their own plan will have greater flexibility and decision-making about the eligibility and scope of services. Stakes of this decision are highest for urban areas in part because of the disproportionate share of targeted children and immigrants in cities.

Alternatively, some states may opt to pass, that is devolve directly to the cities the full burden of welfare reform. If states passed a consolidated block of funds on to cities for welfare, not all localities would be adequately prepared or willing to absorb the full burden of program design, implementation, and monitoring for results, albeit with less resources than necessary. As Annie E. Casey Foundation President Douglas Nelson noted, "It may be fair to predict that the willingness of states to rise to the challenge of making troubled city neighborhoods a priority for innovation and investment will largely determine whether devolution itself succeeds or fails."[10]

RECENT HEALTH AND WELFARE REFORMS: AN URBAN PERSPECTIVE

Managed Care and Medicaid in Cities

Under managed care, the functions of health insurance and health care delivery are carried out through an entity that covers individuals for a defined set of benefits, furnishes covered services to members through a network of providers under contract or employed by the entity, uses prospective utilization controls to manage members' use of services, and monitors the quality of services rendered to members.[16] During the 1990s, state Medicaid agencies have embraced managed care as a mechanism to control costs and ensure access. Women, children, and youth are the populations most quickly moving into managed care, especially through public sector managed care arrangements.[17] Nowhere is this more apparent than in America's central cities, which are prime targets for the growth of Medicaid managed care, given their high concentrations of low-income women and children.[18] In a 1994 national survey of major urban health departments, 61% of city and county health departments serving one or more central cities with at least

100,000 population reported that Medicaid managed care was in place or would be implemented within 1 year.[19] In a 1997 follow-up survey, that proportion increased to 84%, with most urban localities reporting state mandated programs in their cities for Medicaid-enrolled women and children.[20]

Principal concerns about Medicaid managed care for urban women, children, and adolescents include ensuring access to care in a changed provider landscape, ensuring appropriate utilization of primary and preventive services, maintaining quality care given the pressure to control cost, securing the participation of quality providers, helping consumers achieve satisfaction, and managing enrollment and disenrollment as clients move across systems and in and out of eligibility.[21] Urban health departments in jurisdictions where Medicaid managed care was being implemented reported problems in each of these dimensions in the early stages of implementation.[19] The complexities of transition to Medicaid managed care for local health departments and other essential community providers—including public hospitals, publicly funded family planning providers, community and migrant health centers, and minority health physicians—pose even greater challenges to the urban safety net. They often have less revenue to work with and less access to investment capital and feel the brunt of uncompensated care of uninsured patients with short enrollment periods. Essential community providers face a clash between their uncompensated care duties and the principles of managed care.[18]

Several key factors further complicate Medicaid managed care in the inner city: (1) sicker inner city populations, requiring more costly care; (2) lower Medicaid managed care premiums than those paid by commercial insurers, hence lower enrollment or more stringent utilization standards to compensate for an insufficient provider base; (3) special population needs limiting optimal adaptation to a new complex system, including literacy and language barriers; and (4) unstable eligibility and short enrollment periods, limiting the return on managed care plan investments in prevention and primary care.[18] America's inner cities will continue to be the bellwether of consequences and opportunities under Medicaid managed care.

State Children's Health Insurance Program— Title XXI and Cities

The Balanced Budget Act of 1997 (P.L. 105-33) codified a new State Children's Health Insurance Program (CHIP) as Title XXI of the Social Security Act.[22] CHIP is designed to improve children's access to both public and private health insurance through active case finding of eligible children and the provision of financial assistance to states to provide subsidized child health assistance. The key decision each state will have to make by the year 2000 is whether to expand Medicaid. If a state opts for Medicaid expansion, it must follow all Medicaid requirements regarding eligibility (as of June 1, 1996), benefits, and cost sharing. Children who apply and are found eligible are *entitled* to assistance. In addition, assistance is available to qualified alien children who are not citizens only if a state uses Title XXI funds to expand Medicaid, which is exempted from barring aliens.

States also may establish new child health insurance programs, subsidize enrollment into employer-sponsored family insurance plans, or sponsor community-based coverage plans. States that choose to create their own Title XXI insurance plans gain the flexibility to establish the conditions of eligibility, including residency, age, proportion of population covered, disability, and duration of coverage. They may limit coverage to a defined number of children, although they may not exclude children with pre-existing conditions or discriminate against children with certain diagnoses. Unlike the expanded Medicaid option, state-specific Title XXI plans are not considered an entitlement, unless a state establishes their plan as an entitlement under state law by guaranteeing coverage to all who apply and are found eligible. States that use Title XXI funds to establish new programs may not spend federal funds on aid to non-citizen children, as new programs are considered a federal public benefit under welfare reform.[22]

Each state's plan must be approved by the federal government before the state receives the allotted federal dollars. The plans must delineate how the state will do case finding and eligibility screening, which and how many children are proposed for assistance, the level and form of assistance to be provided, the conditions of coverage, and conditions governing insurers. The state's commitment to share costs is critical, and state capacity to secure and sustain required matching funds is of concern.

The CHIP legislation has tremendous implications for urban communities, where the largest numbers of uninsured and immigrant children reside. Safeguards for urban mothers and children may be better ensured in cities where the existing Medicaid program has been successful in reaching currently eligible low-income children and the managed care arrangements have not proven detrimental to ensuring access to preventive health care services. Title XXI requires adherence to existing federal regulations concerning Medicaid eligibility and benefits and prohibits exclusion of qualified alien children who are not citizens—an issue for urban communities with significant immigrant populations. Moreover, in those states where there is incomplete political will to establish a state entitlement to health care for children, and where political sentiment and fiscal reality are likely to shape a new Title XXI insurance program with limited eligibility and benefits, urban uninsured children are the least likely to benefit from insurance reform.

Regardless of options chosen by the state, required outreach and enrollment will need the engagement of the full array of urban safety net providers (disproportionate share hospitals, local health department clinics, federally funded health centers, and other local agencies) to effectively identify eligible children, particularly those hardest to reach. Agreements accompanied by adequate resources and accountability between the state and strategic community partners will be essential to narrow the gap between those urban children who are eligible and those who achieve sustained health insurance coverage.

Of equal importance is the capacity of the health care system to provide all children enrolled through Title XXI with comprehensive, quality primary and preventive health care and to provide those children with special health care needs with the full array of health care services they require. Although an insurance card is necessary to get in the provider door, it is insufficient to ensure utilization of needed care. The challenge for urban communities will be to ensure the seamless connection of outreach, eligibility, enrollment, utilization, and improved health outcomes for more children through comprehensive systems of care.

Welfare Reform's Uncharted Urban Course

Enactment of the Personal Responsibility and Work Opportunity Reconciliation Act of 1996 ended a national policy of entitlement to welfare crafted over a half century ago to cushion the nation's most vulnerable families and children from the adverse effects of poverty. Reform in the nation's welfare system signals a shift in the role of federal public assistance to the poor from a guaranteed safety net of benefits to one of transitional assistance to bridge the gap between welfare and work. It solidifies the continuing devolution of social policy development from the federal to the state level of government. In short, welfare reform changes the rules about whom the government will help, what help will be offered and for how long, and how the help will be administered.

The new federal welfare reform law replaces the long-standing Aid to Families with Dependent Children (AFDC) program with a single cash welfare block grant to states—Temporary Assistance for Needy Families (TANF). It requires adults in families receiving TANF to participate in work activities, imposes a 5-year lifetime limit on receipt of TANF assistance, limits food stamp eligibility for able adults, severs the link between TANF and Medicaid eligibility determination and application, and redefines the eligibility criteria for disabled children to receive Supplemental Security Income (SSI). Unmarried teen parents younger than age 18 must be in school if they have not yet graduated from high school and must live with a parent or responsible adult to receive aid. Initial welfare reform legislation imposed strict regulations on most immigrant beneficiaries, legal or not, precluding eligibility for many benefits; subsequent legislation softened some restrictions for legal immigrants.

Nowhere are changes in state and federal welfare policy being felt more acutely than in America's cities and urban counties, which are home to the greatest concentrations of beneficiaries, and whose infrastructures are absorbing the shock waves of change. Cities have the largest current caseloads of welfare recipients and the largest proportion of long-term recipients who may have more difficulty moving from welfare to work. Child care is an essential ingredient in reform, given the requirements of mothers with infants and young children to work. Quality, affordable child care is in short supply in many urban communities. Jobs to employ those going from welfare to work may not be adequate in number to meet demand. With economic expansion increasingly outside of the inner city, work opportunities for welfare recipients are likely to be located at a considerable distance from residence, adding longer commute times and challenging existing public transportation routes. Cities, the common point of entry for new immigrants, are home to the largest numbers of immigrant populations (both legal and undocumented) whose Medicaid, food stamps, and SSI eligibility changed significantly under welfare reform.

Two surveys by the U.S. Conference of Mayors (USCM) suggest that in the short run, the burden of welfare reform already is being acutely felt in urban communities. The USCM Task Force on Hunger and Homelessness surveyed 29 cities in 1997, of which more than 95% expected requests for emergency food assistance by families with children to increase in 1998. City officials reported that the strong economy has had little or no effect on either hunger or homelessness, and that those jobs obtained are low paying and lack necessary benefits.[23] The mayors' Task Force on Welfare-to-Work reported jobs shortfalls in the 34 major cities and early problems with transportation and child care. Officials estimated that an average of 27% of low-skill jobs in their cities provide health insurance. Four of five cities surveyed reported increased requests for emergency food as a result of welfare changes.[24]

FINDING OPPORTUNITY: RECOMMENDED STRATEGIES FOR SAFEGUARDING CITIES' HEALTH

The combination of managed care, welfare reform, and child health insurance challenges urban communities as never before to rethink the organization, financing, and delivery of health and human services for its most vulnerable populations. The potential ill consequences of these three factors will require state and federal governments to reach out in partnership to the cities to shape and support effective solutions. What must be done to safeguard the health and well-being of urban women, infants, children, and adolescents, given anticipated change in health and social policies into the 21st century?

Seize the opportunity of reform to foster community-wide systems change for healthier children and families. Experience with managed care has helped some cities mobilize better for welfare reform's sweeping changes and be poised to shape Title XXI. The Ramsey County Community Partnership for Welfare Reform developed early consensus on outcomes for families and children in the St. Paul, MN, area. It proposed that people who cannot work or who are working in jobs that do not support their families will be supported by the community, and people receiving cash assistance who can work will be working in jobs that support their families before time limits.[25] Milwaukee's effective working relationship between city and state governments, forged in part through managed care trials, positioned the city to play a major role in the development of BadgerCare, Wisconsin's proposed State Children's Health Insurance Program.[26] Coalitions and collaborative organizations formed in recent years to build healthier cities and communities may have stronger, more timely community-wide responses to welfare reform and Title XXI. The San Francisco Starting Points Initiative, one of more than a dozen Carnegie Corporation of New York funded initiatives to mobilize communities on behalf of young children, provided the city with key information and analysis for local decision-making on welfare reform.[27] Proactively, public health and human services agencies in states and some localities, notably Wake County (Raleigh), NC, are reorganizing for greater efficiency and accountability in anticipation of further reform.[28,29] Reform gives communities the chance to shape lasting, systems-level solutions, to build on their assets, and to achieve desired outcomes. Urban communities that actively embrace the meaning of reform (i.e., social or political improvement; to make better by removing faults or defects) are those best positioned to safeguard the health and well-being of women, children, and families.

Rekindle political will at the local, state and national level to safeguard and promote the health and well-being of all *children and families in America's cities.* As long as social reforms are perceived as being about those different from ourselves, there will be insufficient political will to ensure the health and well-being of those most likely to be affected. As former Housing and Urban Development Secretary Henry Cisneros has asserted, "What this country lacks is not the capacity to end the isolation of the minority poor; it lacks the will."[30] Poor families have long been judged by the majority as weak in their lack of self-sufficiency, undeserving in their dependency on government. The transformation of AFDC into a work-based program may foster new political will for the working poor. Broad sympathies for those now more like "us" may translate to political support for child care, transportation, and other strategies essential for the success of health and welfare reform. Child health insurance under Title XXI gives an opportunity for bridging our efforts between the poorest and the working middle class.

One proposed strategy for breaking the isolation of the urban poor is to link the fates of the cities and suburbs for maternal and child health. It has been argued that, given their interdependence, cities and suburbs do best when they interact and make use of respective and complementary strengths.[31] Suburbs that surround healthy cities tend to be healthier than those that surround sick cities. Only when those in the outer city acknowledge and understand that central city political boundaries do not seal off problems associated with air pollution or childhood poverty or epidemic interpersonal violence among youth can metropolitan alliances be forged to address interconnected concerns.

Another strategy is to have cities advocate for further devolution from the state to the local level of health and human services. Some health policymakers advocate for trading fund flexibility for outcomes accountability as the heart of a new deal between states and localities.[32] Urban governments and equivalent emerging local governance entities will need to prepare for and ensure their readiness to assume the responsibility for local social policy decision-making and accountability. Readiness includes the setting of clear, measurable outcomes and the capacity to develop and use results-based budgets, in the context of community-wide consensus of a vision for children and families.[33]

Strengthen the capacity of the urban public health sector to do its essential governmental roles effectively. Assessment, monitoring, and assurance—the core functions of public health—should prove to be of invaluable service during the continued changes into the next century. With greater capacity in outcomes accountability and in the effective use of data, more urban health departments can become valued and empowered lead agencies to facilitate community-wide consensus on measures and methods for assessing the local impact of managed care, welfare reform, child health insurance, and related social reforms. Indeed, several urban health departments, such as San Diego County, have forged partnerships with managed care organizations to use their capacities in assessment.[34] Critical to this strategy is strong collaboration with state and federal government to ensure compatible methods in monitoring the health and well-being of its women, children, and families in an era of reform. Recent consensus reached on the core functions of public health in maternal and child health, forged among leading public health institutions, gives an excellent framework for moving ahead.[13]

The history of late 20th century health and welfare reform has yet to be written. As was true a century ago, all that is right and wrong in new health and welfare policy will manifest on the stage of urban America. Public health must play an essential advocacy role for systems change that safeguards the health of women, children, and families along the way, for as Ehlinger has noted wisely, "The fate of our cities eventually will become the fate of us all."[35]

References

1. U.S. Bureau of the Census, 1990.
2. Andrulis, D. *Urban social health indicators.* Washington, DC: National Public Health and Hospitals Institute, 1995.
3. Fossett, J.W., and Perloff, J.D. *The "new" health reform and access to care: The problem of the inner city.* Report to the Kaiser Commission on the Future of Medicaid, Washington, DC, December, 1995.
4. Weir, M. Is anybody listening? The uncertain future of welfare reform in the cities. *The Brookings Review.* Winter, 1997;15(1):30–33.
5. Benbow, N., Wang, Y., and Whitman, S. *Big cities health inventory, 1997: The health of urban U.S.A.* Chicago: Chicago Department of Health, 1997.
6. Andrulis, D. The urban health penalty: New dimensions and directions in inner city health care. Washington, DC: The National Public Health and Hospitals Institute, 1996.
7. CityLights 6(3/4). *Special report on low birthweight in U.S. cities, 1993–1995.* Omaha, NE: CityMatCH at the University of Nebraska Medical Center, 1998.
8. Heagarty, M.C. Urban maternal and child health services. In H.M. Wallace, R.P. Nelson, and P.J. Sweeney (eds). *Maternal and child health practices.* 4th ed. Oakland, CA: Third Party Publishing Company, 1994.
9. U.S. Department of Health and Human Services, Health Resources and Services Administration, *Child health USA.* Rockville, MD: 1997.
10. The Annie E. Casey Foundation. *City kids count: Data on the well-being of children in large cities.* Baltimore, MD: Annie E. Casey Foundation, 1997.
11. Times Mirror Center for the People and the Press Poll. Storrs, CT: Roper Center for Public Opinion Research, May, 1991. (Cited in Blendon et al,[12] p 1066.)
12. Blendon, R.J., Altman, D.E., Benson, J., Brodie, M., James, M., and Chervinsky, G. The public and the welfare reform debate. *Archives of Pediatric and Adolescent Medicine.* 1995;149:1065–1069.
13. Grason, H.A., and Guyer, B. *Public MCH programs functions framework: Essential public health services to promote maternal and child health in America.* Baltimore, MD: Johns Hopkins University, 1995.
14. Broder, J.M. Big social changes revive the false God of numbers. *The New York Times.* August 17, 1997, Section 4(1).
15. Watson, K., and Gold, S.D. *The other side of devolution: Shifting relationships between state and local governments.* Washington, DC: The Urban Institute, Assessing the New Federalism, 1997.
16. Rosenbaum, S. Defining, measuring, and enforcing quality in managed care. In R. Stein (ed). *Health care for children: What's right, what's wrong, what's next.* New York: United Hospital Fund, 1997, p. 181.

17. Partnerships for Healthier Families. *Principles for assuring the health of women, infants, children and youth under managed care arrangements.* Washington, DC: Association of Maternal and Child Health Programs, 1996, p iii.
18. Darnell, J., Rosenbaum, S., Scarpulla-Nolan, L., Zuvekas, A., and Budetti, P. Access to care among low-income, inner-city, minority populations: The impact of managed care on the urban minority poor and essential community providers. Report to the Commonwealth Fund by the Center for Health Policy Research, The George Washington University, Washington, DC, December, 1995.
19. Peck, M.G., and Hubbert, E.H. *Changing the rules: Medicaid managed care and MCH in U.S. cities.* Omaha, NE: CityMatCH, at the University of Nebraska Medical Center, 1994.
20. Simpson, P., Garrett-Brown, N., and Peck, M.G. *A second look at Medicaid managed care, MCH, and urban health departments: Changing the rules II.* Omaha, NE: CityMatCH at the University of Nebraska Medical Center, 1998.
21. Fox, H.B., and McManus, M.A. *Medicaid managed care arrangements and their impact on children and adolescents: A briefing report.* Washington, DC: The Child and Adolescent Health Policy Center, 1992.
22. Rosenbaum, S., Johnson, K., Sonosky, C., Markus, A., and DeGraw, C. *Issue brief— An overview of the State Children's Health Insurance Program.* Washington, DC: The George Washington University Medical Center, Center for Health Policy Research, September, 1997.
23. U.S. Conference of Mayors. *1997 Annual status report on hunger and homelessness in America's cities.* Washington, DC: U.S. Conference of Mayor, 1997.
24. U.S. Conference of Mayors. *Implementing welfare reform in America's cities.* Washington, DC: U.S. Conference of Mayors, 1997.
25. Fulton, R. From windows to worries: The Ramsey County experience. Presented at the 1997 Urban MCH Leadership Conference. Atlanta, GA, September, 1997.
26. Nannis, P., Commissioner of Health, Milwaukee Health Department. *Personal communication.* November, 1997.
27. Mihaly, L.K. *Impact of federal welfare reform on children in San Francisco.* San Francisco: Starting Points Initiative, Mayor's Office of Children, Youth and Their Families, May, 1997.
28. Maralit, M., Orloff, T.M., and Desonia, R. *Transforming state health agencies to meet current and future challenges.* Washington, DC: National Governors' Association, 1997.
29. CityLights 6(3/4). *Reorganization, re-engineering, restructuring, right-sizing: Public health leadership in the reorganization of government.* Omaha, NE: CityMatCH at the University of Nebraska Medical Center, January, 1998.
30. Cisneros, H.G. Regionalism: The new geography of opportunity. *National Civic Review.* 1996;85(2):35–48.
31. Savitch, H.V., Collins, D., Sanders, D., and Markham, J.P. Ties that bind: Central cities, suburbs, and the new metropolitan region. *Economic Development Quarterly.* November, 1993;7(4):341–347.
32. Center for the Study of Social Policy. *Trading outcome accountability for fund flexibility.* Washington, DC: 1995.
33. Friedman, M. *A strategy map for results-based budgeting: Moving from theory to practice.* Washington, DC: The Finance Project, 1996.
34. Center for Studying Health System Change. *Issue brief: Tracking changes in the public health system.* Number 2. Washington, DC: September, 1996.
35. Ehlinger, E. Our cities, our future. In CityLights 1(2). Omaha, NE: CityMatCH at the University of Nebraska Medical Center, 1991.

39

Maternal and Child Health at a Critical Crossroads

Karen VanLandeghem and Catherine A. Hess

Major changes in the health and social service system are occurring at a rapid and unprecedented pace and are likely to have a tremendous impact on the overall health and well-being of women, children, and their families. Perhaps the most visible changes have been those caused by recent federal legislation, including the Personal Responsibility and Work Opportunity Reconciliation Act of 1996 (PRWORA) and the Balanced Budget Act of 1997. PRWORA replaces the 60-year welfare system, including the Aid to Families with Dependent Children (AFDC).* The Balanced Budget Act of 1997 not only includes provisions that allow states to expand health insurance coverage for children, but also makes some of the most significant changes to Medicaid since its inception.[†] The vast changes brought by these new laws are further compounded in states and communities by shifts toward managed care delivery systems, state agency restructuring, and an emphasis on greater autonomy in implementing federal laws and reforms. Changes in the health and social service systems have been made most visible at the federal level; however, many of the reforms and changes have already been occurring in states and communities across the country.

In many cases, states and communities have served as the laboratories and proving grounds for change and reform in efforts to cut health care costs, increase access to and availability of health care, and streamline service delivery systems. Perhaps most profound and crosscutting of all the changes are those taking place with shift toward managed care.

Most certainly, mothers and children have unique and often complex health care needs that will need to be considered within the broader context of health and social service system reforms. Women, children, and youth represent the largest population entering into managed care arrangements, primarily because the fastest area of growth in the industry is Medicaid managed care. How systems are

---

*AFDC (Aid to Families with Dependent Children), the former cash assistance welfare program, was a federal entitlement. Those eligible for AFDC were automatically eligible for Medicaid. Under welfare reform, AFDC is replaced by TANF (Temporary Assistance for Needy Families), and the historic link between welfare and Medicaid eligibility is ended. TANF replaces AFDC, JOBS, and Emergency Assistance with a block grant to the states. TANF-funded assistance is not an individual entitlement under federal law. States are required to apply strict work requirements, and there is a 5-year lifetime limit on receipt of benefits funded with federal TANF dollars. (PRWORA, Title I, creates new Part A to Title IV of the Social Security Act [SSA].)

[†]The Balanced Budget Act of 1997 (P.L. 105-33), 111 Stat. 251 (1997), Title IV, Subtitle J. State Children's Health Insurance Program, Sections 4901–4923, includes provisions for establishing separate state children's health insurance programs, expanding Medicaid coverage, implementing presumptive Medicaid eligibility for children, continuing Medicaid eligibility for children losing Supplemental Security Income (SSI) benefits, and creating special diabetes programs for children.

structured and services are delivered to the Medicaid population of women and children may well lay the groundwork for how services are delivered to the general population, with significant implications for how managed care organizations (MCOs) serve all women and children enrolled in managed care.

Clearly, these changes bring new challenges and opportunities for improving the health of all women, children, and youth, including children with special health care needs due to chronic or disabling conditions. Reforms in the health care and social service delivery system are converging at the state and local levels, requiring policymakers and other key stakeholders to make rapid assessments and decisions. State and local health and social service agencies, managed care organizations, community-based organizations, legislators, advocates, consumers, and others all have critical roles in the design and implementation of service delivery systems for women, children, and their families. Specifically, state Title V Maternal and Child Health (MCH) Services Block Grant programs* are at the core of public health agency efforts for women, children, and youth and will play a critical partnership role with these and others in ensuring the health of all women, children, and youth.

Looking Forward, Looking Back: An Historical Context for the Changing Role of Title V Maternal and Child Health Services Block Grant Programs

In 1989, a landmark Institute of Medicine (IOM) study declared public health to be "in disarray."[1] Recent dramatic changes in health and social welfare policies and services have added to the challenges of nearly a decade of efforts to reinvigorate and reinvent public health. For long viewed by much of the public and many policymakers as health care of last resort for the poor, public health agencies, including MCH programs and professionals, have struggled to redefine their images and roles in the mold laid out by IOM. The IOM formulated three core functions for public health—assessment, policy development,

---

*Authorized under Title V of the Social Security Act, the Maternal and Child Health (MCH) Services Block Grant focuses broadly on the health of women, infants, children, and youth. In 1981, Title V's categorical programs were consolidated under block grant legislation, and states were given increased discretion in the use of funds. Amendments in 1989 included important changes that improved accountability while maintaining flexibility.

and assurance. This last function of ensuring the availability of services needed to improve health could be accomplished through a variety of means other than directly providing services.

In 1989, the most significant changes occurred in Title V of the Social Security Act since it was amended to create the Maternal and Child Health Services Block Grant in 1981. Some of the changes, such as linking the purpose of the program to achievement of national health objectives and requiring comprehensive needs assessments, were consistent with the future directions outlined by the IOM. Others, particularly addition of language explicitly stating the program's purpose as one of providing and not just ensuring care, seemed to push the program's thrust more in line with the common perception of public health programs' role as providers of care for the poor.

This tension in roles continued throughout the 1990s. National and state momentum in the first half of the decade toward comprehensive health care reform, including universal coverage, propelled federal, state, and local public health agencies to realign their roles and build their capacities to carry out core public health functions. Anticipating a diminished need, if any, to be providers of last resort, public health agencies focused on how to better articulate and enlist public and political support for core functions. In the aftermath of the failure, in large measure, of these publicly driven, comprehensive reforms, public health had achieved minimal success in gaining such support.

As the focus for reform shifted to the private sector and cost containment–driven managed care arrangements, public health agencies increasingly were confronted by the possibility of losing Medicaid-insured clients, largely women and children. To many, there appeared to be a choice: to focus on strengthening capacities to carry out core public health functions, or to pursue aggressively and competitively a continued role in providing health care services to Medicaid-insured clients.

Yet as the changing health care marketplace took the place of comprehensive public reforms in stimulating redefinition of public health roles, it did not solve one of the fundamental problems in the system—the growing numbers of uninsured. The percentage of uninsured Americans has been steadily increasing since at least 1987. Between 1995 and 1996, the percentage of non-elderly Americans (younger than age 65) without health insurance coverage rose from 17.4% to 17.7%. Further examination indicates that children completely accounted for this increase. In 1995, 13.8% of children and 19% of persons aged 18 to 64 were uninsured, compared with 14.8% of children and 18.9% of persons ages 18 to 64 in 1996.[2] Welfare reform, by denying most benefits to many legal as well as illegal aliens and by severing the link between cash and medical aid, may push those numbers even higher. Counteracting the growing numbers of uninsured are the new child health insurance expansions resulting from the 1997 Balanced Budget Act.

Thus, public health remains on the horns of a dilemma. If it is to ensure that all populations have access to health care, which is one of the factors that contributes to maintaining and improving health status, it must address the remaining needs of uninsured, underinsured, and underserved groups. However, if public health is to address effectively the primary contributors to preventable morbidity and mortality, it must focus on improving capacities and ensuring adequate support for the less publicly visible functions such as research, surveillance, and investigation and control measures on a populations basis or on an individual level, such often non-reimbursable services such as outreach, health education and counseling, or home visiting.

At the present time, public health agencies, and more specifically MCH programs, continue to struggle in a rapidly changing environment with the most appropriate and effective mix of roles and functions to achieve their missions of protecting and promoting health and well-being. This chapter highlights but a few examples of states that have risen to the challenge to reinvent public health services and roles to promote the health and well-being of women, children, and youth, including those with special health care needs. Because managed care is now so pervasive in states, the following examples emphasize the shifting role of public health in working with managed care. Nearly all states are undergoing some type of reform, and, therefore, not all states can be highlighted. The examples here reflect *current* practices by some State Title V Maternal and Child Health Services Block Grant programs; however, it is important to note that many of the systems outlined here remain in flux and continue to evolve, particularly given the recent enactment of the Balanced Budget Act of 1997.

SHIFTING THE MEDICAID POPULATION INTO MANAGED CARE AND THE ROLE OF PUBLIC HEALTH: THE CASE OF VERMONT[3]

In Vermont, public health policy has been strong in supporting a one-tier health care delivery system where nearly all of the providers participate in the Medicaid program and the local health departments provide few services in direct primary care. When the state initiated its Medicaid Early and Periodic, Screening, Diagnosis and Treatment (EPSDT) program nearly 20 years ago, a policy was set that would later have long-standing impact on the respective roles between the state

Medicaid agency and public health. At the time, a Memorandum of Understanding (MOU), which is still in effect today, was signed between the Departments of Health and Social Welfare. The MOU outlined the State Department of Public Health's role, among other responsibilities, of providing outreach activities to the state's Medicaid population.

In 1993, Vermont applied for an S.1115 Medicaid waiver to expand Medicaid coverage to serve pregnant women up to 200% of the federal poverty level and children up to age 18 at 225% of the federal poverty level. This represents at least a third of those groups in Vermont participating now in the Medicaid program. Indeed, the state's Medicaid population has long been a group targeted by the State Health Department through various activities, including its surveillance and services such as the Special Supplemental Food Program for Women, Infants and Children (WIC), immunization, lead screening, and the Vermont Healthy Babies Program.

In the early days of developing the S.1115 Medicaid waiver, the state Medicaid agency was planning to contract virtually all of its Medicaid funding to managed care, with the intent of minimizing carve-outs to other agencies, thereby leaving most decisionmaking to the contracting managed care organizations. The implications of such a plan could have had potentially negative impacts on public health. If managed care organizations did not sub-contract with local public health agencies, it could diminish the existing public health infrastructure. Furthermore, the expertise that public health had in serving the Medicaid population might not be available within the managed care organization.

The state Title V MCH Services Block Grant program had a key role in helping to shape and develop the state Medicaid managed care contract. The end result was a contract that built on what MCOs and public health do best. The Department of Health, particularly the state Title V program, retained its role in core areas including systems oversight, standard setting, case management, and conducting outreach, and the MCOs were able to offer a core set of health services to the Medicaid population. Today, the state has two managed care organizations serving the state's Medicaid population.

Working in partnership, public health and MCOs in Vermont provide critical services and programs to the state's Medicaid population including the EPSDT program. Under the EPSDT program, the Vermont Department of Health provides a variety of activities, including informing families in writing about EPSDT services, setting periodicity screening schedules and standards, providing outreach services, providing consultation on written materials developed by the MCOs, helping families overcome barriers to accessing services and problems, providing administrative case management, and facilitating the participation of the MCOs in local health and human services planning efforts. Vermont's participating MCOs establish a medical home for each EPSDT-eligible child and adolescent, provide medical coordination of care, provide clinical preventive services and screening services, provide other health care as outlined in the benefits package, collect and provide data on utilization, and refer families to and participate in the Vermont Department of Health's Healthy Babies Program.

FLORIDA'S CHILDREN'S MEDICAL SERVICES PROGRAM AND ITS EVOLVING ROLE IN SERVING CHILDREN WITH SPECIAL HEALTH CARE NEEDS[4]

Florida is a state that has had a long-standing commitment to children's issues, particularly in the area of health. Even before Governor Lawton Chiles took office in 1992, there had been discussions at the state level about expanding Medicaid to cover more uninsured children. Indeed, the Florida Healthy Kids program, a county-based program providing school-based health insurance coverage for uninsured children in several counties with plans for expanding statewide, is regarded by many policymakers to be a model program. Congress recognized the merits of the Florida Healthy Kids program when it passed the Children's Health Insurance Program as part of the Balanced Budget Act of 1997, making Florida only one of three states to have their existing children's health insurance program grandfathered in as part of the federal legislation.*

Managed care has been operating in Florida since the early 1980s, but it was not until the early 1990s that Florida, like many other states, turned to managed care arrangements as a way of controlling rising health care costs. Florida's Children's Medical Services (CMS) program, the state's Title V children with special health care needs program, like other key state agencies and programs in Florida, used the influx of managed care to examine their role within the current system and help define how that role might change with the advent of managed care.

---

*The State Children's Health Insurance Program (CHIP) as part of the Balanced Budget Act of 1997 enables states to expand health insurance coverage to children up to 200% of the poverty level (or for states that exceed that threshold, 50 percentage points above their current income ceiling). Florida, Pennsylvania, and New York are the only three states with existing children's health insurance programs that were grandfathered in as part of the 1997 legislation.

In 1993, the Florida CMS program, in consultation with families, the state Pediatric Society, and a network of child experts in clinics and universities across the state, collaborated with the state Medicaid Policy Unit to develop a Medicaid MCO to be managed by CMS for children with special health care needs (CSHCN). This initial effort was later abandoned when it became clear that insufficient data existed to determine appropriate capitation or payment rates. However, this early work would later form the basis for the development of the Alternative Service Network (ASN), a system designed to be complementary to other Medicaid managed care plans in the state.

ASN is a new managed system of care for children with special health care needs who are eligible for Medicaid. As defined in Florida state law, it is an alternative service network which includes health care providers and health care facilities that serve CSHCN. It is designed so that CMS, Florida's State Title V program, will assign a qualified primary care provider to serve as the gatekeeper responsible for providing or authorizing all necessary health services. Services provided through the ASN will be reimbursed on a fee-for-service basis—the ASN is not a risk-bearing entity. The ASN may contract with school districts already participating in the certified school match program for the provision of therapies. The ASN (as managed by CMS and called the CMS Network) competes with managed care organizations to serve the CSHCN population, based on many standards. Rules will be promulgated that specify the referral, enrollment, and disenrollment requirements for Medicaid-eligible CSHCN who are served by the ASN and managed care plans.

With the advent of the federal Children's Health Insurance Program (CHIP), which enables states to expand coverage to uninsured children including CSHCN, the role of the CMS program and ASN is evolving. Current proposals under the state's plan for CHIP, would use the CMS Network to serve CSHCN.

DELAWARE'S DIAMOND STATE HEALTH PLAN[4]

Delaware's statewide Medicaid managed care program, the Diamond State Health Plan, covers all children and adults eligible through the former Aid to Families with Dependent Children (AFDC); pregnant women up to 185% of the poverty level, and all other adults up to 100% of the poverty level. Children who qualify for Medicaid under the Supplemental Security Income (SSI) program* or Delaware's Med-

---

*SSI is a federal program that provides supplemental income to low-income children with disabilities and their families to assist them in purchasing essential items and services they need to care for their child.

icaid Alternatives to Children's Institutionalization (MACI) are also included in the program.

As with Vermont and Florida, the shift toward managed care caused Delaware's Division of Public Health, and more specifically, the state Title V MCH Services Block Grant program, to examine its role in the evolving health care delivery system. After undergoing a structured assessment and planning process, the Division of Public Health decided to offer MCO's a package of services. The package of services emphasized public health's expertise in working with the needs of the Medicaid population. The three public health packages offered to managed care organizations were (1) Early Intervention and Engagement, which included such services as outreach to high-risk populations, health screenings, patient education, and well-baby checks; (2) Enhanced Care for Vulnerable Populations, a package of services for high-risk individuals, including pregnant women, to supplement their primary care services; and (3) Primary Care Partnerships, services designed to monitor chronic health problems in partnership with health plan primary care providers for patients are unable to travel to primary care providers' offices but are able to access public health units. Although DPH offered a capitation or bundled rate payment method, state MCOs were not yet ready to accept this approach, in part because of their lack of experience with public health as a provider. Nevertheless, Title V staff say that this process was crucial in ensuring that public health programs and services were included in the eventual Medicaid managed care contracts.

As is the case in many other states, the role of public health in Delaware continues to evolve. MCH state and local staff as well as the Division of Public Health's managed care coordinator continue to participate in regular meetings with the state Medicaid agency and MCOs. And, MCOs are taking part in statewide public health initiatives such as the Governor's Task Force on Teen Pregnancy.

References

1. Institute of Health. Summary and recommendations. In *The future of public health.* Washington, DC: National Academy Press, 1988, p. 8.
2. Fronstin, P. *Sources of health insurance and characteristics of the uninsured: Analysis of the March 1997 Current Population Survey.* Employee Benefit Research Institute. December, 1997.
3. Presentation to the National Governor's Association meeting by Patricia Berry, MPH, Director of the Division of Community Public Health, Vermont Department of Health, November, 1997.
4. Brown, T.W. *Partnerships for healthier families: Roles for state Title V programs in assuring quality services for women, infants, children and youth in managed care.* Association of Maternal and Child Health Programs, June 1997.

VI

Summing Up

40

Steps for the Future

Vince Hutchins

In the preceding chapters, expert authors have discussed the state of the health and welfare of families at the end of the millennium with a look into the 21st century from each of their viewpoints. This chapter is both a summing up and a focus on looking forward.

30-YEAR CYCLES AND SOCIAL SECURITY

Wilbur Cohen predicted that major social legislation would be enacted in the mid-1990s. Cohen was a teacher and bureaucrat who served under four Presidential administrations and as Secretary of the former U.S. Department of Health, Education and Welfare (HEW) during Lyndon Johnson's administration. After finishing his graduate studies, he became the principal architect of Social Security during the first Roosevelt administration. His foresight in designing the original proposals for the Social Security Act (SSA) in 1935 was later complemented in 1965, through his efforts, with the inclusion of Medicare and Medicaid in the Social Security Act.[1]

Cohen, in 1986, reminded us that social reform in the United States comes in great cycles, a sort of manic-depressive legislative development. "We tend to go a little bit to extremes on this; we go a little bit too fast when we're driving toward that and we go too deeply when we are cutting back." He pointed out that the beginning of the great social reform efforts in this country took place around 1905. The adoption of the Food and Drug Act of 1906, the first White House Conference on Children in 1909, the beginning of Workmen's Compensation, the adoption of Mother's Aid Legislation (which later became Aid to Dependent Children), culminating in the establishment of the Children's Bureau in 1912. It was a tremendous burst of social reform at the height of the Progressive Movement.[1]

Another burst of social legislation occurred in 1935, 30 years later, with the passage of the Social Security Act. Then 30 years later after that—in the midst of the Great Society social legislation—there was the passage of Medicare (Title XVIII of SSA) for the elderly and Medicaid (Title XIX of SSA) for the poor.

Cohen said, "If you analyze the American temperament, . . . attitude and . . . character, social problems may be driven underground for five or ten years, but when they are finally unleashed in a great period of concern about social problems, then people want to do something right away. We have [witnessed this] in 1905, . . . in 1935—thirty years later—and . . . in 1965." He predicted: "It is going to come about in around 1992; I believe that by 1995, thirty years from 1965, we will have in this country a program in which every single person in the United States, will be insured for comprehensive health benefits."[1]

By the spring of 1997, many were losing faith in Cohen's prediction. Social programs for children had deteriorated. Many child advocates thought that elements of welfare reform, enacted within the 30-year cycle in 1996, were harming poor and near-poor children. Social problems were indeed being "driven underground." Then the following August, the State Children's Health Insurance Program (CHIP) was enacted as part of the Balanced Budget Act of 1997[2] (Table 40.1). Codified as Title XXI of the Social Security Act, it did not cover "every single person in the United States" as Cohen predicted, but it was the largest single expansion of children's health insurance since the Medicaid legislation of 1965.

Incorporating the new legislation, CHIP, as Title XXI of the Social Security Act is of major historical interest. Maternal and child health (MCH) advocates have always considered it important that the federal Maternal and Child Health program was enacted as Title V of the Social Security Act. Having Maternal and Child Health as part of the Social Security Act, rather than one of the health laws that tend to be disease focused, is critical to the program. It eliminates the need to reestablish every 3 to 5 years the usual authorization for health legislation; it affirms that children's health requires continuing attention. It draws attention to the need to organize a health program that is responsive to children's total needs, permitting adaptation and modification as needed. It enables the nation to build on the basic structure made possible through the Social Security Act. Placing Medicaid (Title XIX) in the Social Security Act in 1965 with Maternal and Child

---

TABLE 40.1

30-Year Cycle of Social Reform

1905	Food and Drug Act (1906)
	Workmen's Compensation
	Mother's Aid
	Children's Bureau (1912)
1935	Social Security Act
1965	Medicare (Title XVIII of SSA)
	Medicaid (Title XIX of SSA)
1996	Welfare Reform
	State Children's Health Insurance Program (Title XXI of SSA) (1997)

Health (Title V) enhanced the interdependence of these two programs for more than 30 years.

Title V makes possible the organization of an effort in every state* to ensure that children's health needs receive continuing attention based on the need defined by the state. It enables funds to pass from the federal level of government to each state in order to stimulate special attention to children's health. From time to time, as specific health issues or problems affecting children arise, it is possible to incorporate a new and appropriate response. Title V, therefore, is best understood as a mechanism for the development of a capability. It is a commitment. It is a resource. These are critical points in this country's philosophy of children's health. They cross political and administrative approaches for implementing this basic commitment.[3]

In a similar fashion, locating the new State Children's Health Insurance Program (Title XXI) in the Social Security Act has the potential for promoting the same philosophy and processes.

An interesting concept on the protection of children is imbedded within the Social Security Act. A precursor of the Children's Bureau, the 1909 White House Conference had a resolution stating: "Home life is the highest and finest product of civilization. It is the great molding force of mind and of character. Children should not be deprived of it except for urgent and compelling reasons." This concept was further advanced with President Franklin Roosevelt's messages to Congress on June 8, 1934, and January 4, 1935, in both of which he said: "Among our objectives, I place the security of the men, women and children of the Nation first." This placed the welfare of children on a basis of equal importance with the welfare of adults.

The Committee on Economic Security was a temporary agency that Roosevelt created by Executive Order in 1934 to make recommendations for legislation to provide "safeguards against misfortunes which cannot be wholly eliminated in this man-made world of ours." The Committee was even more specific in defining the relationship of children to a general program of economic security for the individual and the family. In its report to the President, the Committee emphasized the fact that "the core of any social plan must be the child" and declared that "Every proposition we make must adhere to this core." The report then proceeded to enumerate the various parts of the plan,

---

*"Every state" includes the 50 states and the nine other political jurisdictions: American Somoa; Commonwealth of the Northern Mariana Islands; District of Columbia; Federated States of Micronesia; Guam; Marshall Islands; Palau; Puerto Rico; and the Virgin Islands.

which became the Social Security Act, and to point out their direct and indirect bearing on the welfare of the child as follows:

Old age pensions are in a real sense measures in behalf of children. They shift the retroactive burdens to shoulders which can bear them with less human cost, and young parents thus released can put at the disposal of the new member of society those family resources he must be permitted to enjoy if he is to become a strong person, unburdensome to the State. Health measures that protect his family from sickness and remove the menacing apprehension of debts, always present in the mind of the breadwinner, are child welfare measures.

Likewise unemployment compensation is a measure in behalf of children in that it protects the home. Most important of all, public job assurance which can hold the family together over long or repetitive periods of private unemployment is a measure for children in that it assures them a childhood rather than the premature strains of the would-be child breadwinner.[4,5]

These two recent legislative amendments to the Social Security Act—Welfare Reform and the State Children's Health Insurance Program—are the most important family policy initiatives in the past 30 years.

END OF THE 20TH CENTURY AND BEYOND

Following Wilbur Cohen's 30-year cycle predictions, the next enactment of major social legislation would be expected around 2025 A.D.—a quarter of the way into the next century. There are a number of issues, discussed earlier in the text, affecting the health and welfare of families that will require our continuing attention before we reach that date. The selection of the handful of issues singled out here for discussion is to emphasize their importance to the health and welfare of families. It is critical to focus on them now and in the near future and not wait for major social change in the distant future.

Women's Health[6]

Women's health issues, long overdue, have slowly moved to the forefront in the past three decades. National and international attention received a burst of activity with 1970's Year of the Woman, which has been further stimulated with subsequent international meetings. Within the U.S. government—although the first Secretary of HEW was Oveta Culp Hobby in the Eisenhower administration, followed later by Patricia Harris in the Carter administration and Margaret Heckler in the Reagan administration—it was not until the appointment of

Bernadette Healy as Director of the National Institutes of Health that major advances were made. Offices for Women's Health had been set up before Healy's arrival, but it was Healy's emphasis on women as principal investigators on research projects, diseases of interest to women as research topics, and women as research subjects that gave women's health a boost in both government and academia, the site of most research projects. This emphasis has continued under Donna Shalala's tenure as Secretary of the Department of Health and Human Services.

In these days of devolution, it is of interest that the new data book of the Jacobs Institute of Women's Health is focusing on individual state data rather than its original compilation of national data only. The text describes women's health in each of the fifty states, incorporating important information on demographics, health status, insurance coverage, risk factors for illness, and health policy issues of particular relevance. The intended audiences are health care providers, policymakers, program administrators, researchers, teachers, and women's health advocates.[6] It will be a rich resource for advocates who plan to keep the movement growing.

Expanded Maternal and Child Health

Related to the topic of women's health is the question of whether maternal and child health should be concerned with more than just the reproductive health of women. An increasing criticism of the MCH program is that it is not interested in the "whole woman" as it is interested in the "whole child." Historically, there has been a three-fold response: (1) women's health has suffered because of the absence of a federal or state government agency that has the responsibility for advocating, programming, and, especially, funding women's health; (2) with a limited amount of MCH funds and a constant need in the field, MCH programs can neither realistically nor ethically dilute the funding base; and (3) the singular and emotional appeal for mothers and children is critical for continued political and public support.

"Where is the male in MCH?" is an increasing refrain. Sometimes this refers to the lack of the father in planning and programming. Is the father included in discussions of bonding, child care, early intervention, and school health? Must the frequently discussed dyad always exclude the father? Sometimes the issue of the male presence refers to adolescent health, which continues to improve its outreach to teen males, although some racial and ethnic teen males may require more attention. Sometimes the question refers to family planning programs, which historically have been seen as having a female focus. However, the reality and perception of male involvement in these programs have changed positively over recent years.

Another frequent suggestion is that the MCH name should be expanded to include families. Families are an integral part of maternal and child health. Since the beginning of C. Everett Koop's tenure as Surgeon General and his work with the Maternal and Child Health Bureau, the involvement of families has been strengthened and institutionalized through their promotion as equal partners in planning, policy, and programs. This was accomplished by working with the public agencies (e.g., state Title V agencies, Early Intervention), the private sector (e.g., American Academy of Pediatrics, March of Dimes), and family associations, such as Family Voices. The objective was attained through policy emphasis rather than a name change.

Ethnic Diversity

Hispanics are the fastest growing minority group in the United States. In 1900, they constituted 9% of the population. As a result of continued immigration and high birth rates, it is estimated that Hispanics will become the largest minority group in the United States by the year 2000. Current projections expect Hispanics to reach 11.2% of the U.S. population by the year 2000 and 13.4% by the year 2010. The Hispanic population in the United States is made up of four major subgroups—Mexican, Puerto Rican, Cuban, and Central and South American. These groups share a common language, yet each has a very distinctive history and experience, differing widely on many demographic traits and cultural dimensions.[7] The challenge is to become conversant with this rapidly expanding population and to meet its health, education, and social needs.

Similar concerns exist for other new arrivals from Southeast Asia, Africa, the Mideast, Eastern Europe, the nations of the former U.S.S.R., and elsewhere.

Immigration

Recent public policy debates have focused largely on the negative effects of immigration on society and particularly on the use of public benefits by immigrant families. Athough the debate remains open concerning immigrants' contribution to society and their relative use of public benefits, the laws affecting immigrants changed substantially in 1996. Despite the restoration of Supplemental Security Income (SSI) and Medicaid benefits for legal immigrants in 1997, many immigrant families remain vulnerable to the effects of reform. The 1997 changes shift the most affected population essentially from the elderly and disabled to working families with children—the population likely to be on food stamps. Before welfare reform, a hard line was drawn between legal and illegal immigrants. The new law moves that line, drawing distinctions between legal immigrants and citizens, rather than between legal and illegal immigrants. The new law also devolves immigrant policy to state and local governments, providing them greater responsibility to determine eligibility for certain federal programs as well as for their own state and local programs.

Immigration proponents argue that these changes have had a chilling effect on immigrant families seeking care from social service agencies. The result, they argue, is that families have turned increasingly to nonprofit organizations to serve their needs. This, in turn, has placed a great strain on the ability of nonprofit agencies to provide effective services.[8] The challenge is to assist both public and private agencies to meet the needs of these families.

Incarcerated Youth

More than 2 million children and adolescents in this country are arrested each year, and more than 600,00 are incarcerated in juvenile or adult correctional facilities. Although these children enter the juvenile justice system with many health care problems, they are, by their detention, further separated from mainstream health care. During the 1990s, a number of efforts have created strong partnerships between providers of public health and the juvenile justice system, but problems remain:

1. Standards for health care services in correctional settings for these young people have been developed but not widely adopted.
2. Health services are often provided on a limited basis or by clinicians with minimal training in adolescent medicine.
3. Service providers are not sensitive to the ethnic and cultural concerns of the population.
4. Financing of health care in correctional settings is problematic for many jurisdictions.[9,10]

A study in the state of Washington revealed that health services differed by facility site. Youth at county facilities had more total visits to emergency rooms and more health care visits per inmate for health problems presenting acutely. More were on suicide watch and on psychiatric medication. Health care used by youth at state facilities tended to be for more chronic conditions.[11]

Meeting the health needs of this population of youngsters will continue to require coordination between the public health and the juvenile justice systems. It also requires advocacy at federal, state, and local levels from those with an interest in social justice and fairness.

Integrated Services and Interdisciplinary Education

During the past decade, there has been a growing national movement to serve the family through integrated service systems supported by programs of interprofessional education. Education, health care, and social work professionals are the leaders in this movement as they collaborate with each other and with families. Corrigan and Bishop described this decade of family-centered activities in a 1997 review: "Family-interprofessional collaboration is no longer an option; it is a necessity and an obligation of professional leadership."[12]

Until recently, the response to children with educational or social care needs has been to develop single-issue or categorical programs. The result was duplication of services for some families, whereas others were unserved or underserved. At the same time, professional responsibility was uncoordinated, overlapping, and often dysfunctional. As human services have moved toward integrated services in response to these problems and to simplify the service system for families, often the professionals are unprepared to collaborate across systems and with families. Professionals serving children need to design training programs to educate a new generation of leaders who are interprofessionally oriented and who can build bridges across professions and agencies. Such preparation must include both preservice and continuing professional education. It will require mobilizing the profession's resources and political power and developing methods to work and learn together to place the well-being of children and families at the top of the social and political agenda.

Children with Disabilities in Poverty

In 1995, the Maternal and Child Health Bureau developed a definition for children with special health care needs.* Because of the lack of

---

*Children with special health care needs are those who have or are at increased risk for a chronic physical, developmental, behavioral, or emotional condition and who also require health and related services of a type or amount beyond that required by children generally.

data for at-risk children, a study by the Child Health Insurance Project looked at only children with "existing" special health care needs in families with incomes below 200% of the federal poverty level. The resultant report[13] estimated that 16.9% of low-income uninsured children had a special health care need in 1994. By comparison, an estimated 6.3% of low-income uninsured children, a third of those with special needs, experienced a disability in 1994, as defined by a limitation in school or play activities due to a chronic condition. In numbers of children nationally, these two estimates translate to 1,210,000 and 460,000 children, respectively.

The 1996 Personal Responsibility and Work Opportunity Reconciliation Act brought a retrenchment in the children's SSI program from a 1990 Supreme Court ruling (Zebley v. Sullivan) that had expanded eligibility of low-income children with disabilities to receive the SSI cash benefit. Because of the new law's disability definitions, it was estimated that 315,000 low-income children would lose or be denied access to benefits between 1997 and 2002.[14] After the public outcry from parent groups and the subsequent implementation of new eligibility rules and an appeal process, the SSI agency predicts that now only about 110,000 children will lose SSI benefits during that time period.

Children with disabilities who are living in poverty will continue to demand our attention. These data indicate that an estimated one in six children in the CHIP-eligible population has an existing special health care need. The American Bar Association created the Children's SSI Pro Bono Project in 1998 to assist families in all states to receive the benefits to which they are entitled. It behooves other child advocates to look carefully at the individual state's benefit package and outreach efforts under Title XXI to ensure that children with special health needs and their families have adequate insurance coverage to meet their special needs.

Child Care

The total number of working women in the United States with preschool children reached 9.6 million by 1994, more than double the total reported in 1970 (4.2 million) and nearly quadruple the count from 1960 (2.7 million). Nearly half of these preschoolers are cared for by parents, grandparents, or other relatives. A significant trend in the last decade has been a decline in home care provided by non-relatives and an increase in the number cared for at child care facilities.[15]

In most families, the schedules of working parents and their children do not mesh. The gap between their schedules can amount to 20 to 25 hours per week. These "latchkey" children, several million in number, require different approaches to child care depending on their age and the availability of family and community resources.

Morgan has described three factors (child-staff ratios, wages, and price) as the "trilemma" of balancing the child care budget. All three must be addressed at the same time, for setting any two of them at a desirable level may have a negative effect on the third factor.[16] Hofferth has stated, "The informal child care market assures that most parents will be able to find someone to care for their children, but not that they will be able to find stable, affordable, high-quality child care."[17] Even if proposed legislation in child care is enacted, adequate age-appropriate slots, extended-care days, career ladders for child care workers, quality, and affordability will remain child care issues to be addressed.

Second-Tier Devolution

The two recent legislative amendments to the Social Security Act—Welfare Reform and the State Children's Health Insurance Program—are in part national experiments in devolution. There is a readiness on the part of many for this development, with considerable discussion of the advantages of moving the decisions and the programs closer to the people. As a consequence, we see both welfare reform and Title XXI, as well as immigration implementation, devolving from the states to cities and local communities—a second-tier devolution.

One of the accompanying federal themes to devolution has been the abandonment of national standards at the federal level, which are often interpreted as one of the "unfunded mandates." While the federal government has steered away from national standards and hastened toward guidelines, models, or less, national professional organizations and others are maintaining national standards to preserve quality and accountability. One of the concerns with second-tier devolution is that states will also move away from standards that could lead to confusion at the community level about the establishment and maintenance of quality of care. The result could be a cacophony of voices with varying agendas and no unifying voice for quality.

LOOKING FORWARD

Enumerating a list of issues to remedy in the next few years may appear daunting. In a time of limited resources or, perhaps, in a time lacking the political will to make the necessary resources available for the alleviation of social and economic problems, it can be disheartening.

John Gardner once said: "Life is full of golden opportunities disguised as irresolvable problems." We need to find as many golden opportunities in this list as we can, leaving only the remainder, with the emerging issues of the next decades, for the next burst of social legislation—near 2025 A.D.

References

1. Cohen, W.J. Jubilees of Social Security. In Monday Comments. Detroit: CHPC-SEM, February 10, 1986.
2. P.L. 105-33, 105th Congress, 1st Session.
3. Cornely, D.A. Service role of pediatric pulmonary centers [speech]. 1983. (Site unknown.)
4. Committee on Economic Security, Social Security Board. *Social Security in America: The factual background of the Social Security Act as summarized from staff reports to the Committee on Economic Security.* Washington, DC: U.S. Government Printing Office, 1937.
5. Hormuth, R. A history of child development centers [speech]. Presented at Region I Child Development Centers Symposium, Rockport, ME, 1980.
6. Jacobs Institute of Women's Health. *State profiles in women's health.* Elsevier Science Inc., New York: 1998.
7. Ooms, T. Latino families, poverty, and welfare reform: Background briefing report. The Family Impact Seminar, The AAMFT Research and Education Foundation, Washington, DC, 1992.
8. Laudencia, A., Morrison, D.R., Rom, M., and Kao, H. Building the future: Strategies to serve immigrant families in the District: Background briefing report. DC Family Policy Seminar, National Center for Education in Maternal and Child Health, Washington, DC, 1997.
9. Thompson, L., and Sheahan, P. *Health care of incarcerated youth: State programs and initiative.* Arlington, VA: National Center for Education in Maternal and Child Health, 1994.
10. Thompson, L.S., and Farrow, J.A. (eds). *Hard time, healing hands: Developing primary health care services for incarcerated youth.* Arlington, VA: National Center for Education in Maternal and Child Health, 1993.
11. Anderson, B., and Farrow, J.A. Incarcerated adolescents in Washington State: Health services and utilization. *Journal of Adolescent Health.* 1998;22:363–367.
12. Corrigan, D., and Bishop, K.K. Creating family-centered integrated service systems and interprofessional educational programs to implement them. *Social Work in Education.* 1997;19(3):149–163.
13. Newacheck, P., Marchi, K., McManus, M., and Fox, H. *New estimates of children with special health care needs and implications for the State Children's Health Insurance Program.* Fact Sheet #4. Washington, DC: The Child Health Insurance Project, 1998.
14. Doolittle, D. Welfare reform: Loss of Supplemental Security Income (SSI) for children with disabilities. *Journal of Society of Pediatric Nurses.* 1998;3(1):33–44.
15. Who's minding the children? *Washington Post Health*, May 12, 1998.
16. Morgan, G.G. *A hitchhiker's guide to the child care universe: A tour for new policymakers.* A Policy Paper. San Diego, CA: The National Association of Child Care and Resource and Referral Agencies, 1992.
17. Hofferth, S.L. Child care in the United States today. Financing child care. *The Future of Children.* 1996;6(2):41–61.

Appendix

APPENDIX A: *Ten Essential Public Health Services to Promote Maternal and Child Health in America* (AMCHP)

1.

Assess the status of maternal and child health at the local, state, and national levels so problems can be identified and addressed.

2.

Diagnose and investigate the occurrence of health problems and health hazards that impact women, children, and youth.

3.

Inform, educate, and empower the public and families regarding maternal and child health in order to promote positive health beliefs, attitudes, and behaviors.

4.

Mobilize community partnerships between policymakers, health care providers, the public and others to identify and implement solutions to maternal and child health problems.

5.

Work with the community to assess the relative importance of MCH needs based on scientific, economic, and political factors, and provide leadership for planning and policy development to address priority needs.

6.

Promote and enforce laws, regulations, standards, and contracts that protect the health and safety of women, children, and youth and that assure public accountability for their well-being.

7.

Link women, children, youth, and families to needed population-based, personal health, and other community and family support services, and assure availability, access, and acceptability by enhancing system capacity, including directly supporting services when necessary.

Source: AMCHP, Association of Maternal and Child Health Programs, 1220 19th Street, NW, Suite 801, Washington, DC 20036.

8.

Assure the capacity and competency of the public health and personal health work force to effectively address MCH needs.

9.

Evaluate effectiveness, accessibility, and quality of personal health and population-based MCH services.

10.

Conduct research and support demonstrations to gain new insights and innovative solutions to maternal and child health-related problems.

....

APPENDIX B: *Web Resources for Health and Welfare for Families*

Section I: *Foundations*

Association for the Care of Children's Health
www.acch.org/ACCH/

Chicago Health Policy Research Council
www.chprc.uchicago.edu/

Child Development Supplement of Panel Study of Income Dynamics
www.isr.umich.edu/src/child-development/home.html

Michigan Panel Study of Income Dynamics
www.umich.edu/~psid

United States Census Bureau
www.census.gov

Section II: *Social Welfare*

Children's Institute International
www.childrensinstitute.org

Idea Central: Welfare and Families
epn.org/idea/welfare.html

National Clearinghouse on Child Abuse and Neglect Information
www.calib.com/nccanch/

National Coalition for the Homeless
nch.ari.net/

Welfare Policy Center
www.hudson.org/wpc/

Welfare Reform and Education in New York State
www.nysed.gov/workforce/welfare.html

Welfare Reform Resource Project
www.welfarereform.org

Section III: *Health Expenditures and Insurance*

Center for Health Care Strategies
www.chcs.org/

Children Now
www.childrennow.org/

Children's Medical Center of Dallas—Managed Care
www.childrens.com/mangcare.htm

HCFA Children's Health Insurance Program
www.hcfa.gov/init/children.htm

State Children's Health Insurance Program
www.aap.org/advocacy/schip.htm

Section IV: *Health Issues and Policy Implications*

American Social Health Association
Sunsite.unc.edu/ASHA/

APHA Maternal and Child Health Section
members.aol.com/Mchapha/index.html

CDC Oral Health Program
www.cdc.gov/nccdphp/oh/

National Maternal and Child Health Clearinghouse
www.circsol.com/mch/

Section V: *Programs and Initiatives*

American Academy of Pediatrics Red Book
www.aap.org/pubserv/redbook.htm

Centers for Disease Control and Prevention National Immunization
Program
www.cdc.gov/nip

Children's Safety Network, National Injury and Violence Prevention
Resource Center
www.edc.org/HHD/csn

Emergency Medical Services for Children (EMSC)
www.ems-c.org

Emergency Nurses Association
www.ena.org

Head Start Bureau
www.acf.dhhs.gov/programs/hsb/

National Conference of State Legislatures The Immigrant Policy
Project
www.ncsl.org/statefed/ipphmpg.htm

The National Immunization Technical Information Service
www.immunization.org

Safe Communities Service Center
www.nhtsa.dot.gov/safecommunities

The Substance Abuse Intervention Programs—Wright State University
School of Medicine
www.med.wright.edu/SOM/academic/SubAbuse/SAIP.html

The Substance Abuse and Mental Health Services Administration
www.samhsa.gov/

General Sites

American Academy of Pediatrics
www.aap.org

Department of Health and Human Services
www.os.dhhs.gov/

Health Care Finance Administration
www.hcfa.gov

Health Resources and Services Administration
www.hrsa.dhhs.gov

Institute for Child Health Policy
www.ichp.ufl.edu

March of Dimes
www.modimes.org/

Glossary

abstinence Abstaining from sexual intercourse.

access initiative A type of innovative programming that improves the availability of and access of individuals to necessary health care services.

acute care A pattern of health care in which an individual is treated for an immediate or severe physical or mental condition.

ADHD (attention deficit hyperactivity disorder) A disorder in children characterized by impulsive behavior, lack of attention, extreme physical activity, and lack of attention.

ADL (activities of daily living) Activities related to basic self-care and functions necessary for independent living, ie. feeding, dressing, walking, bathing, and toileting.

anecdotal evidence Information reported from individuals based on their personal experience, but not obtained from methodologically rigorous research.

assessment One of public health's three core functions, calls for regularly and systematically collecting, analyzing, and making available information on the health of a community, including statistics on health status, community health needs, and epidemiological and other studies of health problems.

battered child syndrome Having a pattern of child abuse, as applied to an individual or a family.

battering Physically abusive behavior.

block grant Method by which government agencies fund states or localities to provide health and welfare services. Although block grants are for specific types of services, they carry minimal regulations and offer considerable flexibility in how the monies are allocated, as compared with categorical or program-specific funding.

cap A specific limitation on funding or services.

capitation Payment to providers of a fixed amount for each person served, regardless of the actual amount and type of services provided, as compared with a fee-for-service reimbursement.

case control design Retrospective study design for the purpose of estimating the cause-effect relationship between suspected risk factor and a disease or condition.

case management A system used by insurance companies and managed care organizations to ensure that individuals receive appropriate, timely, and reasonable services; involves a procedure to plan, obtain, coordinate, and monitor services on behalf of a client or patient.

categorical program Health or social services program supported through funding that must be allocated to very narrowly specified service needs; usually targeted to specific groups at particular risk.

CBO (Congressional Budget Office) The component of the federal legislative branch that provides to Congress fiscal information and economic analysis data and reports.

CDF (Children's Defense Fund) A national advocacy and educational organization focusing on the health and welfare of children.

child abuse/maltreatment The physical, sexual, or emotional maltreatment of a child. Abuse may be overt or covert and often results in permanent physical or psychiatric injury and mental impairment and sometimes can result in death.

child neglect The failure by parents or other caregivers to provide the basic needs of a child by physical or emotional deprivation that interferes with normal growth and development or that places a child in jeopardy.

children with special health care needs Children with physical or developmental disabilities.

CHIP (Children's Health Insurance Program) Federal legislation passed in 1997 that provides funding to states to set up programs to provide health insurance for uninsured children.

chronic disease Long-standing persistent disease or condition.

Continuing Disability Review (CDR) A periodic examination conducted by the Social Security Administration to determine whether the health of a person receiving disability benefits has improved to the point where they are no longer considered disabled.

co-payment A predetermined fee that an individual or family pays for services or goods in addition to what is covered by insurance.

cost shifting Balancing revenue loss or underpayment from certain groups of patients with overpayment or profit resulting from other groups.

cost-based reimbursement Payment for health care services that reflects the actual cost of providing the service.

cost-benefit analysis An approach to evaluation that converts outcomes into monetary terms (dollars) so that both costs and outcomes are expressed in economic terms.

cultural competence The ability to provide services or care that is sensitive and responsive to cultural differences and assumes an awareness of one's own culture, and possession of skills that assist in the provision of services that are culturally appropriate in responding to unique cultural differences, such as race and ethnicity, national origin, religion, age, sexual orientation, and physical or mental disability.

culture of poverty The set of values, norms, motivations, and social and environmental factors that inhibit the ability of poor individuals and families to pursue alternatives that may lead to improved economic independence.

dependent enrollment period Time period during which a health insurance policy holder is allowed to enroll a dependent child for health care coverage.

developmental screening Limited examination or testing of a child by a health care professional for the purpose of determining possible developmental delay and facilitating an appropriate referral.

Disability Determination Services (DDS) agency Agency (usually at state level) that adjudicates the disability claims of applicants for Social Security benefits.

disproportionate share hospitals Hospitals that serve a disproportionate number of low-income patients with special needs. These hospitals may receive supplemental reimbursement as part of the Medicaid program.

early discharge Discharge from inpatient hospital care at the earliest possible time, taking into account key medical factors.

Employee Retirement Income Security Act (ERISA) 1974 federal legislation that regulated private pension plans; also called Pension Reform Act.

employer-based coverage Health insurance available as part of job-related benefits package.

entitlement Financial support, goods, or services to which individuals of groups are entitled by virtue of their specific status. Examples of federally mandated entitlement programs are Social Security and Medicare.

EPSDT (*Early Periodic Screening, Diagnosis, and Treatment*) Program Federal program that supports screening of children for developmental disabilities, and subsequent referral for treatment.

ethnographic Using approaches and methods based in ethnography, i.e., participant observation, case studies; qualitative research.

etiology Underlying causes of a problem or condition.

exclusions Medical services that are either not covered or are limited in an individual's insurance coverage.

federally qualified health centers/CHCs Community health centers, migrant health centers and health care for the homeless clinics which receive federal grants under the Public Health Services Act, Section 330.

fee-for-service A reimbursement mechanism based on payment for a unit of specific services rendered.

fetal alcohol syndrome The various deleterious effects of excessive maternal alcohol consumption on the unborn infant.

frail elderly Older individuals suffering from physical, cognitive, or emotional impairments that may limit their ability to provide entirely for their own needs.

GA (*general assistance*) State or local programs providing public assistance benefits to low-income persons.

gatekeeper A health care provider or case manager who screens and approves specialty care and hospital services.

Government Accounting Office (GAO) The investigative arm of the Congress charged with examining matters relating to the receipt and disbursement of public funds; performs audits and evaluations of government programs and activities.

grandfathered Exempted from a regulation, requirement, or rule change based on the fact that an individual or group of individuals was already engaged in the relevant activity.

hallucinogens The group of drugs that may cause hallucinations when ingested.

Health Care Financing Administration (HCFA) The component within the U.S. Department of Health and Human Services that oversees Medicare and Medicaid and that assesses the nation's health care programs and finances.

health maintenance organization **(HMO)** A common form of a managed care organization; a pre-paid or capitated health care plan in which services are provided by physicians and other health care providers employed by, or under contract to, the HMO.

Healthy People 2000 The national disease prevention and health promotion agenda that includes some 300 national health objectives to be achieved by the year 2000, addressing improved health status, risk reduction, and utilization of preventive health services.

home visiting A health or social service provided in the client's place of residence for the purpose of promoting, maintaining, or restoring health and well-being or for minimizing the effects of illness and disability.

horizontally integrated system A system of linked organizations at the same stage of the production process; examples include hospital–hospital or hospital–nursing home combinations. Mergers occur to achieve economies of scale, improve utilization of resources, enhance access to capital, and extend the scope of the market.

hospital-based home health Home health care services operated directly by a hospital, as opposed to services provided by free-standing (for-profit or non-profit) organizations.

human capital investment Investment in programs and activities directly related to individual productivity and well-being, i.e., education, job development, health promotion, and medical care.

IFA (*individual functional assessment*) An assessment of the effects of an individual's disability on his or her functioning.

in-kind assistance Goods or services that act in lieu of cash, i.e., vouchers, food stamps, matching contributions.

incentive program Programs that use cash or in-kind incentives to encourage participation or to reward positive behaviors.

incidence The number of new cases of a disease or condition in a population over a specific period of time.

indemnity-based insurance With indemnity plans, the individual pays a predetermined percentage of the cost of health care and the insuring company pays the additional percentage; fees for services are defined by providers and vary; individuals retain the freedom to choose any hospital or physician.

indicator A measure of health status or a health outcome.

inhalants Vapors that are inhaled or sniffed (e.g., glue, solvents, gasoline) for the purpose of intoxication.

intentional injury An injury arising from purposeful action, such as interpersonal or self-directed violence.

I&R *databases and services* Information and referral programs designed to link (through hotline, clearinghouses, etc.) individuals with necessary information and services.

long-term care The provision of health and social services over an extended period to individuals who are functionally impaired; typically involves provision of some level of assistance with various activities of daily living.

***low birth weight* (LBW)** Weight at birth of less than 2500 grams, regardless of gestational age.

maladaptive behavior Behavior that is inconsistent with reasonable functioning in the environment and with accomplishing personal goals.

managed care A general term used to refer to the organization of health care providers into systems that accept set fees for services or capitated fees for each patient enrolled.

mandatory eligibility Requiring the eligibility of certain individuals of groups of individuals for benefits or services.

matching funds Money that must be provided by states or localities to match all or some portion of a federal (or state) allocation; these funds must be provided in order to receive the full allocation.

means test An assessment of the income and assets of an individual or family to determine eligibility for certain health and welfare benefits and services.

Medicaid The U.S. federal program, established in 1965, that provides medical care benefits for individuals and families of very low income. Funding is provided by states and the federal government, and programs are typically administered by state welfare departments.

Medicaid agency The specific agency at the state or local level that has responsibility for administration of the Medicaid program.

Medicaid denials Denial of reimbursement to providers for services delivered to Medicaid clients. Denials typically result from fiscal and administrative review of records and determination that services were not necessary.

medical savings accounts A tax-exempt account established by individuals for the purpose of paying for future medical expenses.

Medicare The U. S. national health care insurance program established in 1965 for the elderly.

medically determinable impairment A disability that is identifiable and diagnosable through regular medical procedures.

mental disorder Impaired cognitive or psychosocial functioning resulting from any of a range of causes. Major categories of mental disorder are personality disorders, psychosis, mood disorders, and organic mental disorders.

NCHS (National Center for Health Statistics) The federal government's principal vital and health statistics agency; part of the Centers for Disease Control and Prevention.

negative income tax The concept that if the income of poor families fell below a certain level, they could be reimbursed up to that amount from the federal government as part of the federal income tax system.

non-marital childbearing Giving birth to a child while not being officially married.

Omnibus Budget Reconciliation Act (OBRA) 1989 federal legislation that increased eligibility levels for Medicaid and made significant changes in the design and implementation of the MCH Services Block Grant.

outreach Activities of social welfare and health care workers designed to inform the community of services and to engage eligible target groups to take advantage of services and benefits.

P.L. 104-193 The federal Personal Responsibility and Work Opportunity Reconciliation Act of 1996.

point-of-service **(POS)** *plan* A version of a managed care plan that offers the individual a choice of providers outside of the plan at a higher co-payment rate.

population-based screening The process of discovering characteristics known to be associated with health problems; its purpose is to identify individuals who are at high risk for health problems or who have unrecognized conditions.

population-based public health services Interventions aimed at disease prevention and health promotion that affect an entire population and extend beyond medical treatment by targeting underlying risks such as tobacco, drug and alcohol use; diet and sedentary life styles; and environmental factors.

portability The degree to which health insurance coverage can remain with individuals in an uninterrupted form as their employment and economic status change.

poverty level A measure (taking into account the cost of living index) of the amount of money required by an individual or a family to live at a minimum subsistence level.

poverty by choice theories A set of theories that postulate that those in poverty are comfortable with their situation and will make little or no attempt to change their status.

pre-existing conditions Medical conditions (either chronic or acute) that exist prior to the enrollment into a health insurance plan.

Preferred Provider Organization (PPO) A group of health care providers who have agreed by contract to furnish services to members of a health plan (MCO) at discounted rates.

presumptive eligibility A mechanism for speeding up or eliminating the eligibility determination process for health or welfare services; this process assumes that individuals with certain characteristics are eligible and therefore forgoes any form of means test.

prevalence Measure of the number of individuals or the rate having a disease or condition at a given point in time.

preventive care Services designed to prevent diseases or conditions, or to identify risks for diseases or conditions.

primary care Basic or general health care focused on the point at which a patient ideally first seeks assistance from the medical care system; usually deals with care of the simpler and more common illnesses; the primary care provider should also assume on-going responsibility for the patient in maintaining health and treating disease; such care is generally provided by physicians but is increasingly provided by other personnel such as nurse practitioners or physicians assistants.

primary prevention Prevention strategies that seek to prevent the onset of disease or injury, generally through reducing exposure or risk factor levels; these strategies can reduce or eliminate causative risk factors (risk reduction).

protective factors Characteristics of individuals or their environment that make them less likely to experience certain conditions, illnesses, or experiences.

reduced fertility Reduction in the birth rate.

reproductive health care Gynecologic and obstetric services.

Respiratory Distress Syndrome A lung disorder caused by a lack of pulmonary surfactant, that primarily affects premature infants and causes increasing difficulty in breathing.

risk factors Characteristics of individuals or their environment that put them at greater likelihood of experiencing certain conditions, illnesses, or experiences.

safety net Basic social welfare and health programs that serve individuals without access to other sources of support or care.

sanction A provision that penalizes an individual (or a system) for not conforming.

Section 1902(r)(2) A part of the Medicaid legislation under which states may modify the Medicaid plan to incrementally increase eligibility.

self-efficacy An individual's belief that he or she has the ability to accomplish certain tasks and reach certain objectives.

skilled nursing home care Long-term residential and treatment facilities characterized by intensive health care services provide highly trained and experienced nursing providers.

smokeless tobacco Chewing tobacco and snuff.

social capital Social value; the general value or worth to society, in non-monetary terms, of a resource, commodity, or service.

social insurance Government-operated insurance programs that set aside money in trust (contributions from individuals and employers) to insure individuals in the event of disability, death, unemployment, and retirement.

social networks Links between individuals and other individuals and institutions within their social environment.

SSA U.S. Social Security Administration.

stagflation National economic situation characterized by inflation without economic growth (stagnation).

standard deviation A statistical measure indicating characteristics of the distribution of a data set.

statutory rape Nonsensual sexual relationship with someone younger than the age of consent.

STD Sexually transmitted disease (e.g., syphilis, gonorrhea, chlamydia).

sub-acute care A level of medical care following acute care service, requiring less intensive services; often functions as a transition phase to rehabilitation services or to placement in residential care or return home.

sudden infant death dyndrome (SIDS) Diagnosis given for the sudden death of an infant younger than 1 year of age that, after a complete investigation, remains unexplained.

Sullivan vs. Zebley A 1984 case heard before the Supreme Court that resulted in the development by the U.S. Department of Health and Human Services and the Social Security Administration of a new process of determining disability among children.

supplemental medical insurance Health or long-term care insurance purchased to supplement or expand coverage available through existing health care plan; "Medigap" plans are available to help cover costs not covered by Medicare.

Supplemental Security Income (SSI) The federally supported program that provides cash assistance to individuals with a variety of disabilities; although it is administered primarily by the Social Security Administration, eligibility is not related to previous work record.

surfactant A lipoprotein that when given via direct tracheal instillation to newborns suffering from respiratory distress syndrome favorably alters the lung mechanics and improves oxygenation.

surveillance Systematic monitoring of the health status of a population.

technology dependent Reliant on certain medical equipment (e.g., ventilator, communicator) to perform certain activities of daily living and to maintain quality of life.

Temporary Assistance for Needy Families (TANF) Welfare to work programs established at the state level which comply with 1996 federal legislation.

tertiary prevention Prevention strategies that prevent disability by restoring individuals to their optimal level of functioning after a disease or injury is established and damage is done.

third-party payer An insurance company or government agency that provides payment to providers for services delivered to clients or patients.

three drug cocktails Combination of drugs used in regimen to treat individuals with AIDS.

Title V agency The organization at the state or local level that is responsible for the administration of the Title V Block Grant funds for the designated jurisdiction.

Title XXI Title XXI of the Balanced Budget Act of 1997; creates the State Children's Health Insurance Program (CHIP).

trimester A period of three months (either first, second, or third) during pregnancy.

unintentional injury Injury arising from unintentional events.

U.S. Conference of Mayors Founded in 1932, the official nonpartisan organization of cities with populations of 30,000 or more.

vaginal delivery Childbirth not requiring cesarean section.

vertically integrated system Systems involving the linking of organizations at related stages of the production process (e.g., hospital–insurance company). Vertical integration enables organizations to move toward providing multiple levels and more coordinated and comprehensive services.

very low birth weight **(VLBW)** Weight at birth of less than 1000 grams, regardless of gestational age.

vulnerable populations Groups of individuals that are at risk for certain negative conditions or circumstances.

waiver (1115/1915b) Permissions granted to state Medicaid agencies to attempt innovative pilot programming to encourage Medicaid eligibility and to make systems more efficient.

War on Poverty A series of major health and welfare programs enacted nationally in the 1960s during the administration of President Lyndon B. Johnson.

weight for height The ratio of weight to height; an indicator of infant development.

welfare state A country or jurisdiction where the government guarantees as a right essential goods, services, and opportunities (including income) to its residents.

welfare to work programs The type of welfare/public assistance programs that require recipients to participate in some type of employment in order to maintain their eligibility for benefits.

WIC Program U.S. Special Supplemental Food Program for Women, Infants and Children that provides food assistance to women and children at risk for nutritional deficiency.

workfare An approach to public assistance programming that requires recipients either to work or to receive job training in order to be eligible for benefits.

Year 2000 targets Specific quantitative health objectives for the nation as stated in the document Healthy People 2000.

Index